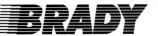

MedEMT
A Learning System
for Prehospital Care

MARK G. WILLS, MD
Director of Emergency Medical Services, Sonoma Valley Hospital, Sonoma, CA
Vice President and Medical Director, Victory Technology, Sonoma, CA

GRANT B. GOOLD, EdD, MPA/MHSA, NREMT-P
Director of EMS Education, American River College, Sacramento, CA
Director of Curriculum Development, Victory Technology, Sonoma, CA

K. LEE WATSON, NREMT-P
Vice President, Eastern Region, Victory Technology, Sonoma, CA

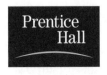

Prentice Hall

Upper Saddle River
New Jersey

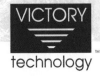

VICTORY
technology™

Sonoma
California

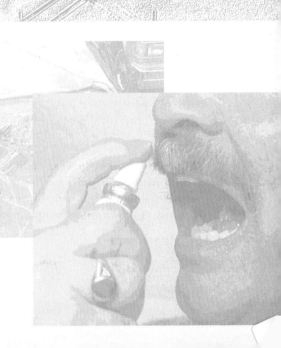

Library of Congress Cataloging-in-Publication Data
Wills, Mark G.
  MedEMT : a learning system for prehospital care / Mark G. Wills, Grant B. Goold, K.
Lee Watson.
    p. ; cm.
  Includes Index.
  ISBN 0-8385-6369-4 (soft cover)--ISBN 0-13-019744-0 (hard cover)
  1. Medical emergencies. 2. Emergency medical technicians. 3. Emergency medical
services. I. Goold, Grant B. II. Watson, K. Lee. III. Title.
  [DNLM: 1. Emergency Medical Services. 2. Emergencies. 3. Emergency Medical
Technicians. WX215 W741lm 2000]
  RC86.7 .W526 2000
  616.02'5--dc21

                                                    00-023111

PUBLISHER: Julie Alexander

ACQUISITIONS EDITOR: Laura J. Edwards

EDITORIAL ASSISTANT: Jeanne Molenaar

DIRECTOR OF PRODUCTION AND MANUFACTURING: Bruce Johnson

MANAGING PRODUCTION EDITOR: Patrick Walsh

MANUFACTURING MANAGER: Ilene Sanford

PUBLISHING CONSULTANT: Elena M. Mauceri

CONSULTING EDITOR: Karen Zabel

INTERIOR DESIGN AND PAGE LAYOUT: Susan Wood
    Design & Production, Inc.

COVER DESIGN: Maria Guglielmo

MARKETING MANAGER: Tiffany Price

MARKETING COORDINATOR: Cindy Frederick

PRINTING AND BINDING: R.R. Donnelley & Sons, Willard, OH

Notice on Care Procedures

It is the intent of the authors and publisher that this textbook be used as part of a formal EMT-Basic education program taught by qualified instructors and supervised by a licensed physician. The procedures described in this textbook are based upon consultation with EMT and medical authorities. The authors and publisher have taken care to make certain that these procedures reflect currently accepted clinical practice; however, they cannot be considered absolute recommendations.

The material in this textbook contains the most current information available at the time of publication. However, federal, state, and local guidelines concerning clinical practices, including, without limitation, those governing infection control and standard precautions, change rapidly. The reader should note, therefore, that the new regulations may require changes in some procedures.

It is the responsibility of the reader to familiarize himself or herself with the policies and procedures set by federal, state, and local agencies as well as the institution or agency where the reader is employed. The authors and the publisher of this textbook and the supplements written to accompany it disclaim any liability, loss, or risk resulting directly or indirectly from the suggested procedures and theory, from any undetected errors, or from the reader's misunderstanding of the text. It is the reader's responsibility to stay informed of any new changes or recommendations made by any federal, state, or local agency as well as by his or her employing institution or agency.

Notice on Gender Usage

The English language has historically given preference to the male gender. Among many words, the pronouns "he" and "his" are commonly used to describe both genders. Society evolves faster than language, and the male pronouns still predominate in our speech. The authors have made great effort to treat the two genders equally, recognizing that a significant percentage of EMTs are female. However, in some instances, male pronouns may be used to describe both males and females solely for the purpose of brevity. This is not intended to offend any readers.

Notice on "Case Studies"

The names used and situations depicted in the case studies throughout this text are fictitious.

Notice on Medications

The authors and the publisher of this book have taken care to make certain that the equipment, doses of drugs, and schedules of treatment are correct and compatible with the standards generally accepted at the time of publication. Nevertheless, as new information becomes available, changes in treatment and in the use of equipment and drugs become necessary. The reader is advised to carefully consult the instruction and information material included in the page insert of each drug or therapeutic agent, piece of equipment, or device before administration. This advice is especially important when using new or infrequently used drugs. Prehospital care providers are warned that use of any drugs or techniques must be authorized by their medical director, in accord with local laws and regulations. The publisher disclaims any liability, loss, injury, or damage incurred as a consequence, directly or indirectly, of the use and application of any of the contents of this book.

10 9 8 7 6 5 4 3 2
ISBN 0-8385-6369-4 (Paper)
ISBN 0-13-019744-0 (Case)

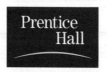
Prentice Hall

Contents in Brief

Contents in Detail

Preface

Welcome to the world of emergency medical services (EMS). You are about to enter an exciting and rapidly changing profession dedicated to providing quality emergency medical service. Emergency Medical Technician-Basic (EMT-B) providers are a dedicated group of people responding to help those in need and providing a unique service to their community. You will soon learn that EMS providers frequently face situations that require quick thinking, clear leadership, and concise communication. Successful completion of an EMT-B course will give you the skills to handle those situations and will allow you to work successfully alongside other out-of-hospital health care professionals. There are many extremely dedicated health care professionals who devote a great deal of their time and energy to providing quality health care. Their skills and talents should serve as examples for your own EMS career, and should provide a yardstick by which to measure your own growing skills.

The career of the EMT is often portrayed as full of energy and life-or-death situations, and in fact there are many situations where your decisions may influence a patient's illness or injury. However, much of an EMT-Basic's time involves preparing for calls and maintaining skills, attending educational programs, or simply waiting for calls. As an anonymous veteran EMS provider once stated, "EMS is 95 percent boredom followed by 5 percent controlled panic." The *MedEMT* system is designed to prepare you to handle not only specific patient complaints, but also crucial situations where you will need to apply intuition, critical thinking, and good judgment. The *MedEMT* system also encourages you to make use of the time between calls, to increase your knowledge and skills, or to help educate your community about emergency medical-related topics. The EMT serves many varied roles in the community, and the *MedEMT* system prepares you for those responsibilities.

This textbook, *MedEMT: A Learning System for Prehospital Care*, is actually one part of a complete learning system designed to prepare you for all of the varied situations you may encounter. All components in this system reflect the required educational materials established by the U.S. Department of Transportation's (D.O.T.) EMT-Basic: National Standard Curriculum (NSC). The text and supporting materials are organized by the D.O.T.'s Module and Lesson outline.

MedEMT includes some additional concepts that have arisen since the publication of the NSC. For example, in 1996, the Centers for Disease Control (CDC) issued Standard Precautions, an updated set of infection control guidelines that effectively replaced the Body Substance Isolation (BSI) guidelines that are referred to in the NSC. To avoid any confusion, *MedEMT* refers to both sets of guidelines. Appendix C, Infection Control, provides detailed information on Standard Precautions from the most recent CDC guidelines.

The *MedEMT* system includes many different learning components designed with both the student's and the instructor's needs in mind. These materials are designed to work together to form a complete and comprehensive learning system. Each component of the system will help you maximize your learning experience and prepare for the demands of emergency medical care. This system uses current EMS curricula, proven field techniques, and state-of-the-art digital technologies to create a rich and varied learning environment. Written by EMS providers and educational experts, the text and the accompanying learning tools are revolutionizing the way EMT-Basics learn their trade and refresh their skills and knowledge.

Providers who excel in EMS look forward to new challenges and are willing to put in the time necessary to achieve success. To build on your existing skills, talents and success in EMS you will need to manage your time wisely. The elements of the *MedEMT* system are designed to work together to maximize your exposure to the key concepts. For example, the text contains references to specific video and animation sections of the *MedEMT* CD-ROM that demonstrate the actual skill procedures. In other sections, you are encouraged to discover exactly how you pronounce technical terms or to practice critical thinking with the Case Studies. The only thing this system is not designed to do is replace the experience and skill your instructor brings to the classroom.

In order to get the most benefit from the elements of the *MedEMT* learning system, you should establish good study habits early in your learning career. Always look at the objectives and read the chapter first. Complete the questions in *MedReview* and at the end of the text chapter, and review the key terms. Complete the case studies in the text and *MedReview*. Afterwards, review the objectives and then revisit any difficult material. MedReview also provides additional exercises to help you review the material. Use the CD-ROM and Companion Website throughout the course to further enrich your studying experience.

The volume of written content and number of EMT-B skills is comprehensive, so be ready to listen carefully to your instructors and come prepared for each class session with meaningful questions and completed assignments. Ask your instructor for clarification on any content or skill procedures that remain unclear as you progress.

Again, welcome to EMS. Your hard work, together with this learning system, will help you provide quality patient care. Good luck!

Acknowledgments

The authors would like to extend our grateful appreciation to the following people who contributed their time and energy to this project.

VICTORY TECHNOLOGY, INC.
John Stalcup, PhD, CEO
Paul M. Hammond, MA,
    Director of Design and Delivery

EDITORIAL TEAM
PUBLISHING CONSULTANT: Elena M.
    Mauceri
SENIOR EDITOR: Karen Zabel, MS
CONTRIBUTING EDITORS: Liz Cragen,
    Victory Technology,
    Michael Shanahan,
    Victory Technology,
    Barbara Acello, MS, RN,
    Innovations in Health Care

DESIGN
Susan Wood Design
    and Production, Inc.

PRODUCTION
Susan Wood
Gina Bostian
Brodie Rich, Victory Technology
Tami Tolpa, Victory Technology
Val Martino

CONTRIBUTING AUTHORS
Barbara Acello, MS, RN, Innovations
    in Health Care
Kathryn Allen, PhD, EMT-B
Gail Altschuler, MD
Heather Davis, MS, NREMT-P
Robert Elling, MPA, EMT-P
Patty Glatt, MD
Alan Jones, EMT-P

Chris Reed, NREMT-P
Michael Shanahan, BA, Victory
    Technology

ILLUSTRATORS
Brodie Rich, Victory Technology
Tami Tolpa, Victory Technology
Tom Sephton
Tad Scheiblich

PHOTOGRAPHERS
Brodie Rich, Victory Technology
Paul M. Hammond, Victory
    Technology
Mark G. Wills, MD
Gary Felder, Story City Productions
Andrew Maley
John White
John Scheiblich
Tim Walton
Jenifer and Shawn Sheppard
Image Perspectives
Dave Carbone, DC Productions

TECHNICAL CONSULTATION
City of Sonoma Fire Department,
    Sonoma, CA
Sonoma Valley Hospital,
    Sonoma, CA
Santa Rosa Junior College, Two Rock
    Campus, Petaluma, CA
American River College,
    Sacramento, CA
American River Fire Department,
    Sacramento, CA
Samaritan Training Center,
    Vacaville, CA
Vacaville Fire Department,
    Vacaville, CA
Glen Ellen Fire Department,
    Glen Ellen, CA

Sacramento Fire Department,
    Sacramento, CA
Sacramento International Airport
    Authority
Merritt College, Oakland, CA
Piner Ambulance Co., Napa, CA
American Heart Association

EQUIPMENT
Heartstream, Inc.
Zoll, Inc.
BLD Medical Products

PHOTO CREDITS
The authors would like to thank the following companies for granting permission to reprint photos and illustrations.
Brent Q. Hafen and Keith J. Karren, Trauma Slides, (Upper Saddle River, NJ, Prentice Hall, 1985.) © 1985 by Prentice-Hall, Inc.
Ch. 1–p. 28, Fig. 1.28
Ch. 8–p. 267, Fig. 8.15
    p. 268, Fig. 8.16
    p. 269, Fig. 8.17
    p. 286, Enhancement Fig. 8.1
Ch. 14–p. 436, Fig. 14.14
Ch. 17–p. 492, Fig. 17.7
    p. 500, Figs. 17.18, 17.19, 17.20
Ch. 18–p. 511, Fig. 18.6
    p. 523, Fig. 18.12
    p. 524, Figs. 18.13, 18.14
    p. 525, Figs. 18.15, 18.16. 18.17
    p. 526, Fig. 18.18
    p. 527, Fig. 18.19
Ch. 20–p. 576, Fig. 20.8
    p. 577, Figs. 20.9, 20.10
    p. 578, Figs. 20.11, 20.12
    p. 579, Figs. 20.11, 20.12
    p. 580, Figs. 20.15, 20.16
    p. 586, Fig. 20.21
    p. 590, Fig. 20.23
    p. 597, Fig. 20.30
    p. 598, Fig. 20.31
    p. 599, Fig. 20.32

Ch. 21–p. 612, Fig. 21.7

Ch. 22–p. 639, Fig. 22.8
 p. 640, Figs. 22.10, 22.11
 p. 641, Figs. 22.12, 22.13

Digital Imagery® copyright 1999 Photodisc, Inc.

Ch. 17–p. 499, Fig. 17.16 (left)

DynaMed

Ch. 21–p. 614, Fig. 21-11

Laerdal Medical Corporation

Ch. 1–p. 11, Fig. 1.11

Ch. 13–p. 391, Fig. 13.2

Steve Lichtman and the Association for Preservation of Historic Ambulances, Mt. Airy, Maryland

Ch. 1–p. 10, Figs. 1.9, 1.10

MedicAlert® Foundation

Ch. 5–p. 169, Fig. 5.21

National Archives and Records Administration

Ch. 1–p. 8, Figs. 1.4, 1.5, 1.6
 p. 9 Fig. 1.7

To the Rescue Museum, Roanoke, Virginia

Ch. 1–p. 6, Fig. 1.2
 p. 9, Fig. 1.8

REVIEWERS

The publisher and Victory Technology would like to thank the following reviewers who contributed valuable feedback throughout the manuscript development process:

Rosemary Adam
The University of Iowa Hospitals & Clinics

Brenda Beasley, BS, RN, EMT-P
Calhoun State Community College

Michael Berg, NREMT-P
Travis County Department of EMS

Sandra Bradley
AMR West/Los Medanos College

Brian Brauer
University of Illinois/Carle Foundation Hospital

Mike Buldra
Eastern New Mexico University

Debra Cason
University of Texas Southwestern Medical Center

Kelly Curry
Cypress Creek EMS

Kim Dickerson, EMT-P, RN
Edison Community College

Bill Drees
The University of Texas Health Science Center at San Antonio

Robert Elling, MPA, EMT-P
Institute of Prehospital Emergency Medicine

Gary Ferrucci, EMTCC, PC
Nassau County EMS Academy

Dianne Fisher, EMT-P

Melissa Franklin, RN

Samuel Gates
Emergency Services Training Center

Marcia Gilson
Philomath Fire Department

Larry Gosdin
Gadsden State Community College

Jack Grandey
Center for Emergency Medicine of Western PA

Jaime Greene
Florida Bureau of EMS

Daniel Griffin, NREMT-P
Alachua County Fire Rescue

Rick Hatton
St. Augustine Technical Center

Jeff Hayes
Austin Community College
Williams County EMS

Richard Hilinski, BA, EMT-P
CCAC Public Safety Institute

Barbara Klingensmith
Edison Community College

Kathryn Lewis, RN, BSN, PhD
Phoenix College

Russ Lewis, RN, MICN
Daniel Freeman Hospital Paramedic School

Dave Massengale
Sacramento County Fire District, Division of EMS

Jeff McBrayer
University of New Mexico, Medic One Training

Scott McConnell
Lima Technical College

Mark McKinnon, NREMT-P

Mike Miller, RN, NREMT-P
West Suburban Hospital Medical Center

Bob Page, AAS, NREMT-P, CCEMT-P
St. John's Regional Health Center

Michael Pante, NREMT-P
Robert Wood Johnson University Hospital

Ted Peterson
Samaritan Training Center

Michael Robinson, MA, NREMT-P
Baltimore County Fire Department

Dan Roline
Gold Cross Education

Bil Rosen, NREMT-P
Capitol Health System/Jersey Shore Medical Center

Bruce Shade, EMT-P
Cleveland EMS

Captain Lee Silverman, NREMT-P
Montgomery County Department of Fire & Rescue Services/Fire & Rescue Training

Wayne Snyder
University of Michigan

Debbie Southerland
Central Texas College

Rob Stohlberg

Walt Stoy, PhD, EMT-P
Center for Emergency Medicine of Western PA

Ann-Mary Thomas
Allegheny University of the Health Sciences

John Todaro
Seminole County EMS Academy

Michael Zemany
Mountain Lakes EMS

To my wife, Denise, and my children, Devyn and Maya, for their love and support, and to my parents for their encouragement. Also, to all the EMS providers I have worked with over the years for their continuous desire to learn and improve patient care.

—Mark G. Wills

My effort is dedicated to every EMS educator who spends countless hours improving the quality of a student's learning experience and ultimately patient care. Your persistence is impressive and your commitment is unwavering. I am blessed to be counted as your peer and friend. Thanks for the journey!

—Grant B. Goold

To Missy, Shelley, Jon, Megan and my family for teaching me to be a husband and a father; and to David, for teaching me to treat people, not just patients.

—K. Lee Watson

Welcome to the Next Generation of EMS Education

We present to you the first fully integrated text and media package for EMT-Basics. This section walks you through the exciting features of the *MedEMT* Learning System. See how integration revolutionizes learning!

Check out the ways the *MedEMT* Learning System integrates content from the text, CD-ROM, and Companion Website:

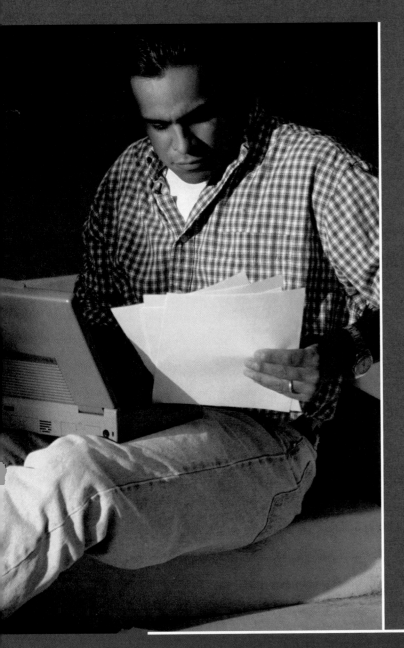

- ▶ Enter the world of the practicing EMT-B with the *Stories from the Field* critical thinking questions on the CD-ROM when you begin each text chapter.

- ▶ Watch full-color videos and animations as you follow the CD-ROM links in the text

- ▶ Discover new ways to learn with the interactive exercises on the CD-ROM

- ▶ Listen to the audio key terms on the CD-ROM

- ▶ Log on to the Internet for further study and research by following the Internet links on the CD-ROM and Companion Website

- ▶ Test your knowledge of each chapter by taking the quizzes on the Companion Website — you'll get instant feedback and scoring

INTEGRATION... SEE HOW IT WORKS!

Chapter-by-chapter, you can make use of the media available in the *MedEMT* Learning System. Here are a few examples:

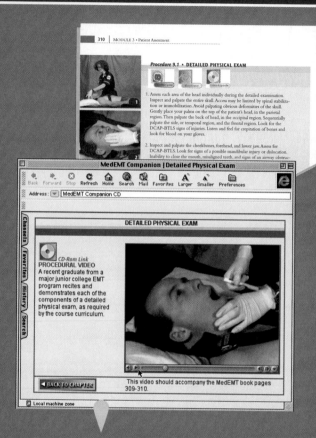

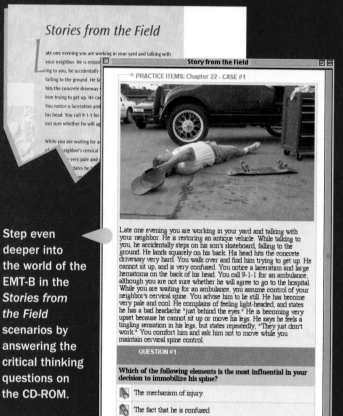

Step even deeper into the world of the EMT-B in the *Stories from the Field* scenarios by answering the critical thinking questions on the CD-ROM.

Follow the CD-ROM links within the Procedures to view videos that put you right in the action! Learning the D.O.T. required procedures is so much easier (and more exciting) when you can see and hear the action!

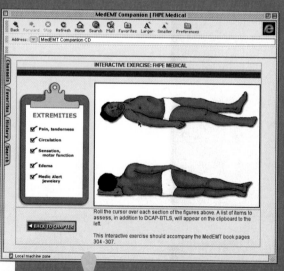

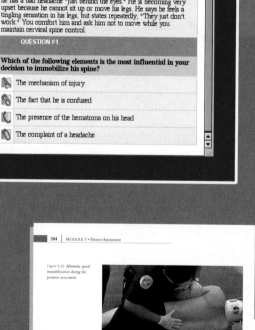

Interactive exercises on the CD-ROM help you to learn by discovery!

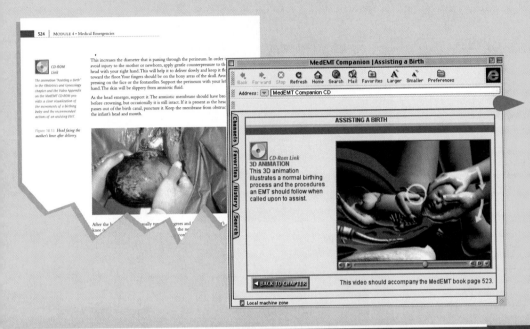

CD-ROM Link

The animation "Assisting a Birth" in the Obstetrics and Gynecology chapter and the Video Appendix on the MedEMT CD-ROM provides a clear visualization of the movements of a birthing baby and the recommended actions of an assisting EMT.

This increases the diameter that is passing through the perineum. In order to avoid injury to the mother or newborn, apply gentle counterpressure to the head with your right hand. This will help it to deliver slowly and keep it from toward the floor. Your fingers should be on the bony areas of the skull. Avoid pressing on the face or the fontanelles. Support the perineum with your left hand. The skin will be slippery from amniotic fluid.

As the head emerges, support it. The amniotic membrane should have broken before crowning, but occasionally it is still intact. If it is present as the head passes out of the birth canal, puncture it. Keep the membrane from obstructing the infant's head and mouth.

Figure 18.11 Head facing the mother's knee after delivery.

After the head usually turns degrees and the knee the ne con

MedEMT Companion | Assisting a Birth

Address: MedEMT Companion CD

ASSISTING A BIRTH

CD-Rom Link
3D ANIMATION
This 3D animation illustrates a normal birthing process and the procedures an EMT should follow when called upon to assist.

◀ BACK TO CHAPTER

This video should accompany the MedEMT book page 523.

Local machine zone

Follow the CD-ROM Links in the margins to view videos and animations that bring the concepts to life!

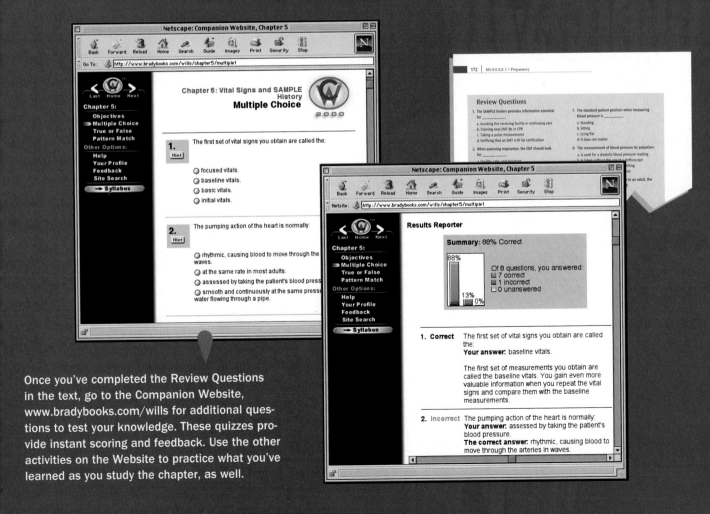

Netscape: Companion Website, Chapter 5

Go To: http://www.bradybooks.com/wills/chapter5/multiple1

Chapter 5:
Objectives
▶ Multiple Choice
True or False
Pattern Match

Other Options:
Help
Your Profile
Feedback
Site Search

▶ Syllabus

Chapter 5: Vital Signs and SAMPLE History
Multiple Choice

1. The first set of vital signs you obtain are called the:
[Hint]
○ focused vitals.
○ baseline vitals.
○ basic vitals.
○ initial vitals.

2. The pumping action of the heart is normally:
[Hint]
○ rhythmic, causing blood to move through the waves.
○ at the same rate in most adults.
○ assessed by taking the patient's blood press
○ smooth and continuously at the same pressu water flowing through a pipe.

Review Questions

1. The SAMPLE history provides information essential for _____
   a. Assisting the receiving facility in continuing care
   b. Training new EMT-Bs in CPR
   c. Taking a pulse measurement
   d. Verifying that an EMT is fit for certification

2. When assessing respiration, the EMT should look for _____

7. The standard patient position when measuring blood pressure is _____
   a. Standing
   b. Sitting
   c. Lying flat
   d. It does not matter

8. The measurement of blood pressure by palpation:
   a. Is used for a diastolic blood pressure reading

Netscape: Companion Website, Chapter 5

Netsite: http://www.bradybooks.com/wills/chapter5/multiple1

Chapter 5:
Objectives
▶ Multiple Choice
True or False
Pattern Match

Other Options:
Help
Your Profile
Feedback
Site Search

▶ Syllabus

Results Reporter

Summary: 88% Correct

88%

Of 8 questions, you answered:
☐ 7 correct
☐ 1 incorrect
☐ 0 unanswered

13%
0%

1. Correct   The first set of vital signs you obtain are called the:
Your answer: baseline vitals.

The first set of measurements you obtain are called the baseline vitals. You gain even more valuable information when you repeat the vital signs and compare them with the baseline measurements.

2. Incorrect   The pumping action of the heart is normally:
Your answer: assessed by taking the patient's blood pressure.
The correct answer: rhythmic, causing blood to move through the arteries in waves.

Once you've completed the Review Questions in the text, go to the Companion Website, www.bradybooks.com/wills for additional questions to test your knowledge. These quizzes provide instant scoring and feedback. Use the other activities on the Website to practice what you've learned as you study the chapter, as well.

Now, let's take a look at the exciting features you'll find in the *MedEMT* text

Stories from the Field

You are dispatched to a multiple-patient car collision one morning at the end of your shift. The incident commander assigns you to assist Carmen in transporting a patient to the hospital. Your patient, who is in serious condition, was driving the blue sedan. She was not wearing a seat belt. Her face hit the steering wheel and windshield. She has a large laceration on her nose and several teeth are missing. There are other minor cuts on her face and chest.

Carmen monitors the patient's airway carefully. Before you arrived, she was immobilized and high-flow oxygen was applied using a non-rebreather mask. Mark is assessing and treating her other injuries. The patient begins to speak to you about the bad luck she has had recently. She vomits a large amount of food mixed with blood. Vomitus pools in her oropharynx, and she begins making gagging, gurgling noises. Carmen immediately asks you to assist her in managing the patient's airway.

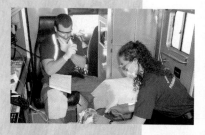

Stories from the Field

Every chapter begins with a case scenario that places you in the role of the practicing EMT-Basic. The stories are written to help you understand why the chapter material is important to your career as an EMT-Basic and to introduce key concepts. Footage of the actual scene puts you right in the action. The stories usually involve one or more EMS peers. Mark, Robin, and Carmen are EMT-Bs who rotate through your shift. Kim is your EMS instructor and a volunteer EMT. Jean is a fellow EMT-B student.

Stories from the Field — Wrap-Up

At the end of each chapter, Stories from the Field—Wrap-Up reviews and applies key concepts to provide closure to the scenario.

Stories from the Field
Wrap-Up

Good airway management skills are essential for providing quality emergency medical care at any level. When uninjured persons begin to vomit, they naturally lean forward or turn their heads to the side. This helps to clear the airway and prevents aspiration. In this situation, your patient is immobilized and cannot clear her airway without assistance. Immediately tilt the backboard to one side. Remove the non-rebreather mask if it restricts the free flow of vomitus. Suction the oropharynx with a large-diameter suction catheter.

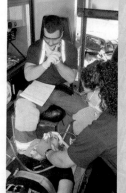

Leave the patient in the tilted position, if possible. After her airway is clear, consider placing an airway adjunct. You must rapidly assess the patient's breathing again. Assisting ventilations with a bag-valve mask device and supplemental oxygen are often necessary. If the patient's breathing is adequate, apply a new non-rebreather mask. Closely monitor the airway and breathing. Consider the patient's injuries life-threatening and transport her to the nearest appropriate facility.

National Registry Examination Tip

This unique feature highlights study tips from veteran instructors to help you prepare for required National Registry or state certification examinations.

EMT Alert

Points out essential information that relate to either your safety as an EMT, or the patient's safety.

D.O.T. Objectives

The knowledge-based, or cognitive, objectives of the D.O.T. (Department of Transportation) curriculum are placed within each chapter immediately before related content. That way, you can see the required objective, then study and learn the material.

Illustrations

Colorful and highly graphic illustrations and photos make understanding important skills and concepts easier and provide realism.

National Registry Examination Tip

Forgetting to take BSI or standard precautions represents an automatic failure on many practical examination checkoff sheets.

Figure 2.7 *Disposable gloves, masks, and goggles.*

EMT Alert

Some patients and healthcare providers develop an allergy to latex. The allergy results from repeated exposure to latex. This can occur during an extended illness or during a healthcare career. The allergy can be severe and can occasionally be life threatening. When obtaining your SAMPLE history data, discussed in Chapter 5, remember to ask patients if they have an allergy to latex.

D.O.T. OBJECTIVE

List the personal protective equipment necessary for exposure to bloodborne and airborne pathogens

Personal Protective Equipment

Using common sense and selecting the correct personal protective equipment will protect you and your patients. Wearing protective equipment to prevent contact with body substances is called barrier precautions. Table 2.1 summarizes the equipment to use in different situations.

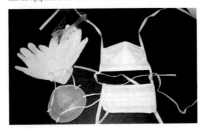

Most of the PPE and patient care supplies used in EMS are disposable (see Fig. 2.7). They are used once, then discarded. However, many items must be cleaned and reused. Follow your agency's infection control plan when disposing supplies and decontaminating equipment.

Vinyl or Latex Gloves

Gloves must be worn any time you might contact blood, body fluids, secretions, excretions, mucous membranes, or nonintact skin. In some areas, local protocol requires EMS personnel to wear gloves for all patient contact. Gloves must always be changed between patients. This is very sound advice. Gloves must also be worn when decontaminating vehicles and equipment because a potential for exposure exists. Always wear utility gloves for cleaning procedures. The chemicals used for cleaning enlarge the pores of disposable gloves, rendering them ineffective.

CD-ROM Link

The "Gunshot Wound" video in the Authentic Emergency Scenes section of the Video Appendix on the MedEMT CD-ROM shows graphic footage of the treatment of a patient who has been shot in the mouth.

Weapons

Weapons that cause penetrating trauma are divided into three categories, based on their initial energy or speed:

- Low-energy weapons, such as knives or other sharp objects
- Medium-energy weapons, such as handguns
- High-energy weapons, such as hunting or military rifles

Always relay information to hospital personnel about the length and type of knife used to inflict the patient's injury. A long kitchen or hunting knife causes more damage than a short pocketknife. However, the external wound may look the same. Never remove an impaled object, such as a knife, from a patient. Removing an impaled object may worsen bleeding. Exceptions to this general rule include impaled objects in the cheek and those that restrict the airway or keep the provider from performing chest compressions. Bring the knife to the emergency department if it is found outside the body. In some communities, law enforcement will transport the weapon. Management of impaled objects is discussed in Chapter 20.

Firearms are medium- and high-energy weapons (see Figs. 8.16 and 8.17). The severity of injuries is determined by the:

- Type of bullet
- Bullet caliber
- Distance fired
- Location of the shooter

If you are unfamiliar with weapons, ask a law enforcement officer about the weapon involved.

Figure 8.16 *Entrance and exit wounds caused by a medium-energy weapon.*

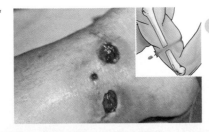

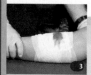

Procedure 21.1 • GENERAL RULES OF SPLINTING

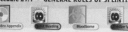

Video Appendix   Stop Bleeding   Bloodborne   Stabilize Spine

1. Although bone and joint injuries may be painful and obvious, never treat these injuries until you have managed the patient's airway, breathing, and circulation.

2. Always practice body substance isolation and standard precautions.

3. Manually stabilize the extremity above and below the injury.

4. Assess the pulse, motor function, and sensory status distal to the injury before splinting. Distal pulses may be difficult to find. If a distal pulse is found, mark the location with a pen for future reference. Record your findings.

5. Expose the injury by cutting or removing clothing. Remove rings distal to the injury.

6. If the extremity is severely deformed, or if the distal extremity is cyanotic or pulseless, notify medical direction. You may be instructed to apply gentle traction to align the limb. This may restore circulation. Stop if you observe increased pain, resistance, or crepitation.

7. Cover open wounds with a sterile dressing. This keeps them free of debris and reduces the risk of infection.

8. If bones protrude through the skin, do not try to move them. They may align themselves when you apply the splint.

9. Pad the splint to prevent pressure and discomfort.

10. Immobilize the joints above and below the injury. This prevents excessive movement.

11. If a patient shows signs of shock, treat for shock and transport immediately.

12. Reassess and record the distal pulse, motor function, and sensation every 15 minutes to ensure that the splint has not compromised circulation.

Procedures

Step-by-step text, photos, and illustrations that are numbered to correspond with the text, guide you through important D.O.T.-required skills. Here is a key to the colorful icons that appear in the "taskbar" area of the procedures:

Video Appendix — Provides links to the *MedEMT* CD-ROM

Request Backup — Highlights important patient and EMT safety issues that are related to the procedure

Oral — Indicates that drug administration is involved, and specifies the route of entry

Airborne — Highlights potential airborne, body fluid, or bloodborne infection control concerns as related to the procedure

---

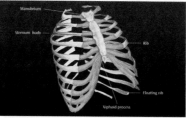

Manubrium

Sternum body

Rib

Floating rib

Xiphoid process

Figure 4.16 *The rib cage.*

The Thorax

The **thorax**, or chest, is a barrel-shaped region containing 12 pairs of ribs and the **sternum**, or breastbone. The upper 10 pairs of ribs are attached posteriorly to the vertebrae and anteriorly to the sternum. The lower 2 rib pairs only attach posteriorly, so they are called floating ribs. The sternum is a flat bone in the center of the anterior chest. The superior portion of the sternum is called the **manubrium**. Clavicles, or collarbones, are attached to each side of the manubrium. The largest region of the sternum is called the body. The inferior tip of the sternum is called the **xiphoid process**. This small bone is very prominent and easy to palpate (see Fig. 4.16).

The thoracic cavity, or rib cage, is the space formed by the ribs, sternum, and thoracic spine. It protects the vital structures of the lungs, heart, aorta, stomach, liver, spleen, and kidneys, and it assists in breathing. Trauma to the chest can injure these organs.

The abdominal cavity is below the thoracic cavity. Unlike the thoracic cavity, it is not protected by a bony case. Consequently, it is most vulnerable in blunt trauma.

The Pelvis

The **pelvis** is a bowl-shaped structure formed from the left and right hip bones, sacrum, and coccyx (see Fig. 4.17). Each hipbone consists of 3 bones that become fused together by adulthood: the ilium, the **ischium**, and **pubis**, or pubic bone.

Paired iliac bones make up the lateral walls of the pelvis. The top portions, which form the palpable wings of the pelvis, are called the **iliac crests**. The pubis is the anterior portion of the pelvis, which lies in front of the bladder.

Thorax | *Part of the body between the neck and abdomen*

Sternum | *Flat bone in the center of the anterior chest, the breastbone*

Manubrium (ma-NEW-bre-um) | *Superior portion of the sternum*

Xiphoid (ZY-foyd) Process | *The inferior tip of the sternum; it is prominent and easy to palpate*

EMT Tip

In blunt trauma, the spleen is particularly vulnerable to laceration injury from the impact of the lower ribs. Injury to the xiphoid process can cause laceration to the liver, heart, or lungs.

Pelvis | *The massive cup-shaped ring of bone at the lower end of the trunk; formed by the hip bones*

Ischium (ISH-e-em) | *One of the bones forming the pelvis*

Pubis (PEW-bis) | *Bony structure forming anterior part of hip bone*

Iliac (ILL-e-ak) Crest | *Upper part of the pelvis*

Key Terms

Definitions are highlighted in the margins next to related content for better comprehension.

EMT Tips

More tips from veteran instructors to help you understand and remember key concepts for real-world application.

Chapter Summary

A quick reference summary of key content covered in the chapter

Key Terms Review

Key terms from the chapter are summarized and page references are provided for quick review.

Case Studies

Realistic scenarios that apply chapter content and encourage critical thinking.

Review Questions

Multiple-choice questions similar to those found on National Registry and state certification / licensure exams.

Chapter Six Summary

- Safely moving your patient to the stretcher and ambulance is an important part of patient care. How you move the patient and the speed of the move affects the patient's condition.
- Lifting, reaching, carrying, pushing, and pulling are frequent sources of injury in EMTs. Always use proper body mechanics when moving patients or other objects.
- Moves are classified as emergency, urgent, and non-urgent, or routine.
- Emergency moves are used when an immediate threat to the patient or rescuers exists. Fire, explosion, an inability to protect the patient from other hazards, or the inability to access other patients are indications for using emergency moves. Using an emergency move increases the risk of aggravating spinal injuries.
- Urgent moves are used when the patient's medical condition is life threatening. An altered mental status or compromised airway, breathing, or circulation are indications for urgent moves. Cervical spine precautions are taken.
- The patient's position may affect the injury or illness. Be aware of special positioning needs.

Key Terms Review

Body Mechanics | page 179	Portable Stretcher | page 195	Stair Chair | page 182
Emergency Moves | page 184	Power Grip | page 180	Urgent Moves | page 184
Flexible Stretcher | page 199	Power Lift | page 180	Vest-Type Extrication
Hyperextension | page 182	Rapid Extrication | page 187	Device | page 197
Long Backboard | page 196	Recovery Position | page 199	Wheeled Stretcher | page 194
Non-Urgent (Routine)	Scoop Stretcher | page 197	Wire Basket Stretcher
Moves | page 184	Short Backboard | page 197	(Stokes Litter) | page 198

Review Questions

1. The leading cause of worker's compensation claims in emergency medical services is:
   a. Workplace stress
   b. Back injuries
   c. Wrist injuries
   d. Disease exposure

2. Body mechanics refers to:
   a. The moving of patients
   b. Principles of posture and lifting
   c. Learning to avoid a back injury
   d. Muscle fatigue in the large muscles

3. When preparing for a non-urgent move, the EMT-Basic should:
   a. Enlist the help of other rescuers
   b. Place the patient in a sitting position
   c. Make sure that the rails on the stretcher are in the up position
   d. Cover the stretcher with blankets to keep the patient warm

4. A key element to remember when lifting is:
   a. Keep your hands at least 18 inches apart
   b. Bend from the waist, not the hips
   c. Use the large muscles of your back
   d. Keep the weight close to your body

CASE STUDIES

Infants and Children

1. You are dispatched to a retail store in an urban part of town. The dispatcher advises you that the patient is a child with respiratory distress. You find a 4-year-old male sitting with his mother. The mother states that the child ate a large leaf from a plastic display plant. The child has noisy, high-pitched breathing and retractions. He appears to be in acute distress.

   A. What is your general impression of the child?

   B. What interventions are appropriate for the signs and symptoms?

   C. You are able to remove some plastic from the patient's upper airway. He is now crying softly and able to talk, but cannot cough. He is irritable and clings to his mother. Should you transport the child to the hospital? How?

   D. If the patient doesn't tolerate a mask, how will you provide supplemental oxygen?

2. Your crew is dispatched to a residence for difficulty breathing. You recognize the address of a 7-year-old girl with asthma. The mother meets you in the driveway with a limp child in her arms. Your initial assessment reveals a 7-year-old female who appears very sick. The girl is lethargic and will not talk to the EMS crew. Her airway is clear and easily opened. Respirations are very shallow, with a rate of 50. The patient makes a grunting noise with each breath and appears blue about the lips.

   A. What is the patient's chief complaint?

   B. If her condition is not stabilized, what might occur?

   C. What treatment is immediately indicated?

3. You are off duty and shopping at a local grocery store. You hear an announcement requesting any doctor in the store to come to the office. You identify yourself as an EMT-B and offer assistance. The manager directs you to a preschool child lying in his mother's lap, apparently sleeping. The mother left the child for a few minutes and returned to find he had opened a bottle of cough syrup. He told her he took some medicine to feel better. Then he fell asleep in the shopping cart.

   A. What should your first action be?

   B. You determine that the child is not breathing and has a slow, bounding pulse. His airway is patent. What should you do to prevent cardiac arrest?

   C. A first responder unit arrives and continues ventilations with supplemental oxygen. How can you be of further assistance?

Beyond the D.O.T....

Enhanced Study

These sections highlight content that goes beyond the D.O.T. curriculum

Examples of other content you'll find in the Enhanced Study sections:

- Gangs
- EMT Code of Ethics
- Respiratory diseases

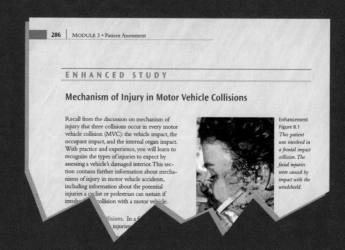

Content Enrichment

MedEMT includes even more cutting-edge content to enrich the student's knowledge:

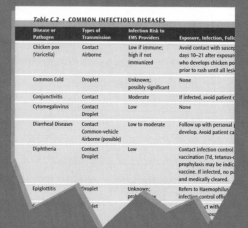

Infection Control

appendix provides accurate, up-to-date coverage of the Centers for Disease Control's latest infection control guidelines.

Spanish Terms and Phrases

reference section provides Spanish translations of key EMS terms and phrases, along with easy pronunciations. Patient questions expect only yes or no answers, for more effective communication with Spanish-speaking patients. The key terms from the text are provided in Spanish on the CD-ROM, as well!

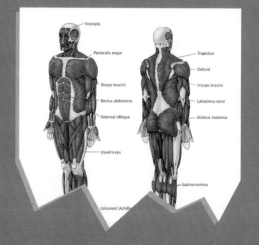

Anatomy and Physiology

content goes beyond the standard, in a well-organized and easy to understand format. Detailed illustrations help reinforce concepts.

Resources for Teaching and Learning

For the Student

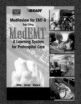

MedReview for EMT-B

This workbook resource provides 1000 new multiple choice questions, in addition to over 150 new case scenarios, plus labeling diagrams, terminology matching exercises, and a summary of key chapter content. Skills competency checklists are also included so you can quickly assess your knowledge of the skills required by the D.O.T. Links to the *MedEMT* CD-ROM are provided throughout.

www.bradybooks.com/wills

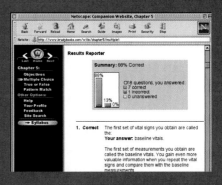

Follow this address to the Companion Website for the *MedEMT: A Learning System for Prehospital Care* text. Tied chapter-by-chapter to the text, this Website reinforces student learning through an interactive study guide and activities as well as links to important EMS-related Internet resources. This site also enables instructors to access instructor resource material and create a customized syllabus that links directly to the *MedEMT* site.

For the Instructor

MedInstruct

MedInstruct is an all-new resource that takes the concept of classroom slides to a new height. Utilizing many of the top-quality videos and animations, pictures, tables, and multi-dimensional illustrations from the text and CD-ROM, *MedInstruct* is the ultimate classroom resource. A dynamic, engaging, Microsoft PowerPoint™ presentation is included for each *MedEMT* chapter. Presentations can be customized by the instructor.

Instructor's Resource Manual for MedEMT

This resource manual provides a lecture outline that mirrors the text, as well as the following items designed to help the instructor teach more effectively, and to make use of limited class time:

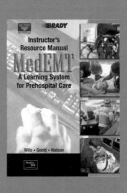

- Interactive discussion of textbook case studies and *Stories from the Field* scenarios

- Teaching Tips sprinkled throughout chapters, from seasoned EMS instructors

- Lecture notes integrated into lecture outline: actual lecture notes from experienced EMS instructors, which help pinpoint important concepts to cover in class

- A plethora of student and instructor activities and discussion questions that provide constant inspiration for spicing up your teaching

- Links to the *MedEMT* CD-ROM, and how to incorporate this new media into your classroom

- Correlation grids to help you transition from your current text to *MedEMT*

- A separate chapter for use in teaching *Spanish Terms and Phrases*

Test Manager

This resource includes over 1000 new multiple-choice questions. All D.O.T. Cognitive Objectives are represented in the questions. Each question includes a difficulty rating. Available in IBM and Macintosh versions.

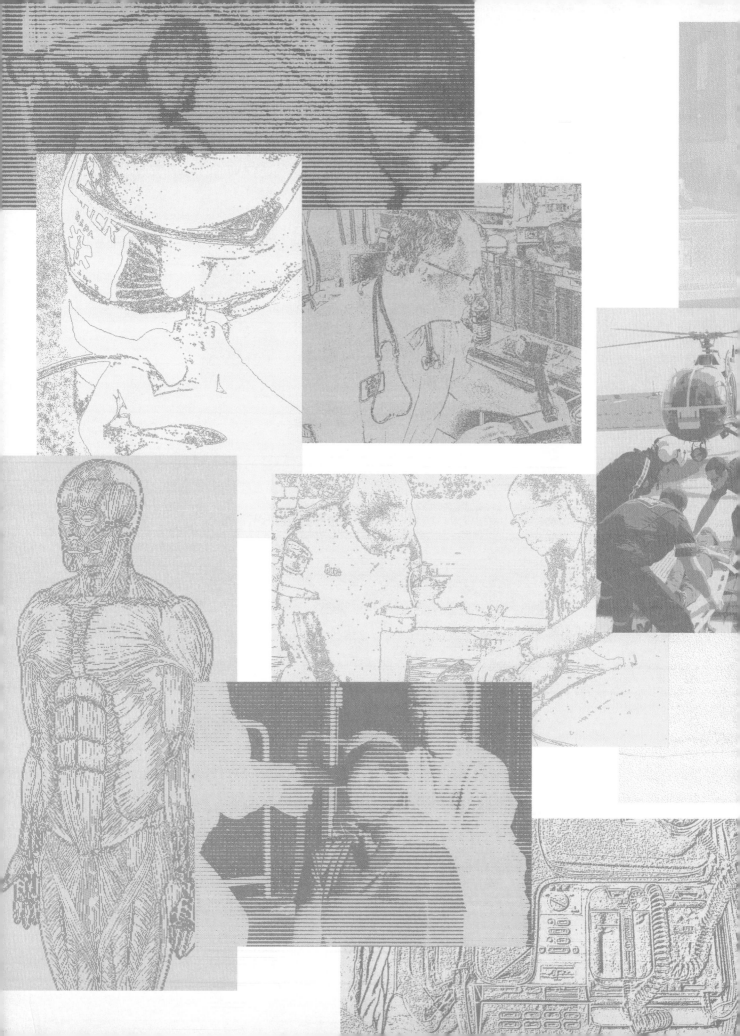

D.O.T. Module
Preparatory

1

Chapter 1

Introduction to Emergency Medical Care

Stories from the Field

You were walking through the mall and saw an elderly man collapse. Mall security came immediately to the man's aid and started CPR. Several minutes later, local firefighters calling themselves EMTs arrived. They placed patches on the man's chest and shocked him. Then an ambulance arrived and whisked the patient away. One of the EMTs did not go to the hospital but helped to comfort the patient's wife nearby. Although you were once certified in CPR, you had never seen anything quite like this before. Less than 15 minutes after the man collapsed, everything at the mall had returned to normal.

Several weeks later, you see the same EMTs at the mall again. This time, they are recruiting volunteers for the fire department. You stop and tell them how impressed you were with the events you witnessed. Bob, Mike, and Kim, the volunteers, invite you to join the fire department. They explain that an Emergency Medical Technician class will be starting soon and that no previous EMS experience is necessary. As you consider enrolling, several questions come to mind: What is an EMT? What are an EMT's responsibilities? How does the EMT relate to other providers, like paramedics? Kim, the instructor, explains that many of your questions will be answered during the first class. With her encouragement, you sign up for the course.

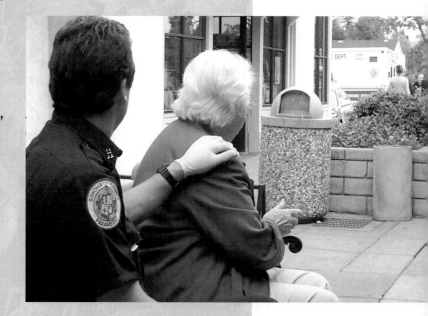

*CD-ROM
Link*

In the video, "Welcome" in Chapter 1 of the MedEMT CD-ROM, a dean from a major junior college EMS training program offers his perspective to those who choose a career in emergency medical care.

Assessment | *Evaluation of a situation or patient; the information is used to determine priorities for management*

*E*ntering the world of the Emergency Medical Services (EMS) can be both the biggest challenge and the greatest reward of your life. The emergency medical profession is constantly changing. Social conditions including violence, poverty, aging, and drug abuse make EMS a stressful profession. Despite these factors, the personal satisfaction you gain from treating patients will be immeasurable.

Your duties as an Emergency Medical Technician (EMT) change with each call. No two calls are ever the same. One moment, you may be delivering a premature infant in a cramped bathroom. During the next call, you may find yourself working systematically, attempting to save the life of a teenage driver whose car has been torn apart by a high-speed collision. You may perform CPR on a young father who collapsed on a basketball court while playing with his children. On some calls, you will simply comfort a chronically ill, elderly patient during transport to the hospital. As an EMT-Basic, your ability to recognize and properly treat an illness or injury may determine whether the patient lives or dies.

On some days, you may respond to one emergency call after another without a break. Other days you will spend your entire shift without a call. Some calls require you to use all your skills and strength. Others involve little more than assisting the patient to the ambulance, performing an **assessment**, and providing transportation to the hospital. Being an EMT is an emotional and physical roller-coaster ride with constant ups and downs.

As an EMT-Basic, you have the opportunity to experience something few others ever do: You will save the lives of those you treat. Any seasoned EMT-Basic will tell you that service to others is the very essence of EMS.

ABOUT THE EMT-BASIC COURSE

People enroll in EMT-Basic (EMT-B) courses for many reasons. Your employer may require you to complete this course. You may be attending so you can become a member of a volunteer fire department or rescue squad. Regardless of the reason you are taking this class, you have one goal in common with your fellow students: You are learning to provide care to sick and injured persons at the scene of an emergency. You will learn how to safely transport the patient to a medical facility. EMTs may work in many other capacities, but caring for sick and injured persons is the core of everything an EMT is and does.

This course is designed to provide you with the knowledge and skills to be an effective Basic Emergency Medical Technician. Developed by the U. S. Department of Transportation, the 1994 EMT-B National Standard

Curriculum provides a standardized course for training EMT students. Many states have increased the length of the program and added content specific to the state or locality. Your instructor will explain the requirements for course completion, and certification or licensure in your state.

In addition to your classroom work, you will participate in clinical or field experiences during your initial education. Your class provides an excellent introduction to patient care, but you will gain most of your experience on the job after certification.

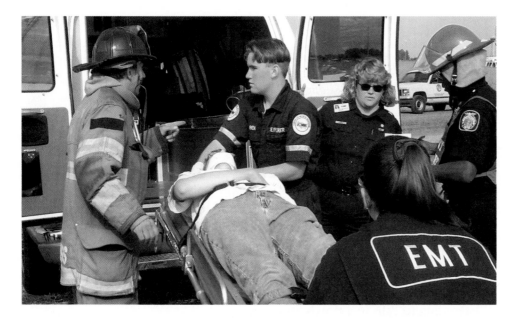

Figure 1.1 *Treatment before and during transport.*

After successful completion of the EMT-B course, you will be qualified to handle many different types of emergencies. First and foremost, you will have the knowledge and skills to manage life-threatening situations. The most important skills involve managing the patient's airway, breathing, and circulation (the ABCs). You will also learn to manage conditions that are not life threatening, such as minor bleeding or injured extremities. These conditions require treatment before or during transport to the hospital (see Fig. 1.1).

The EMT-B course also prepares you to deal with aspects of emergency services not usually thought of as patient care. You must develop ways to deal with personal stress. You will learn methods of helping patients deal with their emotional distress. You will learn how to communicate both verbally and in writing. Good communication is very important. Excellent verbal and written communication protects you from potential legal problems. You will also learn about infection control, equipment maintenance, extrication, and hazardous materials. You will find that the EMT must have knowledge and skills in many different subjects.

The training you receive in your EMT class is not all-inclusive. Preparing you for every EMS situation you will encounter is impossible. However, the judgment and knowledge you develop in class will prepare you to handle most situations effectively. Learning does not end with this class. You are responsible for continuing your education to keep your license or certification current. EMS is a rapidly changing field, and current knowledge will help you provide the best patient care possible. Surprisingly, most of what you will learn in this class has been developed in just the last 30 years.

This chapter introduces many of the concepts, roles, and duties you must know as an EMT-Basic. You will learn these procedures in detail as you progress through the rest of the book.

D.O.T. OBJECTIVE

Define Emergency Medical Services (EMS) systems.

OVERVIEW OF EMS

Every day, countless persons around the world experience traumatic injuries and sudden illnesses outside the hospital setting. These events range from minor problems to life-threatening emergencies. Without speedy intervention, many persons will die. EMS systems provide the link between an emergency in the field and treatment in the hospital. The EMS system is responsible for:

- Responding to calls in a timely manner
- Delivering qualified providers to the scene
- Providing emergency care ranging from basic to sophisticated
- Transporting ill or injured persons to the closest, most appropriate hospital

Figure 1.2 *This wagon served in one of the world's first city ambulance services.*

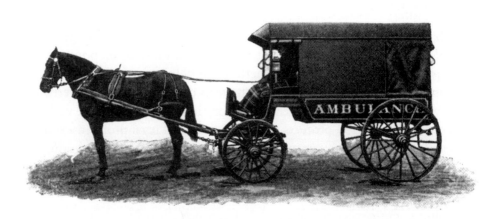

EMS is an extension of the hospital emergency department. EMS systems are credited with saving countless lives each day. They reduce the time between when an emergency event occurs and when a patient receives lifesaving care. The fundamental responsibility of a local EMS system is to provide prehospital care to the citizens of the community. Each community must have a system in place to ensure continual, efficient prehospital care.

EMS has developed from the days when the local funeral home or hospital was the ambulance provider to today's system of coordinated emergency medical response (see Fig. 1.2). Many agencies respond to EMS calls, including fire departments, independent EMS agencies, commercial services, police, rescue squads, and utility companies. In today's EMS system, EMT-Basics work with other healthcare providers to deliver professional emergency medical care (see Fig. 1.3).

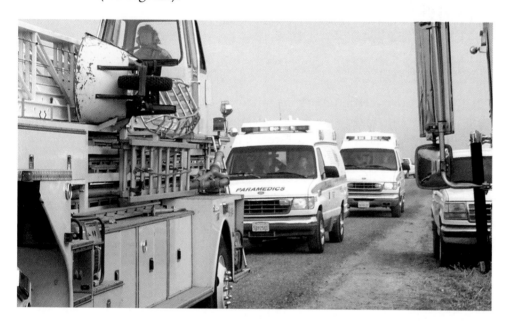

Figure 1.3 *An emergency response to a disaster often involves many agencies.*

The History of EMS

People have been providing care for the sick and injured since man learned to hunt and make war. Although the early methods of controlling bleeding, stabilizing fractures, and providing nourishment were primitive, people recognized that treatment was needed. One of the earliest known medical documents was the Edwin Smith Papyrus, written in 1500 B.C. This document describes the evaluation and organized treatment of a patient. The Bible also provides an example of care in the Old Testament, in which Elisha breathed life into the mouth of a dead child and brought the child back to life.

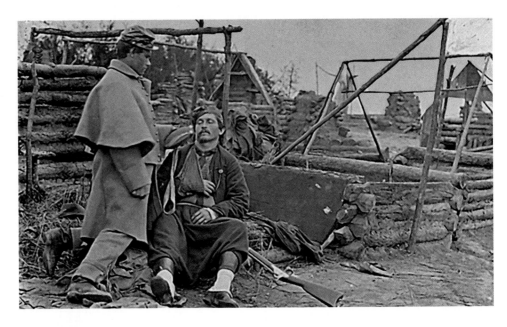

Figure 1.4 *A wounded Civil War soldier waits to be transported.*

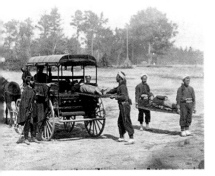

Figure 1.5 *A Civil War ambulance crew removes wounded soldiers.*

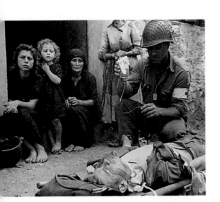

Figure 1.6 *A wounded soldier receives a plasma transfusion at a World War II battle site.*

Battlefield Care

Many of the advances in emergency medical care have been made during times of war. Organized care for the sick and injured outside the hospital had its beginnings on the battlefield. Greeks and Romans had surgeons available to treat the injured during battles. The wounded were transported by chariot from the battlefield to nearby hospitals where surgeons cared for them.

Jean Dominique Larrey, Napoleon's chief military surgeon, was the first to develop the idea of the "flying ambulance." Larrey began treating the wounded on the front lines, then loaded them into a horse-drawn, covered cart and took them to the rear lines for treatment. The first organized ambulance corps was created under his direction.

The first ambulance transportation system in the United States was seen during the Civil War (see Figs. 1.4 and 1.5). After several early catastrophes, the Union Army began training medical corpsmen to treat wounded soldiers in the field. After this initial treatment, the soldiers were rapidly moved to hospitals.

As care continued to improve, fewer deaths due to battlefield injuries were seen (see Fig. 1.6). Field hospitals became the standard of care for treatment during the Korean War. Using helicopters to evacuate injured soldiers also became standard during the Korean conflict (see Fig. 1.7). The ability to treat soldiers immediately, evacuate them quickly, and provide definitive care near the front lines contributed to an increased survival rate.

The Vietnam War saw the use of physician extenders, or medics, who started advanced treatment prior to evacuating the injured to a field hospital. Some of the greatest advances in trauma care were seen during the Vietnam conflict.

Early Prehospital Care in the United States

Early prehospital care in the United States was crude. Few organized systems were available during the first half of the 19th century. The experiences of the Civil War inspired the beginning of urban ambulance services in the United States and England. Edward Dalton, Sanitary Superintendent of the Board of Health in New York City, established a city ambulance service in 1869. Dalton, a former Union Army surgeon, equipped the ambulance with simple medical supplies, such as splints, bandages, and straight jackets. He also supplied a chest of antidotes, anesthetics, brandy, and morphine. By the end of the century, interns staffed the ambulance and provided care on scene. After treatment, the patients were left at home to recover. The ambulance operators of that time had no medical training.

At the turn of the 20th century, most ambulances were operated by hospitals. Care had progressed very little. In 1928, Julian Stanley Wise organized the first all-volunteer rescue squad in Roanoke, Virginia. Wise witnessed a drowning when he was 9 years old. The drowning later provided the inspiration for developing the EMS program. Wise's group was the first to receive training in a combination of Red Cross First Aid, rescue, and life-saving care (see Fig. 1.8). His design for volunteer services was replicated in many other communities throughout the world. His ideas were the foundation of today's EMS system.

The Evolution of Modern EMS

Modern EMS had its early start in Belfast, Northern Ireland, where Dr. J. Frank Pantridge pioneered a system using medical and nursing personnel. These individuals drove from the hospital to remote locations to treat heart attack victims. In Columbus, Ohio, Dr. James V. Warren of Ohio State

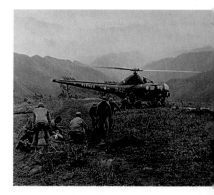

Figure 1.7 *U.S. Marines, wounded in the Korean War, are evacuated by helicopter.*

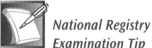

National Registry Examination Tip

Be sure to understand the historical development of EMS in the United States and which federal, state, and local governmental agencies are involved in EMS.

Figure 1.8 *Ambulance from the service founded by Julian Stanley Wise in 1928 in Roanoke, Virginia.*

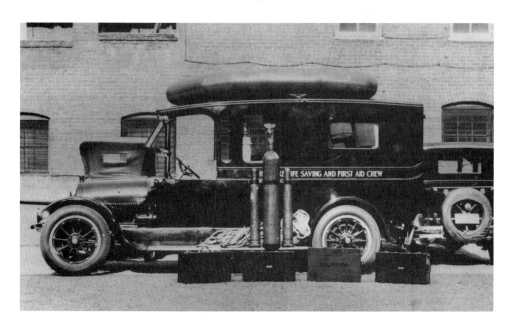

University implemented the Heartmobile, which was a converted mobile home. Each shift was staffed by a cardiologist and three off-duty firefighters from the Columbus Fire Department.

Other early EMS pioneers included Dr. Eugene Nagel, who trained firefighters in Florida to be paramedics. Dr. Leonard Cobb launched the famous Medic I project in cooperation with the Seattle Fire Department. Dr. J. Michael Criley began training firefighters in Los Angeles to be paramedics.

The 1960s

Aside from simple first aid, there was little focus on patient care until the early 1960s. Ambulances consisted of little more than a vehicle-mounted cot, red lights, and a siren. Speedy transportation to the hospital was considered the answer to treating illness or injury. Many funeral home vehicles performed double duty as both hearse and ambulance.

In the 1960s, some ambulance services began to equip their vehicles with oxygen masks (see Figs. 1.9 and 1.10). Some services began delivering a new treatment called cardiopulmonary resuscitation (CPR). These advances met with widespread public acceptance and represent the birth of modern prehospital care.

The National Academy of Sciences published a milestone report in 1966. This report, *Accidental Death and Disability: The Neglected Disease of Modern Society*, declared injury as the neglected disease in America. The report, also called the *White Paper*, documented the inadequate care provided to injured persons outside the hospital setting. The report identified the need for an organized system of prehospital providers to respond to and care for victims of emergencies.

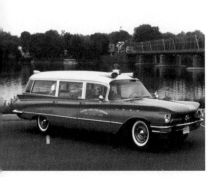

Figure 1.9 *A 1960 Flexible Buick ambulance.*

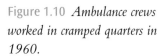

Figure 1.10 *Ambulance crews worked in cramped quarters in 1960.*

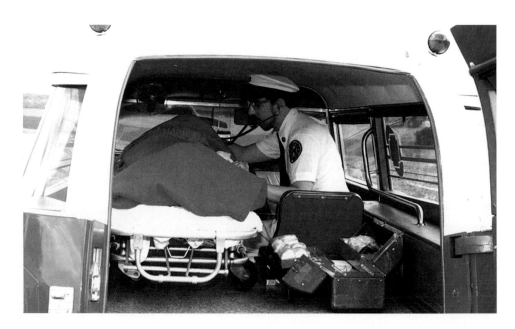

EMS in the 1970s

In the early 1970s, the weekly TV program, *Emergency*, brought prehospital emergency care into the homes of most Americans. This show is credited with the swift acceptance of the paramedic as a healthcare professional. Public demand created by the show led to the rapid increase in the number of EMS systems throughout the country. In 1973, Congress passed the **Emergency Medical Services Systems (EMSS) Act**. This act provided federal funding to begin EMS systems across the United States. The Department of Transportation (D.O.T.) developed training standards for EMTs and equipment standards for ambulances. State and local municipalities began to develop EMS systems. State EMS offices were established. Each state developed certification mechanisms for EMTs. Specialized trauma, pediatric, burn, and neonatal centers were opened. Rapid improvements in technology and equipment facilitated the continued growth of EMS.

Emergency Medical Services Systems (EMSS) Act | *The 1973 Congressional Act that provided federal dollars to begin EMS systems throughout the United States*

EMS in the 1980s

Since the passage of the Omnibus Budget Reconciliation Act in 1981, federal funding for EMS systems has been reduced significantly. Most of the funding for today's EMS systems comes from local and state taxes, revenue generated from ambulance calls, fundraising events, and private contributions. Despite the reduction in funding, the federal government continued to provide direction and leadership for the development of local EMS systems. In 1988, the National Highway Traffic Safety Administration (NHTSA) began the Statewide EMS Technical Assessment program that defined key components for effective EMS systems.

EMS Today

Prehospital emergency care has changed dramatically since the introduction of the *White Paper* in 1966. The television show, *Rescue 9-1-1,* prompted a renewed interest in EMS and raised the public's expectations of the system. Today's EMS agencies bear little resemblance to their predecessors.

In the past few years, EMS professionals have been using drugs and procedures previously limited to the hospital setting. Devices such as the automated external defibrillator (AED) are now being used in public places by lay persons (see Fig. 1.11). As technology advances, many more medical devices will become available to EMS professionals.

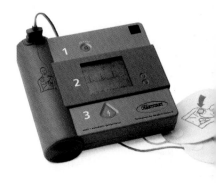

During the last decade, EMS has recognized unique requirements for treating children. Emergency Medical Services for Children (EMSC) provides a variety of training programs that specifically address the needs of children.

Figure 1.11 *An automated external defibrillator (AED).*

The 1990s brought many changes in reimbursement for services. This created a need to reduce healthcare costs. Changes in reimbursement may force EMTs and other providers to expand their traditional responsibilities.

Table 1.1 • **CARE RECEIVED BY PATIENTS IN THE PAST**

	1860s	1950s	1990s
Help Is Requested by:	Someone runs to the hospital to summon help	A family member calls the closest ambulance service by telephone	A bystander who witnesses the incident calls 9-1-1
Agency Responding:	Hospital	Funeral home	EMS agency
Personnel You Would See:	Intern and untrained driver	Certified first aid providers	EMTs and paramedics
Infection Control Measures:	None taken	None taken	Standard precautions
Safety at the Scene:	Not a concern	Relied on law enforcement occasionally, but rarely a problem	Crews responsible for their own safety; also responsible for safety of the patient and bystanders
Training of Personnel:	Usually none; sometimes hospital interns or orderlies were used	Minimal, with a focus on basic first aid	Standardized national curricula for all levels of provider
Care You Would Receive:	Very little care provided. Smelling salts used occasionally; transported to hospital for care (if not dead on arrival of ambulance)	Minimal care, based on "scoop & swoop"; transport was as fast as the vehicle would allow; patient always transported to the closest hospital	Advanced care, including intubation, IV therapy, medications if needed
You Would Be Transported in:	Horse-drawn, covered wagon stocked with brandy, morphine, bandages, and a few other items	Converted funeral coach (hearse) stocked with bandages, splints; oxygen carried in more advanced services	Ambulance stocked with modern equipment and all supplies to manage medical and trauma patients
You Would Be Taken to:	The hospital that sent the ambulance	A hospital determined by your ability to pay, skin color, or personal preference	A hospital determined by specific type of care needed; transported to hospitals with specialized services, such as a trauma center or burn center, according to patient need
Time before You Would Reach the Hospital:	Hours	One hour or less	10 to 20 minutes

Expanded care will increase both the initial and continuing education requirements for providers. In the future, you may not transport every patient to the hospital. You may perform more diagnostic testing at the scene. Tomorrow's EMT will truly be the eyes, ears, and hands of the physician.

Emergency care has progressed significantly in the past hundred years. Imagine falling from a second story window and landing in a pile of leaves.

Table 1.2 • EMS CHRONOLOGY

Year	Event
1797	Jean Larrey, Napoleon's chief physician, implements a prehospital system designed to triage the injured from the field to aid stations
1860s	Civilian ambulance services begin in Cincinnati and New York City
1915	First known air medical transport occurs during the retreat of the Serbian Army from Albania
1920s	First volunteer rescue squads organized in Roanoke, Virginia, and along the New Jersey coast
1958	Dr. Peter Safar demonstrates the efficacy of mouth-to-mouth ventilation
1960	Cardiopulmonary resuscitation (CPR) is shown to be efficacious
1966	The National Academy of Sciences, National Research Council, publishes *Accidental Death and Disability: The Neglected Disease of Modern Society*
1966	Highway Safety Act of 1966 establishes the Emergency Medical Services Program in the Department of Transportation
1972	Department of Health, Education, and Welfare allocates $16 million to EMS demonstration programs in five states
1973	The Robert Wood Johnson Foundation donates $15 million to fund 44 EMS projects in 32 states and Puerto Rico
1973	The Emergency Medical Services Systems (EMSS) Act provides additional federal guidelines and funding for the development of regional EMS systems; the law establishes 15 components of EMS systems
1981	The Omnibus Budget Reconciliation Act consolidates EMS funding into state preventive health and health services block grants and eliminates funding under the EMSS Act
1984	The EMS for Children program, under the Public Health Act, provides funds for enhancing the EMS system to better serve pediatric patients
1985	National Research Council publishes *Injury in America: A Continuing Public Health Problem,* describing deficiencies in the progress of addressing the problem of accidental death and disability
1988	The National Highway Traffic Safety Administration initiates the Statewide EMS Technical Assessment program based on ten key components of EMS systems
1990	The Trauma Care Systems and Development Act encourages development of inclusive trauma systems and provides funding to states for trauma system planning, implementation, and evaluation
1993	The Institute of Medicine publishes *Emergency Medical Services for Children*, which points out deficiencies in our healthcare system's ability to address the emergency medical needs of pediatric patients
1994	EMT-Basic National Standard Curriculum revised
1995	Congress does not reauthorize funding under the Trauma Care Systems and Development Act

Source: National Highway and Traffic Safety Administration, Emergency Medical Services Agenda for the Future, December 1997.

Your head strikes a piece of wood, and you become unconscious. You are two miles from the hospital. What type of care would you have received in the 1860s? 1950s? 1990s? Table 1.1 lists some of the differences you might have experienced. Table 1.2 lists important dates and events in EMS history.

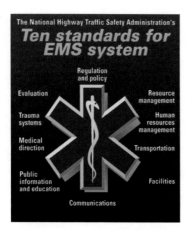

Figure 1.12 *Ten standards for an EMS system.*

EMS Standards

Although each state controls its own EMS system, the federal government provides guidelines and support. The National Highway Traffic Safety Administration (NHTSA) has established ten standards to guarantee high-quality EMS systems everywhere (see Fig. 1.12).

Standards are minimally acceptable requirements. All healthcare professions have standards to use as guidelines for their operations. Healthcare providers must meet or exceed these standards. The level of care and service should never fall below the accepted community, state, or national standards.

The NHTSA EMS standards describe:

- Regulation and policy
- Resource management
- Human resources and training
- Transportation
- Facilities
- Communications
- Public information and education
- Medical direction
- Trauma systems
- Evaluation

D.O.T. OBJECTIVE

State the specific statutes and regulations in your state regarding the EMS system.

Standards for Regulation and Policy

All states have legislation that establishes a lead EMS agency. The state EMS agency is responsible for:

- Determining how prehospital care will be provided in the state
- Establishing and updating EMS legislation
- Setting guidelines for certification and recertification of EMS personnel

- Certification and recertification procedures
- Approving EMS training programs
- Allocating funds to local, regional, and statewide EMS systems
- Enforcing state EMS rules and regulations

Each local or regional EMS agency sets regulations, policies, and procedures to ensure appropriate delivery of prehospital care. The EMS agency also manages local resources and acquires funding to operate the EMS system.

Standards for Resource Management

Each state ensures that all persons with medical problems or traumatic injuries have equal and speedy access to basic emergency medical care and transportation by qualified personnel in approved vehicles.

EMT Tip

Every EMT-Basic must read and understand the state and local statutes, regulations, and policies governing prehospital care. The EMS authorities in many states now publish EMS regulations on the Internet.

The federal Americans with Disabilities Act (ADA) was passed in 1990 to protect disabled persons from discrimination. One of the provisions guarantees equal access to EMS services. In its broadest interpretation, the ADA requires that you, as an EMT-B, provide equal care for all ill or injured patients without regard to any patient's disability. You must communicate with the patient about the problem in a manner that he or she understands. Another provision of the ADA reinforces a disabled individual's right to keep information about his or her condition confidential.

The word "disability" can be applied to many conditions. For example, persons with HIV disease and AIDS are considered disabled under the ADA. Persons with paralysis are also disabled. So are persons with mental or developmental challenges. The ADA does not make distinctions among disabling conditions but mandates that all persons with disabilities be treated equally.

Standards for Human Resources and Training

Many individuals are needed to deliver quality prehospital care. EMS is a team effort. Each state sets requirements for EMS vehicle staffing and training. Most communities require that ambulances be staffed with at least one certified or licensed EMT-Basic. Each state approves educational programs, using a standardized curriculum. The state ensures that instructors are qualified to train individuals to deliver emergency care.

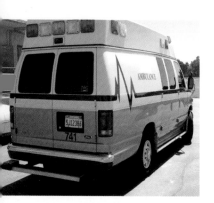

Figure 1.13 *Exterior view of an ambulance from a private ambulance company.*

Standards for Transportation

Safe and effective patient transportation is very important to a properly functioning EMS system. EMS providers will respond to the scene and transport patients by ground or air. All EMS vehicles allow prehospital care providers to respond and transport seriously ill or injured patients quickly. Providing care outside the vehicle may be difficult due to an unsafe environment or bystander interference. The inside of EMS vehicles is a more controlled environment that is used for delivery of care and storage of medical supplies (see Figs. 1.13 and 1.14).

Some communities require response vehicles to be licensed and equipped in a specific manner. Each system has minimum requirements for vehicle design, supply inventory, and maintenance.

Standards for Facilities

Appropriate facilities must be available for the treatment of seriously ill or injured patients. Some patients will need transportation to trauma centers, burn centers, or children's hospitals. The patient is always transported to the closest, most appropriate receiving facility, according to local protocol.

Standards for EMS Communication

Effective communication among all EMS providers is a key to successful patient care. Communication begins with public access to the system. The most widely used method of communication between the public and EMS is the emergency access telephone number, 9-1-1. Important communication takes place among the dispatcher, ambulance crews, and hospitals. Many communities designate special radio channels for EMS communications.

Figure 1.14 *Interior of a typical ambulance.*

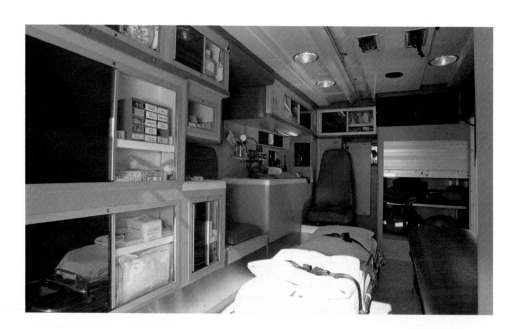

Standards for Public Information and Education

All healthcare workers are responsible for educating others. EMTs are responsible for teaching the public about the EMS system. You will provide information to others about:

- The public's role in the EMS system
- Access to care
- How to contact EMS in your community
- The prevention of illnesses and injuries
- How to help the patient until the ambulance arrives

Standards for Medical Direction

Physicians routinely delegate some tasks to nonphysician healthcare workers. EMS personnel perform these tasks under the remote supervision and direction of the physician. Each EMS system designates a physician to serve as medical director. He or she will be experienced and knowledgeable in prehospital emergency medical care. The medical director oversees EMS personnel in the delivery of patient care.

Standards for Trauma Systems

Each state must have one or more designated **trauma centers**. The EMS systems operating in the state will transport injured patients to these facilities using trauma triage guidelines. Each state also has programs for rehabilitating injured patients, collecting data, and performing mandatory autopsies. The state EMS office will actively participate in disaster planning and coordinating the disaster response of EMTs with other agencies.

Trauma Centers | *Regional facilities having specialized physicians and equipment necessary for treating trauma injuries*

Standards for Evaluation

Your state will have an evaluation program to ensure that the EMS system is providing effective quality care. Regular evaluation identifies problems and makes recommendations for improvement. The evaluation program includes data collection, system management, and quality improvement.

Access to the EMS System

Many communities use the 9-1-1 emergency telephone number. This number is also called the universal access number for police, fire, and EMS. Using the universal access number allows an ill or injured person to call for help quickly, from any location. The universal number reduces stress in a crisis in which the caller may not remember a longer number. A bonus to this system

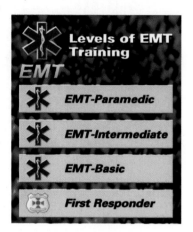

Figure 1.15 *The four levels of emergency medical training.*

is that most young callers can remember the number. Enhanced 9-1-1 systems provide the dispatcher with a visual readout showing the caller's phone number and address. This is invaluable in situations in which the caller is unable to give the dispatcher the location.

Callers in some communities must dial a seven-digit number to access EMS or other public safety services. In these areas, citizens must memorize separate phone numbers for each emergency service. Valuable time is lost if the numbers are not memorized, or if the caller is not familiar with the community. EMS providers are responsible for educating citizens how to access the system. Providing educational programs helps to prepare citizens for emergencies, assures timely entry into the EMS system, and serves as an invaluable public relations tool.

D.O.T. OBJECTIVE

Differentiate the roles and responsibilities of the EMT-Basic from other prehospital care providers.

Levels of EMS Education

Emergency Medical Technicians (EMTs) are responsible for delivering prehospital care. Variations in titles exist from state to state, but the four nationally recognized levels of emergency medical care providers are shown in Figure 1.15.

First Responder

First Responder training prepares the personnel who are first to arrive on the scene of an injury or illness (see Fig. 1.16). First Responders are not trained to care for patients during transport. Students learn to provide immediate care and scene control using little or no equipment. First Responders are trained to recognize various emergencies and can provide CPR, bleeding control, and shock management. They are also taught how to assist the EMTs upon ambulance arrival. The First Responder is usually a police officer, firefighter, industrial safety officer, lifeguard, school nurse, teacher, or other community volunteer.

EMT-Basic

In most states, **EMT-Basic (EMT-B)** training is the minimum level of education for personnel staffing an ambulance. EMT-B classes teach assessment and primary care of ill or injured patients. In some EMS systems, EMT-Bs may be trained in advanced skills, such as performing endotracheal intubation,

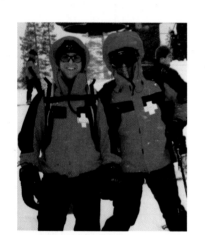

Figure 1.16 *First Responders are the first EMS personnel to arrive on scene.*

First Responder | *One whose training emphasizes immediate care and scene control prior to the arrival of additional EMS services*

EMT-Basic (EMT-B) | *Personnel trained in prehospital techniques including assessment and primary care for the ill or injured patient*

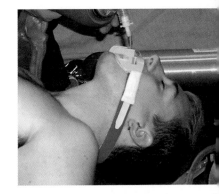

automated or semiautomated defibrillation, and assisting patients with some medications (see Fig. 1.17). Certification at the basic level is necessary to enter an advanced skills training program.

EMT-Intermediate

The **EMT-Intermediate (EMT-I)** has been trained in a variety of advanced life-support techniques. For example, EMT-Is are taught intravenous (IV) line placement, advanced airway techniques, manual defibrillation, and administration of some medications. The skills used by the EMT-I vary widely from one geographical area to the next (see Fig. 1.18).

Figure 1.17 Many EMT-Bs are authorized to provide advanced airway treatment.

Figure 1.18 Many EMT-Is are authorized to operate semi-automated external defibrillators (SAEDs).

EMT-Intermediate (EMT-I) | An advanced EMT trained in intravenous lines, airway techniques, manual defibrillation, and administration of some medications

EMT-Paramedic (EMT-P) | The most highly trained EMT personnel; paramedics perform invasive field care

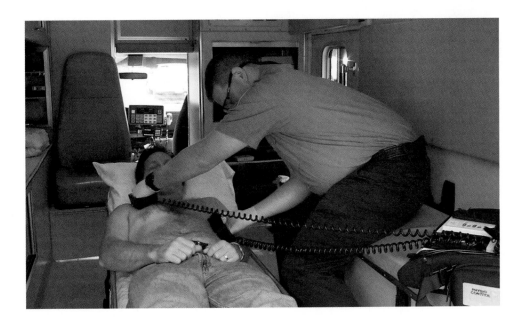

EMT-Paramedic

The **EMT-Paramedic (EMT-P)** represents the highest level of EMT training and licensure. Paramedics work closely with medical direction to provide an advanced level of care in the prehospital environment. The EMT-P performs many advanced skills, including assessment, endotracheal intubation, and manual defibrillation (see Fig. 1.19). Paramedics also interpret electrocardiograms, provide external cardiac pacing, and administer intravenous medications.

Other Components of the EMS System

Although the emphasis of your class is on the responsibilities of the EMT-B, you need to understand how all the different EMS providers work together.

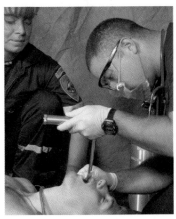

Figure 1.19 EMT-Ps are trained to provide advanced airway management.

Figure 1.20 *EMDs contact EMS services from a command center facility.*

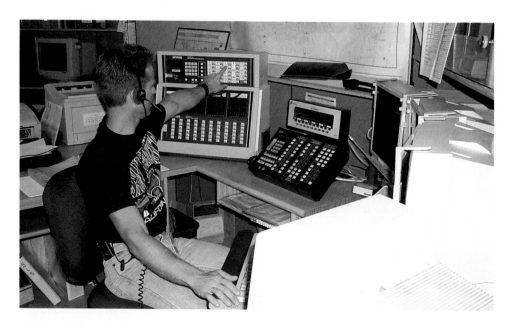

Figure 1.20 *EMDs contact EMS services from a command center facility.*

Emergency Medical Dispatcher

Emergency Medical Dispatchers (EMDS) | Specially trained personnel who answer calls for help, gather essential information, and when indicated, provide pre-arrival instructions over the phone until EMS personnel arrive

In some areas, specially trained personnel called **Emergency Medical Dispatchers (EMDs)** answer calls for help and gather essential information. When indicated, EMDs provide pre-arrival instructions over the phone. The caller uses this information to assist the patient until EMS personnel arrive (see Fig. 1.20).

EMDs are trained to decide what level of response is required. Depending on the situation, Basic Life Support (BLS) or Advanced Life Support (ALS) units may be dispatched. The EMD also determines which unit is closest to the emergency. Some situations require additional resources. For example, the EMD may dispatch police, fire, rescue, or utility companies to the scene.

It is not uncommon for several emergencies to happen at or near the same time. Each EMS system must be properly prepared and have an adequate number of response units. The volume of calls and geographical distances in the community determines the number of units needed. The location of each ambulance is also critical. Rapid response and arrival times are essential for improved patient outcomes. In many EMS systems, ambulances are kept in specific areas to help ensure a timely response to calls for help.

The EMD uses a variety of tools to manage these responsibilities. He or she may use computer-aided dispatch (CAD), medical priority dispatching, and system status management programs. The EMD communicates with EMS crews before, during, and after an emergency response using phone, radio, or computer links.

Other Healthcare Providers

Other EMS providers include physicians, nurses, and other healthcare professionals within the receiving facilities. Local and state law enforcement agencies and fire departments also play a significant role in the EMS system. The various agencies work together to ensure the safety of the EMS responders, the patient, and bystanders.

Specialty Care Centers

The availability of trauma centers, burn centers, children's hospitals, and poison centers varies by region. You must know which facilities are available in your community, their locations, and the protocols for transporting patients to them.

**CD-ROM
Link**

In "The Well-Being of the EMT-Basic" chapter and the Video Appendix on the MedEMT CD-ROM, an EMS instructor emphasizes the importance of BSI and standard precautions.

ROLES AND RESPONSIBILITIES OF THE EMT

During your EMT-B course, you will learn many aspects of your future roles and responsibilities. Understanding your roles and responsibilities will help you manage your patients' needs. These needs can range from providing skilled treatments for a severe illness or injury to comforting the patient with a gentle touch or reassurance. The value of creating a calm environment and reducing stress cannot be overemphasized. In addition, you must attend to the patient's needs without endangering yourself or your crew.

> **D.O.T. OBJECTIVE**
>
> Describe the roles and responsibilities related to personal safety.

Personal Safety

Ensuring your personal safety is always your first priority. There are no exceptions to this rule. Caring for others is impossible if you are injured before arriving or while providing care. Staying physically and mentally fit helps to ensure safety. Be alert to dangerous conditions at the scene. Conditions that can be dangerous include the patient's blood and body fluids, and hazards in or around the location. You may be exposed to violent patients, family members, gang members, or bystanders; animals that bite; unstable buildings or vehicles; fires; explosions; hazardous materials; downed electrical wires; infectious disease; and many other unsafe conditions. You must always follow body substance isolation (BSI) procedures and standard precautions (see Fig. 1.21). This information is presented in Chapter 2 and in later chapters.

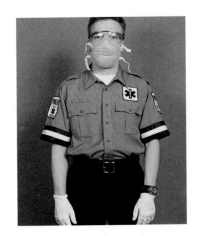

Figure 1.21 *BSI precautions include wearing goggles, gloves, and a mask when appropriate (HEPA mask shown—see Chapter 2, "The Well-Being of the EMT-Basic," for a description).*

Safety of Crew, Patient, and Bystanders

The same hazards that endanger you also endanger others at the scene. Ensuring the safety of everyone is another responsibility of the EMT-B. Limiting bystanders' access to potentially harmful situations reduces the possibility of additional patients. An injured crew member, family member, or bystander can make managing even basic emergencies more difficult.

When you arrive at the scene, you will assess the incident and communicate the information to the dispatcher. He or she will then dispatch other appropriate resources. This might include backup support for multiple patients, response of advanced life-support personnel for critically ill or injured patients, police for traffic control, or the utility company to handle downed electrical wires or leaking gas lines.

Patient Assessment and Care

In addition to safety, patient care is a responsibility of the EMT. All care is based on your assessment of what is wrong with the patient. Completing accurate assessments is one of your most important responsibilities. You will act on your assessment to manage life-threatening injuries and illnesses and relieve patient discomfort.

Figure 1.22 *EMTs frequently work as a team to lift and transport patients.*

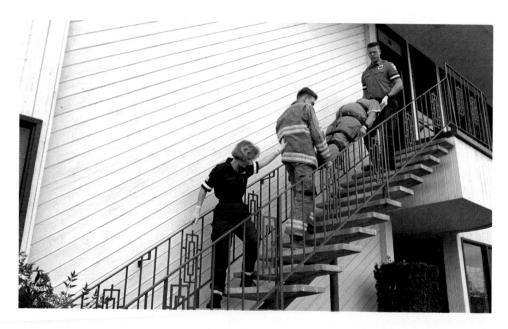

The care you provide will range from applying dressings and bandages to more complicated procedures, such as applying a traction splint or providing spinal precautions. An important aspect of care is recognizing when you have reached the limits of field care, and prompt transport is indicated. While caring for the patient, you may be required to communicate with medical direction. The healthcare provider you speak with may grant permission to administer additional treatments.

An important part of your job is providing emotional support to the patient and others at the scene. Always treat patients with dignity, compassion, and respect. Care for patients the same way you would like your family members to be treated.

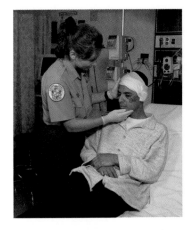

Figure 1.23 *Even after arrival at the hospital, the EMT is responsible for a patient until she is certain that hospital staff will maintain continuity of care.*

Lifting and Moving Patients

Most patients will be lifted and moved before they are transported to the hospital (see Fig. 1.22). Chapter 6 describes safe lifting and moving techniques. You will learn to use various devices to move patients without injuring yourself or aggravating the patient's condition.

Transportation and Transfer of Care

You will continue to care for the patient during the trip to the receiving facility. Safe operation of the emergency vehicle is an important part of caring for the patient. The person driving is responsible for the safety of the patient, crew, bystanders, and the public. Each operator of an emergency vehicle should complete an Emergency Vehicle Operators Course (EVOC) before responding to emergency calls. This training identifies techniques and driving standards unique to emergency vehicle operations. Check with your local EMS agency for requirements and availability of the training.

Upon arrival at the hospital, you will transfer care of the patient to the emergency department staff. You are responsible for maintaining continuity of care so that no patient is inadvertently abandoned due to miscommunication (see Fig. 1.23).

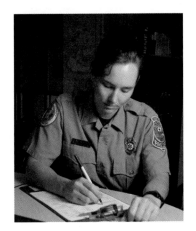

Figure 1.24 *Careful documentation is part of every EMT's job.*

Data Collection

EMS documentation is an important part of the continuation of care (see Fig. 1.24). Your documentation supplies needed information to the emergency department staff. You must accurately complete the run sheet used by your EMS system. Make sure what you have written is legible. Some agencies require EMTs to print the information. Follow your agency policy.

Data collection is important to the funding of most EMS systems. The information gathered is important, even if your agency does not charge for its services. General data may be used to support requests for funding from local

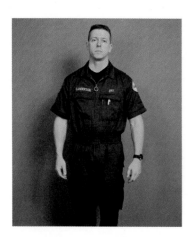

Figure 1.25 *A neat, clean appearance projects a positive image to others.*

EMT Tip

If you want to be treated as a professional, you must look like a professional.

National Registry Examination Tip

Obtain a copy of your local, state, or National Registry requirements for EMT-B recertification and continuing education.

governments or through grant applications. If your agency charges for its services, your documentation is essential to being reimbursed for the services provided.

Patient Advocacy

Your role as the primary care provider requires a unique rapport with the patient. You are responsible for accurately communicating the patient's condition and needs. You may be the only person who is able to speak for your patient's legal rights, privacy, and human dignity.

Patient advocacy can mean gathering the patient's valuables on scene and properly securing them at the hospital, or providing an area that protects the patient's privacy. One of the most powerful methods for patient advocacy is active participation in your local EMS quality improvement program.

Personal Attributes of an EMT

The EMT is a special and unique person. The successful EMT likes people, takes responsibility seriously, and believes in what he or she is doing.

Being an EMT is demanding, physical work. Your job requires both physical and emotional strength. Carrying heavy patients and equipment, performing CPR, or extricating entrapped patients are among the labor-intense activities you will perform. Therefore, you must keep yourself in good physical condition.

A neat, clean appearance projects a positive image to others (see Fig. 1.25). Your appearance promotes confidence in both patients and bystanders. Remember that first impressions are lasting ones. In addition to projecting a professional image, a clean uniform reduces the possibility of contamination.

Continuing EMS Education

Continuing education is a must for EMTs. Emergency medicine is always changing, and you must be willing to change with it. Refresher training is essential for learning about new treatments and regulations. Attending refresher classes also helps you to maintain current knowledge of local, state, and national issues affecting EMS.

Most states require continuing education to keep your certification or license active. Professional journals, conferences, videos, computer-based courses like the MedEMT CD-ROM, and World Wide Web sites such as Victory Technology's MedCollege (www.medcollege.com) are all effective means of reviewing and extending your education (see Fig. 1.26).

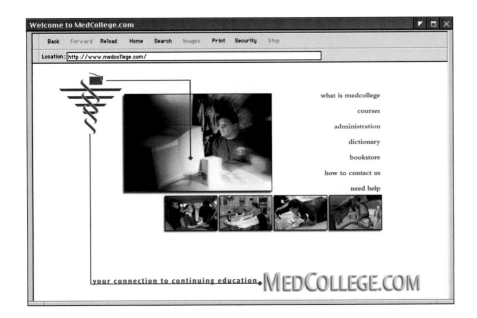

Figure 1.26 *Distance learning through the Internet is becoming a popular option.*

Figure 1.26 *Distance learning through the Internet is becoming a popular option.*

EMT Tip

Read materials on performance improvement from other professions. Discuss how the ideas may be adapted to your EMS system.

D.O.T. OBJECTIVE

Define quality improvement and discuss the EMT-B's role in the process.

Quality Improvement

Continuous self-review helps to meet the **Quality Improvement (QI)** goals of the EMS system. Most EMS systems have a QI system that identifies the strengths and weaknesses of the system. QI activities ensure that the public receives the highest level of prehospital care possible. QI processes can include internal review as well as external activities to monitor service quality. External review may involve customer satisfaction surveys and follow-up phone calls, consultants, and citizen review panels. Your responsibilities for quality improvement include:

- Documentation of events
- Conducting reviews and audits
- Gathering feedback from patients and hospital staff
- Performing preventive maintenance on equipment
- Participating in continuing education
- Maintaining your EMS skills

Quality Improvement (QI) |
Component of an EMS system that identifies the program's strengths and weaknesses and guarantees that the public receives the highest caliber of prehospital care

MEDICAL DIRECTION

Protocols | *Medical orders designed by a physician for a given list of procedures or medications; protocols will vary among localities*

Standing Orders | *Preexisting written plans for treatment of specific complaints, interventions, or medications allowed by protocol without direct contact with medical direction*

National Registry Examination Tip

Be sure to understand how the EMT-B functions under the license of the physician. Be able to distinguish between direct and indirect medical control.

Medical direction assures that all patients receive medically appropriate pre-hospital care. On-line, or direct medical direction, involves active communication between a physician and the EMT crew in the field. Off-line, or indirect medical direction, refers to using **protocols** or **standing orders**. These are written orders designed by a physician for the care of patients with specific conditions. Standing orders will direct you to perform certain procedures or to administer specific medications. Protocols are individualized in each community. Off-line medical control also includes other tasks, such as approving the content of training programs.

Most states require ambulance services and rescue squads to receive medical direction from a physician. The physician is ultimately responsible for the patient care given in the EMS system. Under medical direction, physicians are also responsible for directing continuing education activities and regularly reviewing quality improvement programs.

Relationship of the EMT-B to Medical Direction

The EMT is a designated agent of the physician. The care you provide is considered an extension of the physician's authority. The degree of responsibility varies by state. The medical director in many EMS systems can revoke the extension of authority if the EMT-B is not meeting the minimum standard of care. Your privileges can also be revoked if you function outside your scope of practice. Remember that when you practice as an EMT, you are representing your medical direction physician. Your actions reflect directly upon the physician (see Fig. 1.27).

DUTIES OF THE EMT-B

You will perform the same basic procedures when responding to calls for emergency assistance. The nature of the scene and incident will change, but the procedures are essentially the same in all emergencies. Following is an overview of common EMT-B duties during an emergency call.

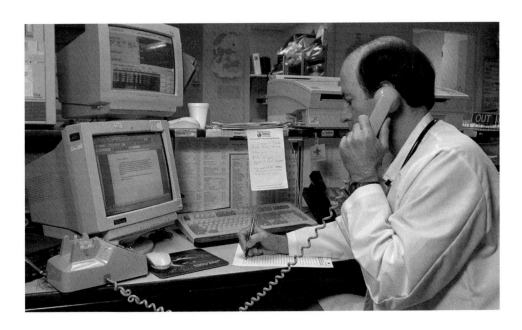

Figure 1.27 *Most states require that ambulance services and rescue agencies receive medical direction from a physician.*

Response to an Emergency Scene

The EMT-B responds to emergency calls, provides efficient and immediate care to the critically ill and injured, and transports the patient to a medical facility. After you are dispatched, you will drive the ambulance or other emergency vehicle to the correct address or location. Always select the safest, most direct route, considering traffic and weather conditions. Observe all traffic regulations governing emergency vehicle operation. Demonstrate due regard for other motorists.

Arrival at the Scene

Upon arrival at the scene of an emergency, you must size up the scene. You will evaluate:

- Scene safety
- The mechanism of injury or nature of illness
- The total number of patients
- The need for additional help

If law enforcement personnel are not present, you might be required to create a safe traffic environment. Place road flares, remove debris, and redirect traffic as needed. These measures protect the patient and emergency responders. Use caution when placing road flares, which can ignite flammable spills at the scene. Be aware that road debris may be valuable as evidence in a crime scene. Do not move vehicles or debris until law enforcement arrives, unless moving things is necessary to provide patient care, is a safety hazard to those at the scene, or is likely to cause additional accidents on the road. If you must remove debris, try to make a simple sketch of the location of items for use by law enforcement.

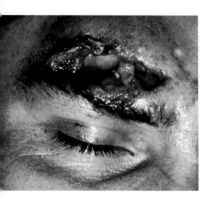

Figure 1.28 *The EMT-B will sometimes encounter patients with severe injuries.*

Assessment

After determining the nature and extent of the illness or injury, you will establish priorities for emergency care. All care is based on your assessment. Your duties include, but are not limited to:

- Opening and maintaining an airway
- Ventilating the patient
- Performing cardiopulmonary resuscitation (CPR)
- Using the automated external defibrillator (AED)

You will learn these procedures in detail later in the class.

Assisting Trauma Patients

EMTs provide prehospital emergency care for a variety of traumatic injuries, ranging from simple abrasions to severe damage to multiple body systems. You will control bleeding, treat shock, bandage wounds, and immobilize painful, swollen, or deformed extremities (see Fig. 1.28).

Entrapment, Disentanglement, and Extrication

When a patient is entrapped, you will assess the extent of the patient's injuries. You are responsible for protecting the patient and for providing emergency care. You will learn to use recognized techniques and equipment to safely extricate the patient. The EMT provides simple rescue services if a specialized rescue unit is not available. If needed, radio the dispatcher for help from special rescue or utility services. During disentanglement and extrication, you will care for the patient without endangering yourself, the patient, or your crew (see Fig. 1.29). You will continue caring for the patient after extrication, using standard emergency procedures.

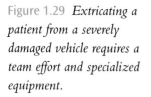

Figure 1.29 *Extricating a patient from a severely damaged vehicle requires a team effort and specialized equipment.*

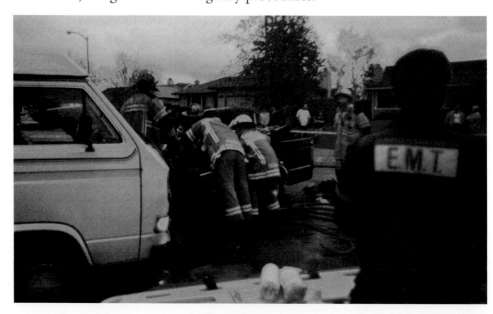

Assisting Medical Patients

The EMT has many responsibilities when assisting medical patients. You will:

- Aid with childbirth
- Manage respiratory emergencies
- Manage cardiac emergencies
- Care for patients with complications of diabetes
- Care for patients with allergic reactions
- Manage behavioral crises
- Care for patients experiencing environmental emergencies, or those related to exposure to heat and cold
- Manage patients with suspected poisoning

Your care is based on an assessment and a history of the patient's medical problems. When assisting patients with medical emergencies, medical direction may instruct you to:

- Assist the patient to take prescribed medications
- Administer oxygen for many types of emergencies
- Administer oral glucose solution for diabetics with low blood sugar
- Administer activated charcoal solution for ingestion of harmful substances

Caring for patients in a confidant, efficient manner provides support and reassurance to the patients and bystanders.

Medical Identification

Some patients have medical problems that require special treatment. These conditions are not always obvious. Patients with serious medical problems such as diabetes, allergies, epilepsy, and heart disease often wear an identification insignia, such as MedicAlert® (see Fig. 1.30). The insignia may be in the form of a bracelet, necklace, or card. Bracelets are recommended because they are easy for rescuers to spot. However, some people are uncomfortable wearing the emblem on the wrist. They may feel that bracelets advertise their medical problems, and instead wear necklaces under their clothing. In some states, the Vial of Life is used to store written records. The vial is kept in the refrigerator where it is safe, accessible, and protected against fire. Always look for medical identification symbols. These items provide vital medical insight if the patient cannot communicate.

Compliance with Regulations

As an EMT, you will abide by all state, local, and agency rules and regulations.

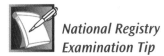

National Registry Examination Tip

Be sure to look for medical ID (usually a necklace or bracelet) while performing patient care skills.

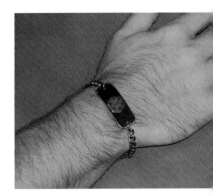

Figure 1.30 *A MedicAlert® bracelet is found on many drugstore shelves.*

Transport to the Treatment Facility

You will transport the patient to the most appropriate facility. A decision regarding which facility to use may be made after consulting with medical direction. Transport decisions are based on the:

- Patient's condition
- Extent of injuries
- Location of receiving facilities
- Capability of receiving facilities

You will work with the vehicle operator to ensure that the ambulance arrives at the destination safely.

Assessment Findings

Some assessment findings will require advice from medical direction. Some findings are relayed to the receiving facility personnel, who will arrange for special professional services upon your arrival.

Reporting to Dispatch

In some EMS systems, you will report directly to the emergency dispatcher or communications center. You will report changes in your availability and your progression through each stage of the call. Most systems require that you report the nature and extent of injuries, the number of patients being transported, and the receiving medical facility. Frequent communication ensures safety. Reporting to the receiving facility helps to ensure that the patient will receive prompt attention upon arrival.

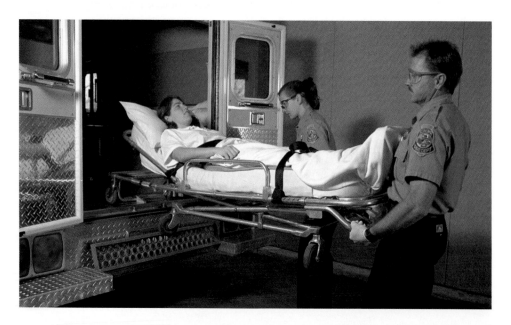

Figure 1.31 *EMTs are responsible for safely moving the patient from the ambulance into the receiving facility.*

Continued Patient Assessment

You will continue to assess the patient during transport and provide care as needed or as directed by medical direction. When you arrive at the receiving facility, you will assist in moving the patient from the ambulance into the facility (see Fig. 1.31). Report your assessment and care of the patient to facility staff verbally and in writing. Assist facility staff in accordance with hospital and agency policy.

Replacing and Cleaning Equipment

After each call, you will restock used linens, blankets, and other supplies. Clean the equipment according to your agency policy. Dispose of single-use supplies. Carefully check all equipment so that the ambulance is completely ready for the next run. Follow your agency policy for reporting, repairing, or replacing defective equipment. Local, state, and federal regulations require decontamination of the ambulance after transporting patients with some infectious diseases, or exposure to certain hazardous materials.

Maintenance of Equipment

For safe, efficient operation, the ambulance must be in good mechanical condition and maintained in a neat, orderly manner. You can determine that the vehicle is in good mechanical condition by following the checklists in the owner's manual. Become familiar with care and maintenance procedures of specialized equipment used by your service.

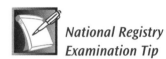

National Registry Examination Tip

Take the National Registry Practical Examination Checklists with you during clinical or field internships. Use these checklists during practice sessions or simulations.

Chapter One Summary

- The Emergency Medical Services system has many elements, including the caller who reports the emergency, the dispatcher, the First Responder, EMS providers, hospital staff, and others involved in the patient's recovery.

- There are four primary levels of EMS training. First Responders are trained to provide care until an ambulance arrives. EMT-Basics are trained to provide basic lifesaving care on the scene of an emergency, and in an ambulance during transport to an appropriate facility. EMT-Intermediates and EMT-Paramedics provide advanced medical care.

- The National Highway Traffic Safety Administration, a part of the Department of Transportation, is the federal agency that over-sees the EMS system at a national level.

- Your roles and responsibilities as an EMT-Basic include:

  Ensuring your personal safety, as well as the safety of the crew, the patient, and bystanders

  Performing a patient assessment and providing care based upon your assessment findings

  Lifting and moving patients safely

  Providing safe transport and transfer of care to an appropriate healthcare facility

  Collecting data and keeping accurate records

  Being a patient advocate

- Quality assurance and improvement is essential to providing high-quality prehospital care. Reviewing patient care reports is a quality-assurance activity.

- The EMT-Basic is an extension of the physician, who provides medical direction through standing orders, protocols, and direct contact during an emergency.

Key Terms Review

Review Questions

1. The Department of Transportation categorizes Emergency Medical Technicians as:

   a. Basic, integral, paramedic
   b. Basic, intermediate, advanced
   c. Basic, integral, advanced
   d. Basic, intermediate, paramedic

2. Which site would be least appropriate to receive a 52-year-old man with severe burns?

   a. Hospital emergency department
   b. Pediatric center
   c. Burn treatment center
   d. Trauma center

3. When responding to any emergency situation, the primary concern of the EMT-B is:

   a. To make sure the media knows the truth
   b. To assist in rescuing victims from dangerous areas
   c. His or her personal safety and the safety of others
   d. To determine the cause of the injury or illness

4. Which of the following is NOT a personal attribute of an EMT-B:

   a. To be neat and clean in appearance
   b. To have a pleasant attitude
   c. To remain in good physical condition at all times
   d. To put the patient's needs above the EMT's own safety

5. Establishing EMS legislation, accrediting training programs, and setting guidelines for certification are the responsibility of the:

   a. Ambulance service director
   b. Local EMS board
   c. State EMS agency
   d. Department of Transportation

6. Enhanced 9-1-1 typically provides which of the following information?

   a. Exact address of incident
   b. Nature of incident
   c. Location of caller
   d. Directions to the incident

7. All of the following providers are trained in the care of medical and trauma patients at the scene of the incident. Which provider listed is NOT trained to care for patients during transport?

   a. First Responder
   b. EMT-B
   c. EMT-I
   d. Paramedic

8. Staffing an ambulance requires which level of minimum training :

   a. First Responder
   b. CPR Training
   c. EMT-B
   d. Paramedic

9. The medical director of an EMS system is a

   a. Nurse
   b. Physician
   c. Paramedic
   d. EMT

10. The 9-1-1 emergency telephone number is sometimes referred to as the

    a. Emergency help line
    b. Enhanced access number
    c. Universal access number
    d. Emergency medical number

11. Trauma centers, burn centers, and children's hospitals are examples of

    a. Advanced life-support centers
    b. Intermediate healthcare centers
    c. Specialty care centers
    d. Primary assistance centers

12. An EMT must provide _____ support as well as physical care when treating a sick or injured patient.

    a. Global
    b. Scene
    c. Standard
    d. Emotional

CASE STUDIES

Introduction to Emergency Medical Care

1 You are just finishing your EMT-B program at the community college. Your class project is to visit a local senior living center to give a presentation on the standards of a high-quality EMS system. You are asked to define Emergency Medical Services, list the standards that a system should meet, and provide a local example of each standard. Approximately 150 people will attend your presentation.

A. Where can you get information on standards for an EMS system?

B. Which of the standards are you contributing to by visiting this group and giving your presentation?

C. What other programs might the system implement to encourage proper use of EMS services in your area?

D. Aside from the proper use of emergency medical services, what other subjects can such presentations address?

2 You begin your shift for the local volunteer fire department by responding to an unresponsive man inside a vehicle. You find the man locked inside a car outside a local bar. As you approach, you look through the car window. You determine that the man is breathing irregularly and has what could be a medical alert bracelet around his wrist. A handgun is visible in the man's lap. Suddenly, the man falls forward and appears to stop breathing. You are the only person on the scene with medical training. A crowd has formed in the parking lot.

A. What is your primary responsibility in this situation?

B. How can you protect the bystanders?

3 The local volunteer EMT-Bs have complained that they are not getting enough patient contact. The local medical director is working to establish relationships with larger EMS systems. This would provide opportunities for internships for those who want more field experience. Unfortunately, this program will take months to start.

A. What are some alternatives for actual patient contact before the internship program begins?

B. Because documentation is so important, how can EMTs participating in a field internship program improve their documentation skills?

Stories from the Field
Wrap-Up

The mall scenario presents EMS at its best. EMS providers worked together, quickly and effectively caring for the patient. Many types of providers work together within the EMS system, including emergency medical dispatchers, First Responders, EMT-Bs, EMT-Is, and Paramedics. Providers have many responsibilities in addition to providing patient care. Many things take place behind the scenes to enable EMS personnel to provide quality prehospital care during a call. You should have a complete understanding of the roles and responsibilities of the EMT-B upon completion of this chapter.

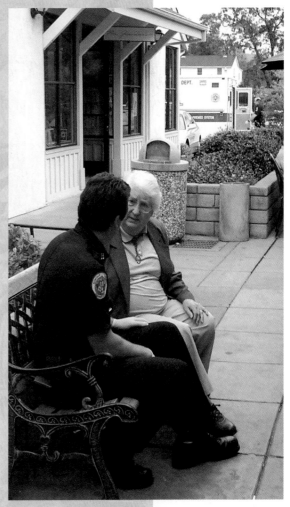

Chapter

2

The Well-Being of the EMT-Basic

Stories from the Field

The fire department assigns you to ride along with Robin and Mark on the BLS ambulance. You are on duty when a call for an unresponsive man is dispatched. You arrive to find family members gathered in a small house in a rural part of your service area. One person directs you to the bedroom, where an elderly man is lying in bed. Mark assesses the patient and finds that he is not breathing, does not have a pulse, and has lost control of his bowel and bladder. The patient is ashen gray, cold, and stiff. Mark informs you and the other rescuers that the patient is dead and that rigor mortis has set in. According to your protocols, no resuscitation will be done. The body will be transported to the emergency department for examination and pronouncement of death. While Mark goes out to the ambulance, you accompany Robin to talk with the family.

When Robin begins to speak with the spouse of the deceased, another family member approaches you. He starts speaking softly, but quickly becomes hostile. He demands that you do something, and not just stand there while his father dies. Robin intervenes and begins talking with him. Mark reappears with the stretcher and asks that you help him remove the body. He hands you a package with a gown, mask, and gloves, and instructs you to put them on.

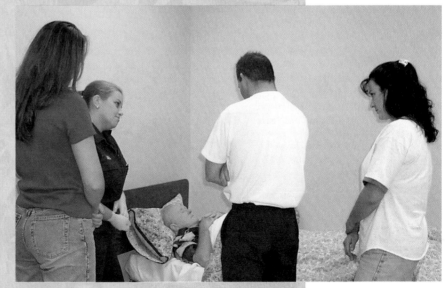

E MT-Basics encounter many unique situations while providing emergency medical care. You will deal with events involving death and terminal illness, amputations, mass casualties, and child abuse (see Fig. 2.1). The death of a coworker, friend, or family member is one of the most stressful events an emergency medical professional will face. EMT-Basics must be prepared to deal with patients and family members who are angry, scared, violent, or seriously injured. You are not immune to the personal effects of stress. In this chapter, you will learn what to expect and how to help yourself, your partners, the patient, and family members during and after stressful situations.

Figure 2.1 *Mass casualty incidents can take a heavy emotional toll.*

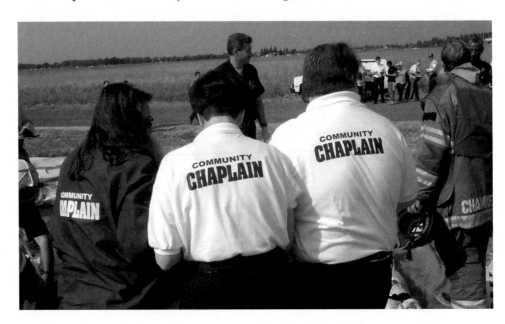

Stress | *Natural emotional and physical reactions to threatening or challenging situations*

Remaining emotionally healthy at work and accepting changes in family life related to your job is challenging. Learning to manage personal stress takes practice. This chapter describes methods of coping with **stress**. Try different techniques until you find those that work best for you. You will also learn how to protect yourself against illness and infection. The information in this chapter is only an overview. Additional concepts related to personal safety are integrated throughout this text.

EMOTIONAL ASPECTS OF EMERGENCY CARE

Emergencies are stressful for everyone. The patient, family members, bystanders, and EMS responders are all affected by emergencies. You will learn to cope with stress while remaining professional on your job. Finding ways to cope with stress is important for your emotional health.

Recognize the signs and symptoms of critical incident stress.

Stressful Situations

Stress is part of life. Anxiety is a natural reaction to threatening or challenging situations. Stress is not always bad. Some experts suggest that certain types of stress cause some individuals to perform more efficiently. Even though positive stressors exist in EMS, this section focuses on negative stress.

Working in EMS brings an additional element of stress to your life. Treating injured, sick, or dying patients is stressful. The stress you face each day will affect you emotionally and physically. Learning effective coping skills is essential to remaining healthy, happy, and effective. Besides personal stress, you will assist patients, family members, and bystanders in stressful situations. Some situations and conditions that cause stress include:

EMT
Tip

Stress in EMS is routine, not the exception.

- Multiple-casualty accidents
- Infant/child trauma calls
- Traumatic amputation
- Infant or child abuse, elder abuse, or spouse abuse
- Death or injury of a coworker or other public safety personnel
- Overwhelming sensory responses (e.g., the smell of a burned patient)
- Regulations
- EMS politics
- Ungrateful, abusive, violent, or impaired patients (whether alcohol or drug influenced or mentally ill)
- Emergency response to the illness or injury of a friend or family member

Warning Signs of Excessive Stress

Stress creates positive and negative reactions. Stress causes the body to release a hormone called adrenaline. In an emergency, the boost of adrenaline may improve your performance. Excessive stress may be the result of a single event, or from repeated exposure to less-stressful events. EMS providers who exhibit signs of excessive stress are said to be experiencing burnout. Burnout is complete mental, emotional, or physical exhaustion. Some warning signs of excessive stress include:

- Irritability with coworkers, family, friends, or patients
- Inability to concentrate

National Registry Examination Tip

During an EMT class, testing is a major cause of anxiety and stress. Gather information on test-taking skills and how to reduce test anxiety. The Internet is a good resource for this type of information.

- Physical exhaustion
- Difficulty sleeping or nightmares
- Anxiety
- Indecisiveness
- Guilt
- Loss of appetite
- Loss of interest in sexual activities
- Isolation
- Loss of interest in work
- Increased substance use or abuse (alcohol, prescription medications, or illegal drugs)
- Depression
- Change in personal appearance or grooming

D.O.T. OBJECTIVE

State possible steps that the EMT-Basic may take to help reduce/alleviate stress.

MANAGING STRESS

Learning to manage personal stress takes practice. Stress reducing techniques include:

- Pre-incident stress education
- On-scene peer support
- One-on-one support
- Disaster support services
- Defusings
- Critical Incident Stress Debriefing (CISD)
- Follow-up services
- Spouse/family support
- Community outreach programs
- Other health and welfare programs such as Employee Assistance Programs (EAPs)

Lifestyle Changes

If you browse through a bookstore or newsstand, you will find a tremendous amount of material related to stress. A lot of research has been devoted to helping people deal with stress. Experts recommend several lifestyle changes to help reduce the negative effects of stress:

- Eat a healthy, balanced diet at regular intervals

- Increase carbohydrates

- Reduce fatty foods

- Avoid caffeine and alcohol

- Reduce sugar intake

- Exercise regularly; exercise relieves stress and improves your strength and endurance (consult with your personal physician before beginning an exercise program)

- Practice relaxation techniques, such as meditation, deep breathing, and visual imagery

- Avoid using tobacco; smoking increases the risk of a fatal heart attack, and increases the chances of cancer and lung disease; smokeless tobacco is also a cancer risk

- Change your work environment or your work schedule to allow yourself more family time; asking for a less busy shift or location may be helpful and is not a sign of weakness

Remember that it takes time to find a balance between work, recreation, family, and health.

EMT Tip

Develop a healthy living plan for the first six months of your professional life in EMS. Include time for exercise, relaxation, and a healthy diet. At the end of six months, honestly evaluate yourself for the signs of stress. Then, change your plan as necessary and practice it for another six months.

D.O.T. OBJECTIVE

State the possible reactions that the family of the EMT-Basic may exhibit due to their outside involvement in EMS.

Support from Family and Friends

Most EMS providers have a strong support group of family and friends. Your family may be the best source of support after a critical incident. Many EMTs gain great support and strength from their spouses, close family members, and willing friends. Talking to a spouse or coworker helps you to release your feelings and emotions and helps to prevent burnout. But remember, when discussing a case, you must maintain patient confidentiality. Learn to discuss your feelings without providing names or identifying details.

**CD-ROM
Link**

*In the "Well-Being" chapter
and the Video Appendix on the
MedEMT CD-ROM, an experi-
enced EMS administrator
discusses the importance of the
CISD process.*

Working in EMS is stressful not only to you, but also to those who support you. Realize that your family may experience negative emotional responses such as:

- Frustration from not truly understanding your feelings
- Fear of being ignored or being second fiddle to your EMS career
- Stress caused by on-call situations
- Anger at interruptions in normal life
- Stress from the inability to plan activities
- Frustration from the inability to share in your experiences
- Frustration from the inability to talk to others about your experiences

To stay healthy, enjoy your job, and keep things in perspective, you must learn to understand, anticipate, and appreciate family members' reactions to stress. Remember that their reactions are normal. Developing healthy solutions to the challenges of working in EMS is hard work.

Critical Incident Stress Debriefing

*Critical Incident Stress
Debriefing (CISD)* | *A meeting
held after a critical incident
that encourages emergency care
workers to discuss their feelings
openly with trained mental
health professionals and peer
counselors*

Critical incident stress debriefing (CISD) is a process designed to help workers identify the stresses of a specific call or several stressful responses. EMS personnel may experience strong emotional reactions after upsetting incidents. Stress related to the incident may interfere with your ability to function effectively. CISD helps participants to identify and understand their feelings. After identifying how you feel, you can develop a plan for managing stress. Trained mental health professionals and peer counselors conduct the meeting. The CISD is conducted within 24 to 72 hours after a critical event. Participating in a CISD gives emergency workers an opportunity to discuss their feelings openly. Meetings are not an investigation or interrogation. The information discussed in the session is strictly confidential.

**EMT
Tip**

*Find out how to access the CISD
program in your area.*

Participating in a CISD Session

The professional conducting the CISD session encourages participants to talk about stressful aspects of the event (see Figs. 2.2 and 2.3). Technical procedures describing management of the incident are not discussed. CISD leaders evaluate the information and offer suggestions for overcoming your feelings of stress. You will not be criticized or judged for talking about your feelings. The session is designed to strengthen the normal recovery process. CISD is effective because you will express your feelings and concerns in an open, nonthreatening environment.

Follow-up to the CISD is crucial. In follow-up sessions, stressed workers and their families are supported and referred to other resources, if necessary. Learning the details of your local CISD program is an important part of your initial EMT-Basic education.

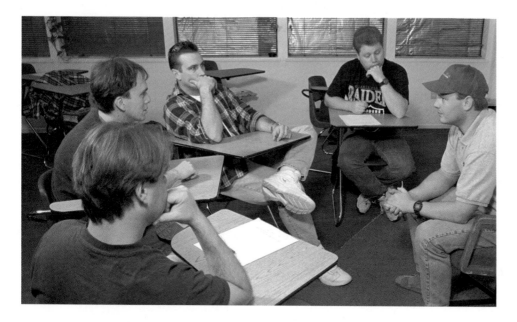

Figure 2.2 *Participants in a CISD session are encouraged to talk about stressful aspects of an emergency event.*

Other Methods of Managing Stress

Participating in classes that teach stress reduction techniques will be helpful to you. Programs are available to help prehospital providers recognize signs of destructive stress. Participating in a class will also help you to identify when to seek peer and professional counseling.

Sometimes the EMT needs on-scene peer support. This type of immediate psychological support is sometimes needed after mass casualty incidents, the death of a partner, or particularly vicious crimes. Other emergency workers at the scene usually give immediate peer support. Your EMS partner, a supervisor, clergyman, or other person willing to listen to your concerns may provide personal or one-on-one support.

After a disaster, specialized disaster support services are available to care for the emotional needs of EMS responders. These team members are trained to act during large-scale disasters. Local CISD team members usually participate in the disaster support team.

Defusing is a specialized process that occurs shortly after a critical incident. Participants are encouraged to express their feelings about the incident, especially feelings of guilt or frustration.

The healing process can take months or years after some incidents. In these cases, participants are given access to long-term therapy and support. These follow-up services also help researchers to measure the total impact of a critical incident.

The CISD program may encourage participants to work with community outreach organizations. These groups provide assistance to individuals affected by the critical event. For example, when a family's house burns to the

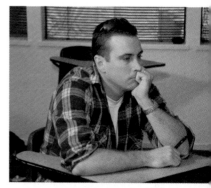

Figure 2.3 *CISD is designed to aid the normal emotional recovery process.*

ground, the CISD team may use an outreach program to find immediate housing and food for the displaced family. Sometimes, helping others to cope with the event helps you to resolve your feelings.

In many EMS organizations, employees with specific challenges are sent to outside specialists who are trained to deal with the issues. For example, individuals experiencing substance abuse, drug addiction, or compulsive gambling are sent to professionals who work directly with these types of problems.

If you decide to seek professional counseling, it does not reflect weakness or inability to do your job. Many employers offer employee assistance programs (EAPs), or counseling programs to help employees manage stress. Professional counseling provides a way of expressing your feelings in a confidential environment. Seeking professional help will help you to cope without depending completely on your support network.

D.O.T. OBJECTIVES

List possible emotional reactions that the EMT-Basic may experience when faced with trauma, illness, death, and dying.

Discuss the possible reactions that a family member may exhibit when confronted with death and dying.

State the steps in the EMT-Basic's approach to the family confronted with death and dying.

DEATH AND DYING

An unfortunate reality of the emergency medical profession is that people die before, during, and after you have cared for them. Learning to recognize, understand, and deal with the issues involved in death and dying are important skills to master early in your career.

Typically, you will deal with two types of situations involving the death of patients. The first situation occurs when death is sudden and unexpected. Emotions run high, and family members may display hysteria, rage, depression, or disbelief. For example, a middle-aged man experiences sudden death or a baby dies of sudden infant death syndrome (SIDS). Without warning, family and friends are confronted with an enormous loss. You may be the first person with whom they interact. They may look to you to provide lifesaving care to bring their loved one back to life. In this situation, most of your attention is directed toward the patient. However, being empathetic and informative with grieving family or friends can greatly reduce their stress. Empathy means understanding how someone else feels. Being empathetic helps family or friends to feel as if they are part of the patient care process. Being informative helps the family to understand that interventions that may look harmful are beneficial to the patient.

The second type of situation occurs when death has been anticipated or when the patient is clearly dead. In this case, you will not attempt to resuscitate. Consoling the family, showing empathy, and performing administrative functions become your priorities. You may help the family contact the treating physician or funeral home. Other ways to help in such cases include notifying law enforcement, collecting telephone numbers, and serving as a gatekeeper for curious people who come to the scene.

The Grieving Process

People experience common reactions when faced with a major loss, such as death. Dr. Elisabeth Kübler-Ross identified the grieving process as a result of her research with dying patients and their families. Although you are not trained to be a grief counselor, understanding the grieving process enables you to recognize the reactions of others as normal and expected. People go through the grieving process when facing a major loss. Losses such as amputation or the death of a loved one or coworker can trigger the grieving process. The grieving person moves through the process at his or her own pace before accepting the loss. The stages of the grieving process are:

- Denial ("Not me…It can't be true.")
- Anger ("Why me?")
- Bargaining ("OK, but first let me…")
- Depression ("OK, but I haven't…")
- Acceptance ("I will make the best of this.")

Reactions to death vary from person to person and from situation to situation. The grieving process has no rules. Do not be surprised to find a patient feeling acceptance one minute, and in the anger stage moments later. This is a normal reaction. Understand and respect the emotional roller coaster the patient and family are enduring. Grieving is a very personal and complex process. The reaction depends on the relationship with the lost loved one, the age and maturity of the survivor, the situation that caused the loss, and many other factors.

Denial

The first reaction to any loss is usually shock, disbelief, or denial. Many people you deal with will be in this first stage. Denial helps to protect a person from the stress of the loss. People in denial may refuse to believe that the information about the loss is true. For example, if your spouse were killed in

EMT Tip

Be aware that others at a scene, especially immediate family members, may have underlying medical problems. The stress of losing a loved one may worsen the problem, creating the need for emergency care. For example, one individual of an elderly couple has died suddenly. The surviving spouse, who has a history of heart disease, may begin to have chest pain. Be prepared to treat or request additional resources for other patients, if necessary.

an airplane crash, your first reaction would be "It can't be true," or "I don't believe it." You hope to be notified later that the information is not true. If the information is wrong, the denial reaction has protected you from painful emotions that follow a loss.

Unfortunately, information about losses is usually true. Family members may have to see the body before believing that the loss is real. Even after seeing the body, reality may not set in for some time. When working with a person in denial, be empathetic but honest. Avoid agreeing with the denial.

Anger

Anger is a common emotion in any loss. Individuals coping with a loss may become angry with or blame the physician, EMS personnel, or family members. A terminally ill patient may be verbally abusive. Family members may respond by directing anger toward the EMT after receiving news of an unexpected death. Avoid taking this anger personally. Be tolerant and patient, and answer each question as honestly as possible. Avoid providing false reassurance, which causes more anger when the truth becomes apparent.

Bargaining

Some people think they can postpone death by negotiating with others. They may try to make deals with doctors, themselves, or religious figures trying to buy more time. For example, you are extricating a patient who is trapped under a tractor-trailer. The patient has experienced a life-threatening crushing injury. During the lengthy extrication the patient repeatedly says, "I know I am going to die, but just keep me alive long enough to see my wife one more time." Listen empathetically when faced with a patient who is bargaining. Avoid providing false hopes or guarantees. Calmly reassure the patient that you are doing everything possible. You cannot guarantee this patient will see his wife again. Offer to relay a message to her. Provide emotional support for the patient.

Depression

Depression is a feeling of hopelessness and helplessness. A dying patient or family of a person who has died may be depressed for a long time. He or she may withdraw from social contacts, mourning unfulfilled dreams, or things left unsaid or undone. A child may regress or lose interest in daily activities after losing a parent or close friend. An elderly person may suffer from insomnia, weight loss, or become isolated. Sadness and despair are normal reactions to the loss, and the feeling will pass over time. If depression persists for years, the person is suffering from a condition called pathological mourning. This is not part of the normal grieving process.

Acceptance

Acceptance is a realization of one's fate. It does not mean that the patient welcomes death. He or she is waiting calmly for death to occur. In this stage, family members often have trouble accepting the inevitable, and may need more support than the patient. Show respect for the situation when working with a patient or family in acceptance. Listening is an important EMT-B skill.

Listening

Listening is one of the best techniques to use when working with death and dying. Compassionate listening allows people to grieve with dignity (see Fig. 2.4). As you deal with dying patients and family members, use a gentle tone of voice. Let them know you will do everything you can to help. Use a reassuring touch when appropriate. In some situations, requesting the services of a pastor or grief counselor may be appropriate.

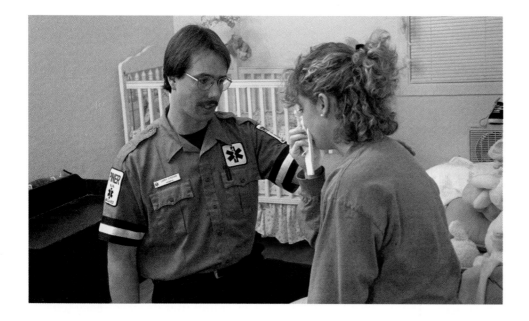

Figure 2.4 *A reassuring touch shows empathy.*

Personal Grief

EMTs are not immune to grief. You will go through the grieving process in times of loss. For example, you may grieve when a patient dies after a difficult extrication, or when a fellow EMS professional is killed in the line of duty. Be aware of your reactions and seek assistance if necessary. Watch for grief reactions in your crew members and be ready to help.

CD-ROM Link

In the "Scene Safety" video in the "Well-Being" chapter and the Video Appendix on the MedEMT CD-ROM, a practicing paramedic and instructor talks about the importance of establishing scene safety for any emergency call.

***Pathogen** (PATH-oh-jen)* | *Microorganism that causes disease*

Body Substance Isolation (BSI) Precautions | *Equipment and standards designed to prevent the spread of communicable diseases*

Standard Precautions (SP) | *The first level of the Centers for Disease Control's revised set of guidelines regarding isolation precautions established in 1996. Replaces BSI and universal precautions*

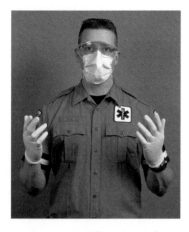

Figure 2.5 *Gloves, a mask, and goggles are components of BSI and standard precautions.*

D.O.T. OBJECTIVE

Explain the need to determine scene safety.

SCENE SAFETY

The greatest dangers to your physical and mental health are usually at an emergency scene. An untrained person responding to an emergency will rush to the aid of the ill or injured patient without considering possible consequences. Remember that personal and crew safety always comes before patient care. To be effective, you must protect yourself and your crew before caring for the patient. Without exception, you must establish the safety of a scene before entering. One wrong decision can suddenly end your career or the career of a crew member.

D.O.T. OBJECTIVES

Discuss the importance of body substance isolation (BSI).

Explain the rationale for serving as an advocate for the use of appropriate protective equipment.

Body Substance Isolation and Standard Precautions

One of the most significant dangers to the EMT-B is invisible. **Pathogens** are microscopic agents that cause infection. Two of the most common pathogens are viruses and bacteria. The threat of infectious disease exists in every patient contact. Taking measures to prevent the spread of infection is your legal and ethical responsibility. The 1994 EMT-B curriculum uses the term **body substance isolation (BSI) precautions** to describe measures to prevent infection (see Fig. 2.5). The term BSI is widely recognized by EMS providers and agencies.

The Centers for Disease Control and Prevention (CDC) are agencies of the federal government that are a branch of the Department of Health and Human Services (DHHS). The CDC are responsible for research and recommendations related to infectious disease. A major focus is the prevention of the spread of infection. In 1996 the CDC published new infection control guidelines called **standard precautions (SP)**. Standard precautions are designed to replace body substance isolation and another system called universal precautions. Standard precautions are easier to remember and provide a higher degree of protection to the worker. The guidelines are discussed further in Appendix C, Infection Control.

Body substance isolation and standard precautions are part of a larger concept called infection control. The precautions are designed to prevent the spread of communicable disease from one individual to another. You must know and follow your agency's infectious disease prevention protocol, whatever it is called.

D.O.T. OBJECTIVE

Describe the steps the EMT-Basic should take for personal protection from airborne and bloodborne pathogens.

Methods for Preventing the Spread of Infection

Pathogens cause disease in many different ways. Different methods are used to prevent the spread of infectious disease. In addition to **personal protective equipment (PPE)**, engineering controls and work practice controls are used to prevent the spread of infection. Engineering controls are ways of making the environment less disease-friendly. Good engineering controls make practicing BSI easier. Examples of engineering controls in EMS are:

- Roll-up flooring, which prevents pathogens from being trapped in joints
- The placement of sharps boxes, which allow providers to dispose of sharps immediately after use
- Placement of personal protective equipment in locations of use, so that EMS providers can readily access the equipment

Work practice controls involve training employees and regulating employee habits to prevent the spread of infection. Examples of work practice controls in EMS are:

- Policies that prohibit recapping of needles to prevent accidental sticks
- Policies that specify how to clean equipment and the ambulance after a call
- Policies that require handwashing immediately before or after patient care

Handwashing, a simple work place practice, is the most effective way to prevent the spread of pathogens from one person to another. Wash your hands for at least 10 seconds before and after patient care. Wash for a longer time if your hands are contaminated or visibly soiled. In cases when handwashing is impractical, the use of a self-drying, no-rinse gel is recommended after every patient. The gel should contain a concentration of isopropyl or ethyl alcohol over 60 percent. The concentration is always listed on the bottle. The CDC do not recommend lower concentrations. Wash your hands with soap and water as soon as it becomes available (see Fig. 2.6).

CD-ROM Link

An experienced paramedic and instructor emphasizes the importance of BSI precautions in the "BSI Precautions" video in the "Well-Being" chapter and the Video Appendix on the MedEMT CD-ROM.

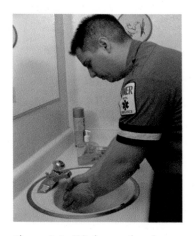

Figure 2.6 *Wash your hands for at least 10 seconds after patient care.*

Personal Protective Equipment (PPE) | *Equipment used by an emergency rescuer to protect against injury and infectious disease*

National Registry Examination Tip

D.O.T. OBJECTIVE

List the personal protective equipment necessary for exposure to bloodborne and airborne pathogens

Forgetting to take BSI or standard precautions represents an automatic failure on many practical examination checkoff sheets.

Personal Protective Equipment

Using common sense and selecting the correct personal protective equipment will protect you and your patients. Wearing protective equipment to prevent contact with body substances is called barrier precautions. Table 2.1 summarizes the equipment to use in different situations.

Figure 2.7 *Disposable gloves, masks, and goggles.*

EMT Alert

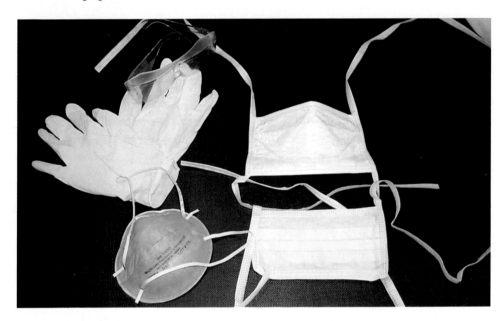

Most of the PPE and patient care supplies used in EMS are disposable (see Fig. 2.7). They are used once, then discarded. However, many items must be cleaned and reused. Follow your agency's infection control plan when disposing supplies and decontaminating equipment.

Some patients and healthcare providers develop an allergy to latex. The allergy results from repeated exposure to latex. This can occur during an extended illness or during a healthcare career. The allergy can be severe and can occasionally be life threatening. When obtaining your SAMPLE history data, discussed in Chapter 5, remember to ask patients if they have an allergy to latex.

Vinyl or Latex Gloves

Gloves must be worn any time you might contact blood, body fluids, secretions, excretions, mucous membranes, or nonintact skin. In some areas, local protocol requires EMS personnel to wear gloves for all patient contact. Gloves must always be changed between patients. This is very sound advice. Gloves must also be worn when decontaminating vehicles and equipment because a potential for exposure exists. Always wear utility gloves for cleaning procedures. The chemicals used for cleaning enlarge the pores of disposable gloves, rendering them ineffective.

Table 2.1 • GUIDE TO PREVENTING BLOODBORNE PATHOGEN TRANSMISSION

Situation	Disposable Gloves	Protective Eyewear	Mask	Gown
Bleeding control with spurting blood	Yes	Yes	Yes	Yes
Bleeding control with minimal bleeding	Yes	No	No	No
Emergency childbirth	Yes	Yes	Yes	Yes
Endotracheal intubation	Yes	Yes	Yes	No
Oral/nasal suctioning; manually clearing airway	Yes	Yes	Yes	Yes
Handling/cleaning instruments with possible contamination	Yes	Yes	Yes	Yes
Measuring blood pressure	Yes*	No	No	No
Giving an injection	Yes	No	No	No
Measuring temperature	Yes*	No	No	No
Cleaning back of ambulance after a routine medical call	Yes	No	No	No

Note: In your area, gloves may not be needed for measuring blood pressure and temperature. Check your local protocols.

Some tips for using disposable gloves effectively are:

- Wear the correct size glove
- Apply gloves before approaching the patient (if this follows your local protocol)
- Wash your hands immediately after using gloves
- Never wash your hands while wearing disposable gloves
- Replace your gloves if they become visibly soiled or torn
- When removing a glove, grasp the wrist end and turn it inside itself to avoid contacting your skin or clothing with blood or body fluids
- When removing especially bloody gloves, avoid allowing blood or body fluids to fly through the air
- Dispose of soiled gloves properly
- Do not reuse disposable gloves
- Wear utility gloves for cleaning

Masks

Wear a surgical mask to protect the mucous membranes of your nose and mouth any time that body substances might spray, splash, or splatter. Airborne diseases are transmitted through the air in tiny droplets. The infected droplets spread disease if the patient coughs, sneezes, laughs, talks, or sings. Normal breathing can spread the pathogen. Tuberculosis, an airborne disease, is particularly troublesome for EMS providers.

EMT Tip

You can read more about infection control in Appendix C. There are also many Internet sites related to infection control. The Centers for Disease Control have the text of standard precautions on the World Wide Web. The guidelines can be found in the hospital section of the CDC web page at www.cdc.gov.

If treating a patient suspected of having an airborne disease, wear a respirator approved by the National Institute for Occupational Safety and Health (NIOSH). The respirators are specially designed to filter out the tiny airborne pathogens. NIOSH certifies that the respirators provide protection against airborne pathogens. Respirators meeting the requirement are the **high-efficiency particulate air (HEPA) respirator**, and N95 and PFR95 respirators (see Fig. 2.8). When purchasing or using an NIOSH-approved respirator, a qualified professional must fit the filter to your face. Check the mask for a tight seal before each use. The patient should wear a surgical mask if an airborne disease is suspected.

Become familiar with the recommendations for airborne disease prevention in your local EMS system. Recommendations are based on state and federal regulations developed by the CDC, the Occupational Safety and Health Administration (OSHA), and other governmental agencies.

Eye Protection

Eye protection is required in certain situations. Always use eye protection if the patient's injuries may splash or spray body substances. A face shield or goggles is used to protect the mucous membranes in your eyes. If you wear prescription eyeglasses, removable side shields may be applied. A mask should always be worn when using eye protection. A good rule to follow is that a mask may be worn without eye protection, but eye protection should not be worn without a mask.

Gowns

Gowns are needed if a risk exists for splashing or spraying body substances (see Fig. 2.9). Examples of such situations are childbirth and major trauma. Changing your uniform is recommended if it becomes contaminated.

The Exposure Control Plan

In organizations in which employees may be exposed to bloodborne pathogens, the employer is required to have an exposure control plan. Ask your instructor, employer, or medical director about your agency's exposure control plan and become familiar with it. Learn the requirements for notification and testing after an exposure incident. Each EMS agency usually designates an infection control officer. This individual can provide information about standard precautions, BSI, immunizations, testing, and documentation.

Immunizations

Some immunizations and testing procedures are recommended for EMTs. Immunizations prevent the spread of common illnesses. Verification of your immune status may be part of the employment process. At the very least, the EMT-B should be immunized against tetanus. Because you have a great deal

High-efficiency Particulate Air (HEPA) Respirator | *A specially filtered mask that is worn when caring for patients suspected or diagnosed with tuberculosis and other diseases caused by airborne pathogens*

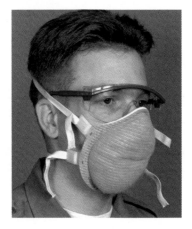

Figure 2.8 *Goggles and a HEPA mask.*

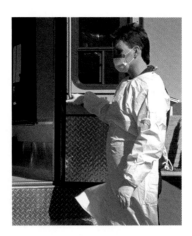

Figure 2.9 *An EMT wearing a gown.*

of contact with blood and body fluids, the hepatitis B vaccine is highly recommended. This vaccine is given in a series of three injections over a six-month period. Tuberculin testing is also suggested. The most effective tuberculin test uses purified protein derivative (PPD). The test will be positive if you have ever been exposed to tuberculosis. If your test is positive, you may be referred to your healthcare provider for preventive care.

EMT Tip

Avoid taking contaminated uniforms to a dry cleaner, to a public laundry or to your home for cleaning. By doing so, you may contaminate other clothing and might transfer pathogens to others in your family or community. Soiled uniforms should be treated in the same manner as soiled stretcher linen and washed at your agency's facility.

D.O.T. OBJECTIVE

List the personal protective equipment necessary for each of the following situations—hazardous materials, rescue operations, and violent situations, as well as crime scenes.

Hazardous Materials

Accidents involving hazardous substances can cause serious illness, death, or lifelong complications if the body is exposed to the substances. Exposure to chemicals can occur by contact, absorption through the skin, inhalation, or ingestion. Chemical spills from truck accidents, explosions, leaks, and other similar situations require special equipment and knowledge (see Fig. 2.10).

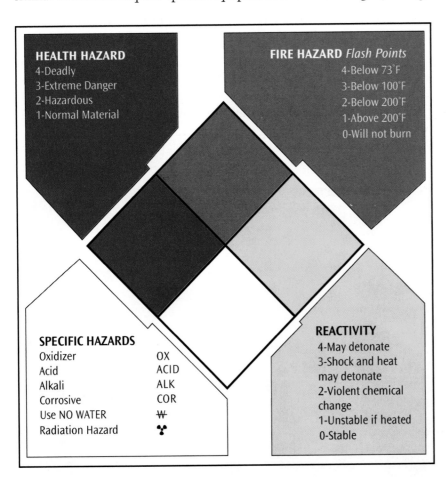

Figure 2.10 *Placards show important information about characteristics of hazardous material.*

EMT Tip

Many EMS agencies have an infection control officer, who has information about immunization requirements and their availability. Another resource for this information is your county public health department.

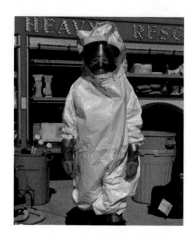

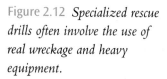

Figure 2.11 *HAZ-MAT suit.*

This is usually beyond the scope of the EMT-B. Your role as a basic provider is to:

- Quickly identify potential hazards
- Protect yourself, patients, and bystanders
- Notify the appropriate authorities, usually a hazardous substance response team

Binoculars are one of the best tools an EMT-Basic can use during a hazardous materials call. Using binoculars helps you to identify signs and placards on vehicles and storage facilities from a safe distance.

Specialized HAZ-MAT teams from state agencies or local fire departments control hazardous materials scenes. A rescue from a hazardous environment requires special equipment, training, and staff. Everyone entering a hazardous scene should be comfortable and efficient in using the self-contained breathing apparatus (SCBA). Other specialized personal protective equipment such as HAZ-MAT suits may also be required (see Fig. 2.11). EMTs provide emergency care only after the scene is safe and patients have been decontaminated. The incident commander will advise you of your responsibilities in this situation. As a rule, EMS personnel do not treat patients until they are removed from the danger zone and have been decontaminated. Specialized classes are available for EMS responders who treat victims of HAZ-MAT exposure. Situations involving hazardous materials are discussed in more detail in Chapter 24.

Rescue Operations

Rescuing patients from fires, explosions, automobile entrapment, and electrocution is inherently dangerous (see Fig. 2.12). The same mechanisms that injured the patient are a threat to the rescuers. Before beginning a rescue

Figure 2.12 *Specialized rescue drills often involve the use of real wreckage and heavy equipment.*

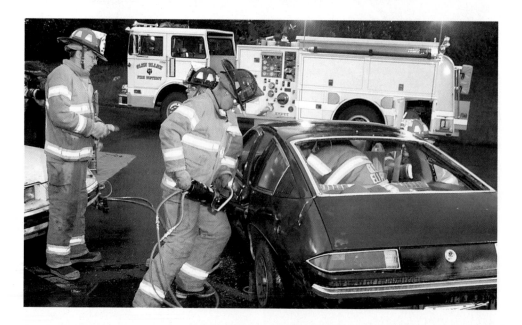

operation, you must identify and reduce potential hazards from electricity, fire, explosion, or hazardous materials. Protective clothing needed for most rescue operations include turnout gear, puncture-proof gloves, helmet, and eyewear. Check with your local rescue team for more information about protective gear. For extensive or specialized rescues, contact your local heavy rescue team (see Fig. 2.13). During extrication, use a blanket to protect the patient from flying glass. Continuing education programs are available for those interested in participating in advanced rescue operations.

Violent Situations and Crime Scene

You may be the first to arrive at a violent situation or crime scene. You will not care for the patient until the scene is under control. Law enforcement personnel are trained to control violent events involving irrational or intoxicated individuals, dangerous pets, weapons, or other threats. The perpetrator, family members, or bystanders may also threaten your safety. Pay close attention to signs of danger and quickly plan your routes of escape. In general, wait for law enforcement to secure any scene with the potential for violence or danger before you enter. Be aware of gang-controlled neighborhoods in your service area. Work closely with your local law enforcement officials to develop plans for answering calls in gang-related areas (see Fig. 2.14). See Chapter 8 for more information on crime scenes.

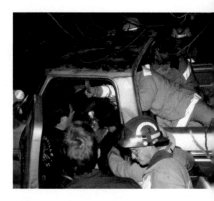

Figure 2.13 *Extrication requires a qualified team of rescuers using specialized equipment.*

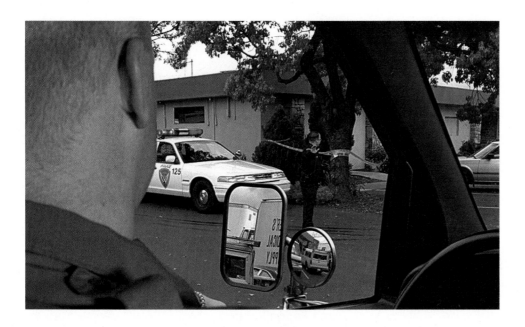

Figure 2.14 *Establish coordination with law enforcement personnel when called to violent situations or crime scenes.*

EMT Tip

Do not attempt to rescue a patient unless you are adequately trained, have the necessary personal safety equipment, and have specialized rescue equipment available.

Chapter Two Summary

- You are responsible for your own well-being. When working as an EMT-B, you are also responsible for the safety of your crew, your patient, and bystanders.

- Death is a normal event. You will work with patients and family members in many stages of grief. Understanding the range of emotions they are experiencing will enable you to help them. Listening empathetically and offering calm, gentle reassurance are effective techniques to use.

- Stress is normal when providing emergency medical care. Certain situations will cause more stress than other situations. Develop healthy methods of relieving the stress of your new duties.

- A healthy lifestyle is essential in dealing with stress effectively. A balanced diet, frequent exercise, and use of relaxation techniques will help. Seek a healthy balance between your duties as an EMT-B, your family, recreational and religious activities, and your health.

- CISD, or critical incident stress debriefing, is a tool to help emergency personnel deal with particularly stressful situations. CISD allows providers to vent their feelings in a nonthreatening, noncritical environment.

- Body substance isolation (BSI) precautions and good handwashing are essential to protect you from exposure to an infectious disease. Assume that all body substances are infectious, and use barrier devices such as gloves, gowns, eye protection, and masks to prevent contact.

- When faced with a hazardous material or rescue situation, never enter the scene unless you are properly trained and equipped to do so.

- Law enforcement should control any scene involving a history of or potential for violence before you provide care.

Key Terms Review

Body Substance Isolation (BSI) Precautions | *page 48*
Critical Incident Stress Debriefing (CISD) | *page 42*

High-efficiency Particulate Air Respirator (HEPA) | *page 52*
Pathogen | *page 48*
Personal Protective Equipment (PPE) | *page 49*

Standard Precautions (SP) | *page 48*
Stress | *page 38*

Review Questions

1. During a critical incident stress debriefing (CISD), emergency care personnel are not given the opportunity to:

   a. Discuss how the job is affecting their families
   b. Get feedback about their fear of making mistakes
   c. Discuss the stressful aspects of a particularly difficult event
   d. File complaints regarding the misconduct of peers in the field

2. BSI equipment and precautions are designed to:

   a. Prevent the spread of communicable diseases
   b. Secure a safe area at an accident scene
   c. Protect the EMT-Basic and patient at a violent crime scene
   d. Test for drug overdose in the patient

3. For emergency childbirth in the field, why should your protective clothing include a gown, gloves, protective eyewear, and mask?

    a. There is danger of a "needlestick" during delivery

    b. No protective clothing is necessary for delivery

    c. You may pass an infectious disease to the infant

    d. There is a risk of spraying/splattering blood

4. You are called to take care of a patient who has symptoms suggestive of an infectious disease. The patient is complaining of a cough, general weakness, and fatigue. The most appropriate personal protective equipment would be:

    a. Gloves and gown

    b. Gown and goggles

    c. Mask and gloves

    d. Goggles and gloves

5. You are a volunteer on a rural ambulance service. You accidentally get blood in your eyes while treating Mr. Johnson's wounds. After you arrive at the hospital, who is the best person to contact regarding the exposure?

    a. A nurse

    b. Mr. Johnson's family physician

    c. Your agency's infection control officer

    d. Your agency's medical director

6. When removing your gloves after a call where no blood or body fluids were present, you should wash your hands for at least how long?

    a. 10 seconds

    b. 30 seconds

    c. 1 minute

    d. 5 minutes

7. You mistakenly enter the scene of a domestic assault in order to treat a patient who has been rendered unconscious. The perpetrator threatens to hurt you in the same manner. Your best course of action would be to:

    a. Retreat from the scene and radio for law enforcement assistance

    b. Notify law enforcement and continue treating the patient

    c. Continue, because the patient is your first priority

    d. Attempt to calm the perpetrator

8. A critical incident stress debriefing is generally held within ___ hours.

    a. 1-2

    b. 24-72

    c. 10

    d. 5

9. Which is the single most effective way to prevent the spread of pathogens from one person to another?

    a. Handwashing

    b. Wearing gloves

    c. Wearing a protective face mask

    d. Wearing a protective suit

10. Protective clothing for vehicle rescue generally includes:

    a. Latex gloves

    b. Turnouts

    c. Turnouts, helmets, and protective gloves

    d. Turnout gear, puncture-proof gloves, helmet, and eyewear

11. Suggested immunizations and tests for the EMT include:

    a. TB

    b. TB, hepatitis

    c. TB, hepatitis, and tetanus

    d. HIV

12. You respond to a call in which the patient tells you he has active TB. What kind of mask should you wear while in contact with this patient?

    a. SCBA

    b. SCUBA

    c. HEPA

    d. DOI

13. Which of the following lifestyle changes can reduce the negative effects of stress?

    a. Keeping your frustrations to yourself

    b. Avoidance of caffeine and alcohol

    c. Eliminating exercise from your routine

    d. Decreasing carbohydrate intake

CASE STUDIES

The Well-Being of the EMT-Basic

1 Your agency is dispatched to a call for a pedestrian struck by a vehicle near the elementary school. A state police officer approaches and tells you that the child is obviously dead. He advises that the area should be treated as a crime scene. When you approach, you recognize the child as the daughter of the mayor.

A. How would you begin to handle this emergency call?

B. What can you do to help minimize the stress that other EMS responders might experience?

C. What other types of EMS calls are commonly associated with stress?

2 The construction foreman is an experienced EMT. He has stressed that if anyone is injured on the job site, you must take BSI and standard precautions before giving first aid. However, you find yourself holding the severely bleeding wound of a fellow worker. You are not wearing gloves. You used and discarded the pair you always carry, so the nearest gloves are in the site office. The foreman arrives on scene and notices your lack of gloves. He begins to give you his lecture on BSI.

A. Are your actions appropriate in this case, or is the foreman correct?

B. Describe some of the basic rules and conditions to follow when using gloves on emergency calls.

C. Are there EMS situations involving direct patient contact that may not require the use of gloves?

3 You are called to the local high school for a gunshot wound. A school security guard arrives on the scene and clears the crowd. You and your partner enter the bathroom. A 15-year-old girl is lying on the floor in a large pool of blood. You kneel down and begin your initial assessment. You determine that the girl does not have a pulse and is not breathing. Her skin is cold to touch. Your exam reveals blood coming from her mouth, nose, and ears. You find a large gunshot wound just behind her right ear. When you look around, you see a large-caliber handgun lying behind a toilet.

A. How should you handle this situation?

B. If the scene is declared a crime scene, what steps will you take when you exit the bathroom?

4 The explosion at the local ice plant was deafening. Dispatch advises that several workers are dead and many more are injured. A strong odor of ammonia fills the air as you leave your station. You know that the plant uses many toxic chemicals to produce ice and that respiratory injuries are probable.

A. Describe your role as an EMT at the site of this hazardous materials event.

B. What specific piece of equipment is very helpful during the scene survey of any hazardous materials event?

C. What local resources are available to help you determine the type of hazardous materials?

D. What types of protective clothing are typically used during a hazardous materials event?

Stories from the Field
Wrap-Up

Providing emergency medical services requires physical and mental strength. Working in EMS exposes you to many hazards to your physical and emotional well-being. Many threats are obvious, but some are not. In this scenario, there are two separate threats to your well-being. The first threat is to your emotional well-being. While speaking with the family, you will deal with a wide range of grief-related emotions. The family's reaction will cause you to feel stressed. You are responsible for helping them deal with the grief of losing a loved one. When you remove the deceased man, you must protect your physical well-being from infectious diseases by using personal protective equipment. The knowledge you have gained from this chapter will help you deal with the emotional aspects of emergency care, as well as the physical threats.

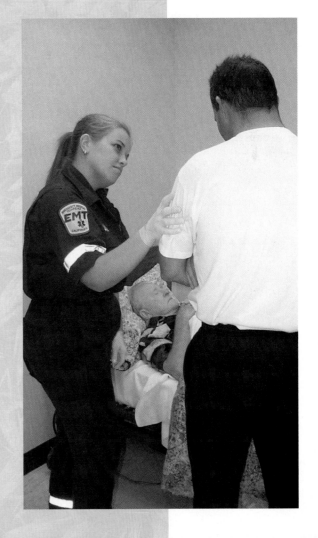

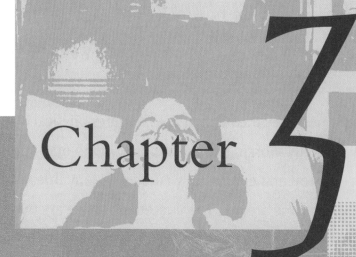

Chapter 3

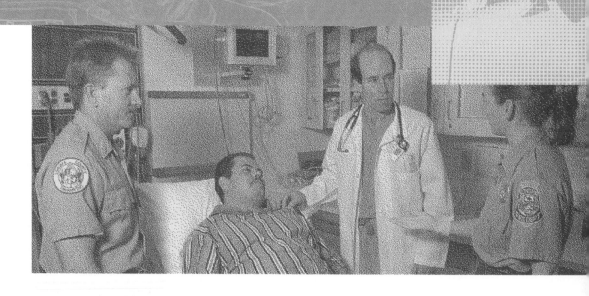

Medical, Legal, and Ethical Issues

Stories from the Field

On the way home from class, you observe a motor vehicle accident. The car has hit a tree and is heavily damaged. You notice that the steering wheel is broken. The windshield is cracked with a starburst pattern. Although you have been on several calls with the fire department, this is the first time you have faced an emergency on your own. You pull off the road, and then begin to question yourself. What should I do? What can I do? Can I get in trouble? What if I do something wrong? Can I get sued?

Fortunately Mark, an EMT from the fire department, pulls in behind you. Mark tells you to call 9-1-1 while he starts to check the vehicle and patient. When you return, you see Mark talking to the patient, who has many small cuts on his face and head. You notice a large knot by his left temple. Mark tells you that the patient is refusing care. While you were gone, he did a quick assessment. The patient does not know who he is or where he is. While you and Mark are talking, the patient tries to start the car. He states he is going to "get out of here before the cops show up."

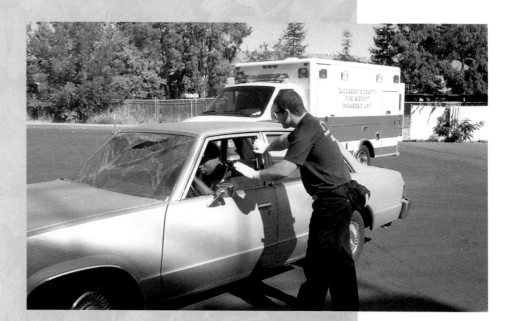

Medical Director | *Physician experienced and knowledgeable in all aspects of emergency care who delegates emergency medical practice to nonphysician providers, such as EMT-Basics and other EMS personnel*

E MTs have many legal and ethical responsibilities. In the normal course of the day, you must make legal and ethical decisions related to patient care. You have obligations to the patient, the **medical director**, and the public. Medicolegal and ethical issues are critical components of every EMS system. This chapter will answer questions such as:

• Should an EMT stop and treat an accident victim when off duty?

• When can patient information be released to the media?

• Can a child with a large laceration on the leg be treated without the parents' consent?

This information will help guide you in making decisions when medicolegal and ethical questions arise.

D.O.T. OBJECTIVE

Define the EMT-Basic scope of practice.

SCOPE OF PRACTICE

Scope of Practice | *A description of the specific care and actions expected and allowed by law*

Local and state laws define the EMT-Basic's **scope of practice** by describing the skills and procedures an EMT-B can use. Laws defining the scope of practice are the foundation for the standard of care. All healthcare workers must maintain a certain standard of care when providing services.

Minimal acceptable standards for an EMT-Basic's scope of practice are outlined in the EMT-B National Standard Curriculum. State and local laws and medical direction will define your responsibilities more specifically. Common skills that are within the EMT-Basic scope of practice are:

• Patient assessment

• Airway management

• Spinal management

• Ambulance operations

• Splinting and basic wound care

• Triage

• Automated external defibrillation

• Basic cardiac life support

When caring for a patient, you are the eyes, ears, and hands of the emergency department physician. Your care is an extension of a physician's care. The medical direction physician is the authority responsible for care given by EMS providers (see Fig. 3.1). Written protocols and standing orders also define your authority to provide care. When caring for patients, you will:

- Follow approved protocols and standing orders
- Maintain telephone or radio contact with medical direction
- Consult medical direction when you have a question or concern
- Care for the patient as instructed by medical direction

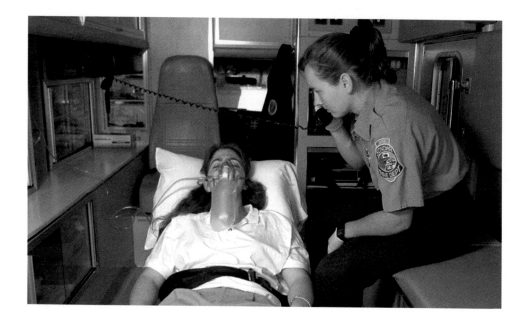

Figure 3.1 *Consulting medical direction.*

Standard of Care

Standards of care describe the minimum acceptable level of care provided in a city, county, community, or EMS region. Standards are set by the actions of the providers in an area. The standard of care is based on:

- Common practices
- Protocols
- Textbooks
- Professional journals
- National curricula
- Public opinion, which may be influenced by the media

You are responsible for your own actions. This means you must provide care according to the standards in your area. In legal action, a jury will determine whether the care you gave met or exceeded the standard of care in your area.

Standard of Care | *The minimum acceptable level of care provided in an EMS system*

When making this decision, your actions will be compared with the actions of others. The jury compares your actions with other EMT-Bs with similar training in a similar situation. You must also learn where EMT-B practice ends and when an advanced provider is needed. Reading your scope of practice and standard of care laws will help you understand your limits.

ETHICS

In some situations, your course of action will not be clearly defined. Ethics is the study of conduct, morality, and standards. Morals are social standards that help clarify behavior that will impact others. Morals arise from community values and opinions. Ethics refer to personal standards and actions that are based on the community moral standards. Your decisions and actions may be reviewed for moral or ethical standards as well as for legality. Ultimately, any ethical decision will be compared against the consequences of that decision.

Understanding ethical responsibilities can be difficult. Imagine that you are returning from a call late at night. You observe your neighbor's house being robbed. Legally, you are not required to notify the police. However, if you asked your neighbor's opinion, she would undoubtedly say that you should have called the police. In this case, calling the police is an ethical responsibility.

In 1978, the National Association of Emergency Medical Technicians published a list of ethical responsibilities for the EMT-Basic. The text of the Code of Ethics is included as Enhanced Study at the end of this chapter. The responsibilities include:

- Make the physical and emotional needs of the patient a priority
- Practice and maintain skills to the point of mastery
- Attend continuing education and refresher programs and courses
- Critically review performance, seeking ways to improve response time, patient outcome, and communication
- Conduct honest and accurate reporting

Never let your personal preferences or bias influence your decisions about patient care. As an EMT-B, you should demonstrate good faith in arriving at your decisions. In some situations, you may be unsure of what action to take. Always consider what is in the patient's best interest. You may also consider a patient's verbal or written statements as well as feedback from the family. Sometimes acting in the patient's best interest will make your job more difficult. For example, a patient asks if she can walk to the ambulance. Allowing her to walk will be easier for you. But ask yourself what is best for the patient. If time permits, contact others for advice. EMS supervisors, medical direction, or law enforcement can help you to make the right ethical decision.

Ethical problems are not limited to patient care issues. Other aspects of your job may require you to make ethical decisions. For example, a coworker comes to work smelling of alcohol. Should you report her? The answers to some ethical questions are elusive at best. Following the guidelines in the Code of Ethics will help you to make the right decisions.

D.O.T. OBJECTIVE

Discuss the importance of do not resuscitate (DNR), advance directives, and local or state provisions regarding EMS application.

ADVANCE DIRECTIVES

Advance directives are documents signed by a patient or the patient's legal representative. Directives state the patient's wishes regarding his or her medical care. The documents provide guidance to those caring for the patient when he or she cannot express these wishes. One example of an advance directive is the do not resuscitate order or DNR.

Do Not Resuscitate Orders

Physicians write **do not resuscitate (DNR) orders** for patients with chronically disabling or terminal illness who do not want resuscitative efforts taken. Persons in long-term care facilities, hospice, and home health care often have DNR orders. The order is usually written at the request of a patient who has issued an advance directive. If a patient has a DNR order, you will not usually provide CPR or other lifesaving care. DNR orders limit the care you can give (see Fig. 3.2). You may care for the patient, but there are limits to the interventions you are allowed to perform. For example, you will not perform CPR or defibrillation. If the patient is still breathing, you may provide comfort measures, such as oxygen.

Review your state laws and local protocols relative to advance directives and DNR orders. If time permits, consult medical direction before following or disregarding a DNR order. When in doubt, or when written DNR orders are not present, begin resuscitation according to local protocol.

Advance Directive | *A legal statement of a patient's wishes regarding his or her health care; used in the event the patient becomes unable to make decisions*

Do Not Resuscitate (DNR) Order | *Written physician's order directing healthcare providers to withhold lifesaving care from a patient in cardiac or respiratory arrest*

Figure 3.2 *Typical prehospital DNR form.*

EMT Tip

Although state or local laws vary, DNR orders are usually only valid in emergencies related to specific medical conditions. DNR orders written for a terminal cancer patient probably will not apply if the patient begins choking in a restaurant or has cardiac arrest after a motor vehicle accident.

EMERGENCY MEDICAL SERVICES
PREHOSPITAL DO NOT RESUSCITATE (DNR) FORM
An Advance Request to Limit the Scope of Emergency Medical Care

I, _____, request limited emergency care as herein described.

I understand DNR means that if my heart stops beating or if I stop breathing, no medical procedure to restart breathing or heart functioning will be instituted.

I understand this decision will not prevent me from obtaining other emergency medical care by prehospital emergency medical care personnel and/or medical care directed by a physician prior to my death.

I understand I may revoke this directive at any time by destroying this form and removing any "DNR" medallions.

I give permission for this information to be given to the prehospital emergency care personnel, doctors, nurses or other health personnel as necessary to implement this directive.

I hereby agree to the "Do Not Resuscitate" (DNR) order.

_____   _____
Patient/Surrogate Signature   **Date**

_____
Surrogate's Relationship to Patient

I affirm that this patient/surrogate is making an informed decision and that this directive is the expressed wish of the patient/surrogate. A copy of this form is in the patient's permanent medical record.

In the event of cardiac or respiratory arrest, no chest compressions, assisted ventilations, intubation, defibrillation, or cardiotonic medications are to be initiated.

_____   _____
Physician Signature   **Date**

_____   _____
Print Name   **Telephone**

_____
Address

THIS FORM WILL NOT BE ACCEPTED IF IT HAS BEEN AMENDED OR ALTERED IN ANY WAY

PREHOSPITAL DNR REQUEST FORM

Durable Power of Attorney for Health Care

Another type of advance directive is the **durable power of attorney for health care** (DPAC or DPOA). Before becoming disabled, a mentally competent person executes a DPAC. The DPAC names a person to make healthcare decisions on the patient's behalf. This person will make decisions only if the patient becomes incapacitated. A family member or close friend is usually designated as the durable power of attorney. In some states, a professional may be appointed as the DPAC. This is illegal in other states, unless the healthcare worker is a relative. Check your local protocol.

The person named durable power of attorney will learn the patient's wishes in advance. He or she will make healthcare decisions for the patient in keeping with these wishes. The authority to make decisions is not permanent. The DPAC is valid only when the patient's decision-making ability is impaired. This could be temporary, such as during an acute illness.

Durable Power of Attorney for Health Care | *A type of advance directive that assigns another person to make medical decisions on the patient's behalf; used only if an individual becomes unable to make decisions*

D.O.T. OBJECTIVE

Define consent and discuss the methods of obtaining consent.

PATIENT CONSENT

Permission for treatment is called consent. Consent must be obtained for all patients before you provide any medical care. One legal concept related to gaining and maintaining consent is the mental competency of the patient. A competent patient is rational and able to make healthcare decisions. A competent patient has the legal right to refuse treatment anytime. Always determine if the patient is competent before beginning care. You will do this as part of your assessment of the patient. Briefly, a patient is considered competent to give consent if he or she is:

CD-ROM Link

In the "Advanced Directives" video in the Medical Legal chapter and the Video Appendix on the MedEMT CD-ROM, an instructor/paramedic points out how advance directives can sometimes relieve certain stresses of patient care.

- Awake
- Alert
- Oriented to person
- Oriented to place
- Oriented to time

You will describe the treatment to a competent patient, using words or signs that he or she understands (see Fig. 3.3). You must also inform the patient of any related risks. If the patient agrees to treatment, he or she is giving informed consent. This means that the patient has been informed of and agrees to the treatment. He or she understands and accepts the risks or consequences.

Figure 3.3 *A competent patient must give you consent before treatment.*

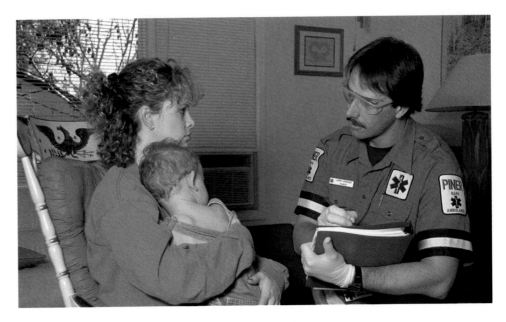

You can treat a patient based on four types of consent:

1. Expressed consent
2. Implied consent
3. Parental consent
4. Consent from a legal guardian of a child or a mentally incompetent adult

> ### D.O.T. OBJECTIVE
> Differentiate between expressed and implied consent.

Expressed Consent

Expressed Consent | Permission for treatment from a patient who is of legal age and is able to make rational decisions; expressed consent is given after the patient is informed of procedures involved in a treatment in a language he or she understands

Expressed consent is given by a patient who is of legal age. He or she must be able to make rational treatment decisions. Verbal consent or affirmative gestures are acceptable forms of expressed consent. You must obtain expressed consent from every conscious, mentally competent adult before providing treatment. Failure to obtain consent can result in charges of assault and battery. This means you have unlawfully touched a person or caused fear of bodily harm.

Implied Consent

Implied Consent | Used for unconscious or mentally incompetent patients requiring emergency intervention; based on the assumption that the patient would give permission to treat life-threatening conditions

Implied consent is an assumed consent for treatment. This type of consent applies to unconscious or incompetent adult patients needing emergency care. Implied consent is based on the assumption that the patient would consent to treatment, if able. In cases of implied consent, the term incompetent refers only to the current illness or injury. In other words, the current condition caused the incompetence. Implied consent is also used for patients who are too ill to respond.

Persons who are considered mentally incompetent may be:

• Irrational from the effects of illness or injury

• Under the influence of alcohol or other drugs

• Mentally ill or deemed incompetent by the court (see the following section)

You may be in doubt about the patient's competence, or whether or not he is able to consent to treatment. If you are uncertain, consult medical direction. If time doesn't allow this, err on the side of caution and care for the patient as a good faith effort. Ask others to continue gathering evidence indicating the patient's mental competency.

D.O.T. OBJECTIVE

Explain the role of consent for minors in providing care.

Consent for Children and Incompetent Adults

Minor is a term used to refer to children under the age of 18. The natural or adoptive parents are the legal guardians for their children, unless another individual has been designated by the court. Adult guardians may be friends or relatives, but the court can appoint any competent adult to look after a child. Individuals appointed by the court are legally responsible for caring for the child if the parents are not available. Parents may also give permission for certain agencies or individuals to authorize care for their child in an emergency. This usually involves school personnel, day care providers, coaches, and similar groups.

Some adults have been declared incompetent by a court. A legal guardian will be appointed to provide consent for these individuals. Consent must be obtained from the guardian unless a life-threatening condition exists.

The person designated as having durable power of attorney can give permission for medical care. An adult may be appointed as the durable power of attorney for one or more children. Always ask for written confirmation from the durable power of attorney.

Implied Consent for Minors

You may be called to care for a minor in a life-threatening situation. Care for the patient based on implied consent if the parent or legal guardian is not available. State laws determine the legal age for giving consent. This usually ranges from the ages of 18 to 21. Become familiar with the protocols and age for consent for treatment in your area.

Emancipated Minors

Some minor children are emancipated minors. Each state has different rules for emancipation. Depending on the state, emancipated minors may be:

• Married

• Pregnant

• Parents of their own children

• Minors living independently in their own homes

• Members of the armed services

Some states do not require parental consent to care for emancipated minors. Other states do not recognize the concept of minor emancipation. A minor who is the natural parent of an infant or child may give consent for that child in most states. Consult with medical direction whenever a question arises regarding consent to treat a minor.

EMS AND THE LEGAL SYSTEM

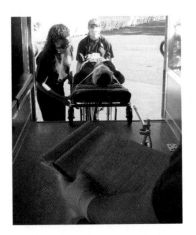

Figure 3.4 *Document your actions to protect yourself from legal action.*

Fortunately, legal action against EMT-Bs is uncommon. It does occur, however, so you must have a basic understanding of the legal system. In order to avoid possible legal action, follow all state and local regulations governing the practice of prehospital care. Become familiar with and follow your standing orders, protocols, and agency policies. Maintain a professional appearance and always conduct yourself as a professional. Use good judgment. Get consent for treatment. Do not exceed the boundaries of EMT-B practice. Provide the best care possible to patients, and never refuse care unless that would place you in immediate danger. Avoid arguing with patients and families. Operate your emergency vehicle safely. Finally, document the care you have provided thoroughly and legibly (see Fig. 3.4).

Two types of law are of specific concern to EMS providers: criminal law and civil law. Criminal law applies to violations of local, state, or federal laws. You may be required to testify in court. You may be asked about events at the scene of an emergency or the actions of a patient or bystander. If proper consent is not obtained before treating the patient, you can be criminally charged with assault and battery or kidnapping. To be convicted, the jury must be convinced beyond a reasonable doubt that a crime was committed.

EMS providers are occasionally involved in civil court cases. Civil cases are also called torts. Most civil suits involve a dispute between two parties over alleged damages. Claims of abandonment and negligence are examples of civil actions affecting EMS providers. Evidence beyond a reasonable doubt is not required in civil cases. Liability, or lack of liability, is determined by a preponderance of the evidence. Simply put, the side that proves its case best wins.

Discuss the issues of abandonment, negligence, and battery and their implications to the EMT-Basic.

Assault and Battery

Assault is threatening or attempting to inflict offensive physical contact. No physical contact is necessary for assault to occur. An assault is often determined to have existed even if battery has not been committed. **Battery** is offensive physical contact or touching of another person without consent. Charges of assault and battery are usually combined, particularly if the parties exchanged threatening words.

Failure to obtain expressed consent from a conscious, mentally competent patient before providing care can result in charges of assault and battery. This also applies to patients who cannot provide consent on their own.

Assault | *Threatening or attempting to inflict offensive physical contact; physical contact is not necessary for assault to occur*

Battery | *Actual offensive physical contact or touching of another person without their consent; usually combined with a charge of assault, particularly if threatening words were exchanged between the parties*

Discuss the implications for the EMT-Basic in patient refusal of transport.

Refusal of Treatment

A competent patient has the right to refuse emergency care or withdraw from treatment anytime. This might occur when an unconscious patient regains consciousness and refuses to be transported to the hospital. All refusals must be made by mentally competent adults following the criteria for expressed consent described earlier. When discussing refusal or withdrawal of treatment with a patient, use terms he or she can understand. If the patient continues to refuse treatment, inform him or her of the consequences. Make sure that he or she fully understands. The patient must accept all risks and consequences associated with the refusal. When patient's intent to refuse treatment is unclear, err in favor of providing care.

CD-ROM Link

The "Release Form" video in the Authentic Emergency Scenes section of the Video Appendix on the MedEMT CD-ROM depicts the problem of a language barrier when trying to obtain consent.

Documentation for Refusal of Treatment

Document all refusals of care. The patient should sign a release from liability form (see Fig. 3.5). If the patient will not sign the form, two EMS workers should witness and document the refusal and the circumstances associated with it.

Figure 3.5 *Release/refusal form.*

Date _____ ALS# _____ Dispatch# _____

Section I   Release at Scene (RAS)

I understand that any evaluation and/or emergency treatment I have received by these EMS person-nel has been on an emergency basis only and is not intended to be a substitute for complete med-ical assessment and/or care. The decision not to accept further care and/or transportation to a hos-pital emergency department has been made by me alone with the understanding that I may have medical complications unknown or unforeseen at this time. I understand that if I change my mind or my condition becomes worse and I decide to accept treatment/transportation by the Emergency Medical Services System, I can call back and they will respond.

Patient's Name (print) _____   Patient Signature _____

Patient/Guardian Signature _____   Relationship _____

Paramedic/EMT Signature_____   Witness Signature _____

Comments: _____

_____

_____

_____

_____

Section II   Refusal of Evaluation/Treatment/Transportation Against Medical Advice (AMA)

I, _____ acknowledge that on

_____
Date   EMT-Paramedic/EMT   License/Cert #   Service Provider Agency
explained my condition to me and advised me of some of the potential risks and/or complications which could or would arise from refusal of medical care. I have also been advised that other unknown risks and/or complications are possible. Being aware that there are known and unknown potential risks and/or complications, it is still my desire to refuse the advised medical care.

I do hereby release EMS personnel from all liability resulting from any adverse medical conditions(s) caused by my refusal of the recommended medical care.

Patient Name (print) _____   Patient Signature _____

Patient/Guardian Signature _____   Relationship _____

Paramedic/EMT Signature _____   Witness Signature _____

Comments: _____

_____

_____

Documenting each patient contact or attempt to provide care is a key factor in protecting yourself from liability. This is particularly true if the patient refuses treatment. Before leaving a scene in which the patient is refusing care, you should:

• Try to persuade the patient to accept treatment or go to a hospital

• Ensure that the patient can make rational, informed decisions

• Inform the patient about the reason that he or she needs treatment or trans-portation to the hospital

- Describe the consequences of the refusal in a manner the patient understands
- Consult medical direction if needed or as specified by local protocol
- If law enforcement personnel are on the scene, ask them to speak with the patient about the consequences of refusing care
- Document your assessment findings, emergency care given, and a detailed account of your attempts to persuade the patient to accept care
- If the patient continues to refuse care, have the patient sign a release from liability form
- Do not refuse to treat or transport a patient unless caring for the patient will endanger you
- Never decide not to transport a patient on your own. Always consult other EMS professionals when a patient is refusing care.

When leaving a person who is refusing care, advise the patient to call again if needed. Tell the patient that he or she can change his or her mind, and you will return. Advise the patient to follow up with his or her physician.

Abandonment and Negligence

An EMT-B can be found legally liable in civil court for emergency care given to patients. Two types of actions are acts of commission and acts of omission. Acts of commission exist when you care for the patient. The care is either inappropriate, or you make a mistake when caring for the patient. Acts of omission occur when you fail to provide care the patient needs. These acts may result in claims of abandonment and negligence.

Once you begin caring for a patient, you must continue to provide the same standard of care until another qualified professional takes over. He or she must provide care at the same level, or a higher level. **Abandonment** is ending patient care without assuring that care is continued at the same or higher level. Patient abandonment can have serious consequences for an EMT-Basic. Actions that imply that you have accepted responsibility for patient care include taking a call from the dispatcher, stopping at a scene, or beginning patient care. Be sure to maintain your level of care until relieved of that responsibility by someone in authority. However, a patient may be initially assessed by an advanced provider who determines that the patient's condition does not require advanced management. In this case, the advanced provider can transfer care to a more basic provider without risking abandonment. Discontinuing care may also be legally acceptable if you must leave the scene for safety reasons.

Abandonment | Termination of care without the patient's consent and without making any provisions for continuing care at the same or higher level

When providing emergency care, you must meet the local standard of care. **Negligence** occurs when the patient is harmed because you acted inappropriately or failed to act. To prevent liability, always ask yourself what another

Negligence | Failure to act as a reasonable, prudent, similarly trained person would act under similar circumstances

EMT-B would do in a similar situation. Then, provide that level of care. To be considered negligent by the court, the jury must consider:

Duty to Act | *A contractual or legal obligation to care for any patient who requests services; does not apply if caring for the patient endangers the EMT-Basic's life*

- Whether the EMT-B had a **duty to act**
- If the EMT-B breached his or her duty to act (care) for the patient
- Whether the patient suffered physical, psychological, or financial harm
- The jury will also consider:
- What another reasonably prudent EMT-B would do in the same circumstances
- Whether the patient's own actions or omissions contributed to his or her injuries

If negligence is proven, the court or jury must also decide what remedy or remedies the patient should receive.

D.O.T. OBJECTIVE

State the conditions necessary for the EMT-Basic to have a duty to act.

Duty to Act

When you are on duty, you have a legal obligation to provide care to any patient who requests your services. The only exception is situations in which caring for the patient would place you in danger. An obligation to provide care may be implied or contractual. An implied obligation exists as soon as you are notified of a request for assistance. As part of the responding emergency team, you have an implied legal obligation to care for the patient. When you begin treatment, you have established an implied contract with the patient.

Formal contractual obligations occur when an agency or system has a written contract to provide services. Formal contracts commonly exist between an EMS agency and a municipality. Some agencies may have contracts with facilities such as sports arenas or long-term care facilities. Specific clauses within the contract will describe when service to a patient can be refused.

Moral and Ethical Obligations

The laws in some states do not require an EMT-B to provide emergency care to patients when:

- The EMT-B is off duty
- The EMT-B is in an ambulance outside his or her service area

In these situations, the duty to act rests on the moral or ethical considerations of the EMT-B. If you decide to provide care while off duty or outside your service area, carefully document the care you give. Your documentation should be the same as if you were on duty. Carefully consider personal risks and legal implications before deciding to provide care when you are off duty. Once you begin care, you must meet the standard of care. This means you must continue caring for the patient until someone of equal or higher training assumes responsibility.

Good Samaritan Laws

Good Samaritan laws are designed to protect individuals from civil liability when providing emergency care. The laws provide immunity from liability if you act in good faith. A person may still be held liable for acts of gross negligence. You must know the extent of your duty to act within and outside your service area. The laws may apply to healthcare providers who are off duty and assist at the scene of an emergency. In some areas, the Good Samaritan law does not offer legal immunity to EMT-Bs. Paid personnel are not protected. Your care must be consistent with the standard of care for your level of training. Familiarize yourself with local or state Good Samaritan laws. Check with your local EMS agency or employer.

EMT Tip

Be aware of the legal requirements for certified or licensed EMT-Bs in your state. Some states or localities require you to provide care in these situations. Your service agency may also have policies or procedures describing your duties.

D.O.T. OBJECTIVE

Explain the importance, necessity, and legality of patient confidentiality.

CONFIDENTIALITY

As an EMT-B, you have access to a great deal of confidential information. You will learn personal information about your patient when completing the history and assessment (see Fig. 3.6). The patient or family may also reveal information that is of a personal or intimate nature. Confidential information includes, but is not limited to, facts about the patient's history, your assessment findings, and any treatment you have provided.

Strict laws and regulations in every state protect a person's right to privacy. Before you can release information, the patient or his or her guardian must sign a written release. Releasing confidential information without permission results in strict penalties in some states. The rules may be more complicated if the patient is a minor. You may not provide information unless legal guardianship has been established.

Figure 3.6 *As part of the medical profession, you are obligated to maintain patient confidentiality.*

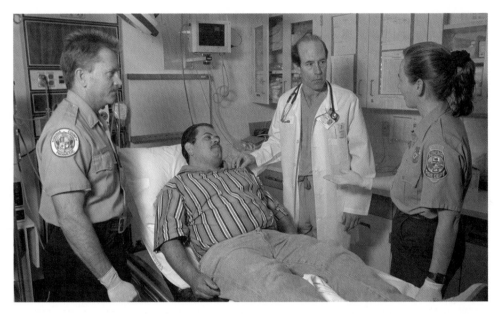

Avoid discussing any details about a patient. You can not release confidential information to anyone, including the patient's family members. You cannot discuss patient information with your own family. Be particularly careful if you are approached by the media. Sometimes reporters will lead you to believe that they already know information about the patient. They do this hoping that you will provide the correct information, which they will publish. If you confirm or deny their statements, you will violate **confidentiality**.

Confidentiality | *An obligation to protect the patient's privacy by not disclosing information to unauthorized individuals*

D.O.T. OBJECTIVE

State the conditions that require an EMT-Basic to notify local law enforcement officials.

When a Release Is Not Required

Confidential patient information may be disclosed without a signed written release in some situations. For example, other healthcare providers need to know information about the patient to continue care. This is particularly true if the patient has an infectious disease. In some states, reporting infectious diseases is required by law.

You may be required by law to provide confidential information. Many states require the EMT-B to report incidents of sexual assault, adult or child abuse, gunshot wounds, dog bites, and other situations to the proper authorities. Some states also require reporting forcible transport of someone against his or her will, or injury of an intoxicated patient. Failure to report such incidents could result in penalties. Become familiar with your state and local reporting requirements.

Insurance agencies may require information before paying for services. If the patient is involved in a lawsuit related to the illness or injury, the court may request your records. If so, court officers will produce a subpoena for the records. The EMS agency must comply with the court's request.

Some states allow the release of patient information for the explicit purpose of educating other healthcare providers. Although you may release information about the medical condition, you must protect the patient's identity. Patient names and other identifying information should be removed from the material. Check with your local EMS system or an attorney for details.

D.O.T. OBJECTIVE

Discuss the considerations of the EMT-Basic in issues of organ retrieval.

ORGAN DONORS

You may care for patients who have chosen to be organ donors. An EMT-B has a limited role in this situation. Be alert for donor volunteers when in the field. Although a potential organ donor is not treated differently from any other patient, your early identification could help save the lives of people waiting for organs. While the patient may not be viable, his or her organs can provide life to others. Providing care such as CPR helps to maintain viable organs. You may wish to notify the receiving facility of a patient's organ donor status. This can be done during the radio report or in person upon arrival.

Signed, legal permission is required before organs can be harvested from a donor. This may take the form of an organ donor card or another legal document (see Fig. 3.7). In some states, a person's intent to be a donor is listed on the back of the driver's license. Family members may consent to organ donation. The laws for family consent vary in each state. Become familiar with your state guidelines.

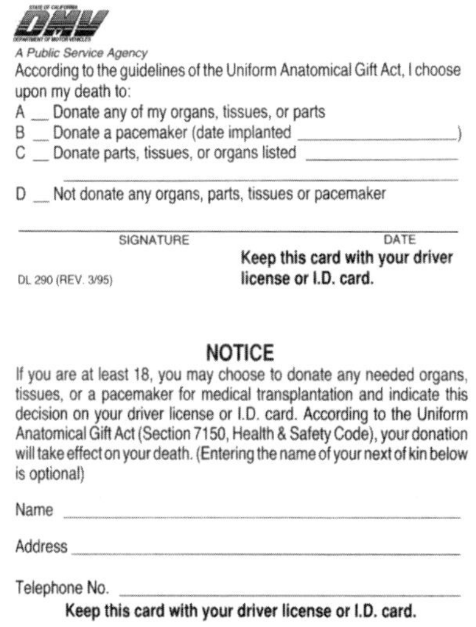

DMV
A Public Service Agency

According to the guidelines of the Uniform Anatomical Gift Act, I choose upon my death to:

A __ Donate any of my organs, tissues, or parts
B __ Donate a pacemaker (date implanted _____)
C __ Donate parts, tissues, or organs listed _____

D __ Not donate any organs, parts, tissues or pacemaker

_____
SIGNATURE   DATE
Keep this card with your driver license or I.D. card.
DL 290 (REV. 3/95)

NOTICE
If you are at least 18, you may choose to donate any needed organs, tissues, or a pacemaker for medical transplantation and indicate this decision on your driver license or I.D. card. According to the Uniform Anatomical Gift Act (Section 7150, Health & Safety Code), your donation will take effect on your death. (Entering the name of your next of kin below is optional)

Name _____
Address _____
Telephone No. _____
Keep this card with your driver license or I.D. card.

Figure 3.7 *California provides for organ donation consent on driver's licenses.*

Differentiate the actions that an EMT-Basic should take to assist in the preservation of a crime scene.

PRESERVATION OF CRIME SCENES

If you suspect a crime is involved, avoid disturbing the scene unless required to provide medical care. Always notify the dispatcher if you suspect a crime. Your primary responsibility is to care for the patient. However, you must preserve potential evidence as much as possible (see Fig. 3.8). Avoid cutting through holes in the patient's clothing caused by gunshot wounds, stab wounds, or other penetrating injuries. Avoid cutting through any knots or ties, because these may provide clues. Observe and document anything unusual at the scene. Do not use an on-scene telephone or bathroom unless given permission by the police. These locations often contain valuable evidence important to law enforcement efforts.

Whenever possible, you must maintain the chain of evidence. The chain provides a documented history or chronology of the exact date, times, and persons having contact with or custody of potential evidence. Check with local law enforcement officers about how to handle potential evidence. The best strategy may be to avoid touching or moving anything at the scene of a potential crime unless it interferes with emergency care.

Figure 3.8 *Keep bystanders away from a potential crime scene to preserve evidence.*

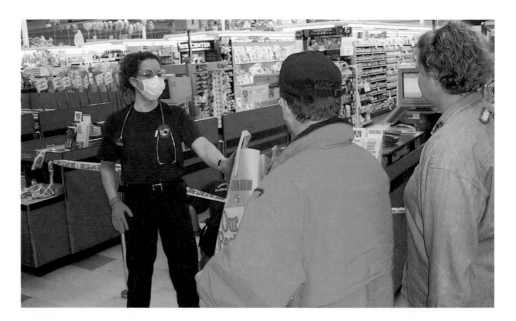

Chapter Three Summary

- You have a legal and ethical responsibility to provide for the well-being of your patient. You must have consent or permission to treat any patient. Expressed consent should be obtained from every conscious, mentally competent adult before caring for the patient. You must explain any procedures and the related risk.

- Implied consent exists when you treat a patient who is unable to give expressed consent and who needs emergency medical care. The consent of a parent or guardian is required for treatment of minors. If the parent or guardian is unavailable, care for life-threatening conditions is based on implied consent.

- A mentally competent adult can refuse treatment or withdraw from treatment at any time. Inform the patient of the risks and consequences of refusing care, and obtain a release from liability. Good documentation is essential to provide legal protection.

- An EMT-B can be charged with assault and battery for:

  Unlawfully touching a patient without his or her consent

  Providing care when a competent patient does not consent to the treatment

- EMT-Bs may become involved in both the criminal and civil court systems. You may be called upon to testify in criminal cases. Claims that an EMT was negligent or abandoned a patient are civil court issues. To prove negligence, the claimant must prove that the:

  EMT-B had a duty to act

  EMT-B breached his or her duty to act

  Patient suffered physical, psychological, or financial harm

  Breach of duty caused the harm

- A duty to act is an obligation to provide medical care. It can be implied or expressed. An implied duty exists when you accept a call from dispatch. An expressed duty may exist because of a written contract with a government agency or business.

- All patient information is confidential and should not be released, except as allowed by law. Certain situations must be reported to law enforcement or other designated agencies.

Key Terms Review

Abandonment | *page 73*

Advance Directive | *page 65*

Assault | *page 71*

Battery | *page 71*

Confidentiality | *page 76*

Do Not Resuscitate (DNR) Order | *page 65*

Durable Power of Attorney for Health Care | *page 67*

Duty to Act | *page 74*

Expressed Consent | *page 68*

Implied Consent | *page 68*

Medical Director | *page 62*

Negligence | *page 73*

Scope of Practice | *page 62*

Standard of Care | *page 63*

Review Questions

1. Which of the following is NOT a case in which an EMT-Basic may release details regarding a patient:

   a. After receiving a written release form

   b. After receiving a subpoena

   c. After receiving verbal permission from the patient himself

   d. In order for other providers to continue care

2. The laws that define the specific care and actions the EMT-Basic is allowed to perform are called:

   a. Scope of Practice Laws

   b. Standard of Care Laws

   c. Good Samaritan Laws

   d. Duty to Act Laws

3. At the scene of a respiratory distress call, you assess the patient, measure vital signs, and administer oxygen prior to calling medical control. The care you provided is allowed based on:

   a. Your duty to act

   b. On-line medical direction

   c. Standard of care

   d. Written protocols

4. You arrive to find Mrs. Holmes pulseless and apneic. Her husband and daughter inform you that she has a DNR order, but they cannot find it right now. What should you for Mrs. Holmes?

   a. Respect the family's wishes and do nothing

   b. Start CPR and transport

   c. Start CPR and call medical direction

   d. Nothing until you contact the patient's private physician

5. Mr. Smith is suffering from colon cancer. He has a valid DNR order, which is present at his home. His hospice nurse has called you because Mr. Smith has choked on a piece of meat. The patient is not breathing upon your arrival. What care would you provide for Mr. Smith?

   a. Do nothing in honor of his DNR

   b. Call medical control for advice

   c. Use BLS obstructed airway skills

   d. Begin CPR and transport

6. You are treating a victim of a fall from a ladder at a construction site. Your patient is reluctant to go to the hospital. He is fully alert and oriented. He finally agrees after you explain the severity of his injuries and the care you are going to provide. What type of consent did the patient give to you?

   a. Expressed consent

   b. Implied consent

   c. Parental consent

   d. Verbal consent

7. The adult driver of a motor vehicle that collided with a tree wants no treatment or transportation from you. She knows her name, the date, the time, and what has happened to her. However, she has a large laceration to her head that is bleeding profusely. What should you do for your patient?

   a. Call her family to take her to the hospital

   b. Treat her wounds despite her protest

   c. Secure her to the stretcher so that you can treat her wounds without interference

   d. Have her sign a refusal of treatment form and advise her of the consequences of refusal

8. You have been called to a day care center for an unconscious infant. The center director begs you to care for the child. She provides you with a form giving consent for emergency care signed by the parents. You can provide care based on:

   a. Expressed consent

   b. Durable power of attorney

   c. Implied consent

   d. Parental consent

9. You are horrified to witness your partner threatening to tape shut the mouth of a loud, drunk patient if he doesn't lower his voice. Your partner has committed what type of violation against this patient?

   a. Slander

   b. Libel

   c. Battery

   d. Assault

10. You arrive at an extended care facility. The patient is in full cardiac arrest. A family member states that the patient has a DNR order. However, the staff and the family cannot locate the DNR order. You should:

    a. Abide by the family's wishes

    b. Begin resuscitation, following your local protocols

    c. Ask your partner what to do

    d. Start CPR and contact medical direction

11. You go on a run for a 15-year-old patient who was hit by a truck from a local trucking company. A newspaper reporter asks you for the patient's name, address, and medical condition while you and your partner are loading the patient into the ambulance. What should you do?

    a. Speak with the reporter, giving her the patient information and his medical condition

    b. Tell the reporter that she is interfering with your care and that you will have her arrested if she continues

    c. Ignore the reporter

    d. Tell the reporter that you are not authorized to release that information

12. In order to give informed consent, a patient must be:

    a. Of legal age

    b. Of legal age and able to make nonrational decisions

    c. Of legal age and able to make rational decisions

    d. Of legal age, able to make rational decisions, and able to understand the possible risks of treatment

13. You respond to a multiple-car motor vehicle collision. A senior EMT directs you to your patient. He is a 32-year-old male, who appears to be sleepy and suffering from an injured right arm. The car is severely damaged, including a windshield impact mark where the patient's head hit the windshield. You note several empty beer bottles in the car and a strong smell of alcohol on the patient. The patient insists on going home to his family doctor to have his arm treated, and refuses transport in your ambulance. What should you do?

    a. Have the patient sign a release form, then release the patient

    b. Release the patient

    c. Involve local law enforcement, and ensure that the patient is treated

    d. Contact medial direction for advice and direction

14. Which of the following is the primary responsibility of an EMT at a crime scene?

    a. Preserve evidence for the police

    b. Don't cut through patient clothing

    c. Emergency medical care of the patient

    d. Assist the police in any way possible

15. Standard of care refers to the _____ acceptable level of care provided in an EMS area.

    a. Minimum

    b. Optimum

    c. Maximum

    d. Standard

CASE STUDIES

Medical, Legal, and Ethical Issues

1
You are required to report to a deposition. During the deposition, the attorney states that he believes that his client's treatment did not meet the local standard of care. He wants details about the 20 minutes during which you managed his client's injuries.

A. Explain the term "standard of care."

B. How does standard of care relate to scope of practice?

2
You are dispatched to an unresponsive patient at a long-term care facility. The long-term care facility is about 15 miles from your station. Winter weather increases your response time dramatically. You arrive to find staff members doing CPR on an elderly woman. The resident has a history of multiple strokes. She has been bedfast for many years. The aides tell you that CPR has been in progress for more than 30 minutes. The patient's family is present and tearfully requests that "everybody stop." The resident does not have an advance directive.

A. How would you act in this situation?

3
Sixteen-year-old Sally has been to a party with her friends. She had a few beers, but is not staggering drunk. A block away from the party, Sally and her friends drive off the road and hit a tree. Sally is the only one injured. She has a large laceration across her forehead. Sally is alert and oriented, with no complaints other than the laceration. She does not want to go to the hospital and is refusing treatment. Her parents are in Europe and will not be back for several days.

A. Given only the facts of this scenario, can Sally legally refuse to be transported?

B. What type of consent must you obtain before treating Sally?

4
The little boy never saw the car as it turned the corner. The vehicle struck the boy and dragged him for several feet. When you arrive, you see the mother holding the 2-year-old boy, rocking his limp body in her arms. The boy appears to be unconscious. He is bleeding profusely from a large scalp wound above his right eye. As you begin to assess him, the mother refuses treatment. She says, "Do not touch my child. My religious beliefs are against emergency medical care. I must have faith in whatever happens to him."

A. What should you do in this situation?

B. Could you take this child away from his mother and begin treatment?

C. What type of consent will you use?

5 During your field internship, you were fortunate to have participated in several extremely informative calls. You kept a copy of each patient report form for your records. Back in class, you make copies of the best calls to review with your classmates.

A. How do you define confidentiality?

B. Have you done anything wrong by sharing these documents with your friends? Why or why not?

C. Can you think of situations in which you would be required to share confidential patient information with others (healthcare workers, law enforcement)? If so, when?

6 Dispatch advises that a highway patrol officer is performing artificial ventilation on the driver of the motorcycle involved in a crash. When you arrive and assume patient care, you observe that the patient has multiple significant injuries, including severe head trauma. As you load the patient into the ambulance, the officer advises you that the driver's license identifies her as an organ donor.

A. How does the donor status of your patient change your treatment?

B. How can you assist in the management of this potential donor's organs?

7 While attending the trading area of a large auto auction, you notice a group of people gathered around a man lying on the floor. As you get closer, you observe the patient acting as if he is drunk or on some type of drug. He does not respond appropriately. The man is breathing normally and has a good, strong pulse. He begins to laugh uncontrollably when you try to check the blood pressure. His skin is moist to the touch. EMS has been notified and is on the way.

A. How could you gather more information about this man's condition?

Stories from the Field
Wrap-Up

As an EMT-B, you should be aware of the laws, rules, or regulations that grant you permission to practice. But you also have ethical responsibilities in addition to legal ones. In this situation, you may not have had a legal duty to act, but you had an ethical obligation to provide care until help arrives. Good Samaritan laws may offer some protection from liability, but these laws are not consistent nationwide. Know the legal criteria for negligence in your state, and become familiar with any legal protections you may have. The best defense against any claim of negligence is thorough, accurate documentation.

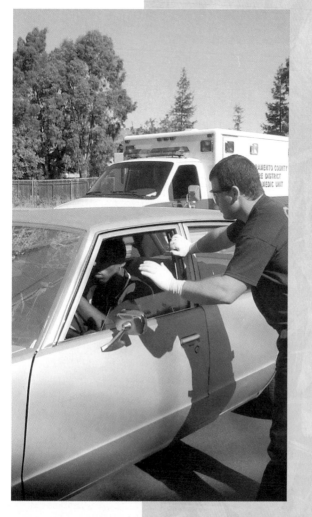

A patient who refuses care also represents a legal challenge to those caring for the patient. Illness, injury, or substance abuse may alter a patient's mental state. In most states, a patient with an altered mental status cannot legally refuse care. However, an EMT-Basic should never treat or transport a patient against his or her will. Consult medical direction or law enforcement if the patient refuses care. Know and follow your agency's policies, procedures, and protocols regarding consent and refusal of care, as well as your local and state requirements.

ENHANCED STUDY

The EMT Code of Ethics

Professional status as an Emergency Medical Technician and Emergency Medical Technician—Paramedic is maintained and enriched by the willingness of the individual practitioner to accept and fulfill obligations to society, other medical professionals, and the profession of Emergency Medical Technician. As an Emergency Medical Technician at the basic level or an Emergency Medical Technician—Paramedic, I solemnly pledge myself to the following code of professional ethics:

- A fundamental responsibility of the Emergency Medical Technician is to conserve life, to alleviate suffering, to promote health, to do no harm, and to encourage the quality and equal availability of emergency medical care.

- The Emergency Medical Technician provides services based on human need, with respect for human dignity, unrestricted by consideration of nationality, race, creed, color, or status.

- The Emergency Medical Technician does not use professional knowledge or skills in any enterprise detrimental to the public well-being.

- The Emergency Medical Technician respects and holds in confidence all information of a confidential nature obtained during professional work unless required by law to divulge such information.

- The Emergency Medical Technician, as a citizen, understands and upholds the law and performs the duties of citizenship; as a professional, the Emergency Medical Technician has the never-ending responsibility to work with concerned citizens and other healthcare professionals in promoting a high standard of emergency medical care to all people.

- The Emergency Medical Technician shall maintain professional competence and demonstrate concern for the competence of other members of the Emergency Medical Services healthcare team.

- An Emergency Medical Technician assumes responsibility in defining and upholding standards of professional practice and education.

- The Emergency Medical Technician assumes responsibility for individual professional actions and judgment, both in dependent and independent emergency functions, and knows and upholds the laws that affect the practice of the Emergency Medical Technician.

- An Emergency Medical Technician has the responsibility to be aware of and participate in matters of legislation affecting the Emergency Medical Technician and the Emergency Medical Services System.

- The Emergency Medical Technician adheres to standards of personal ethics that reflect credit upon the profession.

- Emergency Medical Technicians, or groups of Emergency Medical Technicians, who advertise professional services, do so in conformity with the dignity of the profession.

- The Emergency Medical Technician has an obligation to protect the public by not delegating to a person less qualified any service that requires the professional competence of an Emergency Medical Technician.

- The Medical Technician will work harmoniously with, and sustain confidence in, Emergency Medical Technician associates, the nurse, the physician, and other members of the emergency medical services healthcare team.

- The Emergency Medical Technician refuses to participate in unethical procedures and assumes the responsibility to expose incompetence or unethical conduct of others to the appropriate authority in a proper and professional manner.

Reference: *Written by Charles Gillespie, M.D. Adopted by the National Association of Emergency Medical Technicians, 1978.*

Chapter 4

The Human Body

Stories from the Field

As the rookie on the crew, you are usually asked to take notes while the other EMTs care for the patient. They use your notes to complete the patient report at the hospital. One night, you are assigned to support the local police department's tactical unit on a raid. Unfortunately, things turn sour, and a suspect is shot several times by law enforcement personnel. The patient is brought to the ambulance by two officers and placed in the care of your crew. He is bleeding severely from his chest, but is conscious and screaming for help.

Carmen and Mark immediately begin to care for the patient, and toss you the clipboard. As you note the vital signs and treatments, Carmen asks you to write down the location of the gunshot wounds. The patient continues to complain "I can't breathe." The EMTs seem more interested in treating the wounds than helping you to document the call.

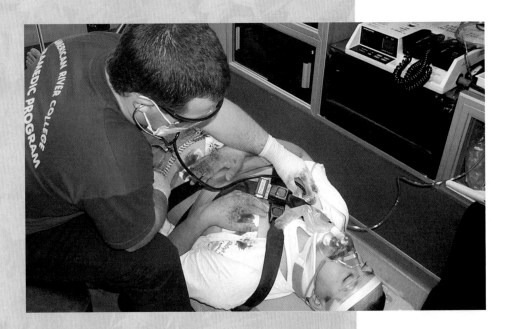

Anatomy | *The study of the structures of the body and how they relate to one another*

Physiology | *The study of the normal functions of the human body*

To assess and manage your patient's condition, you must begin with a working knowledge of the **anatomy** and **physiology** of a healthy human body. Anatomy and physiology are branches of science that describe how the body is functionally organized. Anatomy labels structures of the body and how they physically relate to each other. Physiology describes normal functions and interactions of the body's systems that maintain life and health. A thorough understanding of human anatomy and physiology will give you a strong base from which to build your EMS skills.

Anatomy and physiology use unique terminology. A complete understanding of the terminology is essential for precise and clear communication with medical direction and other healthcare professionals. You must learn the names of specific structures and functions. Learning topographical terms is also important. These terms describe position and direction.

ANATOMICAL TERMS

Knowledge of anatomical terminology is essential to conducting an accurate patient assessment. When reporting patient information to medical direction, your description must be accurate and precise. Anatomical terms describe locations and landmarks of the body and their relationships. Topographical terms describe body positions and directions.

Figure 4.1 *Adult male in standard anatomical position.*

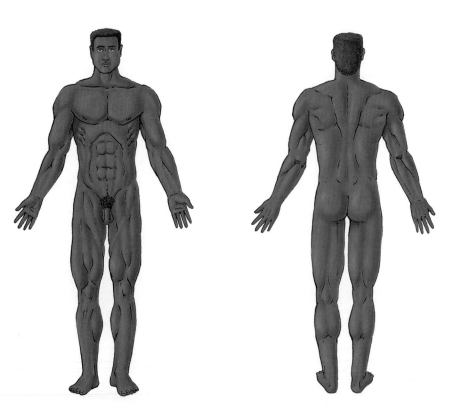

Body Position

Descriptions of direction and position always assume the body is in the anatomical position. This is also called the **standard anatomical position**, or normal anatomical position (see Fig. 4.1). In the normal anatomical position, the body stands upright, facing the observer, with feet flat on the floor, arms hanging at the sides, and palms facing forward.

You must learn the definition of anatomical position because terms such as left, right, up, and down are confusing if the patient's position is not known. To prevent this confusion, anatomists use terms, such as anterior or posterior, that refer to a patient in the standard anatomical position. Using consistent terms improves communication, so when you describe a patient, the word anterior always means toward the front of the body, regardless of the patient's actual position.

A patient may be found sitting or lying in various positions. The **supine** position indicates that the patient is lying on the back, facing up. The **prone** position means the person is lying on the stomach, face down. Patients in the **lateral recumbent**, or lateral position, are lying on the left or right side.

Several positions are used for transporting a patient during a medical emergency. In **Fowler's position**, the patient lies supine with the upper body elevated by a 45- to 60-degree bend at the hips. A patient in the **Trendelenburg position** is supine with the upper body slanted downward. The feet are elevated about 12 inches above the head level. This is also called the **shock position**.

> ### D.O.T. OBJECTIVE
>
> Identify the following topographic terms: Medial, lateral, proximal, distal, superior, inferior, anterior, posterior, midline, right and left, mid-clavicular, bilateral, mid-axillary.

Terms of Direction and Position

Directional or topographical terms describe how the regions and structures of the body relate to one another. Remember that terms of direction and position always refer to the normal anatomical position.

Anatomical Lines and Planes

We can divide the body into regions by drawing imaginary lines and planes that cut through it in different ways (see Fig. 4.2).

The **midline** is an imaginary line drawn vertically through the middle of the body. It extends from the top of the head, through the nose and the navel, and between the legs. This line divides the body into equal right and left sides.

Standard Anatomical Position | *Reference position in which the body is standing upright, facing the EMT with feet flat, arms at the side, palms forward*

Supine (Position) | *Lying on the back*

Prone (Position) | *Lying on the stomach, face down*

Lateral Recumbent Position | *Lying on one side*

Fowler's Position | *Supine position with the upper body elevated by a 45–60° bend at the hips*

Trendelenburg Position | *The supine position inclined with the feet elevated about a foot above the head level*

Shock Position | *See Trendelenburg Position*

Midline | *An imaginary vertical line that divides the body into equal right and left sides*

Figure 4.2 *Body lines and planes.*

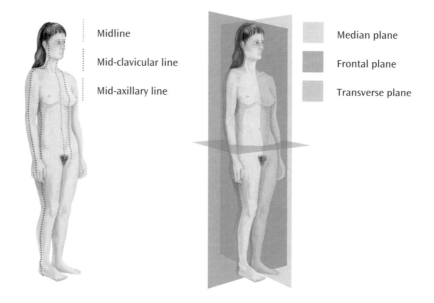

Mid-Axillary (mid-AKS-ul-eh-ree) Line | *Imaginary line drawn vertically through the side of the body, extending from the middle of the armpit to the ankle, dividing the body into front and back sides*

Mid-Clavicular (mid-kluh-VIK-yu-ler) Line | *Imaginary line drawn through the middle of the clavicle (or collar bone), dividing the body into unequal right and left sides*

Figure 4.3 *Lines and planes associated with the thorax.*

EMT Tip

Don't confuse medial, a directional term, with median, a plane.

The body can also be divided from the side. The **mid-axillary line** is drawn vertically through the side of the body, and extends from the middle of the armpit to the ankle, dividing the body into front and back sides.

A sagittal plane is a vertical plane parallel to the midline that divides the body into left and right parts. The median plane or midsagittal plane runs through the midline, dividing the body into equal right and left halves. A vertical plane drawn through the mid-axillary line, dividing the body into front and back halves, is called the frontal plane. A transverse plane extends through a horizontal line, dividing the body into bottom and top segments.

The region between the neck and the waist is called the thorax. The front portion is called the chest, and the rear is called the back. The thorax is divided by its own anatomical lines (see Fig. 4.3). The **mid-clavicular line** is drawn through the middle of the clavicle, or collarbone.

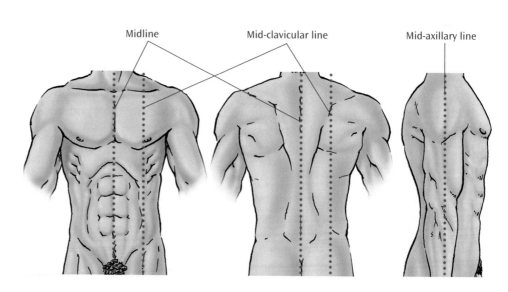

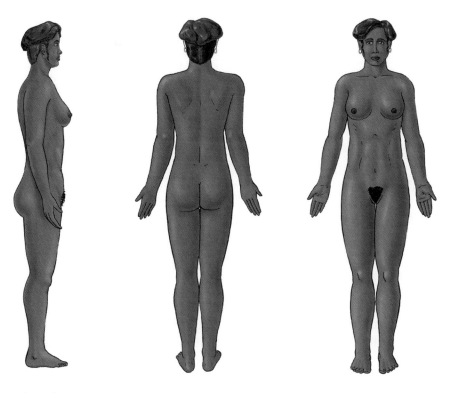

Figure 4.4 *Three views of the body: lateral view (left), posterior view (center), and anterior view (right).*

Medial | *Toward the middle of a body or region*

Lateral | *Away from the midline, to the sides*

Bilateral | *On both sides of the midline (right and left sides)*

Unilateral | *On one side of the body*

Contralateral | *On the opposite side of the body*

Anterior | *Toward the front; front of the body; also called ventral*

Ventral | *Front of the body; also called anterior*

Posterior | *Toward the back of the body; also called dorsal*

Dorsal | *Pertaining to the back of the body; also called posterior*

Superior | *Above another structure*

Inferior | *Below or beneath another structure*

Palmar | *Ventral surface of the hand; the palm of the hand*

Plantar | *Pertaining to the sole of the foot*

Directional Terms

Some terms describe how parts of the body relate to each other in direction and position. Many of these terms can be paired with their opposites or with related terms. Unless otherwise specified, the terms left and right always refer to the sides of the patient, not the EMT–Basic.

Medial is used to describe an area toward the midline or nearer to the midline of the body. **Lateral** means away from the midline or toward the side (see Fig. 4.4). **Bilateral** describes both sides of the body. **Unilateral** means on one side of the body. It may describe either the right or left side. Ipsilateral refers to the same side, either left or right. For example, trauma to the left side of the face might damage the ipsilateral eye (left eye). **Contralateral** means on the opposite side of the body. For example, a stroke in the left half of the brain might paralyze the contralateral or right side of the body.

Other directional terms you will be using are:

- **Anterior** and **ventral** describe the front of the body. **Posterior** and **dorsal** describe the back of the body (see Fig. 4.4).

- **Superior**, cephalic, and cranial are terms used to describe the head or upper part of a structure. **Inferior** and caudal refer to the lower part of a structure, away from the head.

- **Palmar** refers to the palm, or front surface of the hand. **Plantar** refers to the sole, or bottom surface of the foot. The dorsum is opposite the palmar surface of the hand (the back surface). It is also opposite the plantar surface of the foot (the top surface).

Proximal | *Nearer to the head, trunk, or point of origin*

Distal | *Farthest from the head or source; opposite of proximal*

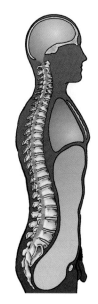

Figure 4.5 *Abdominal cavity shown in red.*

Torso | *The trunk of a body, not including the head or limbs*

Figure 4.6 *Four quadrants of the abdominal region.*

Abdominal Cavity | *The portion of the torso beneath the thorax and above the pelvis; contains the liver, gallbladder, stomach, pancreas, intestines, spleen, kidneys, and ureters*

- Additional terms are used to describe locations along a limb. **Proximal** means nearer to the limb's attachment to the trunk. **Distal** means further from the trunk.

- Illustrative terms also describe depth from the surface of the body. Superficial means on or closer to the surface. Deep means toward the internal aspect of the body, away from the surface.

- Intermediate means between two structures.

Body Regions

The surface of the human body is divided into regions. Each region is characterized by the underlying structures. The major regions are the head, neck, **torso** or trunk, upper extremity (shoulder, arm, and hand), and lower extremity (thigh, leg, and foot).

The torso is the region of the body extending from the neck to the buttock. It is further subdivided into the thorax, or chest, abdomen, and pelvis. The abdomen is the section below the thorax. The navel or umbilicus defines the anterior center of the abdomen. The pelvis lies below the abdomen.

Many visceral, or internal, organs lie beneath the abdominal surface. The **abdominal cavity** contains the intestines, colon, and the thoracic portion of the aortic artery (see Fig. 4.5). Because it is not protected by a bony case, the contents of the abdominal cavity are most vulnerable in blunt trauma.

The abdomen can be subdivided into four quadrants by drawing lines vertically and horizontally through the umbilicus. These are the right upper quadrant (RUQ), left upper quadrant (LUQ), right lower quadrant (RLQ), and left lower quadrant (LLQ) (see Fig. 4.6).

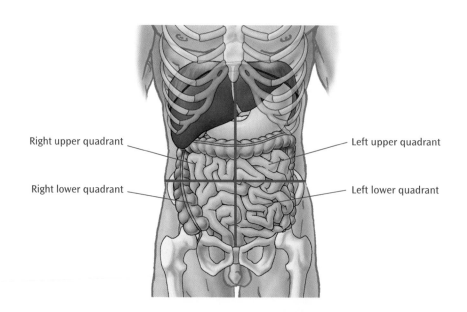

Right upper quadrant — — Left upper quadrant

Right lower quadrant — — Left lower quadrant

Organization of the Body

The body consists of a combination of cells, tissues, organs, and systems. These components can be thought of as organized from simple to complex levels (see Fig. 4.7).

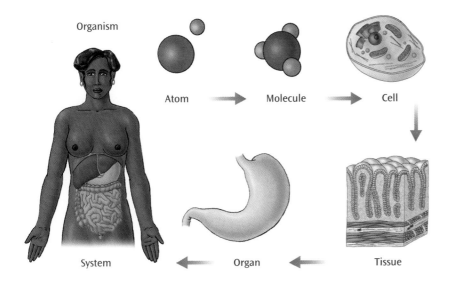

Figure 4.7 *The human body's components are organized from simple to complex.*

Cells are the most basic structural and functional unit found in living organisms. Cells contain specialized structures called organelles that carry out cellular processes such as metabolism and replication (see Fig. 4.8). Many kinds of specialized cells carry out different functions in the body.

Tissues are collections of cells with similar structure and function. The human body consists of four basic types of tissue:

- Epithelial tissue makes up the linings that cover internal and external body surfaces.

- Muscle tissue can shorten, or contract, generating movement. The types of muscle tissue are skeletal, smooth, and cardiac. The action of skeletal muscle is under voluntary control. Smooth and cardiac muscles are involuntary. These muscles act upon impulses sent from the brain.

- Nervous tissue conducts electrochemical nerve impulses that control and coordinate body activities.

- Connective tissue forms structures such as membranes, blood, bone, fat, and cartilage.

Organs are structures made of two or more different types of tissue working together. For example, the heart contains all four basic tissue types:

- Epithelial tissue (lines the chambers of the heart)

- Muscle tissue (causes the heart to contract)

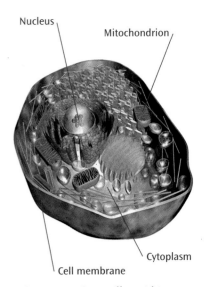

Figure 4.8 *Organelles within a cell.*

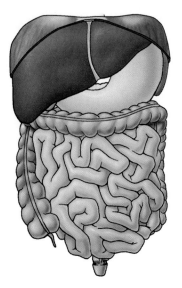

Figure 4.9 *Many organs function as part of the digestive system.*

- Nerve tissue (conducts the electrical signal that triggers a heartbeat)
- Connective tissue (forms the valves between the heart's chambers)

A body system is a group of organs that cooperates to accomplish a particular function. Each organ contributes to the overall function of the system in a different way. For example, in the digestive system, the teeth, tongue, and stomach break up food particles mechanically. The pancreas and gallbladder contribute to the chemical breakdown of food. The intestine absorbs nutrients from the food (see Fig. 4.9).

Other body systems include the respiratory system, the circulatory system, the nervous system, and the endocrine system. The musculoskeletal system is usually referred to as one system. It consists of the muscular system and the skeletal system. A human body functions through the actions and interactions of these systems. The rest of this chapter will introduce you to the structural and functional organization of the major body systems.

D.O.T. OBJECTIVE

Describe the anatomy and function of the following major body systems: respiratory, circulatory, musculoskeletal, nervous, and endocrine.

THE MUSCULOSKELETAL SYSTEM

Musculoskeletal System | Consists of the muscular system and the skeletal system. A human body functions through the actions and interactions of these systems

The **musculoskeletal system** consists of the bony framework of the skeleton and the attached skeletal muscles. Bones provide a core structure to support the body and protect the internal organs. Muscles cause movement of the bones, allowing for locomotion, balance, coordination, and strength. The musculoskeletal system gives the body its shape and enables us to maintain body position or posture. This system also provides an important source of body heat, which is generated during muscle contraction.

The Skeletal System

The skeletal system contains several types of connective tissue.

- Bone is the hard, dense, strong tissue that makes up most of the skeletal system.
- Cartilage is a firm but flexible tissue that allows movement and support between bones. Many bones begin as easily damaged cartilage in early life, hardening into bone tissue as a child develops.
- Tendons attach muscles to bones, causing the bones to move in response to muscular contractions.

• Ligaments attach bones to other bones, increasing the strength of joints. Both tendons and ligaments are made of strong, flexible, fibrous connective tissue.

An adult human body contains 206 bones. Bones function in many capacities, and their shapes differ according to their functions. Much like the steel framework of a building, bones provide structural support for the body. They protect soft tissue structures within the body. For example, the brain is enclosed and protected by the skull. The heart and lungs are encased in the rib cage. Soft tissue in the spinal cord is protected by the spinal column. Bones are essential for movement. By serving as rods to which muscles and tendons attach, bones act as levers to help move our limbs. In addition, blood cells are manufactured in bone marrow. Minerals such as calcium are stored in bone tissue.

The skeleton consists of several regions: the skull, face, spinal column, thorax, pelvis, lower extremities, and upper extremities (see Fig. 4.10).

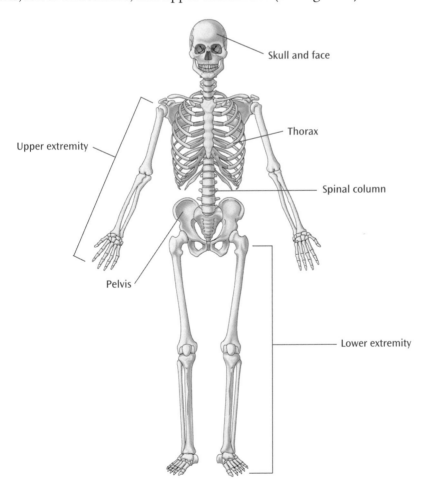

Figure 4.10 *Regions of the human skeleton.*

The Skull and Face

The head consists of the **skull** or cranium. This bone encloses and protects the brain and the facial region. It includes the bones of the eyes, nose, mouth, jaw, and cheeks.

Skull | *Cranium; the bones that comprise and protect the head*

Figure 4.11 *The human skull showing facial and cranial bones. Lateral view (left), frontal view (right).*

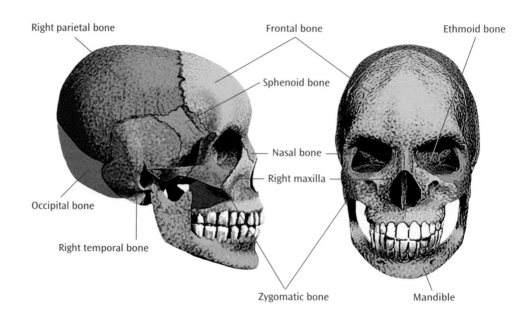

Right parietal bone   Frontal bone   Ethmoid bone

Sphenoid bone

Nasal bone

Right maxilla

Occipital bone

Right temporal bone

Zygomatic bone   Mandible

EMT Tip

You can differentiate the cranial and facial bones by remembering that if a bone touches the brain, it is a cranial bone.

Orbit | *Eye socket*

Maxillae (mak-SIL-ee) | *The two fused bones that form the upper jaw*

Mandible (MAN-di-bul) | *The lower jaw bone*

Zygomatic (ZI-go-MA-tik) Bones | *The cheek bones*

Nasal Bone | *Bone of the nose*

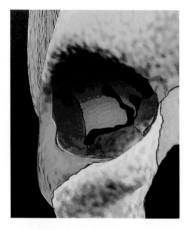

Figure 4.12 *The eye is protected by the bony orbits.*

The cranium consists of 8 cranial bones: the frontal bone, the left and right parietal bones, the left and right temporal bones, the occipital bone, the sphenoid bone, and the ethmoid bone (see Fig. 4.11).

The frontal, parietal, occipital, and temporal bones are named for the parts of the brain they protect. The frontal bone protects the frontal lobe of the cerebrum, or brain, and extends above, below, and to the sides of this portion of the brain. The frontal bone forms the forehead and the superior portions of the bony **orbits**, or eye sockets. Parietal bones make up the sides and roof of the cranium. Temporal bones are below the parietal bones, forming the lower sides of the skull and housing the structures of the inner ear. The occipital bone forms the back of the cranium, protecting the occipital lobe of the brain, called the visual cortex. This bone contains the foramen magnum, a large opening through which the spinal cord passes into the skull.

Fourteen facial bones make up the structure of the face (see Fig. 4.11). The left and right **maxillae** (plural of maxilla) join to form the upper jaw. Sockets in the maxilla hold the upper teeth in place. The **mandible**, or lower jaw, forms the chin. Muscles attach the mandible to the skull to allow for movement when chewing or speaking. The cheekbones are formed from the **zygomatic bones**. The nose consists of the left and right **nasal bones**. Other facial bones are the vomer and the paired inferior nasal conchae, lacrimal bones, and palatine bones. The eyes are protected by the bony orbits, cavities formed by 7 bones that encircle them (see Fig. 4.12).

With the exception of the mandible and the bones of the inner ear, the bones in the skull are not movable, which makes the cranium a rigid container. An injury to the head that causes the brain to swell may result in brain damage. Severe brain swelling can lead to altered consciousness and death.

The Spinal Column

The **spinal column**, or vertebral column, is a chain of bones in the back, extending from the base of the skull to the pelvis (see Fig. 4.13). The vertebral column is strong but flexible. It is designed to protect the spinal cord, support the head, and provide attachment sites for the ribs and many muscles. The structure of the vertebral column allows for flexibility of the trunk of the body. Its curvature provides support and balance.

Spinal Column | *Vertebral column; consists of the cervical, thoracic, and lumbar vertebrae*

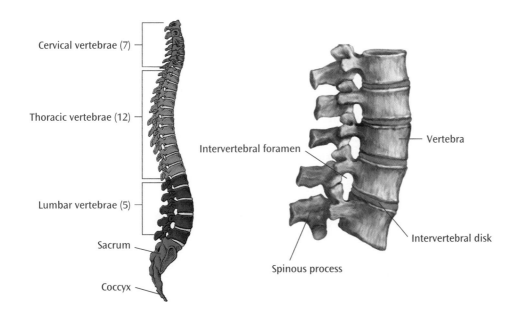

Figure 4.13 *The vertebral column (left) and closeup of the lumbar vertebrae (right).*

Vertebrae (VER-te-bray) | *Plural of vertebra (VER-te-bruh); block-like bones that stack upon one another to form the spinal column*

The spinal column can move in several directions. Bending forward is flexion, and bending backward is extension. Movement to the sides is lateral. Extension also refers to straightening of the spine. The spine can twist by moving the shoulders or hips off the midaxillary plane (rotation).

Vertebrae (plural of vertebra) are block-like bones that stack upon one another to form the spinal column (see Fig. 4.13). In an adult, 24 vertebrae are movable. The other 9 are fused into the rigid sacrum and coccyx at the base of the spine. The vertebrae are categorized by region and structure. Each vertebra has a solid, round vertebral body (see Fig. 4.14).

The spinal cord passes through the vertebral foramen (plural foramina) of each vertebra. The bony vertebral arch protecting the cord forms this space. When the vertebrae are stacked on top of one another, spaces between them form lateral intervertebral foramina, through which the spinal nerves and arteries pass.

Several projections, or spinous processes, extend from each vertebra. Ligaments and muscles are attached at these sites. Ligaments attached to the spinous processes connect the vertebrae, strengthening the posterior aspect of the spinal column. Intervertebral disks are located between the vertebrae.

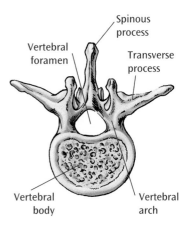

Figure 4.14 *Cross section of a vertebra.*

 EMT Tip

You can remember the number of vertebrae in each area of the spine by thinking of mealtime. We eat breakfast at 7 (seven cervical), lunch at 12 (twelve thoracic), and dinner at 5 (five lumbar).

These fibrous cartilage pads allow for lateral and rotational movement and act as shock absorbers.

Cervical (SUR-vi-kul), Cervical Vertebrae | First 7 vertebrae; the neck

The **cervical** spine, containing the 7 cervical vertebrae, connects the head to the body (see Fig. 4.13). The cervical spine is the most flexible part of the spine, allowing flexion, extension, and rotation. The first 2 vertebrae allow for motion of the head in relation to the neck. They are called the atlas and the axis. Because this is the most movable region of the spine, it is most susceptible to injury.

The thoracic spine is composed of 12 thoracic vertebrae attached to the 12 pairs of ribs. The thoracic vertebrae and the ribs form the upper back and the posterior wall of the thoracic cavity. The ribs prevent much movement of these vertebrae.

Lumbar (LUM-bar), Lumbar Vertebrae | The 5 vertebrae forming the lower back

Five **lumbar** vertebrae form the lumbar spine, or the lower back. These are the largest and strongest vertebrae, because they carry most of the body weight. The larger muscles of the back attach to the lumbar vertebrae. Most back injuries and strains occur in the lumbar region.

Figure 4.15 *The sacrum and coccyx form the back of the pelvis.*

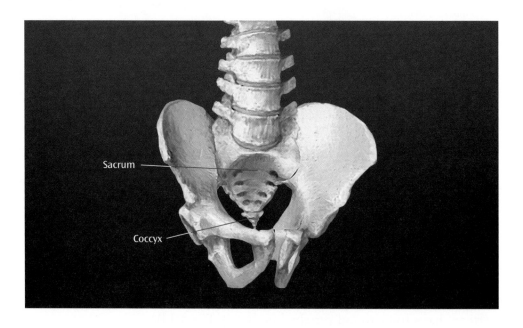

Sacrum, Sacral Vertebrae | The 5 fused vertebrae that form the rigid part of the posterior side of the pelvis

The **sacrum** is a wedge-shaped bone that forms the back of the pelvis (see Fig. 4.15). In late adolescence, 5 sacral vertebrae fuse to form this area. The sacrum provides strong support for the vertebral column, transmitting the weight of the upper body to the pelvic girdle. The base of the sacrum is joined by ligaments to the **coccyx**, which is triangular. It provides an anchor for some muscles of the pelvic floor. Fusion of the 4 coccygeal vertebrae occurs in early adulthood, after sacral fusion.

Coccyx (KOK-siks), Coccygeal Bones | The last 4 vertebrae; the tailbone

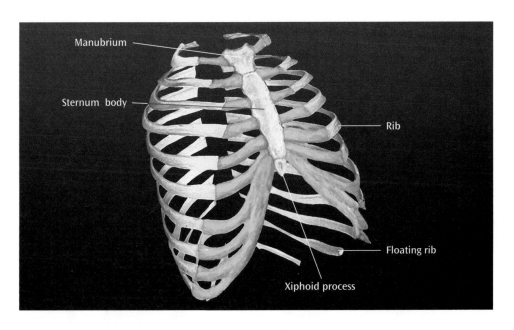

Figure 4.16 *The rib cage.*

EMT Tip

The Thorax

The **thorax**, or chest, is a barrel-shaped region containing 12 pairs of ribs and the **sternum**, or breastbone. The upper 10 pairs of ribs are attached posteriorly to the vertebrae and anteriorly to the sternum. The lower 2 rib pairs only attach posteriorly, so they are called floating ribs. The sternum is a flat bone in the center of the anterior chest. The superior portion of the sternum is called the **manubrium**. Clavicles, or collarbones, are attached to each side of the manubrium. The largest region of the sternum is called the body. The inferior tip of the sternum is called the **xiphoid process**. This small bone is very prominent and easy to palpate (see Fig. 4.16).

The thoracic cavity, or rib cage, is the space formed by the ribs, sternum, and thoracic spine. It protects the vital structures of the lungs, heart, aorta, stomach, liver, spleen, and kidneys, and it assists in breathing. Trauma to the chest can injure these organs.

The abdominal cavity is below the thoracic cavity. Unlike the thoracic cavity, it is not protected by a bony case. Consequently, it is most vulnerable in blunt trauma.

The Pelvis

The **pelvis** is a bowl-shaped structure formed from the left and right hip bones, sacrum, and coccyx (see Fig. 4.17). Each hipbone consists of 3 bones that become fused together by adulthood: the ilium, the **ischium**, and **pubis**, or pubic bone.

Paired iliac bones make up the lateral walls of the pelvis. The top portions, which form the palpable wings of the pelvis, are called the **iliac crests**. The pubis is the anterior portion of the pelvis, which lies in front of the bladder.

The posterior inferior part of the pelvis is the ischium. The acetabulum, or hip socket, is partly formed by the ischium (see Fig. 4.18).

The pelvic cavity, or space within the pelvis, protects the colon, bladder, and internal reproductive organs.

Figure 4.17 *Bones of the pelvis and pelic cavity. Male pelvis (left). The female pelvis (right) is smaller and more bowl-shaped.*

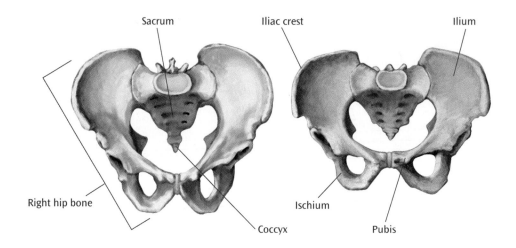

The Lower Extremities

The lower extremity consists of the hip joint, thigh, knee joint, leg, ankle joint, and foot. Each lower limb contains 30 bones used to support the weight of the body. These bones maintain equilibrium and permit locomotion. Because weight bearing is their major function, some mobility is sacrificed in exchange for stability.

Figure 4.18 *The hip joint is a ball-and-socket joint. The acetabulum, or socket, is part of the hip bone (left). The head of the femur (right) forms the ball.*

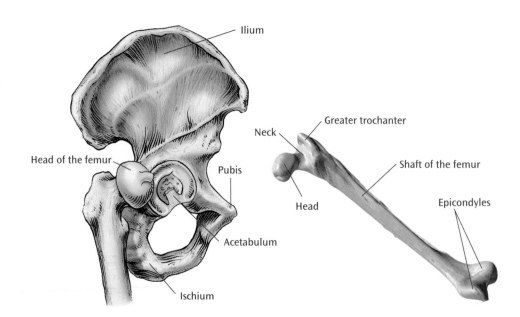

The **femur**, or thighbone, is the longest, strongest, and heaviest bone in the body. It extends from the hip to the knee. The hip joint is a ball-and-socket joint consisting of the ball-like head of the femur, which fits into the cup-shaped acetabulum (see Fig. 4.18). Ball-and-socket joints are described later in this chapter.

Femur (FEE-mer) | *The thigh bone*

The head of the femur narrows into the neck, a frequent site of hip fractures. Fractures are common when an elderly person falls. At the base of the neck is the greater trochanter, a point of attachment for thigh muscles. The long body of the femur is called the shaft (see Fig. 4.18).

At its distal end, the femur widens to form the superior portion of the knee joint (see Fig. 4.19). This is a hinge joint with ligaments and muscles to provide stability. The **tibia**, or shin, forms the inferior portion of the knee joint. The **patella**, or kneecap, forms the anterior part. The action of the patella allows the joint to glide smoothly.

Tibia (TIB-e-uh) | *The shin bone*

Patella (pa-TELL-uh) | *The kneecap*

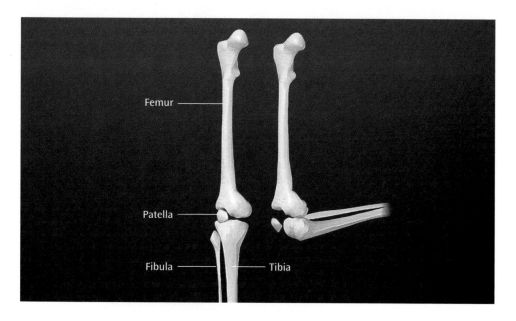

Figure 4.19 *The knee is a hinge joint.*

The lower leg consists of 2 long shaft bones. On the medial side is the tibia and on the lateral side is the **fibula** (see Fig. 4.19). The tibia is the second largest bone in the body. It is designed to bear the weight of the body while walking. At its distal end is the medial **malleolus**, a prominent knobby surface landmark felt on the inner side of the ankle joint. The lateral malleolus is at the distal end of the fibula. It is palpable on the outer side of the ankle joint.

Fibula (FIB-yuh-luh) | *The lateral and smaller bone of the lower leg*

Malleolus (ma-LEE-oh-lus) | *The surface landmark of the ankle*

The foot is made up of many small bones, allowing a wide range of movement and coordination (see Fig. 4.20). The 7 **tarsal** bones of the foot are adapted for weight bearing and locomotion. One of these, the **calcaneus**, forms the back of the heel. The calcaneus is the largest, strongest bone of the foot.

Tarsal (TAR-sul) | *The ankle bone*

Calcaneus (kal-KAY-ne-us) | *The heel bone*

Metatarsals (met-uh-TAR-sulz) | *Foot bones*

The 5 **metatarsals** are the long bones of the foot. The **phalanges** are the bones of the toes. The great toe consists of 2 phalanges, proximal and distal. Each of the other toes consists of 3 phalanges: proximal, middle, and distal.

Figure 4.20 *The bones of the foot.*

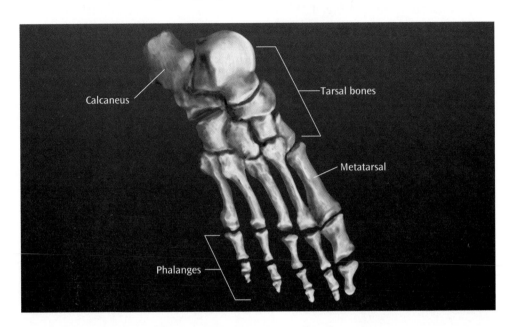

Phalanges (fuh-LAN-jeez) | *Small bones of the fingers and toes*

The Upper Extremities

The upper extremity consists of the bones and joints of the shoulder, arm, and hand. Each upper extremity consists of 30 bones, many of which are structurally similar to bones of the leg.

The upper extremity is attached to the thorax by the pectoral girdle. This area consists of the anterior **clavicle** and the posterior **scapula**, or shoulder blade. The long, thin clavicle can be easily palpated at the top of the anterior chest. This is the bone most frequently broken in the body. The clavicle is attached

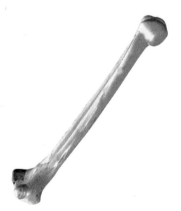

Figure 4.21 *The humerus.*

Figure 4.22 *Cross section of the shoulder joint.*

Clavicle (KLA-vi-kul) | *Bone of the shoulder girdle that joins the sternum to the scapula; collarbone*

Scapula (SKA-pyu-luh) | *The shoulder blade*

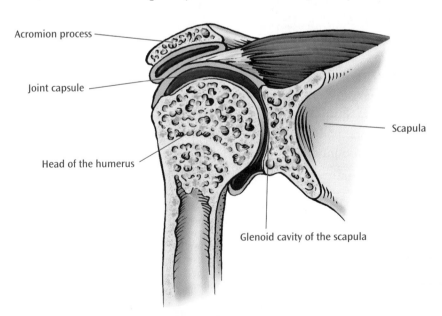

to the sternum. Two scapulae (plural of scapula) are flat, triangular bones that lie on the sides of the upper back. The tip of the scapula, where it is attached to the clavicle, is called the **acromion** process.

The superior portion of the arm consists of the **humerus**, the largest bone of the upper extremity (see Fig. 4.21). The shoulder joint is a ball-and-socket joint similar to the hip joint (see Fig. 4.22). The proximal head of the humerus forms the ball and the glenoid cavity of the scapula forms the socket. This joint permits the arm to move in a wide arc. It is the most flexible joint in the body.

The distal end of the humerus widens to form the elbow joint with the bones of the forearm, the **ulna** and **radius** (see Fig. 4.23). The bony prominence that can be felt as the back of the elbow is called the **olecranon**. The cubital fossa, the fleshy depression in the bend of the elbow, is a common site for insertion of an intravenous line (see Fig. 4.24).

The forearm is the portion of the lower extremity between the elbow and the wrist. It contains two parallel bones. In the normal anatomic position the ulna lies on the medial side and the radius is on the lateral side. When the hand is turned backward, the radius crosses over the ulna. Thus, the radius always lies on the thumb side of the forearm.

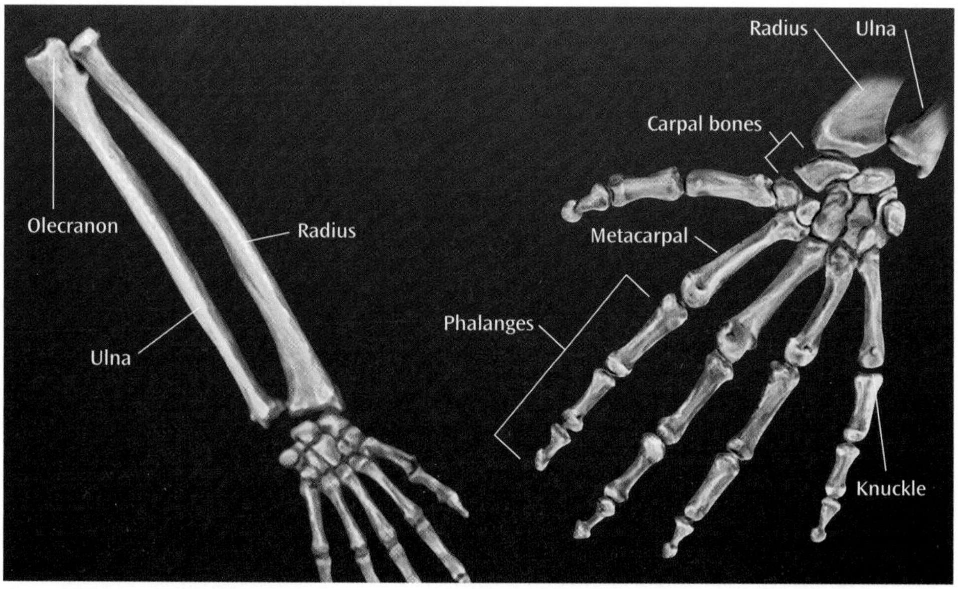

Acromion (ah-KRO-me-un) | *The highest point of the shoulder*

Humerus (HYU-me-rus) | *The upper arm bone*

Ulna | *Bone forming the medial side of the forearm*

Radius | *Bone forming the lateral side of the forearm*

Olecranon (oh-LEK-re-non) | *Elbow bone; tip of the elbow*

Figure 4.23 *The bones of the forearm (left) and hand (right).*

EMT Tip

The front of the elbow is sometimes called the antecubital region, or AC region.

The distal end of the radius widens to form a bony prominence at the wrist, the flexible joint between the arm and the hand (see Fig. 4.23). The wrist contains 8 carpal bones, which are small short bones, arranged in two rows of four and connected to each other by ligaments. Two carpal bones connect with the radius. This allows the wrist to move inward, outward, forward, and back.

Figure 4.24 *The cubital fossa of the elbow.*

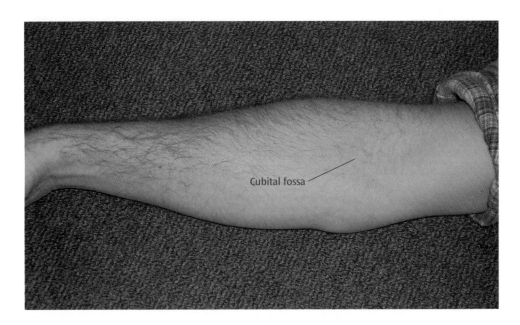

Cubital fossa

The hand is one of the most complex bony structures of the body (see Fig. 4.23). It provides both strength and mobility. The mitt or palm of the hand contains 5 metacarpal bones. These can be described as miniature long bones arranged in an arch. The **metacarpals**, which are attached proximally to the **carpals**, provide grip strength. The distal ends of the metacarpals, known as the knuckles, attach to the finger bones by hinge joints. The 5 fingers consist of 14 small long bones called phalanges. The thumb consists of the proximal and distal phalanges. The other fingers have proximal, middle, and distal phalanges.

Metacarpals (me-tuh-KAR-pulz) | *The hand bones*

Carpals (KAR-pulz) | *The eight bones of the wrist*

Joints

Points of contact between bones are called articulations or joints. Bones can be joined, or can articulate, in several different ways. The structure of a **joint** dictates the range of motion of the bones.

Joint | *A place where bones connect*

In addition to bone, most joints contain other tissue types. Ligaments and tendons, made of tough fibrous connective tissue, increase joint strength. Cartilage provides cushioning between bones in some joints. This is especially important for joints that may sustain an impact, such as intervertebral disks. Synovial joints, such as the shoulder, are surrounded by a joint capsule (see Fig. 4.22). This capsule contains a small amount of synovial fluid that provides lubrication between bone surfaces.

 EMT Tip

Remember "t" for toes in metatarsals so you do not confuse it with the metacarpals of the wrist.

Joints can be classified functionally according to their degree of movement. Some joints are unmovable and hold bones together rigidly. An example is the suture joints of the skull. Other joints permit limited motion. For example, the spinal column is flexible in response to twisting, bending, and compression. Many joints are freely movable, such as the knee, wrist, and shoulder.

Movable joints can move in either angular or circular motions. Angular movements increase or decrease the angle of bones in relation to each other. Flexion causes a joint to bend along a sagittal plane, decreasing the angle between the bones as in bending the knee. Its opposite motion, extension, increases the angle and straightens the joint.

Joint motion along the frontal plane causes lateral movement in relation to the midline of the body. Abduction is movement of a limb away from the midline. Adduction is a motion toward the midline of the body (see Fig. 4.25).

Rotation and circumduction are circular movements in relation to a central axis. Rotation occurs when a bone rotates around its own axis, such as when the head turns. Circumduction describes circular movement from a fixed pivot point, such as an arm drawing circles in the air.

Rotation of the radius and ulna on their axes allows unique motion of the forearm. Rotation of the forearm that turns the palm forward into the anatomical position is called supination. Pronation is the movement that turns the palm backward. Similarly, inversion is rotation of the ankle that turns the sole of the foot toward the midline. Eversion turns the sole outward (see Fig. 4.26).

EMT Tip

When a child is abducted, he is taken away. Abduction of the arm means to pull it away from the midline of the body. Jumping jacks, or flapping your arms like a bird flying, is an example of abduction and adduction.

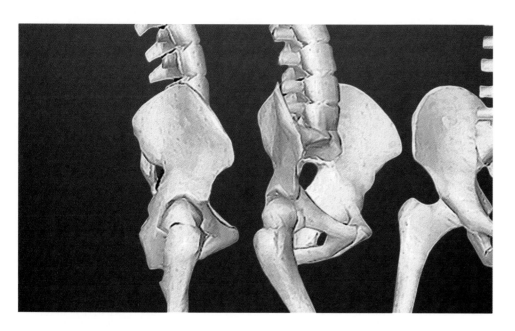

Figure 4.25 *The ball-and-socket joint of the hip showing adduction (center) and abduction (right).*

EMT Tip

Remember the word "up" within "sUPinated." Supinated means palms up, as if holding a bowl of soup.

Six types of joints permit movement of the body:

- **Ball-and-socket joints** consist of a cup-shaped surface that joins with the ball-shaped head of a long bone (see Fig. 4.26). The ball-and-socket joint permits the greatest range of motion of all joints, allowing flexion, extension, adduction, abduction, rotation, and circumduction. The only ball-and-socket joints in the body are the shoulder and hip joints.

Ball-and-Socket Joint | *Cup-shaped surface of a bone that joins with the ball-shaped head of a long bone*

Figure 4.26 *Inversion (left)
and eversion (right).*

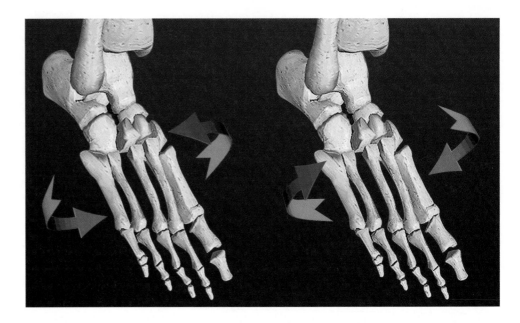

Hinge Joint | *Joint that
allows movement in one plane,
forward and backward*

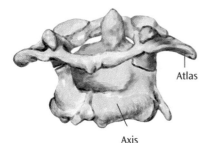

Figure 4.27 *The first two
cervical vertebrae form a pivot
joint.*

Atlas

Axis

- **Hinge joints** occur between the concave surface of one bone and the convex surface of another. These joints permit only flexion and extension. The knee and elbow are hinge joints.

- Condyloid joints form another type of connection between the concave and convex surfaces of two bones. These joints allow movement along two perpendicular planes. The articulations of the metacarpal bones with the phalanges are examples of condyloid joints. The knuckles allow both hinge-like movement of the fingers and sideways movement.

- Saddle joints also have a concave surface opposing a convex surface, but the two surfaces fit together like a rider in a saddle. Like condyloid joints, saddle joints permit movement in two planes. However, they allow for freer angular motion and permit limited circumduction. The articulation at the base of the thumb is a saddle joint.

- Pivot joints only permit rotation around an axis. The articulation of the first cervical vertebra, called the atlas, and the second cervical vertebra, the axis, is an example of a pivot joint that allows the head to turn from side to side (see Fig. 4.27).

- Gliding or plane joints exist between two flat bone surfaces. They permit motion in only one plane. Gliding joints are found between adjoining bones in the wrist and ankle.

The Muscular System

The skeleton provides the body's underlying framework, but it is the muscles that allow us to move (see Fig. 4.28). Muscles have the unique ability to generate physical movement from chemical energy. Muscle tissue can work in a coordinated fashion to perform a wide range of tasks. Besides allowing movement, muscles give the body shape, protect the internal organs, and enable

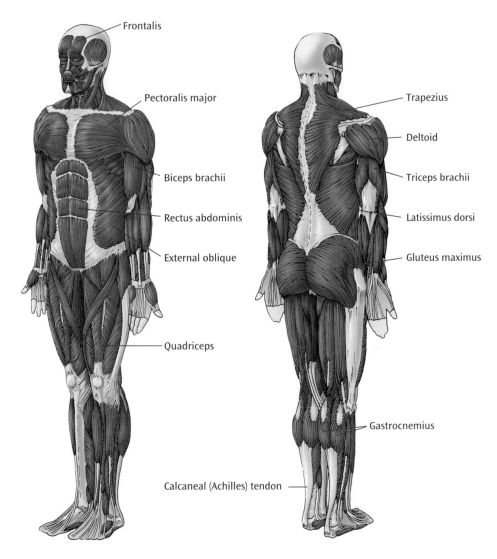

Frontalis

Pectoralis major

Biceps brachii

Rectus abdominis

External oblique

Quadriceps

Calcaneal (Achilles) tendon

Trapezius

Deltoid

Triceps brachii

Latissimus dorsi

Gluteus maximus

Gastrocnemius

Figure 4.28 *Anterior (left) and posterior (right) views of the muscular system.*

them to function. Muscle tissue stores nutrients, and contraction of the muscles produces body heat.

Muscle cells, also called muscle fibers, can stretch and contract because of a property called elasticity. This is an innate tension that allows the cells to return to their normal length and shape. Muscle cells also display excitability, the ability to contract in response to a chemical or electrical signal. Nerve cells provide the excitation impulse that causes the muscles to contract. Only nerve and muscle cells are excitable.

Each of the three types of muscle tissue has its own type of cells and its own mechanisms of control and contraction (see Fig. 4.31). Skeletal muscle is called **voluntary muscle** because it is under conscious control of the nervous system and brain. Skeletal muscle contracts and relaxes through choices made by the individual. We have no conscious control over two types of muscle tissue. Smooth muscles and cardiac muscles carry out the automatic muscular functions of the body. These **involuntary muscles** help to circulate the blood, move food through the gastrointestinal tract, and contract the uterus during childbirth.

Voluntary Muscles | *Muscles that are under conscious control*

Involuntary Muscles | *Muscles that carry out the automatic muscular functions of the body*

Skeletal Muscle

Skeletal muscles, which enable us to move, make up about 40% of body weight and form the body's major muscle mass. Voluntary muscles are responsible for movement of the bones and organs such as the eye and tongue.

Skeletal muscle cells are organized into bundles of long, parallel fibers called fasciculi (see Fig. 4.29). Each fasciculus (singular) is wrapped by a layer of connective tissue. Blood vessels and nerves that supply the muscle travel through this tissue. Connective tissue also encases entire muscles. The connective tissue layers join at the ends of the muscles to form tendons. Tendons attach muscles to bones or to other muscles. Muscle contractions are transmitted through tendons to cause movements of the skeleton.

Figure 4.29 *A skeletal muscle consists of long fibers organized into bundles.*

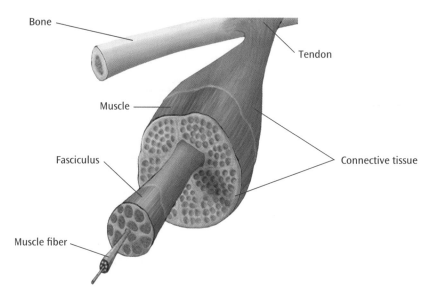

Two types of nerve fibers run through skeletal muscle tissue, carrying signals and information between the muscles and central nervous system (see Fig. 4.30). Motor nerves send signals from the nervous system to the muscles, causing them to contract or relax. Sensory nerves are stimulated by muscle contraction and stretching. They carry data to the nervous system regarding the activity status of each muscle.

Often, the name of a skeletal muscle describes its principal actions. Flexors and extensors decrease and increase the angle of the joint, respectively. Abductors and adductors move bones in relation to the body's midline. Levators produce upward movement, whereas supinators and pronators rotate the palm. A sphincter controls the size of an opening and a rotator moves a bone around its long axis. Muscle names give clues about their locations, shapes, or sizes. For example, the gluteus maximus is the largest muscle in the gluteal region. The gluteus minimus is the smallest. Deltoid means triangular, as in the deltoid muscle (see Fig. 4.28).

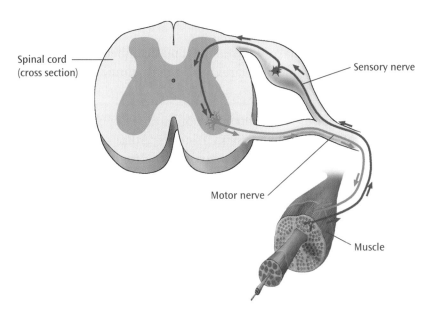

Spinal cord
(cross section)

Sensory nerve

Motor nerve

Muscle

Figure 4.30 *Sensory nerves receive incoming signals (sensation). Motor nerves send signals that make the muscles move.*

Smooth Muscle

Smooth muscle is responsible for muscular control of the digestive, urinary, and reproductive organs, as well as the blood vessels and bronchi. Sheets of smooth muscle tissue comprise the walls of these structures, giving them shape and functionality (see Fig. 4.31). Contraction of smooth muscles controls the flow through tubular structures. This occurs during peristalsis (the movement of food through the intestine), vasoconstriction (the narrowing of the blood vessels), and urination. It also causes the pupils to constrict and hairs on the skin to stand up.

We have no direct control over smooth muscle tissue. Contraction is triggered automatically by the nervous system or by external stimuli such as temperature changes, stretching, hormone release, or changes in oxygen concentration.

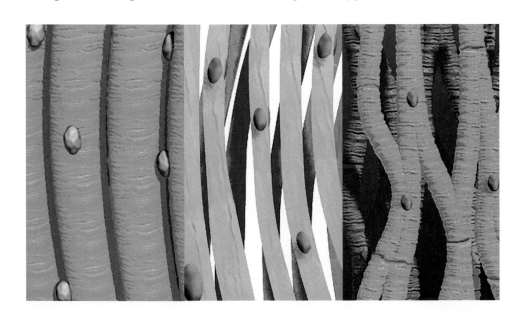

Figure 4.31 *Different types of muscle tissue: skeletal (left), smooth (center), and cardiac (right). Cardiac tissue is found only in the heart.*

Cardiac Muscle

Cardiac Muscle | *Involuntary muscle tissue of the heart that is usually not under conscious control*

Cardiac muscle is the tissue that makes up the walls and chambers of the heart (see Fig. 4.31). It is responsible for the heart's constant, rhythmic beating, and is not found elsewhere in the body.

Unlike skeletal and smooth muscles, contraction of cardiac muscle is not controlled by signals from the nervous system. Instead, cardiac cells have the ability to contract on their own. This property is called automaticity, or autorhythmicity. Specialized cells in the heart's pacemaker send out an electrical impulse that is rapidly transmitted throughout the heart tissue. This causes coordinated contraction of cardiac muscle fibers in a heartbeat. Cardiac muscle contracts quickly and continuously.

Although it is less susceptible to fatigue than skeletal muscle, cardiac muscle requires a constant supply of oxygen. The oxygen is provided by a separate blood supply to the heart: the coronary artery system. Cardiac muscle can tolerate only very brief interruptions of its blood supply before becoming irreversibly damaged.

THE RESPIRATORY SYSTEM

All cells in the body require a constant supply of oxygen (O_2) to fuel their vital processes. Any interruption of the oxygen flow can be life threatening. Brain cells will begin to die about four to six minutes after losing their oxygen supply. In the course of using oxygen, cells produce carbon dioxide (CO_2), a waste product that must be removed from the body. How does oxygen get from the air into all the cells of your body? How is the carbon dioxide removed? These exchanges, facilitated by the respiratory system and the circulatory system, are part of the process of normal breathing, or respiration.

Figure 4.32 *The trachea and lungs (left). Lung tissue is made up of alveoli (right).*

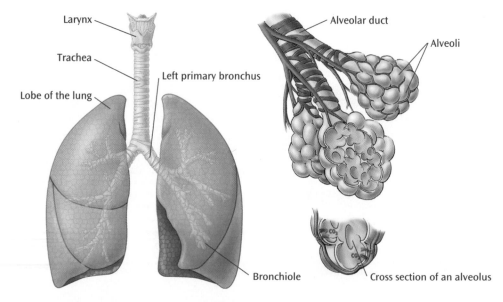

Respiratory Anatomy

The respiratory system consists of a network of branching air passages. This respiratory tree begins at the nose and divides into successively smaller airways, ending in the tiny alveoli of the lungs (see Figs. 4.32 and 4.33). The organs of the respiratory system include the:

- Nose
- Mouth
- Pharynx, or throat
- Larynx, or voice box
- Trachea, or windpipe
- Bronchi (plural of bronchus)
- Bronchioles
- Alveolar ducts
- Alveoli (plural of alveolus)

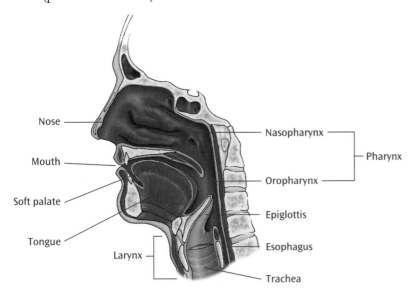

Figure 4.33 *Structures of the upper respiratory tract.*

The Nose and Mouth

During ventilation, air enters the body through the nose or mouth. The incoming air is warmed, humidified, and filtered before moving to the pharynx. The moist, sticky mucous lining of the nasal cavity helps to clean and to moisten the air. Hair-like cilia that line the nose and the respiratory tract sweep foreign particles toward the nose and mouth.

The Pharynx

Air passes through the nose and mouth into a shared passageway, the **pharynx** (see Fig. 4.33). The pharynx is divided into two main parts: the **nasopharynx**

Pharynx (FAIR-inks) | *The throat*

Nasopharynx (nay-zo-FAIR-inks) | *Part of pharynx above the level of the soft palate*

Oropharynx (or-oh-FAIR-inks) | *Part of pharynx between the soft palate and upper end of epiglottis*

Uvula (YEW-vyu-luh) | *The small structure that hangs from the roof of the mouth just in front of the oropharynx; made of connective tissue*

Esophagus (eh-SOF-eh-gus) | *Part of the gastrointestinal tract that joins the pharynx to the stomach*

Larynx (LAIR-inks) | *Part of respiratory tract between the pharynx and the trachea, responsible for the production of voice; also called the voice box*

Cricoid (KRY-koyd) Cartilage | *Ring of cartilage that forms the bottom of the larynx and is an anatomical landmark*

and the **oropharynx**. The nasopharynx is the chamber leading from the nasal cavity. It contains the **uvula**, which helps prevent food from entering the nasal cavity during swallowing.

Both air and food enter the oropharynx through the mouth. The oropharynx contains the base of the tongue and the tonsils. If infected, the tonsils may become enlarged, interfering with breathing. This condition is called tonsillitis. At its inferior end, the pharynx opens into the esophagus and the larynx. The **esophagus** carries food to the digestive system. The larynx leads to the trachea or windpipe.

The Larynx and Trachea

The **larynx**, also called the voice box, forms the entrance to the trachea (see Fig. 4.34). The larynx is constructed mainly of cartilage and muscle. The thyroid cartilage makes up the front of the larynx. This is commonly known as the Adam's apple. Inferior to the thyroid cartilage is the **cricoid cartilage** that forms the bottom of the larynx. This firm ring at the upper edge of the trachea acts as an anatomical landmark during a tracheostomy. A tracheostomy is an opening into the windpipe created by an incision. This procedure is done in some respiratory emergencies.

The **epiglottis**, a leaf-shaped, lid-like structure, is attached to the top of the larynx (see Figs. 4.33 and 4.34). When food is swallowed, the epiglottis covers the larynx. This prevents food or liquid from passing into the respiratory tract. During some medical emergencies, the epiglottis fails to close properly. This could allow food, blood, or vomit to enter the lungs. In some situations, this causes a complete obstruction of the airway. Inhaling food, liquid, or emesis into the lungs is a condition called aspiration.

Figure 4.34 *Larynx and trachea: lateral view (left) and anterior view (right).*

Epiglottis (ep-i- GLOT-us) | *A leaf-shaped, lid-like structure attached to the top of the larynx; closes during swallowing, preventing food or liquid from entering the respiratory tract*

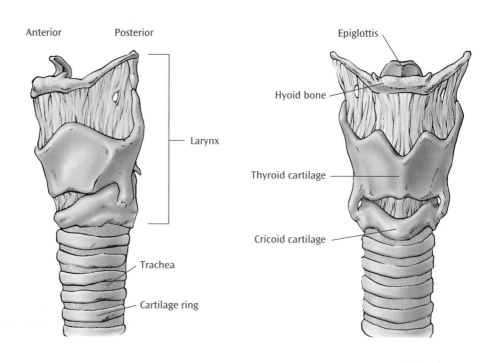

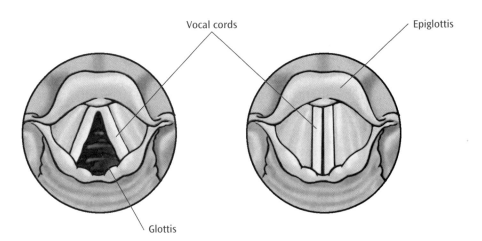

Vocal cords — Epiglottis

Glottis

Figure 4.35 *Cross section of the larynx showing the vocal cords: open (left) and closed (right).*

Glottis (GLOT-is) | *Space between the vocal cords; sound is produced when air passes through opening causing vocal cords to vibrate*

Within the larynx are the vocal cords, two bands of connective tissue held taut by muscles (see Fig. 4.35). The open space between the cords is called the **glottis**. Sound is produced when air passes through the glottis, causing the vocal cords to vibrate.

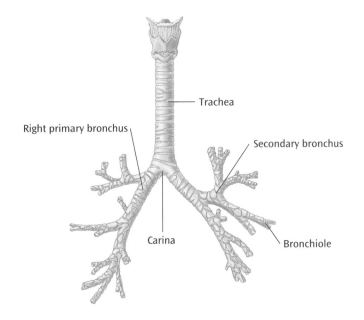

Trachea

Right primary bronchus

Secondary bronchus

Carina

Bronchiole

Figure 4.36 *The trachea and bronchi.*

EMT Tip

The epiglottis should close when we swallow food and should open when we speak. When a person tries to talk and eat at the same time, the epiglottis may not close completely. Food can enter the respiratory tree and obstruct the flow of air. The epiglottis may also fail to close properly in normal activities, such as swallowing.

The **trachea**, or windpipe, is a tube extending beyond the larynx, anterior to the esophagus (see Fig. 4.36). It is formed by C-shaped rings of cartilage that provide a flexible airway. The cartilage keeps the airway permanently open. The trachea is approximately six inches long in an adult. The trachea divides at about the level of the manubrium of the sternum. This division becomes the right and left primary bronchi, the two major branches that begin the bronchial tree leading to the lungs. At the division of the primary bronchi is the **carina** or bifurcation point, a triangular piece of reinforcing cartilage.

Trachea (TRAY-kee-uh) | *The windpipe; main air passage, arising from larynx and dividing into bronchi*

Carina (kah-REE-nuh) | *A triangular projection of the lowest tracheal cartilage; forms the division of the primary bronchi*

The Bronchi

Bronchi (BRONG-kee) | *Plural of bronchus; the two major subdivisions of the trachea*

Bronchioles | *Subdivisions of bronchi; terminate in the alveoli*

EMT Tip

Cigarette smoking paralyzes the cilia, causing loss of the protective sweeping function. When smokers quit, they initially notice more coughing and phlegm. This occurs because the cilia wake up and begin to clean out the accumulated debris.

The primary **bronchi**, the branches of the trachea that enter the lungs, also contain hard cartilage rings that help to keep the larger airways open (see Fig. 4.36). The bronchi are lined with mucus, a thick substance that entraps foreign particles. Cilia are hair-like projections inside the bronchi that sweep material into the throat for elimination. These protective mechanisms keep harmful particles out of the lungs.

The right primary bronchus divides into three secondary bronchi, which lead to the three lobes of the right lung. On the left side, the primary bronchus branches into two secondary bronchi leading to the left lung, which has two lobes. As the bronchi branch and divide closer to the lungs, they have progressively less cartilage. The secondary bronchi further divide into tertiary bronchi, which branch into **bronchioles**.

Of all the conducting airways, the bronchioles have the greatest capacity to regulate airflow. The bronchioles, with little or no cartilage, have a thick, smooth muscle layer, which contracts or relaxes to constrict or dilate the airways. The highest degree of resistance to airflow occurs when the bronchioles are constricted. Asthma, a medical condition characterized by obstructed ventilation and wheezing, is caused by constriction of the bronchioles.

The bronchioles branch into narrower terminal bronchioles, and then into the respiratory bronchioles. These have some cilia, but no mucus is secreted. Each respiratory bronchiole branches into several alveolar ducts. These end in alveolar sacs, or clusters of alveoli assembled around a common air space.

Figure 4.37 *Oxygen exchange between the lungs and the blood occurs in the alveolar sacs.*

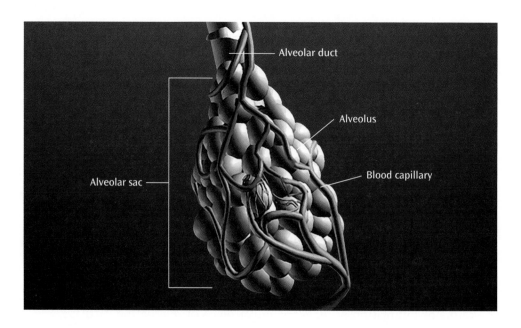

The Lungs

The **lungs** are paired organs in the thoracic cavity. They extend from just above the clavicles to the diaphragm. The volume of the lungs in an average-size adult is 5 to 6 liters.

The microscopic alveoli are the functional units of the lungs, in which gas exchange takes place (see Fig. 4.37). Lungs in the adult contain approximately 300 million alveoli. These are arranged in clusters, like grapes. Their walls are only a single cell layer thick, and they are surrounded by a network of tiny blood vessels.

The thoracic cavity is divided into right and left pleural cavities by a double lining called the pleural membrane. The inside wall of the thoracic cavity is lined by the parietal pleura. The visceral pleura lines the outer surface of the lungs. The pleural cavity is the space between the membranes. Each cavity contains a small amount of lubricating fluid that prevents friction when the lungs expand and contract.

Respiratory Muscles

Ventilation is accomplished through the action of the respiratory muscles. The muscles of respiration include the diaphragm, the intercostal muscles between the ribs, and the smaller accessory muscles of the throat and upper chest. The diaphragm is the main respiratory muscle (see Fig. 4.38). This dome-shaped muscle forms the floor of the thoracic cavity. The diaphragm usually functions under involuntary control, fulfilling the body's need for oxygen. However, it can also perform as a voluntary muscle, such as when we hold our breath or take a deep breath.

Special Considerations for Infants and Children

When working with children or infants, you must remember some important anatomical differences. The mouths and noses of infants and children are smaller than in adults (see Fig. 4.39). The small size means that a child's airway is more easily obstructed than an adult's airway. It can be much more difficult to establish and maintain. Because a child's head is proportionally larger than an adult's head, the tongue takes up more of the space in the pharynx. This can lead to blockage if the tongue swells. The child's trachea is also narrow and more easily obstructed.

An illness or injury that causes swelling or obstruction of any part of the airway could affect a child much more seriously than an adult. For example, a child who accidentally inhaled an object as small as a peanut might block a main bronchus. This situation could become life threatening.

The cartilage in the trachea and chest wall is not fully developed. This causes the airway to be much less rigid than in an adult. A child's trachea is easily

Lungs | *Respiratory organs that exchange oxygen, carbon dioxide, and water between the blood and the outside atmosphere*

Diaphragm

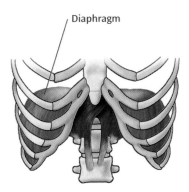

Figure 4.38 *The diaphragm.*

Figure 4.39 *Anatomical differences between adults and children.*

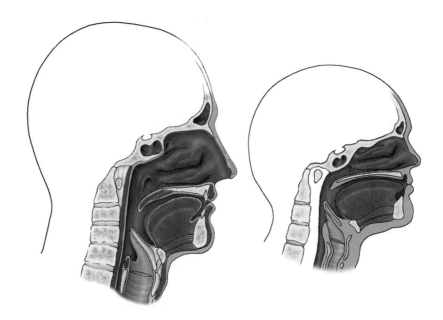

kinked if the neck is hyperextended or hyperflexed. Bending the neck too far in either direction will cause an obstruction. The flexible cricoid cartilage is easily damaged. Because the chest wall is softer, children and infants depend more on their diaphragms for breathing.

Respiratory Physiology

Ventilation | *Exchange of air between lungs and ambient air*

Respiration consists of three phases. In the first phase, **ventilation**, air is transported into the lungs. The next process is gas exchange, in which oxygen is extracted from the air in the lungs and passed into the blood. At the same time, carbon dioxide is released from the blood into the lungs. Finally, during tissue respiration, oxygen is absorbed and used by every cell, and CO_2 is excreted from the tissues into the blood.

Hemoglobin (HEE-muh-glow-ben) | *Protein in red blood cells responsible for oxygen transport*

Specific molecules and chemical reactions in the blood facilitate the transport and exchange of gases. Oxygen, which does not dissolve well in water, is carried in the blood bound to **hemoglobin**, a large protein molecule found inside red blood cells. The amount of oxygen carried in the blood can be measured by the percent saturation of hemoglobin. The normal saturation level is 94% to 96% O_2. Hemoglobin also carries some carbon dioxide, but most of the carbon dioxide in the body is carried in the form of the dissolved bicarbonate ion (HCO_3^-), a product formed from CO_2 and water.

Ventilation

The process of normal breathing is called ventilation. During this process, air moves into the spaces of the lungs where oxygen is released to the blood. Air is drawn into the lungs during inhalation or inspiration. It flows out of the lungs during exhalation or expiration.

Ventilation takes place almost entirely through inhalation. This is an active process requiring muscle contraction. The muscles normally used in inspiration are the diaphragm and the external intercostals (see Fig. 4.40). As the diaphragm contracts, it moves downward and pulls the bottom of the thoracic cavity down. This action makes the cavity larger. At the same time, the external intercostals contract. This causes the sternum and ribs to move upward and outward, increasing the width and depth of the thorax. As the thorax expands, the lungs are pulled toward the chest wall. This movement causes a slight vacuum within the lungs. The negative thoracic pressure draws air in through the respiratory tree and fills the lungs.

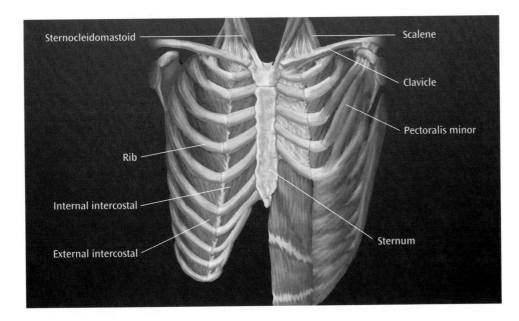

Figure 4.40 *The intercostal and other accessory muscles.*

In contrast to inhalation, normal exhalation is a passive process of muscle relaxation. When the diaphragm and intercostal muscles relax, the thoracic floor moves upward. This causes the ribs to move downward and inward. The size of the thoracic cavity decreases, creating positive air pressure within the thorax. The pressure pushes the air out through the airway.

During deep or labored breathing, the sternocleidomastoid and scalene muscles aid inhalation. This occurs when one is short of breath or during a forced inspiration. These small muscles pull up on the sternum and first two ribs, exerting a maximum pull on the rib cage. Use of these accessory muscles can be seen on the external chest wall. Depressions, known as retractions, appear between the thoracic bones. Retractions are signs of respiratory distress.

During labored breathing, coughing, or obstructed air flow, expiration can also be actively forced. Forced expiration is aided by contraction of the abdominal muscles. When air is forcefully expelled, the contraction of the abdominal muscles pushes the viscera upward against the diaphragm. The internal intercostals pull the ribs closer together.

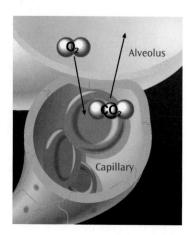

Figure 4.41 *In the lungs, oxygen diffuses into the blood and carbon dioxide is exhaled.*

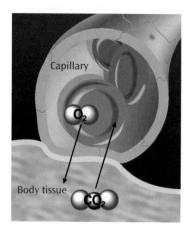

Figure 4.42 *Oxygen is delivered to the tissues and carbon dioxide is removed.*

Regulation of ventilation is involuntary. The central nervous system tells the body when and how to breathe. Specialized cell receptors in the brain and in some blood vessels detect oxygen, carbon dioxide, and hydrogen ions. Low pH or high carbon dioxide concentration stimulates these receptors. When the blood levels of oxygen change, the receptors stimulate ventilation. Although this mechanism is involuntary, it can be overridden by voluntary breathing. The nervous and endocrine systems also exert control over respiration at the bronchioles. Stimulation of certain nerves or the release of some hormones can constrict the bronchioles. When the bronchioles constrict, their resistance to air flow increases. Sometimes stimulation dilates the bronchioles, allowing greater air flow.

Gas Exchange

Gas exchange between air and blood occurs in the thin-walled alveoli (see Fig. 4.41). Because they are so numerous, the alveoli provide an extremely large surface area for gas exchange. Each alveolus is covered by an extensive network of blood capillaries. Oxygen from the air, which is needed by all cells, passes through the alveolar membrane into the bloodstream. Carbon dioxide, an end product of cellular metabolism, moves from the blood into the alveoli for removal from the body.

Oxygen and CO_2 move across the air-blood barrier by diffusion, a passive process for which no energy is required. Air and blood both contain a mixture of gases. During diffusion, the molecules of any gas move from an area of high concentration to an area of lower concentration. This is true whether the molecules are in liquid form, such as blood, or gas form, such as air. Diffusion of oxygen and carbon dioxide occurs because their partial pressures or concentrations on either side of the alveolar-capillary membrane are different. Each gas diffuses to the area where its own concentration is lower.

Blood enters the alveolar capillaries after passing through body tissues. Because cells use oxygen and produce carbon dioxide, the blood is oxygen-poor. This means that the partial pressure of oxygen in the blood is low and the partial pressure of carbon dioxide is high. In contrast, the air in the lungs is oxygen-rich. The oxygen readily diffuses from air in the alveoli into the capillaries. At the same time, the carbon dioxide-rich blood returning to the lungs rapidly gives up its CO_2 to the alveoli. When oxygenated blood from the lungs circulates to the tissues of the body, the principle of diffusion operates in reverse.

Tissue Respiration

Tissue cells have a low partial pressure of oxygen. This is true because oxygen is consumed during metabolism. Carbon dioxide concentration is high in tissues, because the body produces it as a waste product. During tissue respiration, oxygen-rich blood is carried past the cells. Oxygen diffuses into the cells and carbon dioxide passes into the capillaries (see Fig. 4.42). Thus, tissue capillaries release oxygen and receive carbon dioxide. Finally, the blood returns to the lungs. The carbon dioxide is exchanged with oxygen from the air in the lungs, and carbon dioxide is exhaled.

Assessment of Breathing

Normal respiration, or adequate breathing, is regular and relaxed. Normal breathing is called eupnea. A normal breathing rate, regular rhythm, and adequate depth are maintained. Breath sounds are present and equal in both lungs. Chest expansion is full and equal. Breathing takes place comfortably without the use of accessory muscles.

The normal ranges for respiration rates are 12 to 20 breaths per minute for adults, 15 to 30 breaths per minute for children, and 25 to 50 breaths per minute for infants. The depth of breathing is measured by the tidal volume. Tidal volume is the amount of air that moves in and out during a single breath (inspiration followed by expiration). Normal tidal volume is about 500 mL in the adult.

Breathing may be compromised by illness, airway obstruction, or injury. A person experiencing inadequate breathing may complain of shortness of breath, or dyspnea. He or she will display various signs of difficulty breathing, or air hunger. The **respiratory rate** may be outside the normal range, either too fast or too slow. Alternatively, the rate may be normal, but the depth will be shallow, with an inadequate tidal volume. The rhythm may be irregular. Breath sounds may be decreased, absent, or abnormal.

Inadequate breathing leads to low oxygen levels in the tissues, or hypoxia. This causes the appearance of the skin to change. It may look pale or feel cool and clammy. A late sign is cyanosis, a blue coloring of the skin and mucous membranes. It is first noted around the mouth or fingertips.

A person in severe respiratory distress may show an increased effort of breathing, including use of the accessory muscles. You may see retractions of the muscles above the clavicles, between the ribs, and below the rib cage. Retractions are more common in children, who may also show flaring of the nostrils (see Fig. 4.43). Unequal or inadequate expansion of the chest may be seen. Infants may display seesaw breathing, in which the chest and abdominal muscles move in opposite directions. The patient may become exhausted quickly. This is even more critical in children. Finally, agonal respirations, or occasional gasping breaths are seen in the final stage of death.

EMT Tip

Noisy breathing indicates that the patient is having difficulty breathing due to some form of partial obstruction.

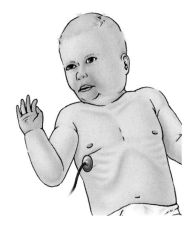

Figure 4.43 *A child in respiratory distress may show cyanosis or retractions.*

Respiratory (RES-pruh-tor-ee) *Rate* | *Breathing rate; measured in breaths per minute*

THE CIRCULATORY SYSTEM

The circulatory or cardiovascular system consists of the heart, blood, and blood vessels. Different types of blood vessels are:

• Arteries

• Arterioles

• Capillaries

• Venules

• Veins

The function of the circulatory system is to transport substances in the circulating blood to every part of the body. Two main circulatory routes or subdivisions are the pulmonary circulation and the systemic circulation (see Fig. 4.44). The pulmonary circulation receives deoxygenated blood from the heart and circulates it to the lung capillaries. Here, carbon dioxide is released to the alveoli and oxygen is picked up. The oxygenated blood is returned to the heart where it is pumped into the systemic circulation. The systemic circulation carries oxygen from the lungs and nutrients from the digestive system to nourish all of the body's cells. The blood returns from the tissues carrying metabolic waste products, ready to pass into the pulmonary circulation again.

Figure 4.44 The pulmonary circulation and systemic circulation. Oxygenated blood is shown in red; deoxygenated blood is shown in blue.

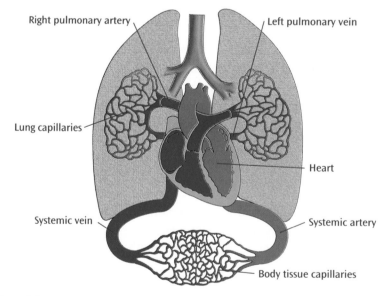

Right pulmonary artery

Left pulmonary vein

Lung capillaries

Heart

Systemic vein

Systemic artery

Body tissue capillaries

The Heart

Heart | *Organ located in the thoracic cavity that receives blood from the veins and pumps it to the arteries*

The **heart** is the pump responsible for moving the blood (see Fig. 4.45). It is a muscular organ found between the lungs within the mediastinum, or middle of the thoracic cavity. Surrounding the heart is a double-lined sac called the pericardium. Similar to the pleural cavity, it contains a small amount of pericardial fluid that enables the heart to expand and to contract with minimal friction. This fluid also acts as a shock absorber during trauma.

The heart wall, or myocardium, is made of thick, contractile cardiac muscle tissue. The myocardium compresses the heart's cavities with great force. This causes blood to pump through the system. Although the heart is a single organ, it functions as two side-by-side pumps. The left and right sides each have two chambers (see Figs. 4.45 and 4.46). The small, upper atria (plural of **atrium**) are the receiving chambers. The lower, larger **ventricles** are the dispensing chambers.

The heart contains four one-way valves that regulate circulation (see Fig. 4.46). **Valves** restrict blood flow to one direction and prevent backflow. The tricuspid valve controls the passageway between the right atrium and right ventricle. The pulmonary valve is found between the right ventricle and the pulmonary trunk artery. The mitral valve, or bicuspid valve, restricts the flow between the left atrium and the left ventricle. The aortic valve regulates the opening of the left ventricle into the aorta.

Atrium (AY-tree-um) | *One of two upper chambers of the heart*

Ventricles | *The two lower chambers of the heart*

Valves | *Structures within the heart and circulatory system that prevent backflow of blood*

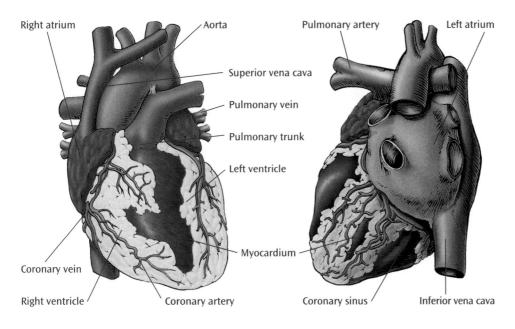

Right atrium — Aorta — Pulmonary artery — Left atrium

Superior vena cava

Pulmonary vein

Pulmonary trunk

Left ventricle

Myocardium

Coronary vein

Right ventricle — Coronary artery — Coronary sinus — Inferior vena cava

Figure 4.45 *Views of the heart: anterior (left) and posterior (right).*

The Cardiac Cycle

The sequence of events involved in a single heartbeat, the cardiac cycle, begins with a relaxation phase. Blood from the tissues drains into the atria during this phase. The right atrium receives oxygen-depleted blood from the systemic circulation, while the left atrium receives oxygenated blood from the pulmonary veins in the lungs.

As the atria fill, they contract, pumping the blood into the ventricles (see Fig. 4.46). This ventricular filling is called diastole. Blood from the right atrium is pumped into the right ventricle. Blood from the left atrium fills the left ventricle. In the next phase, systole, the ventricles contract strongly, forcing the blood out of the heart. The right ventricle pumps oxygen-poor blood into the pulmonary arteries to be oxygenated in the lungs. The left ventricle pumps oxygen-rich blood from the heart to the aorta, where it is distributed throughout the body.

The action of the ventricles can be monitored by listening to the heart's sounds. When you listen through a stethoscope, you hear a "lub-dup" sound made by the closing of the heart's valves. The "lub" is a longer, low-pitched sound that signals ventricular systole. This is the sound of the mitral and tricuspid valves closing when the ventricles start to contract. The "dup" is a quick, snapping sound that is caused by the closing of the aortic and pulmonary valves during ventricular diastole.

Figure 4.46 *Blood flow through the heart.*

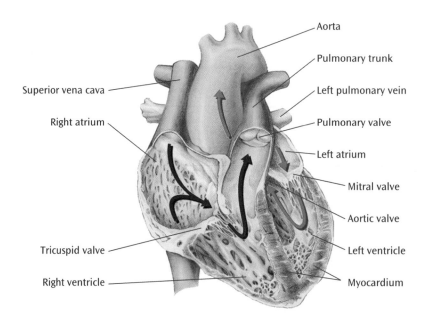

The Cardiac Conductive System

Cardiac muscle is a special type of muscle tissue found only in the heart. The cells contract rhythmically and continuously in a coordinated fashion. This action creates an overall pumping motion that provides a constant flow of blood through the body. Electrical impulses stimulate the heart and synchronize the pumping motions. Specialized cardiac pacemaker cells generate these electrical impulses and conduct them throughout the heart muscle. This is known as the cardiac conductive system (see Fig. 4.47). The ability to initiate and coordinate a complex series of contractions without any stimulation by nerve impulses from the brain is called automaticity of the heart.

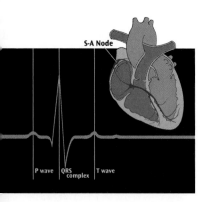

Figure 4.47 *Conduction of impulses through the heart.*

The main pacemaker is the sinoatrial node (SA node), a small mass of cells in the wall of the right atrium. This autorhythmic center triggers contraction of the atria. Part of the impulse is transmitted to the atrioventricular (AV) node, resulting in contraction of the ventricles.

Although the heartbeat is autorhythmic, other body systems can influence its rate. The autonomic nervous system can signal the heart to speed up or slow down. The endocrine system can speed the heart rate during stress. Elevated body temperature from exercise or fever also increases heart rate, whereas the rate decreases if body temperature drops.

The Vascular System

The vasculature is a complex transportation network designed to deliver blood to every cell in the body (see Fig. 4.48). The vessels that channel the blood from the heart to the body's tissues are called **arteries**. Vessels that return blood from the tissues to the heart are **veins**. Arteries branch into smaller vessels called **arterioles**. Small veins are called **venules**. The tiny vessels that carry blood through the tissues are called **capillaries** (see Fig. 4.49).

Arteries | Blood vessels that carry blood away from the heart

Veins | Vessels carrying blood back to the heart

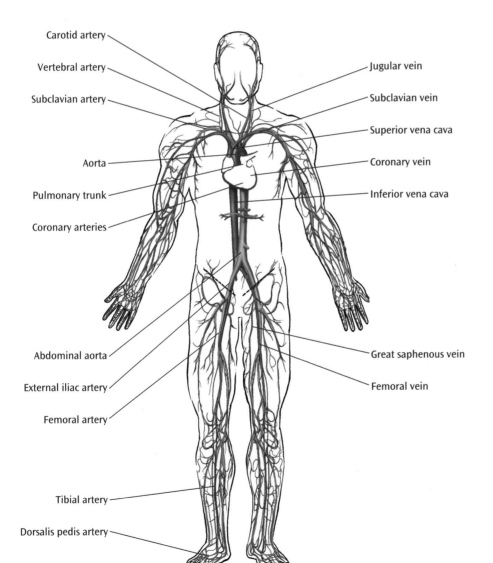

Carotid artery

Vertebral artery

Subclavian artery

Aorta

Pulmonary trunk

Coronary arteries

Abdominal aorta

External iliac artery

Femoral artery

Tibial artery

Dorsalis pedis artery

Jugular vein

Subclavian vein

Superior vena cava

Coronary vein

Inferior vena cava

Great saphenous vein

Femoral vein

Figure 4.48 *The vascular system. Arteries (red) branch into smaller arterioles, then into capillaries. Capillaries join into small venules, which join into veins (blue).*

Arterioles (ar-TEAR-ee-olz) | Smaller vessels that branch off the arteries and lead to the capillaries

Venules | The smallest branches of the veins

Capillaries (KA-pul-air-eez) | Tiny vessels that carry blood through the tissues; the network of capillaries in the tissues and organs is called the capillary bed

Functionally, capillaries are the most important. These vessels carry out a two-way exchange of fluid, nutrients, electrolytes, hormones, waste products, and other substances between the blood and tissue cells. The network of capillaries in the tissues and organs is called the capillary bed. The flow of blood through the capillary bed is called microcirculation.

Arteries

Blood pumped out of the ventricles flows into the arteries (see Fig. 4.50). Because the arteries transport blood under high pressure, they have strong walls that facilitate rapid blood flow. Major arteries distribute the blood to different body regions before branching into distributing arteries, which lead to specific organs and muscles. The smallest branches are the arterioles, which lead to the capillaries. Arteries of the systemic circulation distribute oxygenated blood from the heart to the body's organs. The pulmonary arteries carry oxygen-poor blood from the heart to the lungs.

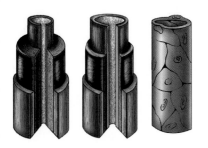

Figure 4.49 *The structure of an artery (left), vein (center), and capillary (right). (Not to scale.)*

Figure 4.50 *Systemic arteries distribute oxygenated blood from the heart to the body's organs.*

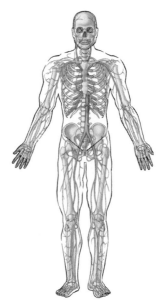

The pulmonary trunk is a large artery that originates at the right ventricle of the heart (see Fig. 4.45). It branches into the left and right **pulmonary arteries** leading to each lung. These carry oxygen-poor blood away from the heart to the alveoli, where it is oxygenated. The pulmonary arteries are the only arteries in the body that carry deoxygenated blood.

The **aorta** is the main artery leaving the heart. It has several sections from which the major systemic arteries branch off to supply various body regions. The left and right coronary arteries are the first major blood vessels to branch off from the aorta as it leaves the left ventricle. Cardiac muscle requires a constant supply of oxygen for its continuous contractions. This is provided by a separate blood supply to the heart: the **coronary artery** system. Any interruption of the heart's oxygen supply will soon result in injury and death of the myocardium, affecting its ability to beat.

Pulmonary Artery | *Originates in the right ventricle and enters the lungs where it branches off and follows the bronchi of the lungs*

Aorta (ay-OR-tuh) | *The main trunk of the arterial system of the body; it leaves the heart from the upper surface of the left ventricle*

Coronary Artery | *Blood vessels that supply the heart with blood*

The next major branches from the aorta are the **carotid** and subclavian arteries. The left and right carotid arteries are the major arteries of the neck. The carotids branch to supply blood to the throat, head, brain, and face (see Fig. 4.51). Pulsations of the carotid arteries are felt on either side of the neck, just below the angle of the jaw.

The right and left subclavian arteries branch out into the shoulder regions. Their vertebral branches supply the posterior portion of the brain. Their axillary branches travel through the shoulders into the arms (see Fig. 4.52). The axillary branches become the brachial arteries, supplying the upper arms. Pulsations of the brachial arteries are felt on the anterior side of each arm between the elbow and the shoulder. The **brachial artery** is used when determining a blood pressure (BP). It is also a common place to measure the pulse of an infant.

Each brachial artery branches distally at the elbow, forming the radial and ulnar arteries. The **radial arteries** are the major arteries supplying the lateral aspect of the forearm (see Fig. 4.52). The ulnar arteries supply the medial aspect. Branches from both vessels deliver blood to the hands and fingers. Pulsations of the radial arteries can be palpated on the thumb side of each wrist. The radial arteries are the site most commonly used for taking the pulse.

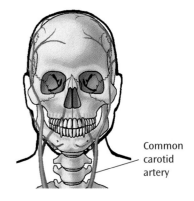

Common carotid artery

Figure 4.51 *The carotid artery supplies the head and neck.*

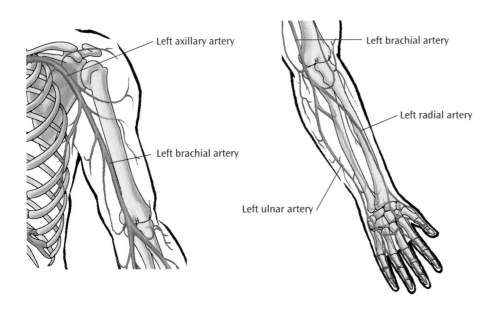

Left axillary artery

Left brachial artery

Left brachial artery

Left radial artery

Left ulnar artery

Figure 4.52 *Arteries of the upper arm (left) and forearm (right).*

Carotid (kah-RAH-tid)
Artery | *Major artery in the neck*

Brachial (BRAY-kee-ul)
Artery | *Major artery of the upper arm*

Radial Artery | *Major artery of the forearm*

After the subclavian arteries branch off, the aorta curves behind the heart and descends anterior to the spine into the thoracic and abdominal cavities. Here, its branches supply the organs and muscles of the thorax, abdomen, and pelvis.

At the level of the navel, the aorta divides into the right and left iliac arteries supplying the lower extremities (see Fig. 4.53). Each side subdivides to form the internal iliac arteries, which supply the pelvic muscles and organs, and the external iliac arteries, supplying the lower legs.

Figure 4.53 *Arteries and veins of the thigh (left) and lower leg (right).*

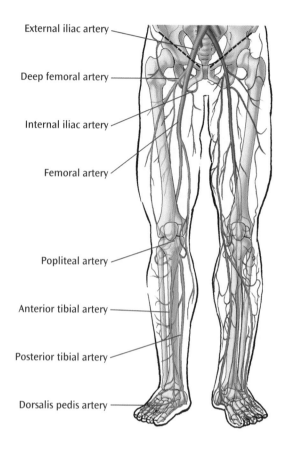

External iliac artery

Deep femoral artery

Internal iliac artery

Femoral artery

Popliteal artery

Anterior tibial artery

Posterior tibial artery

Dorsalis pedis artery

Femoral (FEM-or-ul) Artery | *The major artery in the thigh*

Dorsalis Pedis (dor-SAL-is PEE-dis) Artery | *Artery located on the upper surface of the foot; can be used to assess blood supply distal to a leg injury*

The external iliacs become the left and right **femoral arteries**. These are the major arteries of the thighs. Pulsations of the femoral arteries are felt in the groin area, in the crease between the abdomen and the thigh. At the knee, the femoral arteries become the popliteal arteries, which further branch below the calf into anterior and posterior tibial arteries.

The anterior tibial arteries supply the anterior portion of the lower leg. At the ankle, each anterior tibial artery becomes the **dorsalis pedis artery**. This artery supplies the dorsal aspect of each foot and the toes. Pulsations of the dorsalis pedis arteries can be palpated on the top surface of each foot, toward the big toe. The posterior tibial arteries supply the posterior portion of each lower leg and the heel. Further branches supply the plantar aspect of the feet and toes. Pulsations of the posterior tibial artery can be palpated on the posterior surface of the medial malleolus.

Capillaries

Blood from the heart is pumped through the arteries and arterioles. These vessels further divide into capillaries, the tiny vessels that permeate the tissues throughout the body. Capillaries have thin, permeable walls that allow for the exchange of fluid, electrolytes, hormones, nutrients, wastes, and other substances between the blood and the cells. The peripheral tissues contain approximately ten billion capillaries, with a combined surface area of more than five hundred square meters.

Veins

Following the exchange of nutrients and wastes in the capillaries, the blood flows into venules, the smallest branches of the veins. The venules join into collecting veins from the organs. These further merge into major veins that drain entire body regions. Finally, the venous blood drains into the heart's atria (see Fig. 4.54).

Besides carrying blood back to the heart, veins act as reservoirs for storing large quantities of blood, making it available as the body's needs change. About 60% of the blood in the human body is found in the venous system. Some veins have one-way valves that restrict the direction of blood flow toward the heart. Unlike the arteries, the pressure in the venous system is low. Movement of body muscles helps to propel blood forward. This is called the venous pump.

Oxygen-rich blood from the pulmonary circulation is returned to the left atrium through the pulmonary veins. Blood returning from the coronary circulation of the heart walls drains into the right atrium through the coronary veins. These veins merge into the large coronary sinus. Blood from the rest of the body returns to the right atrium through the superior **vena cava** and the inferior vena cava (see Figs. 4.45 and 4.54).

The superior vena cava collects all the blood that has flowed through the upper body, except blood from the lungs. Blood from the head drains into the right and left jugular veins. In the upper extremities, small veins in the hands and arms combine into the right and left subclavian veins. Blood from the thorax also drains into the subclavians. The jugulars and subclavians merge into the two brachiocephalic veins, which then form the superior vena cava (see Fig. 4.48).

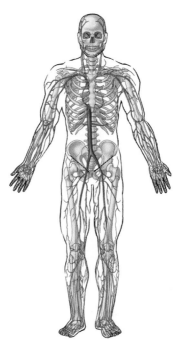

Figure 4.54 *Veins of the systemic circulation.*

Vena Cava (VEE-nuh KAY-vuh) | *Inferior and superior; the final vein of the systemic circulation; it empties into the right atrium of the heart*

Figure 4.55 *Abdominal cavity.*

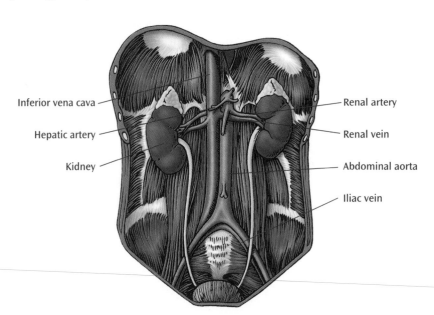

Inferior vena cava

Hepatic artery

Kidney

Renal artery

Renal vein

Abdominal aorta

Iliac vein

**EMT
Tip**

*Varicose veins occur when the
valves in the leg veins become
weak and blood flows backward, causing the superficial
veins to become distended.*

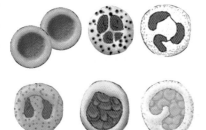

Figure 4.56 *Red blood cells
(upper left) and five types of
white blood cells.*

Plasma | *The serum, or fluid
component, of blood*

Red Blood Cells | *Components
of blood that contain hemoglobin; transport oxygen to the
body's cells and remove carbon
dioxide*

The inferior vena cava collects blood that has flowed through the lower body,
below the diaphragm. The the left and right common iliac veins join to form
the inferior vena cava (see Fig. 4.55). These veins drain smaller veins from the
lower extremities and the pelvis. Blood from the kidneys returns to the inferior vena cava through the renal veins. Blood returning from organs of the
digestive system drains through the hepatic portal circulation. Here, digested
substances that the blood has absorbed are stored or modified by the liver. This
blood passes into the hepatic veins, which then drain into the inferior vena cava.

The Blood

Blood performs three main functions in the body: transport, regulation, and
protection. Blood transports oxygen from the lungs to all cells in the body and
carbon dioxide from the tissues to the lungs. Additionally, it carries nutrients
from the gastrointestinal tract to all areas of the body. It carries waste products
from the cells to the excretory organs, and hormones from the endocrine
glands to the tissues. Blood also helps to regulate and to maintain the body's
temperature, its acidity or pH level, and the water content of cells and tissues.
The clotting system protects the body against blood loss after a blood vessel is
damaged. Finally, specialized blood cells and proteins function as part of the
immune system that protects the body from invading pathogens.

The normal temperature of blood is 38° Celsius (100.4° Fahrenheit). This is
higher than the normal core body temperature, which is 37°C (98.6°F).
Blood has an alkaline pH of about 7.4. The average blood volume is about
5 to 6 liters in adult males and 4 to 5 liters in adult females.

The blood consists of three types of cells suspended in yellowish fluid called
plasma. They are red blood cells (RBCs), or erythrocytes, several different
white blood cells (WBCs), or leukocytes, and specialized blood cell fragments
called platelets (see Fig. 4.56). Most blood cells are produced in the red bone
marrow of certain bones. In addition, many metabolic substances such as
glucose are dissolved in the plasma.

Red Blood Cells

Red blood cells contain hemoglobin molecules that bind to oxygen molecules
for transport in the blood (see Fig. 4.57). As oxygenated blood from the lungs
passes through the body, oxygen is released and diffuses from RBCs into the
tissue cells. Hemoglobin also picks up carbon dioxide created as metabolic
waste, transporting it to the lungs where it is released from the blood and
exhaled. The red hue of oxygenated hemoglobin in RBCs gives the blood its
color. Deoxygenated blood (hemoglobin without oxygen) in the veins and
venules appears dark maroon or bluish in color.

White Blood Cells

White blood cells are part of the immune system and aid in the body's defense against infections. Leukocytes are found primarily in blood vessels, but they also are able to squeeze through capillary walls and pass into the tissues. When this occurs, they travel directly to a site of infection. An increase in WBC levels in the blood normally indicates an infection. Six cell types perform specific protective functions, including:

- Production of antibodies
- Destruction of invading microbes
- Destruction of cancerous cells
- Protection against allergic responses
- Protection against inflammation

White Blood Cells | Cells in the blood responsible for controlling disease conditions, such as infections caused by microorganisms

Platelets

Platelets are specialized cell fragments that are essential for the formation of blood clots. Hemostasis is stopping bleeding after tissue damage. This involves three processes. First, the smooth muscle forming the blood vessel walls contracts, restricting blood flow in the damaged area. Seconds later, platelets stick to the damaged vessel in a process called platelet adhesion. As more platelets stick to each other, a plug is formed over the damaged area, slowing blood flow out of the vessel. Finally, chemicals called clotting factors that are released from the plasma and platelets trigger coagulation, or blood clotting. The platelet plug becomes interwoven with strands of the protein fibrin, resulting in a clot that blocks the injury.

Platelets | Component of blood essential for clotting

Plasma

Plasma is the fluid portion of the blood that carries the blood cells and dissolved nutrients and wastes. In a normal sample of whole blood, plasma accounts for 55% of the volume. The plasma is about 90% water. Components in the plasma are involved in immune responses, blood clotting, and regulation of the circulation and the body fluid balance. Plasma can pass through capillary walls into the spaces between the cells in the tissues. Here it is known as tissue fluid.

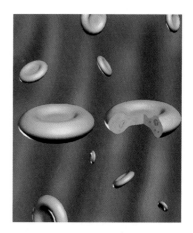

Figure 4.57 *The red blood cell carries oxygen bound to hemoglobin.*

Physiology of Circulation

Circulation is the rhythmic cycling of blood through the vessels and tissues, driven by the continuous pumping of the heart. The amount of blood pumped by the heart into the vessels each minute is called the cardiac output. This amount varies with the body's requirements. For example, muscles, which use oxygen for their energy production, require more blood flow during active periods. Proper functioning of the circulation can be checked by measuring physiological effects such as the pulse and blood pressure.

Circulation | Flow of blood from the heart through arteries to capillaries and returning to the heart through veins

The Pulse

The pulse results from rhythmic waves of blood sent out by the strong contractions of the left ventricle. The frequency of the pulse shows the heart's rate of beating. The quality of the pulse is also noted as an indication of cardiac output. The pulse is described as strong, full, weak, or thready (irregular). The pulse can be palpated in places where an artery lying near the skin surface also passes over a bone. The peripheral pulses are an indication of blood flow through the extremities. These are palpated in the radial, brachial, posterior tibial, and dorsalis pedis arteries. The central pulses, located closer to the heart, can be felt in the carotid and femoral arteries.

Blood Pressure

Blood Pressure | *Force of the blood on the vessels; systolic pressure is the working pressure; diastolic pressure is the resting pressure*

As blood is rhythmically pumped out of the left ventricle, it exerts force against the walls of the blood vessels. This force is another indication of cardiac output. A **blood pressure** reading measures the pressure at two points in the cardiac cycle. When the left ventricle contracts, pressure in the arteries rises to a maximum amount. This is the systolic pressure, or the working pressure of the heart. The blood pressure falls as the ventricular muscle relaxes. The diastolic pressure is the steady level the system returns to when the ventricle is at rest.

Perfusion

Perfusion (per-FEW-zhun) | *Microcirculation of blood within the organs and tissues, when oxygen and nutrients are delivered to the cells and their waste products are removed*

Perfusion refers to the microcirculation of blood through all of the organs and tissues. As blood circulates, oxygen and other nutrients are delivered to the cells and waste products are removed. The body shifts the blood flow to different tissues in response to its changing needs. This process is known as shunting.

Hypoperfusion (HY-po-per-few-zhun) | *Shock; inadequate cardiac output causing a decrease in the delivery of oxygen and clearance of carbon dioxide*

With proper circulation, perfusion is complete. The nutritional and energy needs of each cell are met. However, if the circulation is inadequate for any reason, the tissues do not receive enough oxygen. This state is called **hypoperfusion**. Inadequate perfusion can cause permanent organ damage, so the condition must be identified and treated quickly. When hypoperfusion is profound, it can lead to a state of depression of the body's vital processes. This state is commonly called shock.

Shock is characterized by signs and symptoms such as:

• Rapid, weak pulse

• Rapid, shallow breathing

• Subnormal temperature

• Restlessness, anxiety or mental dullness, altered mental status

• Nausea and vomiting

• Reduction in total blood volume

• Pale, cool, clammy skin

As shock progresses, the skin becomes cyanotic, or blue-gray in color. This is a late sign of shock. Low or decreasing blood pressure is also a late sign of shock.

THE NERVOUS SYSTEM

The nervous system controls the voluntary and involuntary activity of the body. It senses changes within the body and in the outside environment. The system analyzes the details, then integrates all of this to determine the response to be made by the body.

Neurons are specialized nerve cells, capable of transmitting electrical impulses (see Fig. 4.58). Neurons can relay information over distances as short as one millimeter, or as long as a meter or more. For example, a single neuron carries sensory information from the toes to the base of the brain. Information from sensory receptors throughout the body is carried to the spinal cord and brain by sensory nerves. Outgoing impulses that cause muscles to contract or glands to function travel through motor nerves.

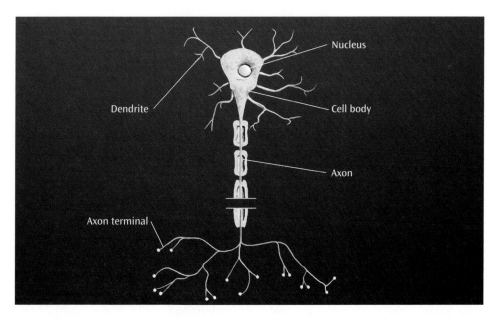

Figure 4.58 *A single nerve cell.*

The nervous system is divided into two anatomical divisions, the **central nervous system** and the **peripheral nervous system** (see Fig. 4.59). The central nervous system (CNS) includes the brain and spinal cord. The peripheral nervous system (PNS) consists of long nerve fibers that carry information between the CNS and the muscles and organs. The nervous system can also be divided according to function. The somatic nervous system (SNS) is involved in conscious perception of the environment and voluntary movements of the body.

Central Nervous System | *The brain and spinal cord*

Peripheral Nervous System | *The sensory and motor nerves that extend from the spinal cord throughout the body*

Figure 4.59 *Posterior view of the nervous system.*

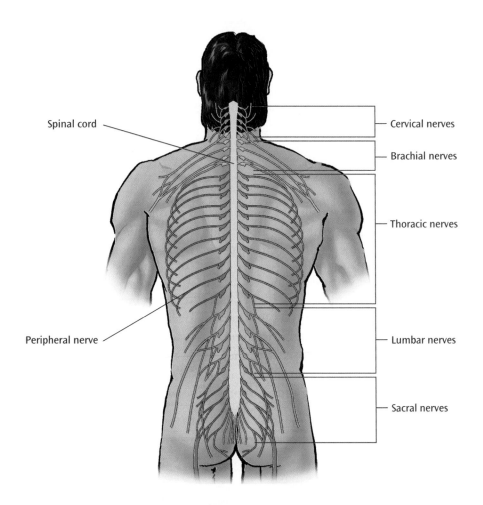

Spinal cord

Peripheral nerve

Cervical nerves

Brachial nerves

Thoracic nerves

Lumbar nerves

Sacral nerves

The autonomic nervous system (ANS) senses the body's internal environment. This system controls involuntary functions such as heart rate, gastrointestinal contractions, and glandular secretions.

The Central Nervous System

The central nervous system consists of the brain and spinal cord. This system integrates all sensory input and motor output exchanges with the peripheral nervous system. The CNS is the seat of memory, emotion, and intellect. The central nervous system is encased in a membrane called the meninges. A cushion of cerebrospinal fluid bathes and protects the spinal cord and brain.

Cranium (KRAY-nee-em) | *The skull*

The brain is the most complex and least understood organ in the body. About 20% of the body's entire blood supply goes to the brain. This ensures an ample supply of oxygen and nutrients for its cells. The brain is located within the **cranium** for protection (see Fig. 4.60). It has three main subdivisions: the **cerebrum**, **cerebellum**, and medulla oblongata.

Cerebrum (seh-REE-brem) | *The largest part of the brain; consists of two hemispheres*

The cerebrum makes up most of the brain mass. It controls all voluntary movement, stores memory, and is the seat of intelligence, reasoning, and creativity. The cerebrum is partially separated into left and right cerebral hemispheres

Cerebellum (seh-reh-BEL-em) | *Portion of the brain that coordinates voluntary muscular movements*

by a deep sagittal groove. The hemispheres of the brain have anatomical and functional differences. The right side of the brain controls the left side of the body. Likewise, the left side of the brain controls the right side of the body. For most people, the left side of the brain is important for language, math, scientific skills, and reasoning. The right side of the brain is involved in spatial and pattern recognition, insight, and creativity.

The cerebellum is in the posterior and inferior aspect of the cranium. It helps to maintain posture and balance, and governs coordinated, skilled movements such as running or speaking. The medulla oblongata is part of the lower brain known as the brainstem. It exerts control over autonomic (involuntary) functions. The medulla regulates blood pressure, body temperature, hunger and thirst, sleep and waking cycles, and respiration.

The spinal cord is contained within the vertebral column, or spinal cavity. The cavity also contains blood vessels and cerebrospinal fluid (CSF), which is a clear, colorless liquid that resembles blood plasma. Adipose tissue in the cavity acts as a cushion for the spinal cord. The spinal cord runs from the base of the brain to the level of the lumbar vertebrae. It transports information about the entire body to and from the brain.

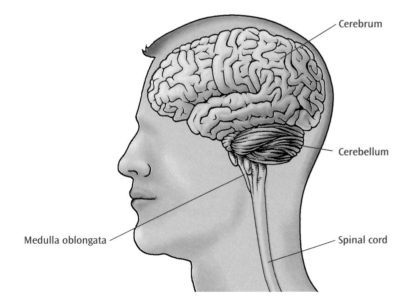

Figure 4.60 *The brain.*

The Peripheral Nervous System

The peripheral nervous system (PNS) consists of the nerves located outside of the brain and spinal cord. The PNS carries impulses between the CNS and various receptors, muscles, and glands in the extremities and internal organs. Sensory nerves carry information from the body to the brain and spinal cord. Motor nerves carry information from the brain and spinal cord to the body's structures.

Functional Divisions of the Nervous System

The two functional divisions of the nervous system are the somatic nervous system (SNS) and the autonomic nervous system (ANS). The SNS regulates voluntary control of the body, and the ANS governs involuntary functions. Structures of the SNS and ANS exist in both of the anatomical divisions. Nerves in the central nervous system and the peripheral nervous system carry both somatic and autonomic information. Somatic and autonomic functions rely upon both sensory and motor neurons.

Somatic Nervous System

The somatic nervous system functions in conscious perception and voluntary control of the body. An example is voluntary movement of the limbs. Somatic sensory nerves carry general sensations of pain, touch, temperature, and proprioception, or sense of body position. They also transmit information from the special senses: hearing, equilibrium (balance), gustation (taste), olfaction (smell), and vision. Somatic motor neurons control voluntary skeletal muscles.

Autonomic Nervous System

The autonomic nervous system controls the involuntary actions of cardiac muscle, smooth muscle, and glands. Autonomic sensory nerves monitor internal body conditions such as oxygen and carbon dioxide levels in the blood. They also detect presence of food in the digestive tract. The motor portion of the autonomic nervous system is divided into sympathetic and parasympathetic divisions. These divisions have opposite effects upon the smooth muscle, cardiac muscle, and glands that they innervate.

The sympathetic division increases the body's available energy, and is active when a person is under increased physical or emotional stress. It is thus named the fight or flight system. During stress, the fight or flight response of the sympathetic division initiates a characteristic set of physiological changes. These include:

- Dilation of the pupils
- Increased heart rate and blood pressure
- Constriction of blood vessels of the skin and some organs
- Dilation of blood vessels in organs such as skeletal muscles, cardiac muscle, liver and adipose tissue
- Rapid and deep breathing as the bronchioles dilate
- Rise in blood glucose levels
- Release of epinephrine and norepinephrine
- Decrease in processes that are not essential for the stress response, such as digestion

The parasympathetic system is responsible for maintaining normal body functions. This system also restores and conserves energy during recovery periods. Parasympathetic activity tends to slow the heartbeat. It enhances smooth muscle contractions for activities such as glandular secretion, the digestion and absorption of food, and the elimination of wastes. It is sometimes called the rest and repair system. Intense fear can increase the activity of this system so much that one loses control over bodily functions.

THE INTEGUMENTARY SYSTEM

The skin is the body's largest organ, weighing 10 to 11 pounds and covering an area of about 22 square feet in an average-sized adult. This integument, or covering, is composed of skin tissue, nerve endings, and blood vessels (see Fig. 4.61). The skin together with the hair, nails, and glands comprise the integumentary system. These structures protect the body, aid in temperature regulation, permit sensation of the environment, excrete wastes, and produce vitamin D.

Skin cells produce keratin, a tough protein that helps to keep moisture in and bacteria out. Skin cells also produce melanin, a pigment that blocks the sun's ultraviolet (UV) rays, preventing damage to the skin's underlying tissues. Racial differences in skin tone are due to variations in melanin content. Body temperature is regulated by sweat glands and blood vessels in the skin that dilate and constrict. Nerve endings in the skin sense heat, cold, touch, pressure, and pain. The sensory nerves transmit information about the environment to the brain and spinal cord. Vitamin D, an essential aid in calcium absorption, is produced from a compound in the skin when exposed to ultraviolet rays in sunlight. Finally, some waste products are excreted in sweat.

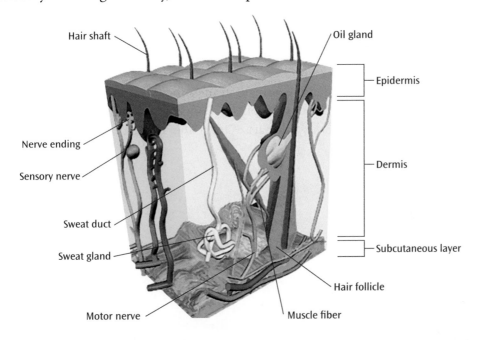

Figure 4.61 *Three-dimensional section of the skin.*

Hair shaft

Oil gland

Epidermis

Nerve ending

Sensory nerve

Dermis

Sweat duct

Sweat gland

Subcutaneous layer

Hair follicle

Motor nerve

Muscle fiber

Epidermis (ep-i-DER-mus) | *Outermost layer of skin*

Dermis (DER-mus) | *Layer of skin located beneath the epidermis that supplies the skin with nutrients*

Subcutaneous (sub-kew-TAY-ne-is) Layer | *Third layer of skin located under the dermis; attaches the skin to underlying structures*

The skin is made up of three layers: the **epidermis**, the **dermis**, and the **subcutaneous layer**. The outermost layer of the skin, the epidermis, is a thin, protective layer containing many dead cells. The epidermis is thicker on the palms and soles of the feet, where friction and wear are heavy. Blood vessels do not pass through the epidermis, so it relies on the underlying dermis for nutrients and oxygen.

The second layer, the dermis, is thicker, living tissue capable of supplying the skin with nutrients. Hair follicles, muscle fibers, sweat glands, and sebaceous, or oil, glands are embedded in the dermis. Fibroblasts are cells in the dermis responsible for wound healing and scar formation. The dermis also contains papillae, skin ridges found on the palms and soles that form finger, hand, and footprints.

Beneath the dermis is the subcutaneous layer. This layer attaches the skin to underlying structures. Fat formed and stored in the subcutaneous layer is an important energy source and a heat insulator. It also serves as a form of protection for underlying structures. The characteristic male and female body shapes result from varying patterns of subcutaneous fat storage.

The skin contains four accessory structures. These are the hair, nails, oil glands, and sweat glands. Hair prevents heat loss from the head, protects against foreign objects entering the eyes, and enables the sensation of touch. Sensitive touch receptors in the skin are activated by movement of the hairs. Nails help to protect the ends of the fingers and toes from injury, and aid in gripping. Oil glands in the dermis secrete sebum, an oily substance rich in proteins, fats, and cholesterol. Sebum helps to prevent hair from becoming too brittle, keeps the skin from becoming too dry, and discourages the growth of some bacteria and fungi. During puberty, hormones cause the sebaceous glands to manufacture excessive amounts of sebum, causing acne.

Sweat, or perspiration, functions primarily in cooling the body through evaporation (see Fig. 4.62). Two types of sweat glands secrete sweat. Eccrine sweat glands originate in the dermis, and open directly onto the surface of the skin through pores. The open pores release sweat consisting of mostly water and salts. Apocrine sweat glands originate in the subcutaneous layer, and release a viscous sweat secretion into hair follicles concentrated around the pubic area, armpits, and nipples. Body odor arises from apocrine sweat glands.

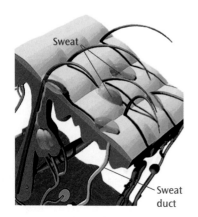

Figure 4.62 *Sweat glands in the skin.*

THE ENDOCRINE SYSTEM

The **endocrine system** is a collection of glands that secrete substances called **hormones** (see Fig. 4.63). These hormones are secreted internally into the bloodstream and cause specific effects at distant organs and tissues of the body. The functions of the endocrine system are to regulate the growth and development of the human body, to maintain a balanced metabolism, and to regulate physical responses to stress.

The endocrine glands include the:

- Pituitary gland
- Thyroid gland
- Parathyroid glands
- Adrenal glands

Besides these glands, some organs perform endocrine functions. These include the hypothalamus, pancreas, gonads, heart, intestines, and during pregnancy, the placenta.

Endocrine System | *Collection of ductless glands that internally secrete hormones into the bloodstream*

Hormones | *Biologically active substances secreted by an endocrine gland; travel through the bloodstream to exert an influence on distant organs or body tissues*

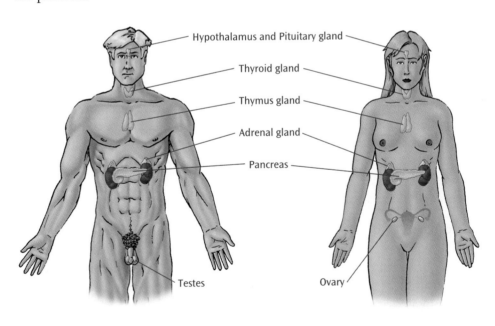

Figure 4.63 *Glands and organs of the endocrine system.*

The hypothalamus is found at the base of the brain. The hypothalamus is often called the master gland, because it receives many cellular signals and responds by secreting a variety of hormones that regulate many other endocrine glands.

The pituitary gland is just below the hypothalamus. This gland is divided into two portions, the anterior and the posterior pituitary glands (see Fig. 4.64). The anterior pituitary gland regulates growth. It also oversees the regulation of the thyroid, parathyroid, and adrenal glands, the pancreas, and the gonads.

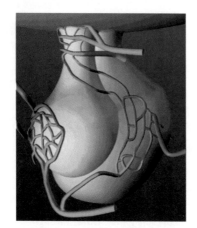

Figure 4.64 *The anterior and posterior lobes of the pituitary gland.*

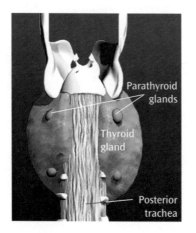

Figure 4.65 *The thyroid and parathyroid glands.*

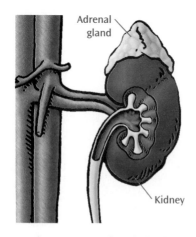

Figure 4.66 *Adrenal gland.*

The posterior pituitary gland stores and releases two hormones produced by the hypothalamus. These hormones are oxytocin, which is active in the mother during childbirth and breastfeeding, and antidiuretic hormone (ADH), which regulates the body's water level.

The thyroid gland is found in the neck, in front of the trachea (see Fig. 4.65). The thyroid gland releases hormones that regulate metabolism, or the rate of energy use in the body. The hormones also regulate normal growth and development. Diminished production of thyroid hormones is called hypothyroidism. An abnormally high level of thyroid hormones is called hyperthyroidism. Hyperthyroidism is often identified by a visibly enlarged thyroid gland, called a goiter.

The parathyroid gland consists of four small glands located on the posterior surface of the thyroid (see Fig. 4.65). The parathyroids regulate the metabolism of calcium and phosphorus in the bones and blood.

The paired adrenal glands are found in the abdominal cavity, resting on top of each kidney (see Fig. 4.66). These glands have two functionally different parts. The outer layer is called the adrenal cortex and the inner part is the adrenal medulla. The adrenal cortex secretes hormones called glucocorticoids, which provide for adaptation of the body to stressful situations. Glucocorticoids cause the body to reduce its protein supplies, growth, and inflammatory and immune system responses. The adrenal cortex also secretes hormones called mineralocorticoids that regulate salt and water balance.

The adrenal medulla produces adrenaline, or epinephrine, and norepinephrine, which regulate the body's fight-or-flight response. This response readies a person to deal with stressful or physically taxing situations. It causes an increased heart rate, stronger heart contractions, increased blood pressure, dilation of blood vessels leading to the skeletal muscles and lungs, and constriction of blood vessels feeding the skin and intestines.

The pancreas is found in the abdominal cavity. The pancreas produces insulin and glucagon, which regulate sugar metabolism. The pancreas also secretes enzymes that assist in the digestion of food. The medical condition resulting from insufficient insulin is called diabetes mellitus. When untreated or inadequately treated, it leads to uncontrolled high blood sugar levels. Endocrine emergencies are most commonly seen in diabetic patients.

The gonads are the testes in the male and ovaries in the female. The sex glands produce the hormones that regulate sexual development and normal sexual functions.

Chapter Four Summary

- Knowledge of the human body and how it works is important to you as an EMT-B. It enables you to communicate with other health-care professionals effectively and allows you to perform a competent assessment. You must understand the normal to recognize things that are wrong with the patient.

- Each system has specific purposes, although they all work together to keep us healthy.

  Musculoskeletal system—Gives the body shape, allows movement, and protects internal organs

Respiratory system—Provides oxygen to the bloodstream and removes waste gases

Circulatory system—Transports blood cells, plasma, and platelets throughout the body

Nervous system—Controls the voluntary and involuntary activities of the body

Integumentary system (skin)—Protects the body from the environment, bacteria, and other organisms

Endocrine system—Secretes chemicals responsible for regulating body activities and functions

Key Terms Review

continued

Key Terms Review (cont.)

Review Questions

1. Which of these means "toward the midline"?

   a. Lateral

   b. Medial

   c. Proximal

   d. Distal

2. The term lateral is best defined as:

   a. Toward the midline of the body

   b. Away from the midline of the body

   c. Toward the transverse plane of the body

   d. Away from the frontal plane of the body

3. Posterior is best described as:

   a. Farthest from the point of attachment

   b. Toward the upper surface of the body

   c. Toward the front surface of the body

   d. Toward the back surface of the body

4. The term superior most nearly means:

   a. Larger

   b. Closer to the head

   c. Stronger

   d. Closer to the point of attachment

5. The individual bones of the spinal column are known as:

    a. Spinous processes
    b. Spinal bones
    c. Cervical bones
    d. Vertebrae

6. The xiphoid process, an important landmark for CPR, is located on the inferior tip of the _____ .

    a. Manubrium
    b. Tubercle
    c. Sternum
    d. Floating ribs

7. How many pairs of ribs are there?

    a. 10
    b. 12
    c. 13
    d. 14

8. The trachea connects:

    a. The pharynx and the larynx
    b. The larynx and the bronchi
    c. The esophagus and the larynx
    d. The bronchi and the lungs

9. The bones of the ankle are called:

    a. Tarsals
    b. Phalanges
    c. Carpals
    d. Metaphalanges

10. The term metatarsal refers to the:

    a. Hand bones
    b. Foot bones
    c. Wrist bones
    d. Ankle bones

11. Tissues of the skeletal system include all of the following, except:

    a. Cartilage
    b. Tendons
    c. Muscles
    d. Connective tissue

12. The shoulder blade is also known as:

    a. The clavicle
    b. The acromion
    c. The scapula
    d. The sternum

13. The ribs are attached to the 12 _____ vertebrae.

    a. Cervical
    b. Thoracic
    c. Lumbar
    d. Sacral

14. Muscle that makes up the walls of organs and is under involuntary control is:

    a. Skeletal muscle
    b. Smooth muscle
    c. Striated muscle
    d. Cardiac muscle

15. The condition of low oxygen levels in the tissues is called:

    a. Hypothermia
    b. Hypotension
    c. Hypocalcia
    d. Hypoxia

16. The term vein refers to:

    a. Any vessel carrying blood away from the heart
    b. Any vessel carrying oxygenated blood
    c. Any vessel carrying blood toward the heart
    d. Any vessel carrying unoxygenated blood

17. The right side of the heart receives blood from:

    a. The left side of the heart
    b. The superior and inferior venae cavae
    c. The pulmonary circulation
    d. The aorta

18. The skin is the body's largest:

    a. Tissue
    b. Fascia
    c. Organ
    d. Muscle

CASE STUDIES

The Human Body

1 You are dispatched to the scene of a motor vehicle accident. Upon arrival, you find a pickup truck on the side of the road next to a dead deer. The driver is not injured, but his friend, who was riding in the bed of the truck, was thrown forcefully against the cab. According to the driver, the passenger struck the cab sideways at armpit level. The rear of the cab is slightly deformed from the impact. The patient is in the bed of the truck, unconscious.

A. Using anatomical terms, describe the area of the body that impacted the cab.

B. What internal organs may have been affected by the trauma?

C. What musculoskeletal structures may have been injured?

2 Your EMS unit works in an urban area with a high rate of violent crime. Shortly after midnight, you are dispatched to an assault call. Upon arrival, you see that police have secured the scene. You find a 27-year-old female sitting on the steps of the house, spitting up blood. The police advise you that she has been uncommunicative but awake and responsive since their arrival. The only information that bystanders can provide is that an assailant struck the victim in the throat several times with a baseball bat, causing discoloration and swelling below the Adam's apple.

A. Describe the patient's injury using anatomical terms.

B. Given the presence of contusions to the neck, what internal structures may be injured?

C. The spitting of blood (hemoptysis) and the inability to speak would lead you to believe there is damage to what structure? Why is this significant?

Stories from the Field
Wrap-Up

A working knowledge of anatomy and physiology is very important to the EMT-Basic. Before you can recognize what is wrong with a person, you must understand normal anatomy and physiology. Carmen and Mark focused on treating the chest wound because it could be the reason the patient was having difficulty breathing. The better your understanding of how the body works, the easier it is for you to understand how the body reacts to illness and injury.

Knowledge of anatomy and physiology is also important so you can communicate effectively with other healthcare personnel. Emergency medical providers must be able to clearly and effectively describe a patient's condition both verbally and in writing. Use only medical terms that you fully understand. Relay information in simple English when possible.

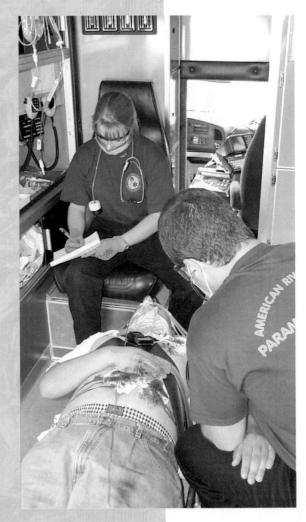

Chapter 5

Vital Signs and SAMPLE History

Stories from the Field

You are dispatched to an unknown illness call. When you arrive, you find a young woman who has been complaining of nausea and abdominal discomfort for several days. The patient is very pale and sweaty. Robin begins to prepare the patient for transport, and helps her to assume a comfortable position on the stretcher. The patient is requesting transport to a hospital across town. She tells you that she has no other transportation available. Robin checks the vital signs and obtains the patient's medical history and chief complaint. The receiving hospital is about 20 minutes away. Robin asks you to repeat the vital sign measurements two more times en route. This is difficult, because the patient is laughing and talking. The patient is in no acute distress, but Robin has instructed you to ask history questions and take vital signs.

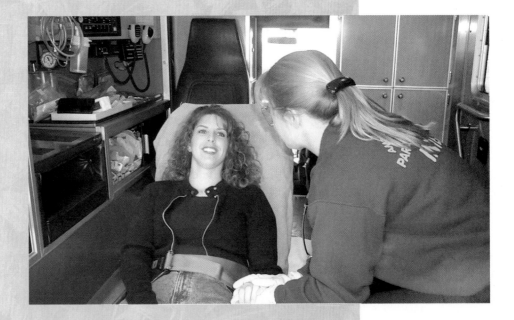

Vital signs and a medical history are obtained on almost every patient you will encounter. Vital signs provide valuable information for your overall assessment of a patient. In future chapters, you will learn more about specific treatment pathways and how baseline and ongoing vital sign measurements help you to identify the need for additional interventions. Taking the vital signs several times during transport will help to identify changes in the patient's condition. This information is valuable in the continuum of care.

The SAMPLE history is a brief, organized summary of the patient's relevant medical history. Obtaining this information will help to guide your actions, and will assist the receiving facility in providing care. The SAMPLE history is taken early in the evaluation of a conscious patient. If the patient is unconscious, attempt to obtain the same information from family members or bystanders. In some cases, the mnemonic OPQRST will help you to evaluate the signs and symptoms of a patient's chief complaint.

CHIEF COMPLAINT

Chief Complaint | Patient's self-described worst or most serious concern at this time

Determine the patient's **chief complaint** soon after you arrive at the scene. The chief complaint is the primary reason that you were called today, even though the patient may have other problems or injuries. For example, a patient with a history of high blood pressure and diabetes mellitus calls EMS because of a sudden bout of severe chest pain. The existing medical conditions must be addressed in the patient's total care. However, the chief complaint is acute chest pain.

Chief complaints often provide clues to treatment. Knowing the chief complaint will help you to learn the nature of the patient's problem. Using this information, you can quickly decide which treatment pathway to use. Be prepared to learn the chief complaint by doing a thorough assessment even if the patient is unresponsive. While performing your assessment, have a crew member ask family members, bystanders, or others on scene for any valuable information they know.

The symptoms of the chief complaint may progress, change, or even subside. For example, a patient calls an ambulance because of shortness of breath and pain. Although the patient has had slight chest pain for several days, the shortness of breath is new. The chest pain has changed, and now radiates down the arm.

Along with the chief complaint, you will record some general information about the patient, including age, race, and gender. As an EMT-B, you must recognize that patients experience a wide range of emotions in emergencies. Many patients are anxious and upset. The best response to a patient's concerns is to provide a careful explanation of what you are doing and the reason.

EMT Tip

Treat the patient based on his or her chief complaint and signs or symptoms, not only the vital sign measurements.

D.O.T. OBJECTIVE

Identify the components of vital signs.

VITAL SIGNS

Vital signs are outward expressions of internal processes. When taking vital signs, you will measure skin temperature, pulse, respirations (breathing), and blood pressure. A pupil check is also part of routine vital signs in some agencies. Checking vital signs, or vitals, provides information about how the body's key systems are functioning (see Table 5.1). Evaluating vital sign values provides a quick overview of the patient's condition.

Vital Signs | Pulse rate and quality, breathing rate and quality, blood pressure, skin color, skin temperature, skin condition, pupil size and quality, and capillary refill in children

Table 5.1 • **RANGES OF AVERAGE VITAL SIGNS BY AGE**

Age	Pulse (beats per minute, at rest)	Respirations (breaths per minute, at rest)	Systolic Blood Pressure (mmHg) at rest	Diastolic Blood Pressure (mmHg) at rest
Adult	60–100	12–20	90–150	60–90
15 Years	55–105	12–20	100–120	66–80
10 Years	70–110	20–30	80–120	53–80
5 Years	80–120	20–30	80–110	53–73
3 Years	80–130	20–30	–	–
1 Year	80–140	20–30	–	–
Newborn (Birth to 1 month)	120–160	30–50	–	–

Blood pressure is not usually measured in children under 3 years of age.

EMT Tip

Listening to lung sounds with your stethoscope is covered in detail in Chapter 9–Patient Assessment.

Baseline vital signs are the first set of readings taken when you arrive. You will use these values to compare with subsequent vital signs. Taking vital signs several times and comparing the values will help you to detect changes in the patient's condition. You will measure:

- Breathing rate and character
- Pulse rate and character
- Skin color, temperature, and condition
- Pupil size and reaction

D.O.T. OBJECTIVES

Describe the methods to obtain a breathing rate.

Identify the attributes that should be obtained when assessing breathing.

Differentiate between shallow, labored, and noisy breathing.

Respiration (res-per-AY-shun) |
Breathing; process through which air enters and leaves the lungs

Inspiration | *Taking air into the lungs (inhalation)*

Expiration | *Expelling air from the lungs (exhalation)*

Respirations

Respirations are measured by observing the rise and fall of the chest. A single **respiration** consists of one **inspiration**, or inhalation, and one **expiration**, or exhalation. The rate and quality of breathing are both important when assessing respirations. Record the respiration rate and quality so that you do not forget the findings. Also record the appearance of any secretions the patient coughs up, such as sputum and blood.

Counting the number of breaths in a 30-second period and multiplying by 2 will give you the number of respirations per minute. The normal rate for an adult is 12 to 20 breaths per minute. This range varies slightly, depending on age. If the respirations are irregular, slow, or appear abnormal, count the rate for one full minute. If you have difficulty counting respirations, fold the patient's arm across the abdomen. Count each rise and fall of the abdomen as one respiration.

EMT Tip

Patients may consciously alter the respiratory rate when being watched. Avoid telling the patient you are counting respirations. You can do this by measuring the pulse rate, then continuing to hold the wrist while glancing at the chest and counting the respirations.

Quality of Respirations

You will evaluate the breathing quality while you are assessing the respiratory rate. Four categories of respiration characteristics are:

- Normal breathing
- Shallow breathing
- Labored breathing
- Noisy breathing

Normal breathing is easy and effortless, not labored. The average person's chest wall expands approximately one inch during inspiration. The patient does not use the accessory muscles, and the rhythm is regular. Breathing is silent and not painful. You will not hear wheezing or gurgling sounds.

The chest and abdominal wall move only slightly during shallow breathing. You will hear or feel very little air movement as the patient breathes.

Labored breathing is an effort for the patient. He or she may use the accessory muscles, such as the trapezius and sternocleidomastoid. You may observe nasal flaring and retraction of the skin between the ribs or above the collarbone (see Fig. 5.1). These are intercostal and supraclavicular retractions. The patient may gasp for air. You may hear grunting or noise during forceful exhalation. The patient may also have **stridor**, a harsh or high-pitched sound during inhalation. Stridor is an indication of upper airway obstruction.

EMT Alert

In children with labored breathing, you may see significant use of the abdominal muscles. This is characterized by seesaw motions of the chest and stomach.

Stridor | *Harsh, high-pitched sound during inspiration*

Figure 5.1 *Nasal flaring is one sign of labored breathing.*

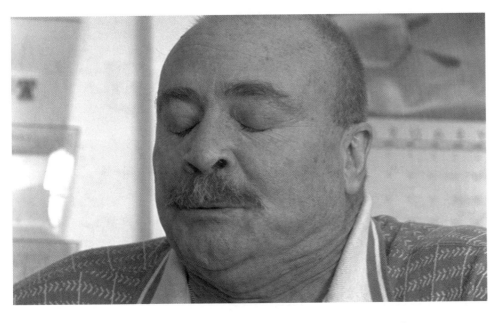

CD-ROM Link

The video, "Vital Signs—Breathing," in the Vital Signs chapter and the Video Appendix on the MedEMT CD-ROM shows examples of abnormal breathing signs.

Noisy breathing is characterized by an increase in audible sounds. You may hear snoring, wheezing, or gurgling. Crowing, a turbulent sound, may be present during inspiration. Noisy breathing is not normal and suggests a disruption in the flow of air.

Listen for breath sounds near the mouth and on both sides of the chest. If the patient has a penetrating injury to the chest wall, gurgling sounds may be heard through the hole or wound.

D.O.T. OBJECTIVE

Describe the methods to obtain a pulse rate.

Pulse

The **pulse** is a wave of pressure passing through the circulatory system as the heart contracts. This wave is palpated, or felt, in places where an artery lies near the skin and over a bone. Several locations are used to measure the pulse (see Fig. 5.2).

The peripheral pulses can be measured at the:

- Radial artery
- Brachial artery
- Dorsalis pedis artery
- Posterior tibial artery

Figure 5.2 *Pulse locations.*

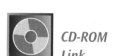

CD-ROM Link

The video, "Vital Signs– Circulation," in the Vital Signs chapter and the Video Appendix on the MedEMT CD-ROM demonstrates the steps in checking and recording a patient's pulse.

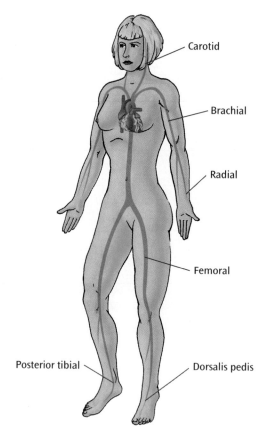

The presence of a peripheral pulse is an important finding. This tells you that the heart is circulating blood to the extremity. If an extremity is injured, the presence of a pulse suggests that the blood vessels are not severely damaged.

Two pulse points are close to the trunk of the body:

- Carotid artery
- Femoral artery

These central pulses are used if you cannot feel the pulse at other sites. In severe shock, you may be unable to feel the pulse in the extremities. The central pulses are palpable longer than other sites due to their size and location.

- The **radial pulse** is palpated on the anterior lateral surface of the wrist, proximal to the thumb (see Fig. 5.3). This pulse is used for evaluating circulation in the upper extremities. Always check the radial pulse first when assessing concious adults and children more than one year old.

- The **brachial pulse** is palpated on the medial aspect of the biceps brachii muscle. It also indicates the quality of circulation in the upper extremities. The brachial site is the preferred site for checking the pulse of a child less than one year old (see Fig. 5.4).

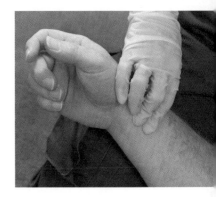

Figure 5.3 *Checking the radial pulse.*

Figure 5.4 *Measure the brachial pulse in an infant.*

Radial Pulse | *The flow of blood through the radial artery; palpated on the anterior lateral surface of the wrist, proximal to the thumb*

Brachial Pulse | *The flow of blood through the brachial artery, palpated in the medial aspect of the upper arm*

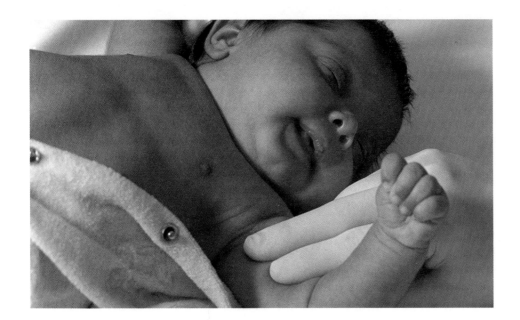

- The pedal, or dorsalis pedis pulse, is palpated on the dorsum of the foot (see Fig. 5.5). This pulse provides information about circulation in the lower extremities.

- The posterior tibial pulse is palpated posterior to the medial malleolus, or ankle bone. It also helps to evaluate circulation in the lower extremities.

- The carotid pulse is palpated just lateral to the larynx and trachea. It is medial to the sternocleidomastoid muscle of the neck (see Fig. 5.6). If you cannot feel a peripheral pulse during your initial pulse check, evaluate the carotid pulse. Because of its proximity to the heart, the carotid pulse is the best indication that the heart is circulating blood.

- The **femoral pulse** is palpated in the upper thigh, but can be very difficult to assess. The presence of a femoral pulse helps to evaluate circulation in the lower extremities.

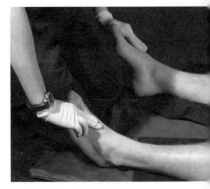

Figure 5.5 *Assessing the pedal pulses.*

Femoral (FEM-or-ul) Pulse | *The flow of blood through the femoral artery in the upper thigh*

Figure 5.6 *Assessing the carotid pulse.*

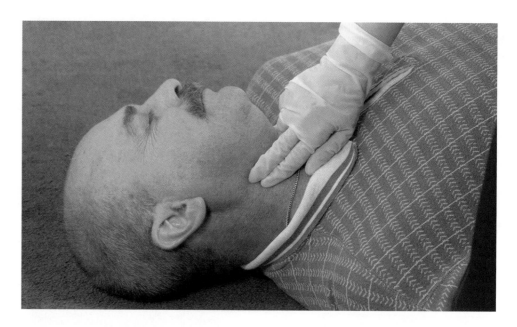

Measuring the Pulse

In patients older than one year, take the initial pulse at the radial artery, on the thumb side of the wrist. For patients younger than one year, palpate the pulse at the brachial artery, on the thumb side, slightly superior to the bend of the elbow (see Table 5.2).

Apply gentle pressure when checking the pulse. Pressing hard will cut off arterial circulation. Place the tips of your first two or three fingers over the artery. Avoid using your thumb, which has a pulse of its own. If the peripheral pulses are not palpable, check the carotid pulse. Avoid palpating both carotid arteries at once. This could inadvertently block blood flow to the brain. Use caution when measuring carotid pulses in an elderly patient or any patient who has a compromised vascular system. These patients may have atherosclerosis, a condition that causes narrowing of the arteries. Pressure on a single carotid could be enough to stop the blood flow to the brain. Pressure could also cause a clot to break free and travel to the brain, causing a stroke. Applying excessive pressure to the carotid artery can also cause the patient's heart rate to slow dramatically.

Table 5.2 • PULSE SITES

Age Group	Pulse Site	Notes
Adults and Children Older than One Year	Radial Pulse	Primary site for evaluating peripheral pulse and circulation in upper extremities
	Carotid Pulse	Primary site for evaluating central pulse if radial pulse not present
	Pedal/Posterior Tibial Pulses	Sites for evaluating circulation in lower extremities
	Brachial Pulse	Site for evaluating circulation in upper extremities
	Femoral Pulse	Additional site for evaluating a central pulse
Children Younger than One Year	Brachial Pulse	Primary site for evaluating peripheral pulse
	Carotid Pulse	Primary site for evaluating central pulse if brachial pulse not present

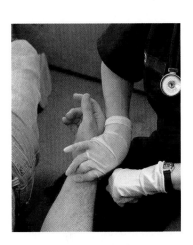

Figure 5.7 *Count the beats for 30 seconds.*

D.O.T. OBJECTIVES

Identify the information obtained when assessing a patient's pulse.

Differentiate between a strong, weak, regular, and irregular pulse.

Pulse Rate and Quality

When checking the pulse, you will assess its rate and quality. To determine the rate, count the number of beats in 30 seconds, then multiply by 2 (see Fig. 5.7). This will give you the number of beats per minute. If the pulse is irregular, weak, or slow, count the pulse for one full minute. The normal pulse rate in adults is 60 to 100 beats per minute. **Bradycardia** is a heart rate below 60 beats per minute. A heart rate above 100 beats per minute is **tachycardia**.

Bradycardia (bray-deh-KAR-de-uh) | *Slow heart rate*

The quality of the pulse is determined by the volume and rhythm of each beat. Volume is determined by the force of contractions. The volume is felt as the strength with which the blood is pushed through the arteries. It is characterized as strong or weak. A normal pulse is easily palpated and is characterized as strong. An abnormally forceful pulse, called a bounding pulse, may be caused by hypertension or cardiac abnormalities. An abnormally weak, or thready, pulse suggests hypovolemia, or low blood volume. This may be caused by shock, heart failure, or vascular disease.

Tachycardia (tak-eh-KAR-de-uh) | *An unusually rapid heart rate*

The pulse rhythm is characterized as regular or irregular. A normal pulse has a regular rhythm. The pulse rhythm corresponds to the rhythm of a normal heartbeat. An irregular pulse is felt at uneven intervals. Heart arrhythmias, shock, and other factors can cause the pulse to be irregular.

Skin Assessment

Evaluating the skin color will help you to determine how well the tissues are perfused with oxygenated blood. You will evaluate the skin for color, temperature, and condition. In children under six years old, you will also check the capillary refill time.

Conjunctiva (kon-junk-TIE-vuh) | *Membrane lining the eyelids and the surface of the sclera of the eye*

Oral Mucosa | *Pink membrane lining the inside of the mouth*

Cyanosis (sy-uh-NO-sis) | *Blue coloring of the skin; may indicate poor oxygen uptake or reduced perfusion*

Skin Color

Normal skin tone is determined by a pigment called melanin. People with dark skin have more melanin than people with light skin. The nail beds, **conjunctiva**, and **oral mucosa** do not contain melanin. Checking the skin color in these areas will provide a true picture of the patient's oxygenation. Skin color is an important finding. Well-perfused skin with a good supply of oxygenated red blood cells has a healthy, pink tint. In infants and children, examine the palms of the hands and the soles of the feet.

Patients whose skin appears pale may not be receiving an adequate supply of red blood cells. Because red blood cells carry oxygen, the patient may be perfusing poorly. Impaired blood flow may be caused by:

- Anemia
- Hemorrhage
- Nervous system damage
- Anxiety
- Low cardiac output
- Shock

Skin that is blue or blue-gray is cyanotic (see Fig. 5.8). **Cyanosis** suggests poor oxygenation of the blood and tissues. It may also be caused by reduced perfusion from slow-moving blood. Common causes of cyanosis are:

- Cardiac arrest
- Airway obstruction
- Respiratory distress

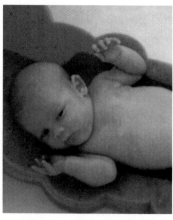

Figure 5.8 *Signs of cyanosis are a blue-gray tint around the extremities, lips, and mouth.*

- Shock
- Heart disease
- Blood clots
- Vascular disease
- Cold exposure

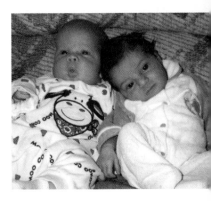

Red skin is flushed with blood. This is a normal reaction if the patient has been exposed to heat, or has just come in from the cold. The red color is caused by relaxation of the blood vessels, increasing blood flow to the face and hands. Flushing is caused by fluctuating hormones in some women. Patients with carbon monoxide poisoning may have a flushed appearance. A very bright, cherry red complexion is a late sign of carbon monoxide poisoning. This is caused by carbon monoxide binding with the patient's hemoglobin.

Figure 5.9 *Jaundiced skin in an infant (left).*

Jaundice is yellow-appearing skin (see Fig. 5.9). Abnormal yellowing may also be seen on the mucous membranes of the mouth and tongue. The **sclera**, or whites of the eyes, appear yellow. The color is caused by excessive levels of liver metabolites, such as bilirubin. Jaundice suggests:

- Liver abnormalities, such as hepatitis or alcoholic cirrhosis
- Excessive destruction of red blood cells
- A blocked bile duct from gallstones or a tumor

Jaundice (JAWN-dis) | *Yellow deposits in skin and whites of the eyes caused by increased bilirubin in the blood; indication of liver abnormality*

Sclera | *Outermost layer of the eyeball; whites of the eyes*

D.O.T. OBJECTIVES

Identify the normal and abnormal skin temperature.

Differentiate between hot, cool, and cold skin temperature.

Identify normal and abnormal skin conditions.

Skin Temperature and Condition

The relative skin temperature is measured by placing the back of your hand against the patient's skin (see Fig. 5.10). Normal skin is warm to the touch. Abnormally hot skin suggests fever, infection, or overexposure to heat. Skin that feels cool to the touch suggests poor circulation, poor perfusion, or exposure to the cold. In extreme cases of cold exposure, the skin will also feel stiff.

The normal skin condition is dry. Moist or wet skin suggests an abnormality. Skin may be cool and moist due to hypovolemic shock or anxiety.

Figure 5.10 *The forehead is a common area to assess skin temperature.*

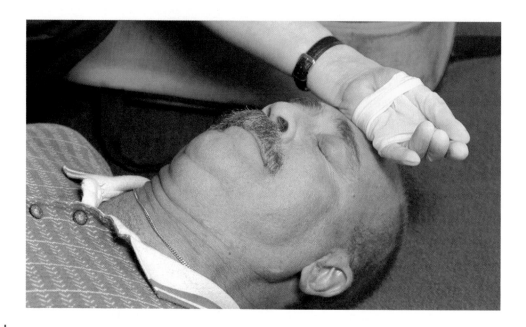

> **D.O.T. OBJECTIVE**
>
> Identify normal and abnormal capillary refill in infants and children.

Capillary Refill Time

You will measure the capillary refill time in infants and children younger than six years of age. To do this, press on the skin or nail beds, then release (see Fig. 5.11). Pressing forces blood out of the capillaries, causing the skin to blanch, or become pale. The time it takes for normal color to reappear is a rough indicator of perfusion.

Figure 5.11 *Pressing on the nail empties blood from the capillaries (left). When the nail is released, measure the time for the capillaries to refill (right).*

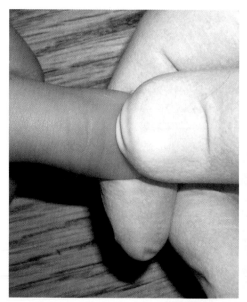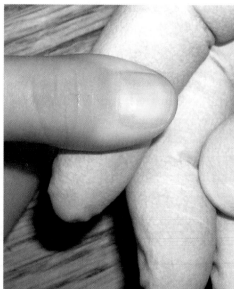

Normal capillary refill time in infants and children is less than 2 seconds. An abnormal, prolonged capillary refill time suggests poor perfusion. This is commonly due to shock or cold exposure. Current EMS literature suggests that capillary refill is a good measurement of circulatory status only in patients younger than 6 years of age. Checking capillary refill in adults may provide a false sense of circulatory stability. Capillary refill may be normal in adults experiencing the early stages of shock.

D.O.T. OBJECTIVES

Describe the methods to assess the pupils.

Identify normal and abnormal pupil size.

Differentiate between dilated (big) and constricted (small) pupil size.

Differentiate between reactive and nonreactive pupils and equal and unequal pupils.

Pupil Assessment

Assess the patient's **pupils** for size, reactivity, and equality. Normal pupils are round and regular, equal in size, and reactive. Tiny red vessels are normally seen in the sclera. Bleeding should not be visible. The cornea and **lens** should be clear, not cloudy.

The pupils control how much light enters the eyes (see Fig. 5.12). In bright light, a normal pupil constricts, or becomes smaller. This change in size

Pupil | *Circular opening in the iris that allows passage of light into the eye*

Lens | *Refracting structure of the eye located directly behind the pupil*

Figure 5.12 *A cross section of the eye.*

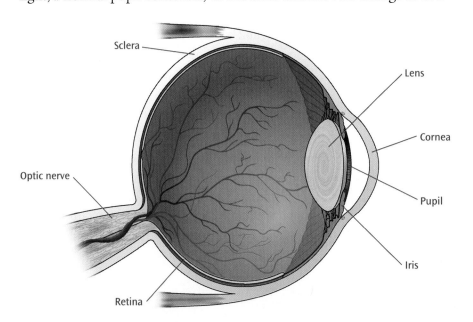

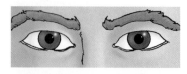
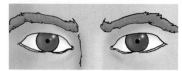
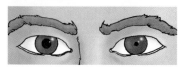

Figure 5.13 *Dilated pupils (top), constricted pupils (center), and unequal pupils (bottom).*

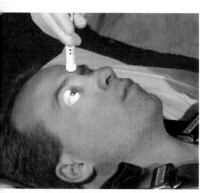

Figure 5.14 *Checking pupil response to light.*

EMT Tip

If you are not sure whether a patient's pupils are reacting normally given the ambient light, try comparing the pupil reaction to another person's on scene.

protects the retina from damage caused by excessive light. The pupils dilate, or become larger, in the dark or in diminished light. This allows more light to enter. The change in pupil size enables us to discriminate objects more clearly. Pupils should be evaluated in normal or slightly dim lighting.

When checking pupils, you will determine how quickly they react to light. Pupil reactivity is described as:

• Reactive—normal muscle response to light source variations

• Sluggish—abnormally slow response to direct light

• Nonreactive—no muscle response to direct light sources

Normal pupils are 2 to 6 mm in diameter and respond equally to light. Dilated pupils can suggest decreased blood flow to the brain, cardiac arrest, or drug use. Constricted pupils may suggest head trauma, opioid drug use, or excessive ambient light. Some eye drops also cause the pupils to constrict (see Fig. 5.13). Pinpoint pupils are less than 2 mm in diameter and suggest a lesion or compression of the pons in the brainstem.

Pupils are described as unequal when they differ in size. Unequal pupils suggest stroke, head injury, another neurological problem, or an artificial plastic eye that does not react to light. Surgery to remove cataracts may cause the pupils to become irregular in shape. A few people have chronic, unequal pupils.

Checking Pupil Response

Shine a penlight into each eye to check pupil response (see Fig. 5.14). Cover one eye, then quickly bring the light from the side of the face directly over the pupil. Hold for a second, then remove the light. Repeat the procedure with the other eye. When checking pupils, make sure the patient is not looking directly at another light source. This is usually the case when assessing a patient in a supine position outdoors.

The size of a reactive pupil changes when exposed to light. The normal response is for both pupils to constrict when a light is shined into one eye. A direct light reflex causes the lighted pupil to constrict. Concurrent constriction of the other pupil is called a consensual light reflex. These reflexes should occur even if the patient is asleep or unconscious. Watch for changes in pupil size and the speed of changes.

Nonreactive pupils do not react to light and are fixed in midposition. The shape may be irregular or slightly ovoid. Nonreactive pupils suggest midbrain swelling or lesions, such as in head injury or stroke. Fixed, dilated pupils indicate medullary dysfunction, which may be caused by stroke, intracranial swelling, bleeding, profound hypoxia, or brain death.

Blood Pressure

Blood pressure is the force of blood exerted on the walls of the vessels and organs of the body (see Fig. 5.15). Blood pressure is influenced by heart function and the total blood volume in the cardiovascular system. Heart function controls the amount of blood pumped with each heartbeat, and the number of beats per minute. The cardiovascular system is a closed loop, like a radiator. Blood loss causes decreased blood pressure. High blood pressure, low blood pressure, or rapidly changing blood pressure can all be indicators of underlying disease or traumatic injury.

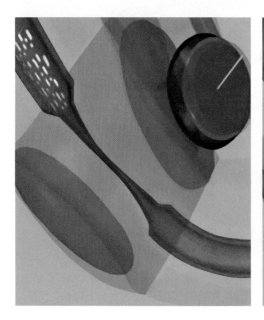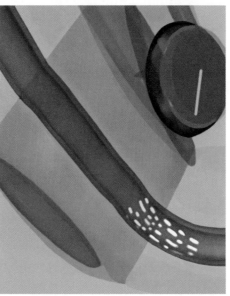

Figure 5.15 *Bloodflow is blocked when the cuff is inflated (left). Bloodflow resumes when the cuff is deflated (right).*

Blood pressure is measured using an instrument called the **sphygmomanometer** (see Fig. 5.16). Values are recorded in millimeters of mercury, or mmHg. Blood pressure is recorded as two numbers (see Fig. 5.17). The first number is the **systolic pressure**, which is the working pressure of the heart. The second number, the **diastolic pressure**, is the resting pressure. You may want to review the physiology of circulation in Chapter 4 to help you understand the action of the heart.

Sphygmomanometer (sfig-mo-mah-NOM-eh-ter) | *Blood pressure cuff*

Systolic (sis-TALL-ik)
Pressure | *The pressure in the arterial system when the left ventricle contracts; first sound heard when assessing blood pressure by auscultation*

Diastolic (di-uh-STALL-ik)
Pressure | *The pressure exerted on the walls of the arteries when the heart is at rest; when assessing blood pressure by auscultation, it is measured when the sound stops*

Figure 5.16 *A standard sphygmomanometer.*

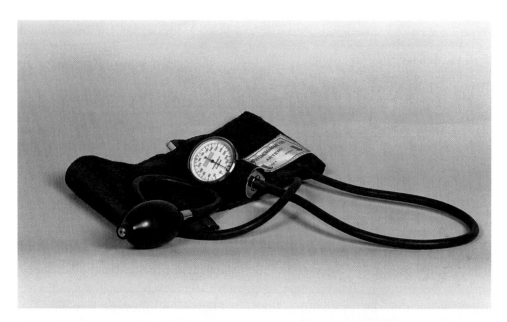

Figure 5.17 *Healthy systolic and diastolic blood pressures.*

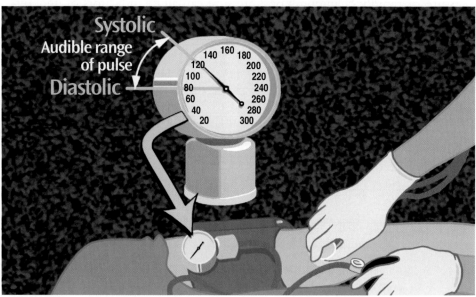

D.O.T. OBJECTIVES

Describe the methods to assess blood pressure.

Explain the difference between auscultation and palpation for obtaining a blood pressure.

Blood Pressure Measurement

Apply the blood pressure cuff securely around the arm. Center the bladder over the brachial artery. Some cuffs have arrows showing exact placement.

The blood pressure cuff is a sleeve containing an inflatable bladder. Before taking the blood pressure, measure the length of the bladder. For an accurate reading, the bladder must be equal to at least 80% of the circumference of the patient's arm.

Measure blood pressure in patients older than three years of age. When working with children, treat the patient, not the pressure. For an infant or child younger than age three, the physical assessment is more valuable than specific vital sign numbers. Important observations include the child's overall appearance, responsiveness, and respiratory distress.

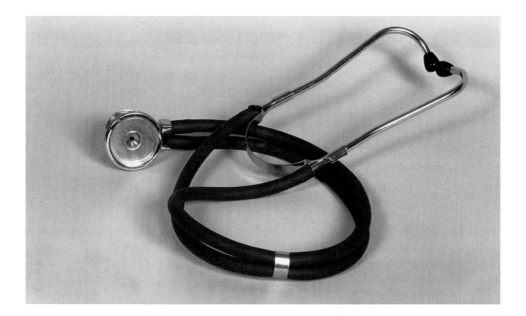

Figure 5.18 *Standard stethoscope.*

Two methods are used for measuring blood pressure. When using the **auscultation** method, you will listen for the systolic and diastolic sounds using a stethoscope (see Fig. 5.18 and Procedure 5.1). When measuring blood pressure by **palpation**, you will palpate the radial pulse. The systolic pressure is felt as the blood pressure cuff is deflated. You cannot determine the diastolic pressure by palpation. You may rely on palpation when the surrounding noise makes auscultation impossible. Using both methods to get an accurate reading is best, if practical.

Auscultation | *Listening for sounds with a stethoscope*

Palpation | *Assessment by touch or feel*

Palpation Method of Taking Blood Pressure

You can measure the systolic blood pressure by palpation.

1. Select and position the cuff as you would for auscultation.
2. Close the screw on the handset.
3. Locate and palpate the radial pulse with one hand.

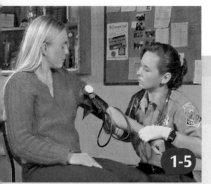

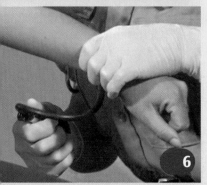

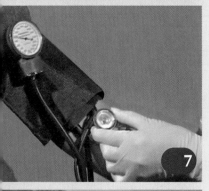

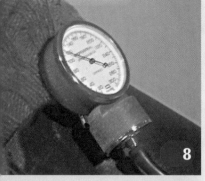

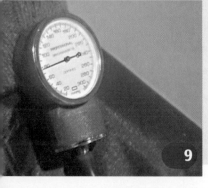

Procedure 5.1 • BLOOD PRESSURE BY AUSCULTATION

Video Appendix

1. Assist the patient into the sitting position. Advise him or her to relax one arm. If this position is not practical, take the pressure with the patient lying or standing. Record the patient's position when the reading is taken.

2. Select the correct size blood pressure cuff for the patient.

3. Position the cuff securely around the upper arm, about one inch above the elbow. Center the bladder over the brachial artery.

4. Palpate the radial pulse with your first two fingers.

5. Close the screw on the handset.

6. Inflate the cuff until you can no longer feel the radial pulse. At this point, the pressure in the cuff matches the pressure needed to close the brachial artery, stopping the flow of blood. Continue to inflate the cuff 20 to 30 mmHg above this point.

7. Place the stethoscope in your ears. Insert the diaphragm under the distal part of the cuff, over the brachial artery.

8. Watch the gauge. Release the screw on the handset slowly, deflating the cuff at 2 mm per second. As the pressure drops, blood begins to flow through the artery. The turbulent blood flow through the partially compressed vessel will be heard through the stethoscope. When you hear two consecutive beats, remember the pressure reading. This represents the systolic blood pressure.

9. As you continue to release pressure, you will reach a point at which the artery is no longer compressed. At this point, the sounds disappear. Remember the number. This is the diastolic pressure.

10. Fully deflate the cuff, but leave it in place for sequential readings.

11. Record your measurements immediately. The reading is recorded as systolic/diastolic, or "120/80."

12. Repeat the readings periodically to check for changes in blood pressure.

4. While palpating the radial pulse, inflate the cuff to 20 to 30 mmHg above the point where the pulse disappears.

5. Open the screw, and slowly deflate the cuff. When the radial pulse returns, observe and remember the number on the gauge. This is the systolic pressure.

6. Leave the deflated cuff in place so you can recheck the blood pressure.

7. Record the reading as "120/P by palpation."

Factors Influencing Blood Pressure

Many factors, including the patient's age and gender, influence blood pressure. Think of blood pressure as a range of values, rather than a single ideal value. Pressures within this range are called normal resting blood pressures.

Size and placement of the blood pressure cuff affects the accuracy of the reading. A cuff that is too large will lead to a false low value. An undersized cuff will cause a false high reading. Large cuffs are available for obese or muscular patients. An oversized cuff is called a thigh cuff, because it is designed for placement on the thigh of a normal-sized patient. Use a small cuff, called a pediatric cuff, for children and small adults.

When checking blood pressure, remember:

- The patient's position affects the value. Blood pressure is normally measured when the patient is seated (see Fig. 5.19). The value will be different if the patient is lying or standing. Make a note if pressure is taken in a position other than sitting.

- Blood pressure is usually, but not always, equal in both arms. A substantial difference suggests a narrowed or occluded artery in one limb. Note which arm is used for measurement.

- Anxiety is a common emotion in emergencies. This causes a release of adrenaline, increasing blood pressure.

- Exercise causes a physiologic increase in blood pressure. This is a normal process by which increased blood flow brings more oxygen to the muscles. Make a note if the patient was involved in strenuous activity just before assessing this vital sign.

- Bacterial or chemical toxins can affect blood pressure by changing the diameters of blood vessels.

Changes in blood pressure can also be caused by:

- Changes in cardiac output

- Heart disease

- Valve disease

- Ruptured aneurysm

- Significant blood loss

CD-ROM Link

The series of animations entitled, "Vital Signs–Blood Pressure," in the Vital Signs chapter and the Video Appendix on the MedEMT CD-ROM illustrates how a blood pressure cuff actually affects the blood vessels while measuring pressure.

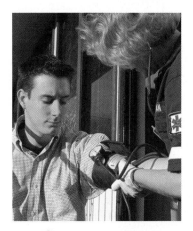

Figure 5.19 *Make sure the patient is comfortable and relaxed to ensure a proper reading. The seated position is preferred.*

CD-ROM Link

The video, "Vital Signs– Measuring Blood Pressure," in the Vital Signs chapter and the Video Appendix on the MedEMT CD-ROM demonstrates the steps in taking a patient's blood pressure.

**EMT
Tip**

A person's normal blood pressure may vary based on physical size. Medical history also influences the value. Some patients have normal blood pressures as low as 90/50. Others may have normal values that seem unusually high. If a reading appears abnormally low or high, ask the patient about his or her normal blood pressure. Ask about a history of blood pressure problems.

High Blood Pressure (Hypertension)

Hypertension has many causes. The exact cause is often unknown. Ask the patient or family about blood pressure history and current medications. Providing this information will help the emergency department staff to differentiate chronic hypertension from an acute episode.

Common causes of hypertension are:

• Vascular diseases, such as atherosclerosis, which causes narrowing of the blood vessels. Narrow vessels increase vascular resistance. The heart must work harder to move the same amount of blood through a narrow vessel.

• Kidney disease, which causes fluid retention. This increases the blood volume, leading to elevated blood pressure.

• Sodium retention, which can lead to water retention.

• Metabolic disturbances.

High blood pressure, or hypertension, can damage the vasculature. Sustained high blood pressure readings can result in:

• Blood clots

• Stroke

• Myocardial infarction, or heart attack

• Ruptured aneurysm

• Hemorrhage

Low Blood Pressure (Hypotension)

The blood flow in the vessels must be adequate to nourish the tissues with oxygen. Vital organs such as the brain, heart, and kidneys need a constant supply of oxygenated blood. Hypotension suggests a serious condition. Closely monitor blood pressure that drops rapidly. This often indicates a serious medical emergency. Look for a source of external bleeding and signs of internal bleeding.

Common causes of hypotension are:

• A decrease in circulating blood volume. This is caused by a direct loss of blood from bleeding or hemorrhage. External hemorrhage is usually visible, although the blood may be hidden by clothing. Hemorrhage may be internal and not visible upon simple inspection of the patient. In this case, the blood pressure reading may be low, or successive readings may decrease over time.

- A change in the diameter of the blood vessels. For example, in neurogenic shock, changes in neural activity cause the vessels to dilate. This expands the space normally occupied by the blood. The blood volume does not increase, causing a drop in blood pressure.

- Cardiac tamponade, a condition in which the heart muscle cannot contract or fill properly. A tamponade is generally caused by fluid build-up between the cardiac sac and the cardiac muscle tissue. This results in low systolic pressure with rising diastolic pressure.

- Head trauma or brain injury can cause increased systolic pressure with stable or falling diastolic pressure.

Common conditions in which the blood pressure can drop rapidly are:

- Shock

- Cardiac failure

- Toxins or poison in the blood

***EMT
Alert***

Reevaluate vital signs after any change in the patient's mental status or condition.

***National Registry
Examination Tip***

Review the normal vital sign values until you can cite them from memory. Pay close attention to pediatric values. You must be able to recognize normal blood pressure values or ranges for a patient's age and size. Practice quickly determining a treatment plan when blood pressure is outside the normal range.

D.O.T. OBJECTIVE

State the importance of accurately reporting and recording the baseline vital signs.

Vital Sign Reassessment

You will continue to reassess the vital signs while you are caring for the patient. Comparison of new measurements with the baseline values will alert you to changes in the patient's condition. Changes may affect how you treat the patient. A record of vital signs is used by the emergency department staff to help detect the underlying problem.

Reassess and record vital signs:

- At least every 15 minutes in a stable patient

- At least every 5 minutes in an unstable patient

- After every significant medical intervention you provide

- When requested by advanced life support personnel

D.O.T. OBJECTIVE

Identify the components of the SAMPLE history.

SAMPLE HISTORY

After measuring the baseline vital signs, you will obtain the patient's medical history (see Fig. 5.20). Knowing the history will help you to learn the cause of illness. Use the information to guide your treatment. In an emergency, you may not have time to take a full medical history. Obtaining as much relevant information as possible helps to ensure good care.

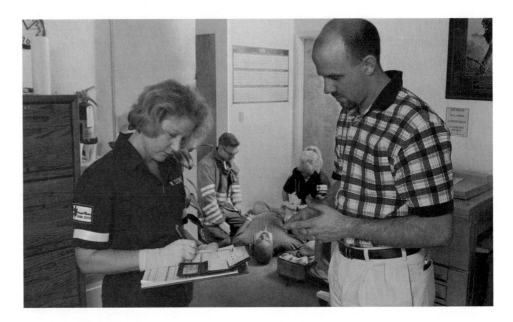

Figure 5.20 *Obtaining a patient's medical history.*

The medical history is best obtained from the patient. If he or she is unable or unwilling to provide the information, family members or bystanders may be able to provide some details. If the patient is uncooperative or combative, explain that you are an EMT who is there to help.

The **SAMPLE history** provides a brief, organized summary of the patient's relevant medical history and conditions that may affect his or her care. SAMPLE is an acronym for the information you will obtain and record:

S | Signs and symptoms

A | Allergies

M | Medications

P | Pertinent past history

L | Last oral intake

E | Events leading up to the current medical problem

SAMPLE History | *Mnemonic used to summarize a patient's relevant medical history (Signs/symptoms, Allergies, Medications, Past history, Last oral intake, Events leading to injury or illness)*

These items are described in the following sections for the general case. More specific information that relates to specific conditions will be covered throughout the book. When taking the SAMPLE history, note pertinent negative findings, or things the patient denies. A pertinent negative finding is anything you would normally expect to find, hear, or see, but do not. For example, record that a patient with abdominal pain "denies nausea and vomiting" or that a cardiac patient "denies shortness of breath or dizziness."

EMT Tip

You cannot measure anxiety objectively. You can measure signs associated with anxiety, such as rapid heart rate or breathing.

D.O.T. OBJECTIVE

Differentiate between a sign and a symptom.

Signs and Symptoms

A **sign** is an identifiable condition displayed by the patient. An observer can objectively measure signs. Examples of signs include:

- Respiratory distress or wheezing, which you can hear
- Bleeding or hemorrhage, which you can see
- Skin temperature (cold or warm), which you can feel

Sign | An observable indication of illness or injury

A **symptom** is a condition felt and described by the patient. Symptoms are subjective and cannot be measured objectively by an observer. Examples of symptoms are:

- Feeling short of breath
- Anxiety
- Nausea

Symptom | Condition described by the patient that can't be observed

---

D.O.T. OBJECTIVE

Discuss the need to search for additional medical identification.

Allergies

Patients can be allergic to many substances. Examples are:

- Medications, such as penicillin, MRI contrast fluid, or anesthetics
- Foods, such as eggs
- Environmental allergies, such as pollen, grasses, ragweed
- Toxins, such as bee venom

An allergic reaction may have caused the chief complaint. You must also consider allergies before treating the patient. Exposure to an allergen can cause anaphylactic shock. This is a serious condition. It may result in respiratory distress and cardiovascular failure. Respiratory and cardiovascular emergencies are covered in Chapters 12 and 13. Inadvertently exposing the patient to an allergen during your care creates a great risk. For example, wearing latex gloves while caring for a patient with a latex allergy will cause a severe reaction. Asking about allergies is imperative. This is particularly true if you will be administering medications. Note that some vaccines are prepared from chicken eggs, which can cause a food allergy. If the patient is unresponsive, look for a medical identification emblem, or ask family members about allergies.

Medications

Knowing what medications the patient is taking, or has taken, is valuable in assessing the potential causes of an emergency. If the patient is unresponsive, medication information may be your only link between the current chief complaint and an underlying cause. Always check for information about medications on a medical identification bracelet, tag, or necklace. Ask about current and recent use of both prescription and nonprescription medications. Questions to ask include:

- What medications are you currently taking?
- Is the medication prescribed for you?
- Why are you taking it?
- How long have you been taking it?
- Have you taken any other medications in the past few weeks or months?
- What time did you take the last dose?

Carefully examine medication containers. The label will show the date that the prescription was filled, the amount to take, and the directions for taking the medication. By evaluating this information, you will learn if the patient is taking the medication correctly. If the patient has taken the medication for a long time, he or she probably has a chronic, or recurring, medical problem. New medications may be ordered because of changes in the patient's condition, or for the current illness. Some medications may be given for more than one disease. For example, Lasix® is a common drug used for several conditions. Ask the patient, "Why are you taking Lasix?" or, "Are you on Lasix for your blood pressure, or is there another medical reason?" Be sure to ask about other medications. The patient may fail to mention birth control pills and over-the-counter drugs, such as cold medications, aspirin, or allergy medications.

Street Drug and Alcohol Use

If appropriate, ask the patient about illicit drug or alcohol use. Explain that you are an EMT, not the police. Inform him or her that knowing about any drug and alcohol use is important to the care you provide. Obtaining a history of drug or alcohol use can be important when determining the patient's ability to consent or refuse medical care.

Pertinent Past Medical History

Ask the patient about past medical conditions, surgical conditions, and trauma. For example:

- "Do you have a heart condition, thyroid problem, diabetes, or other past or ongoing medical conditions?"
- "Have you ever had surgery or an injury that could be related to this incident?"
- "Are you currently under a doctor's care?"

Look for a medical identification tag during your assessment. Finding a medical identification emblem can provide vital patient information. One type of tag or medallion is the MedicAlert® medical identification emblem★ (see Fig. 5.21). MedicAlert® Foundation has a toll-free number, (800) 633-4260, through which you can obtain the patient's basic medical record, allergies, and medications.

In some parts of the country, patients also maintain valuable medical information in a Vial of Life. Usually, the Vial of Life emblem is found on the door of the refrigerator. This location keeps the vial protected against fire. Some patients now keep emergency medical information on a plastic credit card. Check with your local EMS agency to determine what types of identification are common in your area.

Last Oral Intake (Solid or Liquid)

A history of food and fluid ingestion is important in some conditions. Ask the patient when he or she last ate solid food. When was the last time he or she had any liquids? How much did the patient ingest? What was it? Did the patient vomit?

Events Leading to Injury or Illness

A good open-ended question for this category is, "Tell me what happened." Also, ask:

- "Has this ever happened before?"
- "Are you taking any medications that could cause this?"
- "What makes your condition worse?"
- "Is there anything that helps to relieve the pain (or other symptom)?"
- "What is the last thing you remember?"

If the patient has a chronic condition, ask:

- "This has been going on for a while, but what made you call today? Did it become worse? Did something change? Was there a new symptom?"

For a patient with chest pain, ask:

- "Is the chest pain worse with exertion? Is it still present when you rest?"

★ MedicAlert® is a federally registered trademark and service mark.

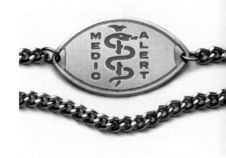

Figure 5.21 *MedicAlert® Medical Identification Bracelet.*

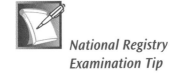

National Registry Examination Tip

Be sure to look for a medical identification tag during your assessment of any patient.

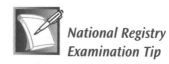

OPQRST History

OPQRST is a mnemonic used to evaluate signs and symptoms of the patient's chief complaint. This is especially true when patients complain of any type of pain. Taking an OPQRST history will help you to understand the patient's signs and symptoms:

O | Onset. "When did the problem start? Do you know what caused the problem?"

P | Provocation. "What caused the symptoms? What makes them worse? What makes them better?"

Q | Quality. "Describe the problem. What does it feel like?" (Sharp or dull pain, burning, tearing?)

R | Radiation. "Is the sign or symptom isolated or generalized? Where is the pain? Where does it go?"

S | Severity. "On a scale of one to ten, with one being the least, and ten being the worst pain/discomfort/difficulty, how severe is it?"

T | Time. "How long have you had the problem? How long does it last?"

Your ability to accurately assess a patient's medical history and gather vital signs is essential to good patient care. The mnemonic SAMPLE provides a simple mechanism for obtaining an overview of the current illness and past medical history. Use OPQRST questions to further evaluate a patient's chief complaint. Always ask questions that the patient can understand. Sometimes, you may ask the same question three different ways, getting three different answers from the patient. All may be correct. Questioning patients is an art. Practice so that you obtain a clear picture of the patient's history.

Obtaining vital signs and history information is the first step in your thorough assessment of the patient's condition. Patient assessment procedures are discussed in more detail in Chapters 8 and 9.

Chapter Five Summary

- Obtaining baseline vital signs and a SAMPLE history is an important part of the assessment process you will learn in Chapters 8 and 9.

- Vital signs include general information and evaluation and measurement of the patient's breathing, pulse, skin, pupils, and blood pressure.

- Obtain the chief complaint, age, and gender of every patient.

- Determine the respiratory rate, and evaluate quality as normal, shallow, labored, or noisy.

- Check for peripheral pulses (radial in adults, brachial for patients less than one year old). If you cannot find a peripheral pulse, check for a carotid pulse. Count the pulse rate and evaluate the pulse as strong or weak, regular or irregular.

- Evaluate the skin color in the nail beds, oral mucosa, and conjunctiva. Characterize the skin color as pale, cyanotic, flushed, or jaundiced. Evaluate the skin temperature as normal, hot, cool, or cold. Also note whether the skin is wet, moist, or dry.

- Assess the pupils by briefly shining a light into the patient's eyes. Determine pupil size and reactivity. Note whether pupils are equal in size; whether they react equally to light; and whether they are dilated, constricted, or normal.

- Obtain a blood pressure reading by auscultation. If you cannot hear the blood flow, use the palpation method.

- Obtain the SAMPLE History:

Signs /symptoms

Allergies

Medications

Past medical history

Last oral intake

Events leading to the injury or illness

Key Terms Review

Auscultation | *page 161*
Brachial Pulse | *page 151*
Bradycardia | *page 153*
Chief Complaint | *page 146*
Conjunctiva | *page 154*
Cyanosis | *page 154*
Diastolic Pressure | *page 159*
Expiration | *page 148*
Femoral Pulse | *page 151*

Hypertension | *page 164*
Inspiration | *page 148*
Jaundice | *page 155*
Lens | *page 157*
Oral Mucosa | *page 154*
Palpation | *page 161*
Pulse | *page 150*
Pupil | *page 157*
Radial Pulse | *page 151*
Respiration | *page 148*

SAMPLE History | *page 166*
Sclera | *page 155*
Sign | *page 167*
Sphygmomanometer | *page 159*
Stridor | *page 149*
Symptom | *page 167*
Systolic Pressure | *page 159*
Tachycardia | *page 153*
Vital Signs | *page 147*

Review Questions

1. The SAMPLE history provides information essential for _____.

   a. Assisting the receiving facility in continuing care
   b. Training new EMT-Bs in CPR
   c. Taking a pulse measurement
   d. Verifying that an EMT-B is fit for certification

2. When assessing respiration, the EMT should look for _____.

   a. Rate and moisture
   b. Rate and quality
   c. Rate and rhythm
   d. Quality and strength

3. The normal respiration rate for an adult is _____ breaths per minute.

   a. 12 to 20
   b. 15 to 25
   c. 20 to 25
   d. 25 to 30

4. An adult's central pulse may be assessed at:

   a. The carotid artery
   b. The apex of the heart (apical pulse)
   c. The brachial artery
   d. The dorsalis pedis artery

5. The normal pulse rate for an adult is _____ beats per minute.

   a. 40 to 60
   b. 60 to 100
   c. 80 to 100
   d. 100 to 120

6. A normal relative skin temperature should feel _____ against the back of your hand.

   a. Cold
   b. Cool
   c. Warm
   d. Hot

7. The standard patient position when measuring blood pressure is _____.

   a. Standing
   b. Sitting
   c. Lying flat
   d. It does not matter

8. The measurement of blood pressure by palpation:

   a. Is used for a diastolic blood pressure reading
   b. Is taken without the use of a stethoscope
   c. Is useful only in the hospital setting
   d. Is complicated by excessive noise

9. When measuring blood pressure in an adult, the stethoscope is commonly placed:

   a. Over the brachial artery
   b. Over the radial artery
   c. Over the carotid artery
   d. Over the coronary artery

10. In which of the following cases would the EMT-B measure blood pressure by palpation alone?

    a. When the patient is violent
    b. When the patient is unconscious
    c. In cases of suspected spinal injury
    d. When there is excessive ambient noise

11. Knowledge of a patient's history of illness and injury _____.

    a. Is useful to doctors and paramedics only
    b. Is often the key to correct assessment and treatment
    c. Rarely affects the EMT's decisions for treatment
    d. Is a violation of the patient's privacy

12. The "M" in SAMPLE refers to:

    a. Medical identification tag
    b. Moving the patient
    c. Medications
    d. Multiple injuries

13. An uncontrolled hemorrhage will eventually cause the blood pressure to _____.

    a. Increase
    b. Decrease
    c. Remain the same
    d. Hemorrhage has no effect on blood pressure

14. Blood pressure should be measured in all patients who are more than _____ years of age.

    a. 6
    b. 4
    c. 3
    d. 1

15. The pedal pulse gives circulation information about the _____.

    a. Upper extremities
    b. Skull
    c. Torso
    d. Lower extremities

16. Yellow skin may suggest:

    a. Hepatitis
    b. Carbon monoxide poisoning
    c. Lack of oxygen
    d. Exposure to cold

17. Red skin may suggest the presence of _____.

    a. Excess blood
    b. Carbon monoxide
    c. Excess oxygen
    d. Lack of oxygen

18. _____ vital signs are first measurements that serve as a point of comparison for subsequent vital sign readings in order to detect changes in the patient's condition over time.

    a. Advanced
    b. Beginning
    c. Baseline
    d. Primary

19. When measuring the "pupil" vital sign, what else is measured in addition to pupil size?

    a. Level
    b. Color
    c. Width
    d. Reactivity

20. A single breath consists of one full cycle of inspiration and _____.

    a. Ventilation
    b. Inhalation
    c. Expiration
    d. Respiration

21. The two methods of measuring blood pressure are palpation and _____.

    a. Acquisition
    b. Percussion
    c. Auscultation
    d. Orientation

22. The _____ history provides a brief, organized summary of the patient's relevant medical history and conditions that may affect his or her care.

    a. INITIAL
    b. ONGOING
    c. PERTINENT
    d. SAMPLE

CASE STUDIES

Vital Signs and SAMPLE History

1 The local coal plant is burning a new coal fuel. Residents of a nearby mobile home park have been calling EMS frequently. You have had several calls from residents complaining of shortness of breath in the past week. You are dispatched to the mobile home park again today. When you arrive on scene of another shortness of breath call, you see the elderly female patient sitting on her porch. She is using her neck muscles to breathe and appears exhausted. Her lips are slightly blue, and she is smoking a cigarette. She can only speak in four to five word sentences.

A. Given this information, how would you categorize this patient's breathing?

B. What signs and symptoms will you look for to confirm your findings?

2 Your EMS pager sounds. You recognize the address of the call. The older man living on the farm retired a few years ago due to failing health. When you arrive, family members tell you they found the patient lying in the bathroom, unable to communicate. You find him wedged between the shower and the toilet. He is breathing but cannot speak. The right side of his face is drooping. You cannot find a palpable pulse in his upper extremities.

A. What other location(s) will you use to check for a pulse?

B. What is the normal pulse value and quality in an elderly patient?

C. What complications will you suspect if the patient's pulse rhythm is irregular?

3 Your search and rescue crew has been looking for a young boy for more than three hours. With the snowfall last night and freezing temperatures, you need to find this boy quickly. Your partner calls you over to a small tool shed almost covered by bushes. He has found the small boy lying curled up next to his dog. His clothing is insufficient for the weather conditions. He is lethargic and very slow to respond.

A. How will you assess this patient's skin when obtaining vital signs?

B. If the patient has dark skin, how will your skin assessment change?

C. What conditions cause the skin to feel cool to the touch?

4 The shift has been slow. You have just about run out of material to study and review. You are dispatched to the kidney dialysis center. While you are en route, dispatch updates the call information and advises your crew that the patient weighs more than 250 kilograms (500 pounds). You know that you cannot measure the patient's blood pressure using a regular cuff.

A. How will you measure this patient's blood pressure?

B. What other assessment information can you use to evaluate the patient's blood pressure or perfusion status?

Stories from the Field
Wrap-Up

O btaining vital signs is an important part of basic emergency medical care. A set of vital signs provides useful information. Unfortunately, taking one set may not provide a true indication of the patient's condition. Changes that occur over successive sets of vital signs are important, and can help you to detect hidden injuries. Taking vital signs periodically will also help you to detect subtle changes in the patient's condition. Always take at least two sets of vital signs on every patient, regardless of the chief complaint. More than two sets of vital signs will be indicated in some patients.

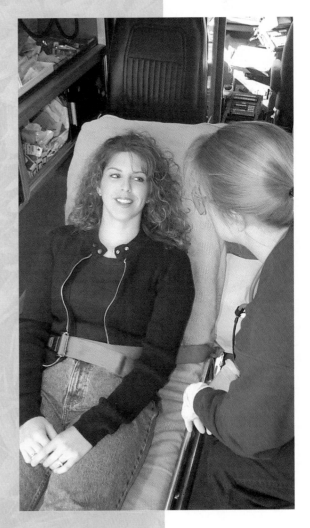

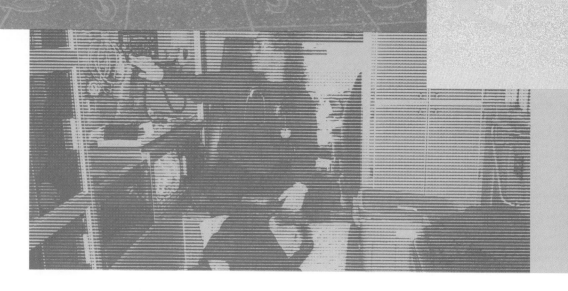

Chapter 6

Lifting and Moving Patients

Stories from the Field

You and your partners, Carmen and Robin, are dispatched to a small apartment complex. The call is for a woman who is in respiratory distress. The entryway that leads to the patient's apartment is very narrow and you have to hold your gurney on end to make it fit through. Inside is a 56-year-old woman who weighs more than 250 pounds. She is in severe respiratory distress and is unable to speak. Her sister tells you that she is having one of her asthma attacks and needs to be seen by a doctor.

After Carmen and Robin place the patient on oxygen and obtain a SAMPLE history, you attempt to move the patient to a wheeled stretcher for transport. You soon realize that she is too large for you to maneuver the stretcher through the doorway and hall. The patient is unable to lie flat and her breathing difficulty is growing worse. The fire department has not arrived yet and Carmen and Robin ask you to help formulate a plan.

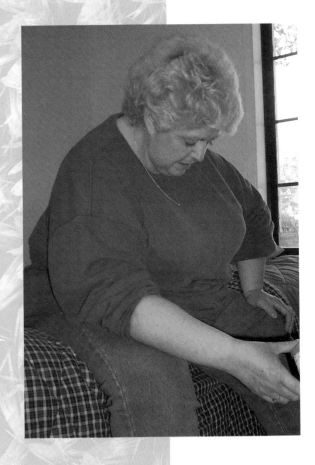

**CD-ROM
Link**

The videos in the series "Lifting and Moving" in the Lifting and Moving chapter and the Video Appendix on the MedEMT CD-ROM demonstrate the elements of lifting and moving techniques that will reduce back injury.

Safely moving patients from the scene to the hospital is what EMTs do on all calls. It is at the very core of what you are called upon to do in EMS. Proper lifting and moving techniques are an extension of the EMT's responsibility for scene safety. As we have learned, scene safety extends to both the safety of the patient and to the EMT.

Back injuries are one of the most common injuries suffered by healthcare workers. Many EMS workers injure their backs on the job each year. In some cases, the injuries result in long-term disability and premature retirement. Back injuries are the leading cause of worker's compensation insurance claims in the emergency medical services field. Most back injuries are caused by lifting and moving patients improperly. The most common causes of back injuries in EMS workers are:

- Poor posture
- Being in poor physical condition
- Using improper body mechanics
- Lifting and moving patients and heavy objects incorrectly
- Doing jobs that require high energy
- Lifting and moving patients from confined spaces, such as cars, bathrooms, or cluttered areas

Back injuries are painful, and may cause permanent disability. Caring for your back is important. Prevention is the key to reducing your risk of back injury. You will learn good body mechanics and proper lifting and moving techniques during your initial training (see Fig. 6.1). Consistently using these techniques will protect your back and help to lengthen your EMS career.

Figure 6.1 *Proper lifting techniques must be practiced to avoid injury.*

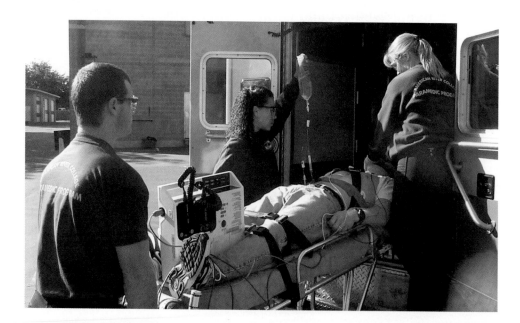

BODY MECHANICS

Body mechanics are principles and applications for lifting and moving. They describe ways of using your body correctly to prevent injury. This chapter focuses on safe and efficient methods of using your body while lifting and moving (see Fig. 6.2). Following these guidelines will protect you, your partner, and your patients from injury. Apply these principles and techniques during every call.

There are three key elements of body mechanics. Applying these techniques when lifting and moving patients or heavy objects will reduce your risk of serious back injury:

- Use the large muscles of your legs, hips, and buttocks when lifting. Contract your abdominal muscles. Avoid using your back muscles, which are small, weak, and easily injured.
- Stand in good body alignment with your back straight. Your head and shoulders should be centered above the hips. The hips should be centered over your feet. Never twist when lifting. Maintain a wide base of support by keeping your feet at least 12 inches apart.
- Keep the weight of the object you are lifting as close to your body as possible.

Body Mechanics | Moving your body correctly while lifting and moving to prevent injury

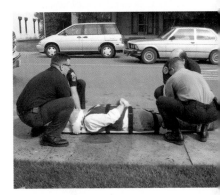

Figure 6.2 *Maintain good body alignment when lifting.*

D.O.T. OBJECTIVE

Discuss the guidelines and safety precautions that need to be followed when lifting a patient.

Lifting Techniques

Some general safety guidelines should be observed when lifting:

- Consider the size and weight of the patient. Determine whether you will need extra help to safely accomplish the lift.
- Know your own physical abilities and limitations and those of your coworkers.
- Communicate clearly and frequently with your partners when lifting (see Fig. 6.3).
- Position your feet properly and safely, approximately 12 inches apart.

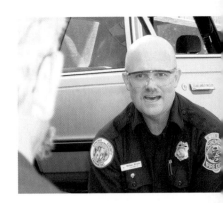

Figure 6.3 *Communicate with your partner throughout the lift.*

• Assess the ground for obstructions, slippery conditions, or other potential hazards.

• Keep yourself in good physical condition.

Many healthcare workers wear back support belts when on duty. Most feel better when wearing the belt during lifting. Your physician or physical therapist may recommend that you use one, or this may be a policy of your employer. Back support belts are controversial. Studies have shown that workers wearing support belts have fewer back injuries. Other studies have shown no difference in the rate of injuries. However, wearing the belt reminds you to keep your back straight and to use good body mechanics. Because using improper body mechanics when wearing the belt is difficult, the belt is beneficial. You are less likely to become injured if you are using good body mechanics.

Some workers believe that wearing the support belt enables them to lift heavier loads. This is not true. Believing the belt protects you increases your risk of injury if you lift more weight than you would without a belt. At the time of this writing, there is no proof that wearing a back support increases the amount of weight that you can lift or carry.

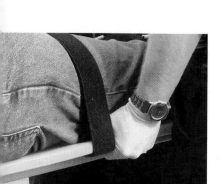

Figure 6.4 *Proper gripping technique.*

Power Grip | *Gripping items with palms and fingers in complete contact with the object; fingers bent at the same angle and hands 10 inches apart*

Power Grip

Your hands are the only part of your body in contact with the object you are lifting. A strong, secure grip is important to prevent injury. Using the **power grip** gives you a strength advantage (see Fig. 6.4). Always use this grip when lifting and moving. Proper hand position for the power grip is:

• Palms and fingers in complete contact with the object

• All fingers bent at the same angle

• Hands 10 inches apart

Power Lift | *A specialized lifting and moving technique that uses the large muscles of the legs to lift and carry the weight*

Power Lift

Using the **power lift** or squat lift position prevents injury (see Procedure 6.1). When using this position, your back remains stable in its normal curvature. The power lift is the best position to use for lifting. This technique is particularly helpful for individuals with weak knees or thighs.

Procedure 6.1 • POWER LIFT

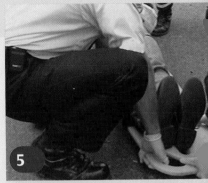

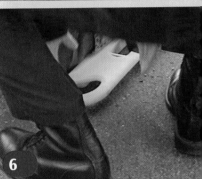

1. Keep your feet flat on the floor, comfortably spaced, and turned slightly outward.

2. Tighten your back and abdominal muscles, which locks your back into a slight inward curvature.

3. Straddle the object to be lifted, if possible.

4. Bend at the knees to assume a squatting position. Flex your hips, keeping your waist straight.

5. Grasp the object, using the power grip.

6. Distribute your weight on the balls of your feet or just behind them.

7. Lift as you stand up, raising your upper body before your hips. Keep your back locked in position.

8. Hold the weight you are lifting as close to your body as possible.

9. When lowering the object, reverse the steps of the power lift. Keep your back locked, and avoid bending or twisting at the waist.

D.O.T. OBJECTIVES

Describe the safe lifting of cots and stretchers.

Discuss the guidelines and safety precautions for carrying patients and/or equipment.

 EMT Tip

When lifting or moving a patient, always explain what you are going to do and what you expect of the patient. Clarifying expectations and crew roles before a lift will avoid painful mishaps.

Lifting Cots and Stretchers

Always use good body mechanics and observe proper lifting techniques when lifting cots, stretchers, spine boards, or other transport equipment. In particular:

• All equipment has weight limitations. Know or approximate the weight to be lifted. Never exceed the limitations of the equipment. Plan a safe alternative method for moving patients who exceed the limitations.

- Never lift patients or heavy objects by yourself. At least two people are needed for a lift. An even number of people should stand on each side to balance the lifting device. During the move, all personnel should move smoothly and in unison.

- Use the power grip and power lift for strength and safety.

Carrying Techniques

Avoid carrying patients except when absolutely necessary. Instead, use wheeled transport devices, such as a stretcher or stair chair. Carrying the stretcher over small obstacles and rough terrain may be necessary occasionally. The precautions for safely carrying a stretcher are the same as for safe lifting, with some additional considerations:

- Estimate the weight to be carried, and know your crew's limitations

- Coordinate the move and communicate with your partners

- It is best to work with people whose height and strength is similar to yours

- Use proper lifting techniques

- Keep the weight close to your body when carrying stretchers and equipment

- Tighten your abdomen, lock your back, and avoid twisting

- If you must bend, use your hips and knees, not your waist

- Avoid **hyperextension** of your spine caused by leaning back from the waist

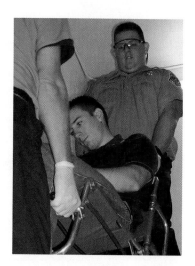

Figure 6.5 *Whenever possible, use a stair chair to transport a patient down a flight of stairs.*

Hyperextension | *Extension of a joint beyond its normal limit during movement*

> **D.O.T. OBJECTIVE**
>
> Discuss one-handed carrying techniques.

One-Handed Carrying

Although not generally preferred, occasionally you may have to carry a transport device with one hand. If this is necessary, make certain that you keep your back locked when lifting and carrying. Avoid the tendency to lean to one side to compensate for the unbalanced weight.

> **D.O.T. OBJECTIVE**
>
> Describe correct and safe carrying procedures on stairs.

Stair Chair | *Specialized device used for transportation of patients down stairs or through narrow spaces; may have wheels*

Stairs

Whenever possible and medically appropriate, use a **stair chair** for carrying patients on stairs (see Fig. 6.5). This device is preferred to a stretcher. Follow all lifting precautions, and use good body mechanics. Lock your back, bend your knees, and flex your hips. Always avoid bending at the waist. Keep the weight and your arms as close to your body as possible. Ask another person to stand at your back and serve as a spotter when moving down stairs (see Fig. 6.6). The spotter should steady your back and tell you the number of steps and any other hazards.

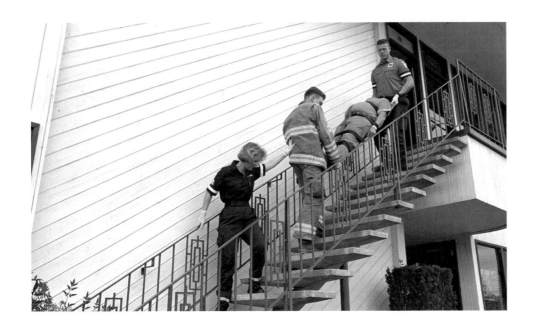

Figure 6.6 A spotter should be used whenever moving down stairs.

National Registry Examination Tip

Review proper lifting techniques and safety considerations. Be able to recognize signs and symptoms of back injuries associated with lifting.

D.O.T. OBJECTIVES

State the guidelines for reaching and their application.

Describe correct reaching for log rolls.

Reaching Techniques

Reaching for patients and objects increases the risk of injury. Guidelines for injury-free reaching are:

- Keep the muscles in your back locked in the correct position.
- Avoid twisting.
- Avoid reaching more than 15 to 20 inches in front of your body (see Fig. 6.7).
- Avoid reaching overhead or other positions that require bending backward.
- Avoid standing in positions that require strenuous reaching for longer than one minute.

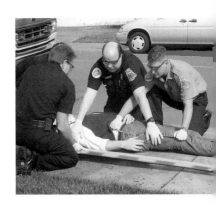

Figure 6.7 Proper reaching technique when log rolling a patient.

- You must reach over patients during the log roll procedure (described in Chapter 22). Keep your back straight (see Fig. 6.8). Use your shoulder muscles. Lean from the hips.

D.O.T. OBJECTIVE

State the guidelines for pushing and pulling.

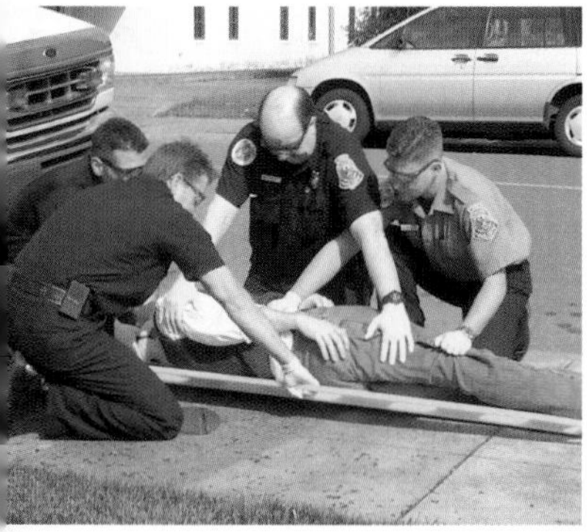

Figure 6.8 *Remember to keep your back locked when lowering the patient.*

Pushing and Pulling Techniques

Sometimes you have to decide whether to push or pull a piece of equipment or other heavy object. Pushing a heavy object is safer for your back than pulling it, as long as you follow these guidelines:

- Keep your back locked in a straight position. Bend your elbows, keeping your arms close to your sides.
- Bend your knees to keep the pull line through the center of your body. Keep the weight close to your body.
- Push by using the muscles between your waist and shoulders.
- If the weight is below your waist, work from a kneeling position.
- Avoid pushing or pulling items above your head.

D.O.T. OBJECTIVE

Discuss the general considerations of moving patients.

Emergency Moves | *Specific extrication or lifting and moving techniques used when immediate danger threatens the EMT or the patient*

Urgent Moves | *Techniques for moving a patient whose condition is life-threatening; cervical spine procedures are taken*

Non-Urgent (Routine) Moves | *Lifting and moving patients when there is no immediate threat to life*

MOVING PATIENTS

In an emergency, you must decide how quickly to move the patient. You will make your decision based on your assessment of scene safety and the patient's medical condition. Patient moves are classified into three categories:

- **Emergency moves**, in which the patient must be moved immediately
- **Urgent moves**, in which the patient should be moved quickly
- **Non-urgent** or **routine moves**, in which the patient can be moved whenever ready for transport

Avoid moving patients with suspected spinal cord injuries until the spine is fully immobilized. Aggravating a spinal cord injury is one of the greatest threats to a patient requiring an emergency move. In Chapter 22, techniques for specific immobilization procedures are fully described. If you believe that your life or the patient's life is in imminent danger, an emergency move is necessary. During an emergency move, it is difficult to manually stabilize the spine while you are extricating or moving the patient. Quickly and properly place an interim immobilization device before the move, if possible. If you can't place one, maintain as much spinal immobilization as you can under the circumstances. Provide spinal immobilization before an urgent move. Rule out the possibility of spinal cord injuries before performing non-urgent moves.

Whenever possible, move the patient into alignment with the long axis of his or her body. This measure limits the risk of further injury to the spine. Keep the long axis movement in mind when quickly removing a patient from a vehicle. Minimize side-to-side movements of the spine.

D.O.T. OBJECTIVE

State three situations that may require the use of an emergency move.

Emergency Moves

Move a patient immediately only when your crew or the patient are in immediate danger. Emergency moves may be necessary if:

- Fire, or the danger of fire, is present.

- Explosives or other hazardous materials are at the scene.

- You cannot protect the patient from life-threatening hazards at the scene (e.g., imminent building collapse, threatening or violent situations, or dangerous flood conditions).

- The patient is blocking access to other patients who require lifesaving care.

- The patient's position prohibits lifesaving emergency care. For example, a patient who is upside down in a car, wedged between a toilet and wall, or suffering cardiac arrest while lying in bed.

This list does not and cannot cover all cases that may require emergency moves. You must apply the principles you learn here to quickly decide if an emergency move is appropriate.

When you must quickly move a patient who is on the floor or ground, use one of the following methods to drag him or her to safety. Remember to stabilize the spine as much as possible and move the patient along the long axis of the body.

Clothing drag. Pull on the patient's clothing in the neck and shoulder area. Keep the patient's head between your forearms if possible.

Armpit-forearm drag. From the back, place your arms under the patient's armpits and grasp the forearms. Grasp the left forearm with your right hand. Use your left hand to grasp the right forearm (see Figs. 6.9 and 6.10).

Figure 6.9 *Grasp the patient's forearms from behind (left). Align your back as you rise to your feet (right).*

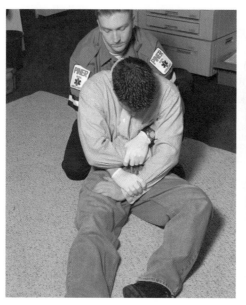 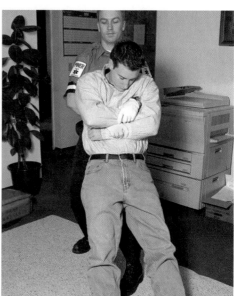

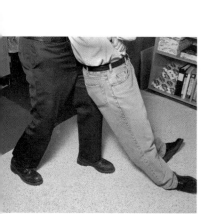

Figure 6.10 *Reduce the strain of the armpit-forearm drag by placing one leg against the patient's lower back for support.*

Foot drag. Drag the patient by the ankles. Avoid impacting the patient's head with the ground.

Blanket drag. Carefully roll the patient onto a blanket, time permitting. Drag the blanket (see Fig. 6.11).

Figure 6.11 *Blanket drag. Try an alternate carry if the terrain is rocky.*

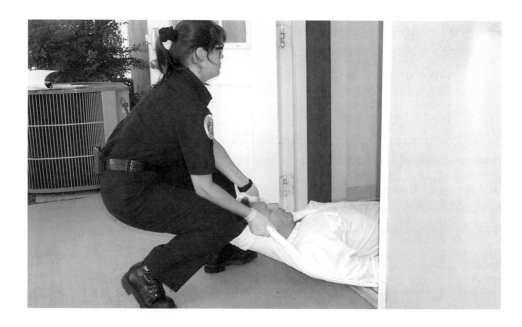

One-rescuer assist. Drape the patient's arm around your neck, grasping it with your hand. Slide your other hand around the waist for further support (see Fig. 6.12).

Two-rescuer assist. If two EMTs are available, place one of the patient's arms around each EMT's shoulder. The EMTs grip the patient's hands and place their free arms behind the patient's back, holding the waist (see Fig. 6.13).

Urgent Moves

Urgent moves are reserved for patients with critical injuries or illnesses. Move the patient quickly if you believe his or her medical condition presents an immediate threat to life. Situations in which urgent moves are necessary include:

- Airway compromise
- Inadequate breathing
- Major bleeding
- Shock (hypoperfusion)
- Altered level of consciousness

You will take cervical spine precautions, even if minimal, before moving the patient. In this type of move, applying a short spine board or extrication vest could result in dangerous delays.

Rapid Extrication

Rapid extrication is a specific technique used for patients who must be urgently removed from a vehicle. EMS systems use several versions of rapid extrication. Know and follow your local protocols.

Ensuring that the patient's spine is not compromised is a key to rapid extrication. One EMT must always maintain control of the patient's cervical spine. Do not let go until someone else's hands take over. Move the patient using short, well-coordinated moves. Communicate and coordinate your actions with other rescuers for safety. Coordinating each step reduces the risk of additional injury to the patient and the response team. Rapid extrication is a three- or four-person procedure that is described in Procedure 6.2.

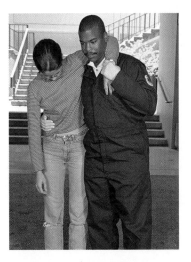

Figure 6.12 *Be careful not to injure yourself when performing a one-rescuer assist.*

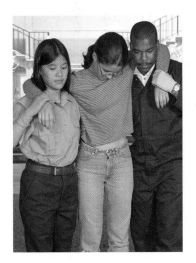

Figure 6.13 *Communicate with your partner and the patient about any obstacles during a two-rescuer assist.*

Rapid Extrication | *Specialized techniques for quickly removing a patient from a vehicle without compromising the cervical spine*

Procedure 6.2 • **RAPID EXTRICATION FROM THE DRIVER'S SEAT**

1. EMT #1 positions herself behind the patient in the vehicle. She brings the head into a neutral in-line position, supporting the head and manually immobilizing the neck.

2. EMT #2 applies a cervical immobilization device to the patient. He then assumes control of the thorax.

3. EMT #3 places a long spine board near the car door.

4. EMT #3, or a fourth EMT, moves to the passenger seat and frees the patient's legs.

5. EMT #2 uses clear and concise communication to direct the next step. Rotate the patient as a unit. Stop when EMT #1 (holding the head) encounters the "B" post between the vehicle doors.

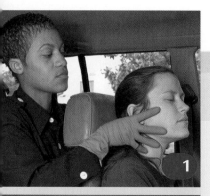

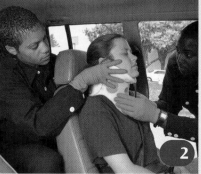

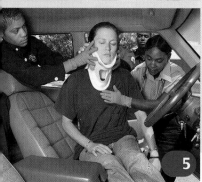

Non-Urgent Moves

After assessing the patient and environment, if you decide that there is no immediate threat to life, move the patient when your team is ready. You will complete your assessment and provide necessary treatment before preparing the patient and ambulance for transport. In this situation, you will use a non-urgent technique. The patient is moved from the place where he or she was evaluated onto a carrying device. In a non-urgent situation, avoid moving patients with suspected spinal injuries until the spine is fully immobilized. Techniques used for moving patients without spinal injuries include the direct ground lift, extremity lift, direct carry, and draw sheet methods.

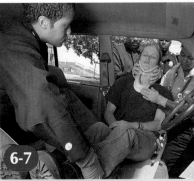

6-7

6. EMT #3 moves the patient's legs onto the seat. He moves to the driver's side of the vehicle and, from outside, assumes responsibility for cervical spine immobilization from EMT #1.

7. EMT #2 continues to support the thorax. EMT #1 moves to control the patient's pelvis and lower extremities. At this point, the patient's back is in the open doorway, feet are on the seat, and all the EMTs have full control of the patient's body.

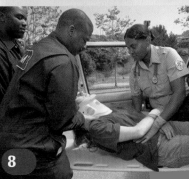

8

8. The fourth EMT places one end of the backboard on the driver's seat, next to the patient's buttocks, using the car seat to support the board. If necessary, ask bystanders to support the sides of the board until the patient is fully moved.

9. On a signal from EMT #3, all EMTs gently slide the patient onto the long spine board. Two moves may be necessary to get the patient to the head of the board. Move the patient completely onto the board, then immediately immobilize the head and neck.

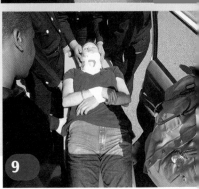

9

Moving a Patient from the Ground

Use the direct ground lift or extremity lift for moving a supine patient from the floor or ground onto a stretcher. The direct ground lift is a two- or three-person technique used when no spinal injury is suspected (see Procedure 6.3). Use the two-rescuer extremity lift only after you have ruled out injuries to the spine and the extremities (see Procedure 6.4).

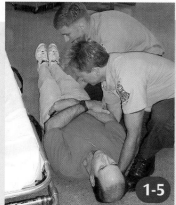

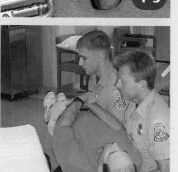

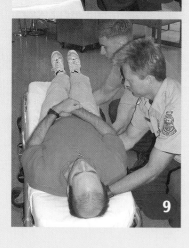

Procedure 6.3 • DIRECT GROUND LIFT

Back Safety

1. Position the stretcher as close to the patient as possible. Lower it to the lowest possible position. Secure the wheels so they will not roll.

2. Two or three EMTs position themselves on one side of the patient, each facing the patient, with one knee on the ground.

3. Cross the patient's arms over the chest or abdomen, if possible.

4. EMT #1, who is closest to the head, slides an arm under the neck and grasps the patient's opposite shoulder. This supports the head and neck during the move. Position the free arm under the lower back.

5. EMT #2 slides one arm under the patient's back above the buttocks. Place the other arm under the patient's knees.

6. EMT #3, if present, kneels between EMTs #1 and #2, with both arms under the patient's waist. The other rescuers reposition their arms further up or down the back, as appropriate.

7. On a signal from EMT #1, all EMTs roll backward, using their leg force to lift the patient onto their braced knees. All EMTs pull the patient close to their chests.

8. On a second signal from EMT #1, all EMTs stand in unison and carry the patient to the stretcher.

9. On a third signal from EMT #1, all EMTs drop to one knee and gently roll the patient onto the stretcher.

Procedure 6.4 • EXTREMITY LIFT

Back Safety

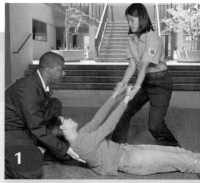

1. Two EMTs gently raise the patient to a sitting position.

2. The two EMTs kneel beside the patient, one at the head and the other next to the knees. EMT #1, at the head, slips his arms under the patient's shoulders and arms. He grasps the left forearm with his right hand. His left hand grasps the right forearm.

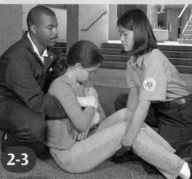

3. EMT #2 slips her arms under the patient's knees.

4. On signal from EMT #1, both EMTs rise to a squatting position. On a second signal from EMT #1, both EMTs stand up simultaneously.

5. EMT #2 changes arm positions, allowing her to turn around and walk forward. Both EMTs carry the patient to the stretcher.

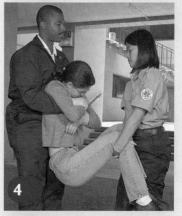

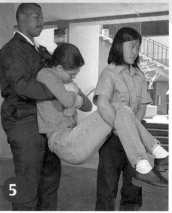

Moving a Patient from a Bed

Two techniques are commonly used for moving a supine patient between a bed and a stretcher. These are the direct carry and the draw sheet method. At least two EMTs are needed to perform these procedures. Neither method is appropriate for a patient with spinal injury. In a direct carry (see Procedure 6.5), the EMTs lift the patient directly. For the draw sheet method (see Procedure 6.6), the bottom sheet is used as a tool for moving the patient.

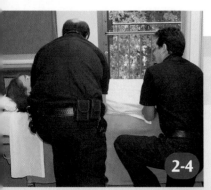

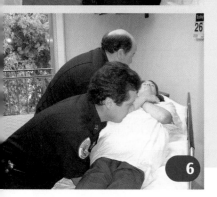

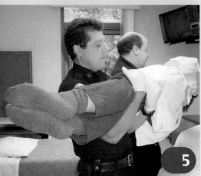

Procedure 6.5 • DIRECT CARRY

Back Safety

1. Position and prepare the stretcher by adjusting the height to equal the height of the bed. Lower the rails, and unfasten the straps. Place the stretcher perpendicular to the bed, with the head of the stretcher at the foot of the bed.

2. The EMTs stand between the bed and stretcher, facing the patient. EMT #1, at the head, slides his arm under the patient's neck. The other hand cups the patient's opposite shoulder.

3. EMT #2 places his hand under the patient's hip, lifting slightly.

4. EMT #1 slides his free arm under the patient's back, while EMT #2 supports the hips and lower legs.

5. On signal, both EMTs slide the patient to the edge of the bed. Using a movement similar to a weight-lifting curl, they lift the patient, curling him or her to their chests.

6. Holding the patient securely, the EMTs rotate simultaneously. They gently place the patient on the stretcher.

Procedure 6.6 • DRAW SHEET METHOD

1. Loosen the bottom sheet of the bed. Roll the sheet inward from both sides, toward the patient, until it is next to the patient's body.

2. Prepare the stretcher. Adjust the height, lower the rails, and unbuckle the straps.

3. Hold the stretcher securely against the side of the bed with your body.

4. Carefully reach across the stretcher and firmly grasp the sheet. Hold the sheet taut with an underhand grasp. Position your hands at the patient's head, chest, hip, and knees.

5. On a signal, gently slide the patient onto the stretcher.

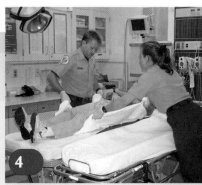

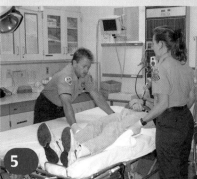

PATIENT TRANSPORT EQUIPMENT

Various types of stretchers, cots, and boards are used for moving patients into the ambulance, in preparation for transport. You must select the right equipment for the scene and the patient's condition. The procedures for using, inspecting, cleaning, maintaining, and repairing the equipment are different for each model. Follow local protocol and the manufacturer's directions.

Always use proper lifting techniques when loading a patient into the ambulance. If your agency uses hanging stretchers (a stretcher that is hung from the ceiling of the ambulance above a cot), these should be loaded before a wheeled stretcher. Before moving the ambulance, make sure that each cot and stretcher is secured and locked in place.

Any patient with a suspected spinal injury must be immobilized using proper equipment and techniques before being moved. Immobilization is described more fully in Chapter 22.

EMT Tip

Be sure to use good body mechanics even while practicing moving.

National Registry Examination Tip

Review the indications and steps for completing all of the emergency moves.

Wheeled Stretchers

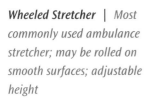

Wheeled Stretcher | Most commonly used ambulance stretcher; may be rolled on smooth surfaces; adjustable height

The most common device for moving and transporting patients is the **wheeled stretcher** (see Fig. 6.14). It can be rolled on smooth surfaces. One EMT guides the stretcher from the head, while another pulls from the foot of the stretcher. Rolling the stretcher protects your back.

If the terrain is unstable or uneven, it may help to roll the stretcher in its lowest position. When rough terrain or other conditions prohibit rolling the stretcher, two or more EMTs must carry it. Using four EMTs in this situation is ideal. Position one EMT at each corner to provide maximum stability and strength. Space limitations or a shortage of personnel may limit the number of carriers to only two. In this case, remember that the stretcher might become unbalanced easily. Significantly more strength will be required to move the patient. For better stability, the EMTs should face each other from opposite ends of the stretcher.

Figure 6.14 *Wheeled stretcher.*

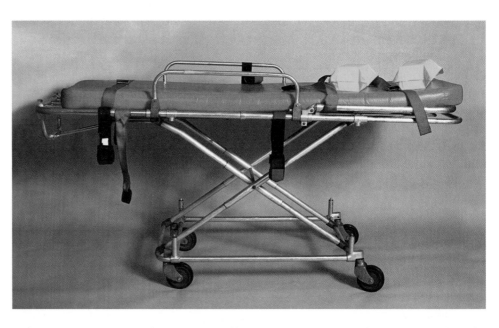

When carrying a stretcher, avoid walking in exact step with the EMT directly in front of you. Follow all the guidelines for safe lifting and carrying, including having enough help available.

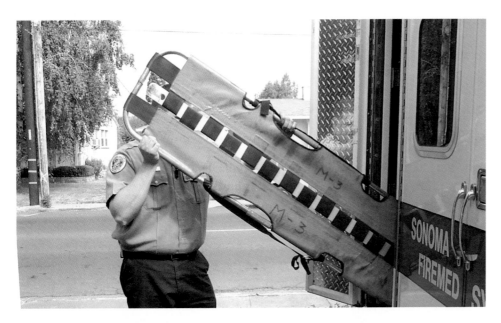

Figure 6.15 *Portable stretcher.*

Portable Stretcher | *Light, collapsible stretcher useful in small spaces*

The **portable stretcher** is useful when a patient must be moved from a space that is too small for a wheeled stretcher (see Figs. 6.15 and 6.16). Most ambulances use the stretcher as an auxiliary device, in case more than one patient must be carried. The portable stretcher is light and strong and usually folds or collapses for easy storage.

Stair Chair

A stair chair is a collapsible device used for moving patients on stairs or in confined spaces (see Fig. 6.17). They are useful in tight elevators. Many models have wheels and can be pushed like a wheelchair on smooth ground. Patients with shortness of breath or nausea may be more comfortable in the sitting position. In these situations, the stair chair may be used. Avoid using

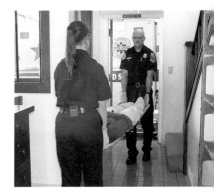

Figure 6.16 *Portable stretcher in use.*

Figure 6.17 *Stair chair.*

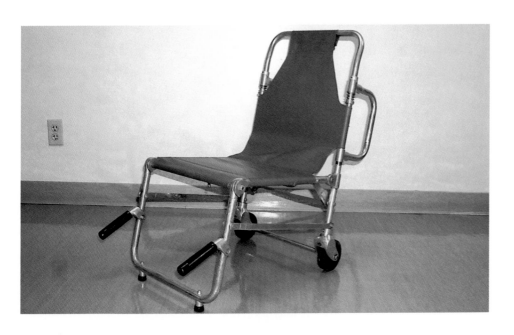

the stair chair for patients with altered mental status, suspected spinal injury, or injuries to the lower extremities.

Backboards

Backboards are made of wood or plastic and come in long and short sizes. Backboards are important pieces of emergency equipment.

Long Backboard | *Device used for full spinal immobilization*

The **long backboard** is also called a **long spine board** or **long board** (see Fig. 6.18). The board can serve as a spinal immobilization device, or as a firm surface on which to perform CPR or to protect the patient from cold or irregular ground. The long backboard can be applied while the patient is standing or lying down.

Figure 6.18 *A long spine board.*

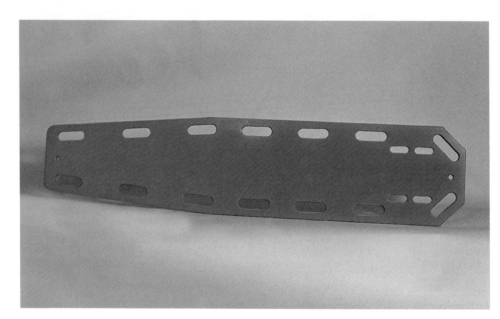

Figure 6.19 *A short backboard.*

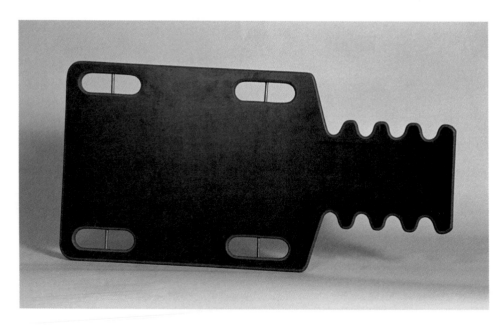

The **short backboard**, or **short board**, is used to immobilize the head, neck, and trunk (see Fig. 6.19). It is used for removing a patient with suspected spinal injury from a vehicle when rapid extrication is not indicated. First, apply a rigid cervical collar to the patient's neck. This is described in Chapter 22. Then place the short board between the patient and the seat. After the patient is strapped securely to the short board, he or she is moved to a long spine board.

Vest-Type Devices

A **vest-type extrication device** may be used instead of a short spine board (see Fig. 6.20). This device is useful when the patient is in a small car, bucket seat, or other confined space (see Fig. 6.21). The vest device is flexible and may be easier to place than a short board if environmental obstructions are present. Chapter 22 describes the use of a vest-type extrication device.

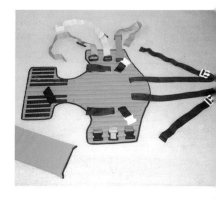

Figure 6.20 *Kendrick extrication device (KED).*

Figure 6.21 *The KED's flexible design makes it easier to place in tight spaces.*

Short Backboard | *Device for immobilizing the upper part of the spine when a long board cannot be used*

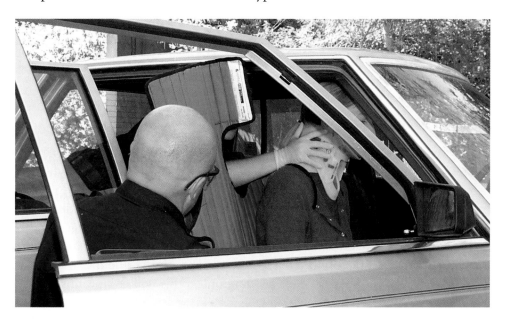

Scoop (Orthopedic) Stretcher

The **scoop** or **orthopedic stretcher** separates vertically into two halves that are assembled around the patient (see Fig. 6.22 and Procedure 6.7). This is a good device to use in confined areas. The scoop stretcher offers no spinal support and is not recommended for patients with suspected spinal injuries.

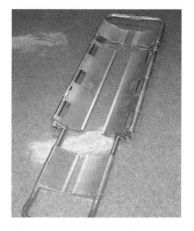

Figure 6.22 *Scoop stretcher.*

Vest-Type Extrication Device | *A flexible device used to help immobilize the spine in confined spaces*

Scoop Stretcher | *Device used to move patients with no suspected spinal injuries from confined areas*

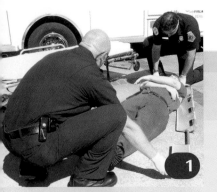

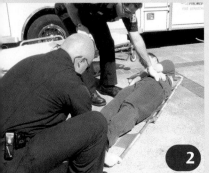

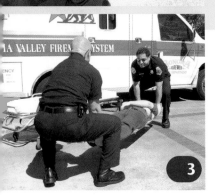

Procedure 6.7 • USING A SCOOP STRETCHER

Back Safety

1. After adjusting the stretcher for the height of the patient, spread the sides and place them on each side of the patient.

2. Collapse and lock the stretcher sides together under the patient, taking care not to pinch the patient or catch any clothing.

3. On a count, lift the stretcher together, using proper lifting techniques.

4. Transfer the stretcher to the bed, gurney, or wheeled stretcher using smooth, coordinated movements.

Wire Basket Stretcher (Stokes Litter)

The **wire basket stretcher** is also called **basket stretcher**, **Stokes litter**, or **Stokes basket** (see Fig. 6.23). This device is used for moving patients over rough or irregular terrain (see Fig. 6.24). It can accommodate a long backboard if immobilization is necessary. Using the basket helps to protect the patient from tree branches and other hazards while being carried. Wire basket stretchers are lighter than wheeled stretchers and are useful in many rescue situations. Lying on the wire may be uncomfortable for the patient. Always line the inside of the stretcher with a sheet or other padding unless this will compromise patient or rescuer safety.

Figure 6.23 *A wire basket stretcher with long board in place.*

Wire Basket Stretcher (Stokes Litter) | *Carrying device used for patient transport over rough or irregular terrain*

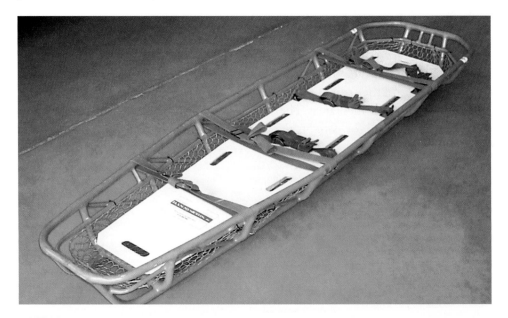

Flexible Stretcher

The **flexible stretcher** is made of flexible canvas or synthetic material. It has three large carrying handles on each side. This stretcher is especially useful for moving patients in narrow or confined areas, or for patients who are too large for more traditional devices.

PATIENT POSITIONING

Patients with certain conditions must be positioned in specific ways before and during transport. Whenever possible, position the patient in the **recovery position** for transport (see Fig. 6.25). This is also called the lateral recumbent position. Roll a patient with no suspected spinal injury onto one side without twisting the body. The left side is preferred, because this allows easier access by EMTs. In an ambulance with a driver-side stretcher mounting system, the patient will face the aisle.

If a patient is unwilling or unable to assume the recovery position, allow the patient to assume any position of comfort, unless the position could cause harm or interferes with your care. Pay particular attention to how the position affects your ability to manage the airway.

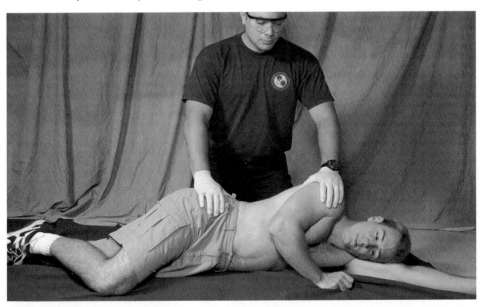

If the patient has an altered mental status or is not able to protect the airway, use the recovery position. An unresponsive patient without suspected spinal injury should also be positioned in the recovery position.

Unless an emergency or urgent move is indicated, a patient with a suspected spine injury must not be moved until the head, neck, and spine have been completely immobilized. The patient is positioned on a long backboard with as little spinal movement as possible.

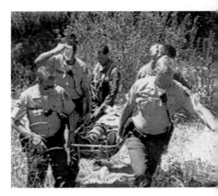

Figure 6.24 *Wire basket stretcher used in an environmental emergency.*

Flexible Stretcher | *Carrying device made of flexible materials with large carrying handles; used for moving patients in narrow or confined spaces*

Figure 6.25 *The recovery position.*

CD-ROM Link

The video "Climber's Descent" in the Authentic Emergency Scenes section of the Video Appendix on the MedEMT CD-ROM shows the transport of a fallen rock climber across rugged terrain.

Recovery Position | *Standard transportation position for a patient without spinal injury; patient is rolled onto one side, usually the left*

A patient with chest pain or difficulty breathing should be positioned in a sitting, or Fowler's, position. Sitting upright makes breathing easier and relieves pressure on the chest. A patient experiencing shock should be placed in the Trendelenburg position (supine with the legs elevated 8 to 12 inches above the head) to increase blood flow to the heart and other vital organs (see Fig. 6.26).

Figure 6.26 *The Trendelenburg position increases blood flow to the vital organs when a patient is in shock.*

National Registry Examination Tip

Review the indications, uses, and capabilities of each type of stretcher and cot. Recognize which devices are designed for transport, which are designed for immobilization, and which are used for both.

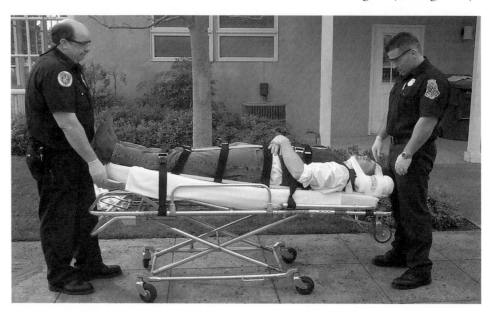

Low blood pressure sometimes occurs in pregnant patients. This is caused by the weight of the fetus compressing the large blood vessels in the chest and abdomen. This compromises circulation for both the mother and the fetus. Positioning the patient in the left-side-lying position relieves the pressure (see Fig. 6.27).

Figure 6.27 *The left-side-lying position relieves the pressure of the fetus on the maternal blood vessels.*

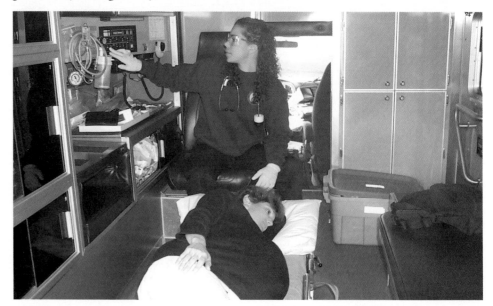

A patient with nausea or vomiting can be placed in a position of comfort. Position yourself so you can intervene immediately if vomiting occurs. If the patient is immobilized, elevate one side of the backboard to help maintain the airway.

Chapter Six Summary

- Safely moving your patient to the stretcher and ambulance is an important part of patient care. How you move the patient and the speed of the move affects the patient's condition.

- Lifting, reaching, carrying, pushing, and pulling are frequent sources of injury in EMTs. Always use proper body mechanics when moving patients or other objects.

- Moves are classified as emergency, urgent, and non-urgent, or routine.

- Emergency moves are used when an immediate threat to the patient or rescuers exists. Fire, explosion, an inability to protect the patient from other hazards, or the inability to access other patients are indications for using emergency moves. Using an emergency move increases the risk of aggravating spinal injuries.

- Urgent moves are used when the patient's medical condition is life threatening. An altered mental status or compromised airway, breathing, or circulation are indications for urgent moves. Cervical spine precautions are taken.

- The patient's position may affect the injury or illness. Be aware of special positioning needs.

Key Terms Review

Body Mechanics | *page 179*
Emergency Moves | *page 184*
Flexible Stretcher | *page 199*
Hyperextension | *page 182*
Long Backboard | *page 196*
Non-Urgent (Routine)
  Moves | *page 184*

Portable Stretcher | *page 195*
Power Grip | *page 180*
Power Lift | *page 180*
Rapid Extrication | *page 187*
Recovery Position | *page 199*
Scoop Stretcher | *page 197*
Short Backboard | *page 197*

Stair Chair | *page 182*
Urgent Moves | *page 184*
Vest-Type Extrication
  Device | *page 197*
Wheeled Stretcher | *page 194*
Wire Basket Stretcher
  (Stokes Litter) | *page 198*

Review Questions

1. The leading cause of worker's compensation claims in emergency medical services is:

   a. Workplace stress
   b. Back injuries
   c. Wrist injuries
   d. Disease exposure

2. Body mechanics refers to:

   a. The moving of patients
   b. Principles of posture and lifting
   c. Learning to avoid a back injury
   d. Muscle fatigue in the large muscles

3. When preparing for a non-urgent move, the EMT-Basic should:

   a. Enlist the help of other rescuers
   b. Place the patient in a sitting position
   c. Make sure that the rails on the stretcher are in the up position
   d. Cover the stretcher with blankets to keep the patient warm

4. A key element to remember when lifting is:

   a. Keep your hands at least 18 inches apart
   b. Bend from the waist, not the hips
   c. Use the large muscles of your back
   d. Keep the weight close to your body

Review Questions *(cont.)*

5. When required to reach, an EMT-Basic should:

   a. Reach no more than 30 inches

   b. Only flex in the center of the back

   c. Use and tighten the abdominal muscles

   d. Reach no more than 20 inches

6. Wheeled stretchers should be guided from the:

   a. Left side

   b. Foot end

   c. Head end

   d. Right side

7. Emergency moves are used:

   a. Only when airway compromise is present

   b. After the dangerous conditions have cleared up

   c. Only when immediate danger is present

   d. After the airway has been managed

8. During rapid extrication events, which person usually controls movement of the patient?

   a. The EMT-Basic controlling the patient's thorax

   b. The EMT-Basic who is the strongest

   c. The EMT-Basic at the feet of the patient

   d. The EMT-Basic at the head of the patient

9. Which improper lifting technique is most likely to cause a back injury to you or your partner?

   a. Feet shoulder width apart

   b. Hips aligned over feet

   c. Keeping back straight

   d. Weight far in front of you

10. Which lifting technique is best and safest to use when raising and lowering a stretcher or cot?

    a. Power lift

    b. Direct ground lift

    c. Direct carry

    d. One-handed carry

11. What piece of equipment is best used to move an unresponsive patient up a narrow basement stairwell?

    a. Wheeled ambulance stretcher

    b. Stair chair

    c. Short backboard

    d. Scoop stretcher

12. Which position is most appropriate to transport an unresponsive patient without suspected spinal injury?

    a. Fowler's position

    b. Position of comfort

    c. Trendelenburg position

    d. Recovery position

13. You are transporting a chest pain patient with shortness of breath and fatigue. In what position should you transport this patient?

    a. Supine on the stretcher

    b. Trendelenburg position

    c. Fowler's position

    d. Recovery position

14. When moving a patient on stairs, the stair chair should be used:

    a. Always

    b. Whenever it is safe and the patient's condition allows it

    c. If the stairs are not too steep

    d. Never

15. The three categories for classifying the urgency of moving patients are urgent, non-urgent, and:

    a. Expectant

    b. Hasty

    c. Sudden

    d. Emergency

16. Which is the greatest threat to a patient who requires an emergency move?

    a. The patient may suffer extremity injury

    b. The patient's cardiac function may be compromised

    c. The patient may suffer spinal injury

    d. The patient may suffer thoracic injury

17. Which is an example of a situation requiring an urgent move?

    a. A patient with a fractured fibula

    b. A patient with an altered level of consciousness

    c. A patient with a fractured hip

    d. A patient on fire from a burning building

CASE STUDIES

Lifting Techniques

1 You find a 36-year-old man complaining loudly of right hip pain. He is alert and oriented. He denies any other injuries or significant medical history. He tells you that he was injured when he slipped on the carpet, landing on his side. During your assessment, you find shortening and medial rotation of the right leg. The right hip area is swollen. The patient, who weighs at least 330 lbs (150 kg), lives in a second-floor apartment with no elevator access.

A. **What safety precautions will you take to lift and carry this patient?**

2 Despite the partial collapse, the chief foreman says that the building is structurally sound and safe. You agree to enter and search for one last employee. You and your partner find a 27-year-old female about 200 yards inside the building. She appears to have fallen approximately 30 feet. The patient has an obvious fracture of her left femur. You also suspect potentially significant internal abdominal injuries. As you prepare for extrication, you notice a distant section of the building beginning to shift. You and your partner decide there is imminent danger.

A. **What will you do immediately in this situation?**

B. **List other situations that may require using emergency moves.**

C. **Besides proper lifting and carrying techniques, what other important precaution should you take while using an emergency move for this trauma patient?**

D. **List the three methods commonly used for emergency moves.**

3 The crash tore the telephone pole completely out of the ground. According to the utility workers, the scene is safe now. Power to the lines has been shut down, so they are not a danger. You park the rescue vehicle and approach the scene. You observe that the vehicle has sustained only moderate damage to the front end and that the airbags have deployed. The driver of the vehicle is a 55-year-old male who is alert and oriented. He is complaining of chest pain. He states, "I think I was having a heart attack just before the crash." The patient's skin is cool, pale, and moist to touch. You see no signs of additional injuries during your physical exam.

A. **What steps will you take to remove this patient from his automobile?**

B. **Is an emergency move called for in this situation? Justify your answer.**

Stories from the Field
Wrap-Up

There are many potential roadblocks when moving this patient to the Emergency Department. The patient's location, size, and general condition are all factors to be considered before a move. Perhaps the most important lesson to be learned is that you may not be able to move a patient at all, until proper help arrives. It is your responsibility to make sure you have adequate assistance. Until then, you must give supportive care and prepare to make the move as easy as possible. This might include moving furniture out of the way, scouting out possible alternative routes, and obtaining equipment to assist with the move such as a stair chair or a long spine board. When the fire department arrives, they will assist you in moving the patient, possibly by removing the doorway. The patient might be placed on a board and moved down the hallway. The patient could then be strapped onto a gurney for transport to the ambulance. When you have enough assistance, you will be able to assure the safety of all concerned.

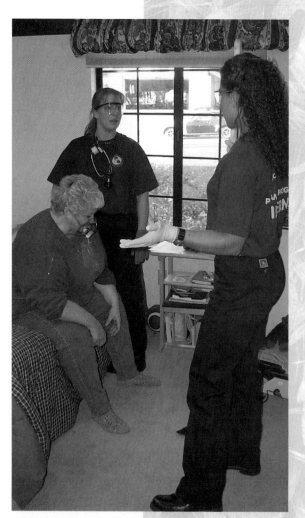

D.O.T. Module
Airway

2

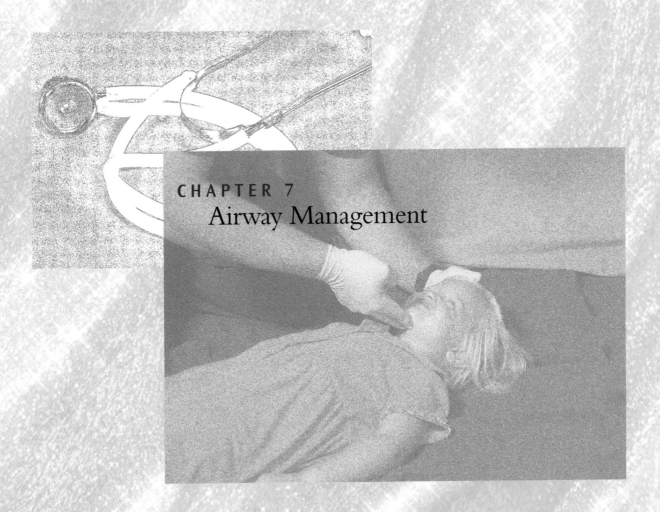

CHAPTER 7
Airway Management

Chapter 7

Airway Management

Stories from the Field

You are dispatched to a multiple-patient car collision one morning at the end of your shift. The incident commander assigns you to assist Carmen in transporting a patient to the hospital. Your patient, who is in serious condition, was driving the blue sedan. She was not wearing a seat belt. Her face hit the steering wheel and windshield. She has a large laceration on her nose and several teeth are missing. There are other minor cuts on her face and chest.

Carmen monitors the patient's airway carefully. Before you arrived, she was immobilized and high-flow oxygen was applied using a non-rebreather mask. Mark is assessing and treating her other injuries. The patient begins to speak to you about the bad luck she has had recently. She vomits a large amount of food mixed with blood. Vomitus pools in her oropharynx, and she begins making gagging, gurgling noises. Carmen immediately asks you to assist her in managing the patient's airway.

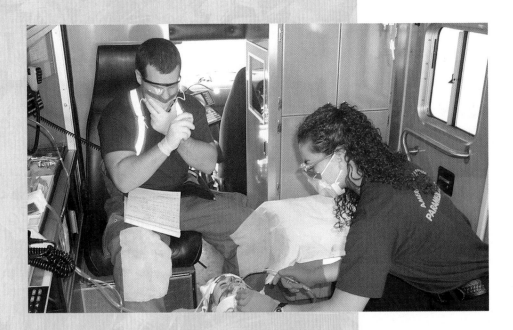

Patent (PAY-tent) | *Open; accessible*

Every patient must have a **patent**, or open, airway to survive. Every cell in the body needs a constant supply of oxygen to carry out vital processes. This is supplied by the rhythmic exchange of oxygen and carbon dioxide during inhalation and exhalation. Whenever a patient's airway is obstructed, you must clear it immediately. After the airway is open and clear, you must determine whether breathing is present and adequate. You will decide if supplemental oxygen is needed, based on your assessment. If so, you will select an appropriate oxygen delivery device and flow rate. If a patient is not breathing, or is breathing inadequately, you must provide assistance. You will use a mouth-to-mask technique, a bag-valve mask device, or a flow-restricted, oxygen-powered ventilation device.

This chapter covers techniques for assessing, intervening, and maintaining a patient's airway and breathing. Information about respiratory emergencies will be presented in Chapter 12.

D.O.T. OBJECTIVE

Name and label the major structures of the respiratory system on a diagram.

RESPIRATORY SYSTEM REVIEW

As you learned in Chapter 4, the respiratory system serves three main functions. It extracts oxygen from the air for transport to the body's tissues. Simultaneously, carbon dioxide (CO_2), a cellular waste product, moves to the lungs for excretion into the air. Movement of air past the vocal cords produces the voice.

The respiratory tree includes the anatomical airway structures necessary for exchange of air in the lungs, called ventilation. The upper airway consists of the nose and mouth, pharynx, larynx, and epiglottis. The lower airway consists of the trachea, bronchi, bronchioles, and alveoli. The lungs allow the exchange of oxygen between the air and the blood (see Fig. 7.1 and Figs. 4.32–4.37 in Chapter 4). Oxygenation and perfusion cannot occur if any part of the respiratory tree is obstructed.

Anatomy of the Airway

Aspiration | *To draw foreign material, a foreign body, or fluid into the respiratory tract while inhaling*

Air enters the body through the nose and mouth. Here it is warmed, humidified, and cleaned. Trauma to the nose or mouth may cause bleeding. This can lead to **aspiration**, or inhalation of foreign material into the respiratory tract.

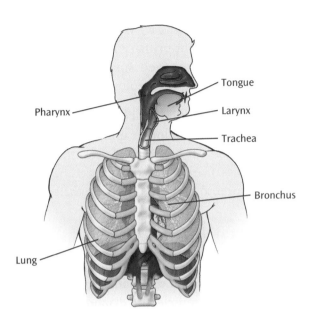

Figure 7.1 *Anatomy of the respiratory system.*

After leaving the oral or nasal cavity, air passes into the throat or pharynx. Airway obstruction often occurs because the pharynx is blocked. The tongue can fall to the back of the throat, obstructing the airway in an unconscious patient. Other causes of pharynx obstruction are:

- Accumulation of vomitus or secretions

- Tissue swelling from trauma or an allergic reaction

- Destruction of the airway

- Occlusion by a foreign object

The larynx permits speech and helps to prevent food from entering the respiratory tract. The larynx contains the vocal cords. The portion of the larynx called the thyroid cartilage is also called the Adam's apple. The lower portion of the larynx contains a firm cartilage ring, the cricoid cartilage. The ligament between the cricoid cartilage and the thyroid cartilage is called the cricothyroid ligament, or cricothyroid membrane.

The epiglottis is a flap-like structure that prevents food and liquid from entering the trachea during swallowing. An unresponsive patient can lose this protective mechanism. This greatly increases the risk for aspiration. The epiglottis can swell rapidly in a condition called epiglottitis, a life-threatening condition that may occur in young children.

Below the larynx, air continues through the trachea or windpipe, a tube formed by 16 to 20 C-shaped cartilage rings. Some patients with neurologic or advanced respiratory disease have a tracheostomy tube surgically inserted by a physician. The tracheostomy tube is placed directly into the trachea for breathing or the removal of secretions.

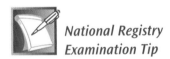

National Registry Examination Tip

Study the basic airway structures in your textbook. You must be comfortable with the anatomical location and function of each structure. Be sure you study the nares and the nasopharynx.

As the trachea descends into the chest cavity, it divides into two major branches. These are the left and right primary bronchi. The bronchi branch into passageways that become progressively smaller, called bronchioles. These end in millions of tiny **alveoli** (plural of alveolus) that comprise the lung tissue.

The alveoli are arranged in clusters around common air spaces, which are surrounded by an extensive network of blood capillaries. Oxygen diffuses through the walls of the alveoli. From there, it enters the bloodstream for transport to the body's tissues. Carbon dioxide carried back from the cells diffuses out of the bloodstream into the alveoli to be exhaled as waste.

The Process of Breathing

Movement of air into and out of the lungs is called respiration. The structures of the lower airway are located within the **thoracic cavity**, which is surrounded by the ribs. A thin, dome-shaped muscle, the **diaphragm**, is at the lower border of the ribs. This muscle separates the chest cavity from the abdominal cavity. Movement of the diaphragm permits breathing. Inhalation is the process of drawing air into the lungs. This occurs when the volume of the thoracic cavity expands. Exhalation is the process of moving air out of the lungs. It occurs when thoracic volume decreases.

Ventilation

Inhalation, or inspiration, requires contraction of the diaphragm and the **intercostal muscles** between the ribs (see Fig. 7.2). As the muscles contract, they increase the width and depth of the thoracic cavity so that it fills the entire rib cage. The lungs, which are very elastic, expand inside the thoracic cavity. When the volume of the thoracic cavity increases, air pressure in the lungs drops below atmospheric pressure. The negative pressure inside the chest causes air to flow into the lungs.

Alveoli (al-VEE-o-li) | *Termination of the respiratory passages; the functional units of the lungs, across whose walls gas exchange occurs*

Thoracic (tho-RAS-ik)
Cavity | *Body cavity enclosed by the sternum, ribs, and vertebral column*

Diaphragm | *Primary muscle of breathing; forms the bottom portion of the thoracic cavity*

Intercostal Muscles | *Muscles located between the ribs; involved in breathing*

Figure 7.2 *During inhalation (left), muscle contraction creates a larger space within the chest, allowing room for the lungs to expand. During exhalation (right), the diaphragm and intercostal muscles relax, moving up and in, respectively.*

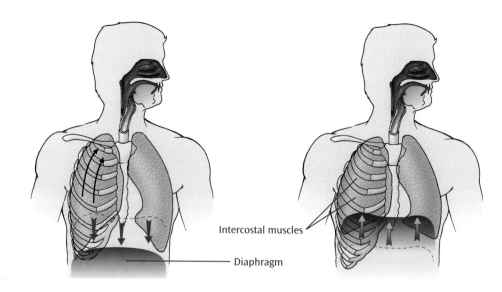

Intercostal muscles

Diaphragm

Exhalation, or expiration, occurs when the diaphragm and intercostal muscles relax (see Fig. 7.2). The diaphragm moves upward passively. The ribs move downward and inward. Thoracic cavity size decreases. This causes the pressure around the lungs to increase. As the thoracic volume decreases, air pressure in the lungs rises above atmospheric pressure. The higher pressure results in air movement out of the lungs.

When breathing is inadequate or labored, additional thoracic muscles assist with inspiration. These are the sternocleidomastoid and scalene muscles (see Fig. 7.3 and Fig. 4.40 in Chapter 4). The extreme use of these accessory muscles is called **retractions**. The patient tires quickly because a great amount of energy is needed for breathing. He or she may deteriorate rapidly. In some respiratory diseases, normal expiration is impaired. In these cases, active use of thoracic muscles is required to expel air from the lungs.

Respiratory failure occurs when normal breathing is interrupted. Oxygen intake is not sufficient to support life. Respiratory arrest is the condition when breathing stops completely.

Retractions | *Depressions in the neck, above the shoulder blades, between and below the ribs; indicates extensive muscle use during breathing due to respiratory distress*

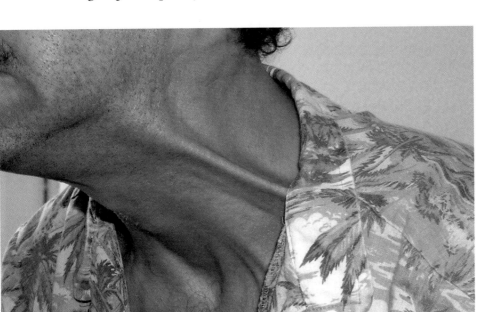

Figure 7.3 *Assessment of this patient reveals use of accessory muscles of the neck. The man is clearly in respiratory distress.*

 EMT Tip

Think of the circulatory system as a train with the red blood cells as cars. Oxygen boards the train in the alveoli and is carried through the body. When an oxygen passenger gets off the train in the cells, a carbon dioxide passenger gets on. When the train returns to the alveoli, carbon dioxide disembarks and another oxygen boards.

Oxygen passes from the air into the blood by gas exchange. It moves into the body's cells, while carbon dioxide moves out. Gas exchange occurs by diffusion, which is a passive process. The gas molecules move from areas where they are more highly concentrated to areas of lower concentration.

Oxygen-rich air moves into the alveoli during inhalation. Here, alveolar/capillary exchange takes place (see Fig. 4.41 in Chapter 4). The oxygen passes from the alveoli into the capillaries. Simultaneously, carbon dioxide passes from the blood into the alveoli. It will be removed as waste during the next exhalation.

The oxygen-rich blood from the lungs is carried to all of the body's cells. Oxygen passes from the capillaries into the cells during capillary/cellular exchange (see Fig. 4.42 in Chapter 4). Carbon dioxide, the end product of metabolic functions, passes from the cells into the blood. The blood is now low in oxygen and high in carbon dioxide. It returns to the lungs where carbon dioxide is again exchanged for oxygen.

MANAGEMENT OF THE AIRWAY

EMT Alert

No airway procedures should be performed without adequate BSI and standard precautions.

Before beginning your thorough assessment, you must ensure that your patient is breathing adequately. The airway must be patent for breathing to take place. Care of the patient's airway and breathing is your highest priority. The rest of this chapter explains techniques for evaluating and managing airway problems.

The first step in direct patient care is assessment of the airway. An airway obstruction is a life-threatening condition requiring immediate intervention. Use emergency procedures to open and maintain the airway. After maintaining a patent airway, you will assess the adequacy of the patient's breathing. Assisted artificial ventilations or supplemental oxygen may be needed before the patient is out of danger. Carefully assess the need for assisted ventilations if an obstruction or other condition compromises the airway. If assisted ventilations are not necessary, provide high-flow oxygen by non-rebreather mask.

Body substance isolation precautions are very important during airway management. Vomitus, secretions, or other potentially infectious materials may be expelled from the airway. Wear gloves, mask, and eye protection. A gown may be needed in some situations.

Airway Obstruction

The first step in assessing the airway is to check for any obstruction. Open the patient's mouth and look for blood, vomit, secretions, or foreign bodies. Common causes of airway obstruction are:

- The tongue (the most common cause in adults)
- Small foreign objects
- Incompletely chewed food
- Alcohol consumption while eating
- Teeth, dentures, or dental appliances
- Trauma

An airway obstruction may be complete or partial. A patient with complete airway obstruction is unable to speak, cough, or gag. The appearance of the skin changes quickly, especially in infants and children. Rapid onset of cyanosis in the face and fingers is a good indication of airway obstruction. Patients usually grab their throats. This is called the universal choking sign. The patient will also appear very anxious. You must remove the foreign body immediately.

Some air can pass through the vocal cords and into the lungs if the airway is partially obstructed. Signs of partial obstruction are coughing, gagging, or attempting to clear the airway forcefully. Stridor, a high-pitched sound, may be heard. The patient can usually speak, but may utter only a word or two. The patient can probably clear a partial obstruction without intervention. Be alert, however, because a partial airway obstruction can quickly become a complete obstruction.

If a patient has an upper airway foreign body obstruction, clear the object using abdominal thrusts and finger sweeps (see Fig. 7.4). Review the procedures for foreign body airway obstruction (FBAO) learned in your Basic Life Support (BLS) course. This information is reviewed in Appendix B. Complete three cycles of the FBAO procedure. If the obstruction persists, transport immediately. Continue the FBAO procedure while en route.

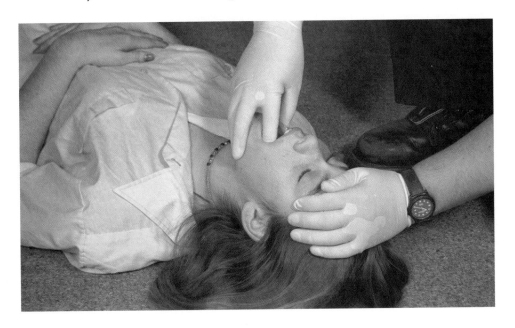

Figure 7.4 Use your finger to sweep grass, teeth, food, or other foreign bodies from the upper airway.

National Registry Examination Tip

Several practical exam stations require you to open and maintain a patent airway. You must be able to open the airway using different methods. You may also be required to assess another person's ability to open the airway. Make sure you are comfortable using the head-tilt/chin-lift and jaw-thrust maneuvers.

Opening the Airway

If you continue to observe signs of obstruction after removing all foreign bodies, immediately attempt to open the airway. For an alert medical patient, use the head-tilt/chin-lift maneuver. If the patient is unresponsive or shows signs of head, neck, or spinal injury, use the jaw-thrust maneuver. These techniques were presented in the Basic Life Support course and are summarized in the following sections. Some CPR courses teach the cross-finger technique for opening the airway of an unconscious patient without suspected spinal injury. The head-tilt/chin-lift maneuver is a more appropriate technique for EMT-Basics to use.

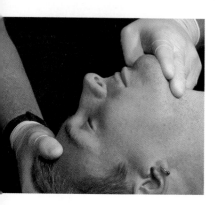

Figure 7.5 *Avoid hyperextending the neck when performing the head-tilt/chin-lift maneuver.*

Figure 7.6 *The tongue is a very common airway obstruction in adult patients (left). The head-tilt/chin-lift procedure lifts the tongue off the back of the throat (right).*

Head-Tilt/Chin-Lift Maneuver | *The preferred method for opening and maintaining an airway in a patient without suspected neck injury*

D.O.T. OBJECTIVE

Describe the steps in performing the head-tilt/chin-lift maneuver.

Head–Tilt/Chin–Lift Maneuver

The **head-tilt/chin-lift maneuver** is only used for patients without suspected spinal injury (see Figs. 7.5 and 7.6).

1. Place one hand on the patient's forehead and firmly tilt it back.
2. Place the fingertips of the other hand under the bony portion of the lower jaw.
3. Lift the chin so that the lower teeth almost touch the upper teeth. Avoid compressing the soft tissues under the jaw.
4. Keep the mouth open. If dentures are secure, leave them in place. Intact dentures help to maintain the airway. If dentures are loose, remove them.

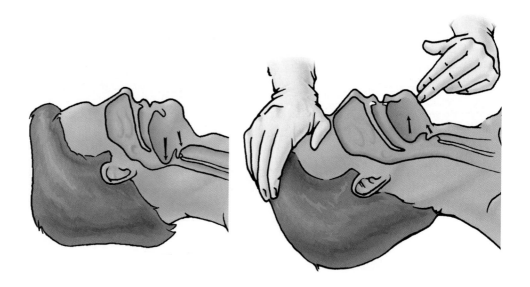

D.O.T. OBJECTIVES

Relate the mechanism of injury to opening the airway.

Describe the steps in performing the jaw-thrust.

Jaw–Thrust Maneuver

The **jaw-thrust maneuver** is used to open the airway when there is a possibility of spinal injury. You might suspect this based on your assessment or on the mechanism of injury for a trauma patient. It is a safe procedure that can be used for any patient. Follow these steps (see Fig. 7.7):

1. Kneel behind the patient's head. Stabilize your elbows on the floor, bed, or other surface. Position your hands on each side of the patient's lower jaw.

2. Gently grasp the angles of the lower jaw. Stabilize the head with your forearms.

3. Push the angles of the patient's lower jaw forward, using your index fingers.

4. Use your thumb to retract the lower lip if closed.

Jaw-Thrust Maneuver | The preferred method for opening and maintaining an airway in a patient with suspected spinal injury

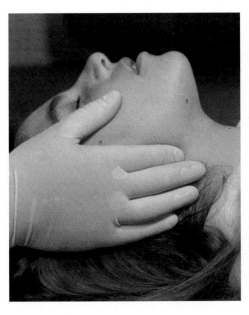 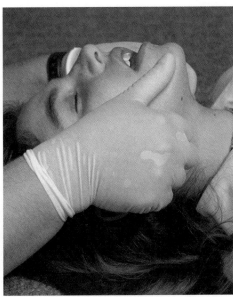

Figure 7.7 *For the jaw-thrust maneuver, gently grasp the angles of the lower jaw (left). Use your index fingers to push the lower jaw forward and open the airway (right).*

 CD-ROM Link

The videos "Head-Tilt/Chin-Lift" and "Jaw-Thrust" in the Airway Management chapter and the Video Appendix on the MedEMT CD-ROM demonstrate techniques for opening an airway.

D.O.T. OBJECTIVE

State the importance of having a suction unit ready for immediate use when providing emergency care.

Suctioning

After the airway is open, assess the need for suctioning. Suctioning is a procedure for removing blood, vomitus (emesis), fluids, secretions, and food particles from the airway. Removal of solid foreign material, such as teeth, may require a powerful suction unit.

 EMT Alert

The jaw-thrust maneuver should be used in patients with any possibility of a spinal injury.

Suction equipment must be available when you are managing a patient's airway or assisting ventilations. Inserting an oral or nasal airway may cause vomiting, so suction must be ready. The quality of the patient's breathing provides clues about the need for suction. Immediate suctioning may be indicated if gurgling sounds are present, or if the patient sounds like he or she is choking.

Suction Units

Suction units consist of:

- Vacuum source
- Collection container
- Tubing
- Suction tips or catheters

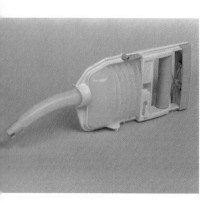

Figure 7.8 *Portable suction units can be taken to the patient's side in case there is vomit or blood in the airway. Hand-held units are used once, then discarded.*

Suction devices may be either wall-mounted or portable (see Figs. 7.8 and 7.9). Mounted devices are installed in the ambulance near the patient's head. These units are powered by the vehicle's electrical system. Portable suction devices are lightweight, convenient, and easily carried. They are available in two styles. The battery-operated unit is rechargeable. Hand-operated units are convenient and disposable. These are used for one patient, then discarded.

Figure 7.9 *Battery-operated suction units are lightweight for use in or away from the ambulance.*

 CD-ROM Link

Suctioning technique is demonstrated in the video "Airway Management–Suctioning" in the Airway Management chapter and the Video Appendix on the MedEMT CD-ROM.

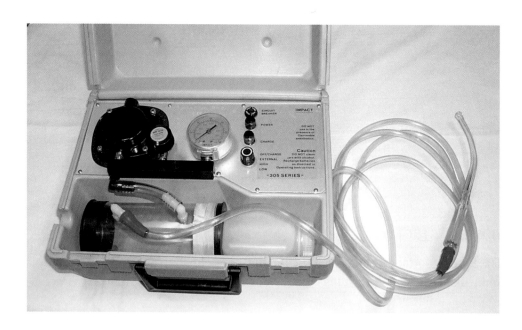

A suction device, like all equipment, must be inspected regularly. The device must be ready and immediately available. The battery must be recharged immediately after use, so that it is fully charged when needed. The gauge on a suction unit should generate 300 mmHg of vacuum when the hose is blocked.

Two types of suction catheters are used. The hard or **rigid suction catheter** is commonly called a tonsil tip, or tonsil sucker. This tip is used to suction the mouth and oropharynx of an unresponsive patient. A rigid suction catheter is inserted only as far as you can see.

The French or **soft suction catheter** is used for suctioning the nasopharynx (see Fig. 7.10). It is also used for clearing an endotracheal tube or nasopharyngeal airway, and other times when a rigid catheter cannot be used. Measure the French catheter so that it is inserted only as far as the base of the tongue. For suctioning the nasopharynx, measure the catheter from the tip of the nose to the tip of the ear. When suctioning the mouth and oropharynx, measure the catheter from the corner of the mouth to the tip of the ear. Some French catheters have a port. This is a small, plastic tunnel. Suction is applied by covering the port with a gloved fingertip. This method of suctioning is safer and gives the EMT more control than catheters without a port.

D.O.T. OBJECTIVE

Describe the techniques of suctioning.

Procedure for Suctioning

Always observe body substance isolation and standard precautions when suctioning may be required. A patient who needs suction might cough, vomit, or bleed. Selecting the correct personal protective equipment will reduce your potential for exposure to these substances. At a minimum, use eye protection, a mask, and gloves. If splashing is a possibility, a gown is indicated. If you suspect the patient has been exposed to tuberculosis, use a NIOSH-approved HEPA respirator (see Chapter 2).

Follow these steps for suctioning a patient:

1. Turn the unit on. Check to see that the suction is working.

2. Select and attach an appropriate catheter.

3. Insert the catheter into the oral cavity with suction turned off. Avoid inserting the catheter beyond the base of the tongue (see Fig. 7.11).

4. Apply suction. Turn the unit on or cover the port in the catheter.

5. Move the catheter tip from side to side as you withdraw it.

6. The patient is not receiving oxygen while you are suctioning. Avoid suctioning adults for longer than 15 seconds at a time. In infants and children, suction for 5 seconds.

Rigid Suction Catheter | *Non-flexible catheter used to suction an unresponsive patient*

Soft Suction Catheter | *A soft catheter used for suctioning the nasopharynx and in other situations where a rigid catheter cannot be used*

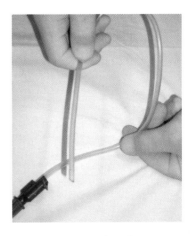

Figure 7.10 *French catheters are made of soft, flexible plastic.*

National Registry Examination Tip

Whenever you are managing a patient's airway, state that you have suction available nearby. Always suction when necessary. Never hesitate.

EMT Tip

Mastery of suction devices is an important skill. Practice with as many different types of devices as possible. Learn to use, clean, and troubleshoot each device.

Figure 7.11 *Measure a suction catheter before inserting it (left). The tip should be inserted only as far as the base of the tongue (right). This figure shows a rigid catheter.*

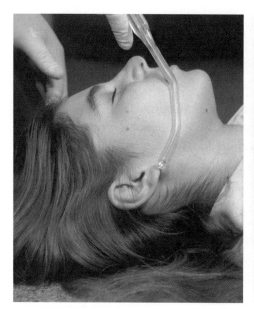 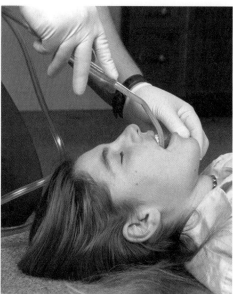

EMT Tip

Airway adjuncts do not prevent aspiration.

7. Carefully observe the patient during suctioning. The patient may deteriorate quickly. Careful observation is especially important in children. A slow, rapid, or irregular heart rate suggests a dangerous decline in oxygen. This may be caused by the suction or by stimulation of the airway by the catheter. If the patient is in distress, remove the catheter immediately. Ventilate with oxygen for at least 30 seconds.

8. Watch the suction tubing to make sure that foreign objects pass directly into the collection canister. Do not let the tubing become clogged. If necessary, rinse the catheter by suctioning water through the tubing (see Fig. 7.12). Cleaning the catheter prevents obstruction by dried or thick material.

9. Dispose of single-use suction equipment correctly. Clean and disinfect reusable parts with an EPA-approved disinfectant after each use. Follow your agency protocol.

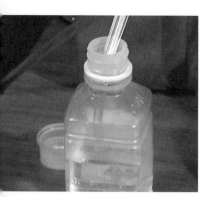

Figure 7.12 *Sterile water or normal saline can help to clear suction tubing clogged with thick secretions, blood, vomit, or food.*

If secretions or emesis cannot be removed quickly, log roll the patient and clear the oropharynx with a finger sweep. If the patient produces frothy secretions as rapidly as you can remove them, suction for 15 seconds. Stop and artificially ventilate for 2 minutes. Suction again for 15 seconds. Continue treating the patient this way. Consult medical direction.

Sometimes a patient's airway continues to fill with fluid or foreign objects. Consider placing the patient in the recovery position (see Fig. 7.13). This allows material to flow from the mouth by gravity. The airway of a trauma patient may be full of blood, vomit, and other fluids. After you have taken full spinal precautions, tilting the spine board slightly may keep the airway clear.

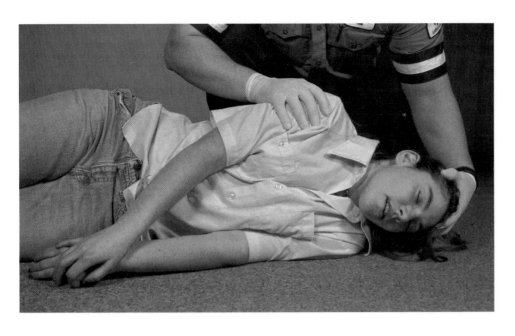

Figure 7.13 *A nontrauma patient can be placed in the recovery position if he or she continues to have heavy secretions, bleeding, or vomiting. The fluid should drain naturally from the mouth.*

Airway Adjunct | *Device that helps keep the airway open by keeping the tongue away from the back of the throat*

Oropharyngeal (or-oh-FAIR-en-GEE-ul) Airway | *A curved plastic device with a flange inserted in the patient's mouth; used to keep the tongue from blocking the pharynx*

Nasopharyngeal (NAY-zoh-fair-en-GEE-ul) Airway | *A soft rubber airway device inserted through the nose; designed to maintain an open airway by displacing the tongue off the pharynx*

Maintaining Airway Patency: Airway Adjuncts

Airway adjuncts are devices that help to maintain an open airway. If you believe that a patient cannot maintain the airway, consider using an adjunct.

Using an adjunct is essential for all unconscious patients. Monitor the level of consciousness carefully. If you attempt to insert an airway and the patient gags, he or she may not need the airway adjunct. Presence of the gag reflex is an indication that the body's normal airway protective mechanisms may be sufficient. Remove an **oropharyngeal airway** if the patient becomes responsive and begins to gag. The **nasopharyngeal airway** is the only airway that can be safely used for a conscious patient.

> **D.O.T. OBJECTIVE**
>
> Describe how to measure and insert an oropharyngeal (oral) airway.

Oropharyngeal Airway Adjunct

The oropharyngeal airway adjunct (OPA) is used to help maintain an open airway. It is used for unresponsive patients with no gag reflex. The OPA is a curved plastic device with a flange at the mouth opening. The flange prevents the device from slipping into the patient's airway. When properly fitted, the flange rests between the lips. The tip of the airway ends at the angle of the jaw (see Fig. 7.14).

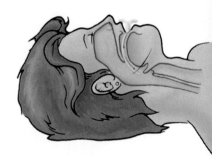

Figure 7.14 *Properly sized OPA.*

Figure 7.15 *Oropharyngeal airways come in many sizes for properly fitting newborns to large adults.*

CD-ROM Link

The technique for inserting airway adjuncts is demonstrated in the OPA and NPA videos in the Airway Management chapter and the Video Appendix on the MedEMT CD-ROM.

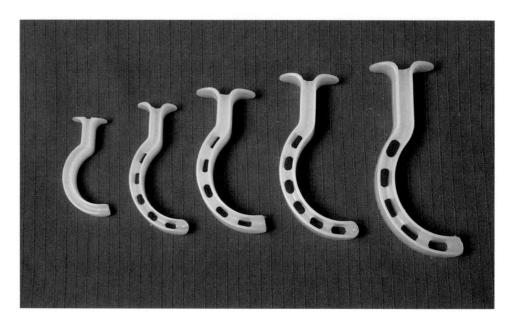

Insertion of an oropharyngeal adjunct does not guarantee an open airway. It must be used together with manual techniques and suctioning to maintain the airway. An OPA will cause patients with a gag reflex to vomit. Do not be afraid to remove an oral airway if the patient gags or cannot tolerate the airway. Always have suction ready when placing or removing an adjunct. Removal triggers the patient's gag reflex. This usually results in vomiting.

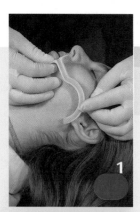

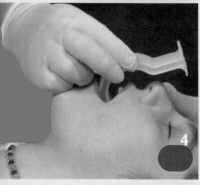

Procedure 7.1 • INSERTING AN OROPHARYNGEAL AIRWAY

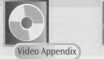

Video Appendix   Body Fluids

1. Select the proper size airway adjunct. Measure from the corner of the patient's lips to the bottom of the ear lobe or the angle of the jaw. An airway that fits correctly will fill this space. It will not be too short or too long.

2. Open the patient's mouth.

3. Avoid obstructing the airway with the tongue.

4. Insert the airway upside down, with the tip facing toward the roof of the mouth.

Size is an important consideration when selecting an oral airway (see Fig. 7.15). An oropharyngeal airway that is too large may obstruct the airway or traumatize airway structures. An OPA that is too small or inserted incorrectly can push the tongue back into the throat, blocking the airway.

Procedure 7.1 describes how to insert an oropharyngeal airway in an adult.

In an infant or child, inserting the airway right side up may be preferable (see Fig. 7.16). This prevents damage to the soft palate, which could interfere with the infant's ability to suck and feed. To insert an oropharyngeal airway in an infant:

1. Select the proper size airway adjunct by measuring from the corner of the mouth to the earlobe.

2. Position yourself at the patient's head.

3. Open the mouth.

4. Press the tongue down and forward with a tongue depressor. This prevents damage to the soft palate.

5. Insert the airway with the curved end facing down.

6. Advance the airway until the flange comes to rest between the lips.

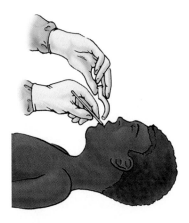

Figure 7.16 *The OPA can be inserted in infants and children by following the curvature of the tongue. This prevents damage to the mouth.*

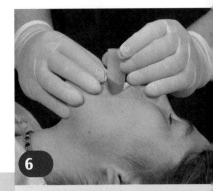

Procedure 7.1 • Oropharyngeal Airway *(cont.)*

5. Advance the airway gently until resistance is encountered.

6. Turn the airway adjunct 180 degrees.

7. Continue inserting until it comes to rest with the flange on the patient's teeth.

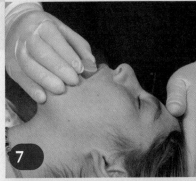

8. If placed correctly, the OPA will allow air to pass freely. Listen and feel for air movement.

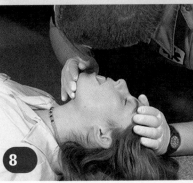

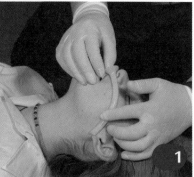

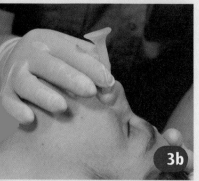

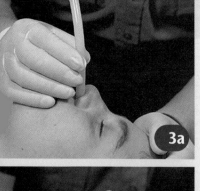

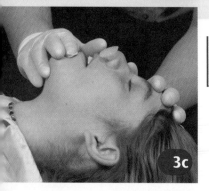

D.O.T. OBJECTIVE

Describe how to measure and insert a nasopharyngeal (nasal) airway.

Nasopharyngeal Airway Adjunct

Nasopharyngeal airway adjuncts (NPAs) are less likely to stimulate vomiting (see Fig. 7.17). They are used for responsive patients who need assistance to maintain their airways. The airway is lubricated before it is inserted. Despite the lubricant, insertion may be a painful or uncomfortable process. The nose and face have many blood vessels. Expect a small amount of bleeding when an NPA is inserted. Never force a nasopharyngeal airway into place.

To insert a nasopharyngeal airway, follow Procedure 7.2.

Procedure 7.2 • INSERTING A NASOPHARYNGEAL AIRWAY

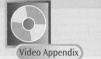

Video Appendix

Body Fluids

1. Select the proper size airway adjunct. Measure from the tip of the nose to the tip of the ear. Also compare the diameter of the tube with the size of the patient's nostril.

2. Lubricate the airway with a water-soluble lubricant.

3. Insert the adjunct posteriorly. The bevel end should point toward the base of the nostril or nasal septum.

4. If the airway adjunct cannot be inserted into one nostril, try the other side.

D.O.T. OBJECTIVES

List the signs of adequate breathing.

List the signs of inadequate breathing.

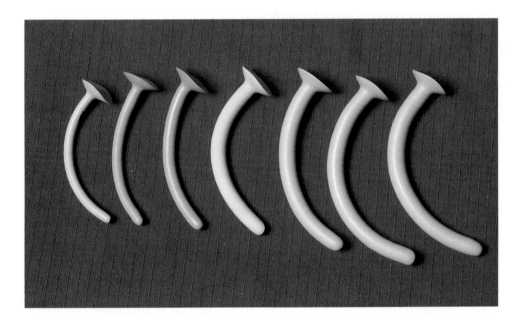

Figure 7.17 *Like OPAs, nasopharyngeal airways are manufactured in many sizes to properly fit any patient.*

EMT Tip

While inserting an NPA, gently rotate the device. Turn it back and forth slightly while applying gentle pressure. Never force the airway into place.

Assessing Breathing

After assessing airway patency and intervening if necessary, you must assess the patient's breathing. Breathing may be compromised due to illness, obstruction, or injury. If a patient complains of difficulty breathing, consider the situation serious until proven otherwise. Difficulty breathing is a critical consideration in all pediatric patients.

When a patient's breathing requires conscious effort, something is wrong. Many patients will wait a long time before calling EMS. During this time, breathing becomes more difficult, and the patient may tire quickly. Some patients give up trying as soon as you arrive and go into respiratory arrest.

Assess breathing by:

- Measuring the respiratory rate
- Observing the rhythm of respirations
- Determining the quality of respirations
- Evaluating the depth of respirations
- Observing chest wall movement
- Listening to breath sounds

During your assessment, a primary concern is the presence or absence of breathing. You also monitor the adequacy of respiration (see Tables 7.1 and 7.2). You will perform a more detailed evaluation of breathing for a patient with a respiratory emergency. Assessment of breathing is described further in Chapter 9.

Observe the rise and fall of the patient's chest during a complete cycle of inhalation and exhalation. Normal adult breathing is relaxed and regular. The

National Registry Examination Tip

Learn the indications, contraindications, and potential complications associated with using airway adjuncts. Practice until you are comfortable and familiar with using them. Practice measuring oral and nasal airways on patients of different sizes. Practice until you can use the adjuncts while performing the other skills listed on the evaluation forms.

Table 7.1 • ADEQUATE VS. INADEQUATE BREATHING

Characteristic	Adequate Breathing	Inadequate Breathing
Rate (breaths per minute)	Adult—12 to 20 Child—15 to 30 Infant—25 to 50	Adult—Less than 8 or greater than 24 Child—Apnea, or breathing absent
Rhythm	Regular	Irregular or labored Seesaw breathing Agonal respirations
Effort of Breathing	Minimum effort; no use of accessory muscles	Increased effort with use of accessory muscles
Breath Sounds	Present and equal	Diminished, absent, or noisy
Chest Expansion	Adequate and equal	Inadequate or unequal
Depth (Tidal Volume)	Full, easy breaths	Shallow or inadequate
Chest Wall Movement	Equal, full, and symmetrical	Retractions
Skin	Normal color Warm	Pale or cyanotic Cool and clammy

Table 7.2 • RESPIRATION SIGNS

Characteristic	Adequate Respiration	Inadequate Respiration
Rate	Normal	Rapid
Effort of Breathing	Easy, effortless	Labored
Breath Sounds	Quiet	Stridor, crowing, or noisy
Grunting	Absent	Present on exhalation
Chest Expansion	Equal and symmetric	Asymmetric
Nasal Flaring	Absent	Present (especially in children)
Retractions	Absent	Present
Body Position	Relaxed	Sitting upright or leaning forward

patient does not use accessory muscles. Monitor the respirations to see if the chest expands and contracts easily. The chest expansion should be equal for each breath. At the same time, measure and record the respiration rate. Compare your findings with the normal value for the patient's age group.

Use a stethoscope to listen for the presence of equal, normal breath sounds. Listening to breath sounds with a stethoscope is discussed in more detail in Chapter 9. Listen to both the anterior and posterior chest (see Fig. 7.18). Compare the sounds of the right and left lungs at their apices (tops), middles, and bases. Also note the **tidal volume**, the amount of air inhaled and exhaled

Tidal Volume | *The amount of air inhaled and exhaled in a single breath*

with each breath. Tidal volume is reduced in illnesses that cause narrowing of the lower airway structures. Feel for movement of air at the nose or mouth, if necessary.

If the breathing rate is outside the normal range, ventilation may or may not be adequate. You might observe signs of inadequate ventilation, or air hunger, such as:

- Retractions
- Nasal flaring (see Fig. 7.19)
- Irregular rhythm
- Unequal or inadequate chest expansion
- Shallow tidal volume (shallow breathing)
- Abnormal, diminished, or absent breath sounds
- Pale, cool, and clammy skin

A late sign of **hypoxia**, or low oxygen levels, is cyanosis, a blue-gray coloring. It is usually first noted around the lips or fingertips. Occasional, irregular gasping breaths called **agonal respirations** may be seen just before death.

Assisted Artificial Ventilation

If the patient's breathing is inadequate or absent, you will assist him or her using artificial ventilation. Assisted artificial ventilation includes several techniques for forcing air into the lungs. You must provide assisted artificial ventilation if a patient is not breathing sufficiently to maintain good oxygenation. Assisted artificial ventilation may be indicated if the patient has:

- Inadequate tidal volume
- Respiration rate that is too slow or too fast
- Signs of respiratory compromise
- An altered level of consciousness

Different skills and equipment are used for each method of artificial ventilation. Each has advantages and disadvantages. Select a method based on the requirements of the clinical situation and the equipment available. In general, the techniques used by EMT-Basics, in the order of preference for use, are:

- Mouth-to-mask
- Two-person bag-valve mask
- Flow-restricted, oxygen-powered ventilation device
- One-person bag-valve mask

Suctioning the airway may be necessary during artificial ventilation. Consider using an oropharyngeal or nasopharyngeal airway.

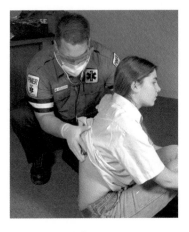

Figure 7.18 *The posterior thorax is the best place for listening to lung sounds. Listen at the apex and the base of each lung.*

Hypoxia (high-POKS-e-uh) | *Deficiency of oxygen*

Agonal (AY-gun-ul) Respirations | *Occasional gasping breaths that may occur in the final stage of death*

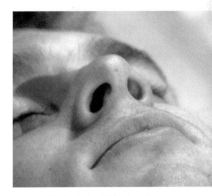

Figure 7.19 *Nasal flaring is a sign of respiratory distress, even in adults.*

The risk of exposure to blood, vomitus, and secretions is high during assisted artificial ventilation. Protect yourself by using body substance isolation (BSI) precautions. Apply PPE before beginning the procedure.

• Wear gloves, eye protection, and a mask at all times.

• Wear a NIOSH-approved respirator if you suspect the patient has tuberculosis.

• Wear a gown if splashing of body fluids is likely.

When ventilating a patient, maintain a rate of at least 12 breaths per minute in adults and 20 per minute in infants and children. Continually assess the effectiveness of assisted ventilation (Table 7.3). Ventilation is adequate if the patient's chest rises and falls with each ventilation, and the heart rate returns to normal. Ventilation is inadequate if the chest does not rise and fall, the rate of ventilation is too fast or slow, or the heart rate does not return to normal.

Table 7.3 • EFFECTIVENESS OF ARTIFICIAL VENTILATION

Adequate Ventilation	Inadequate Ventilation
Chest rises and falls with each ventilation	Chest does not rise and fall with each ventilation

Rate of ventilation is sufficient
    Adult—12 breaths per minute
    Child—20 breaths per minute
	Rate of ventilation is too slow or too fast

Heart rate returns to normal	Heart rate does not return to normal

Mouth-to-Mouth Ventilation

Mouth-to-mouth ventilation can be performed by a single rescuer with no special equipment. It provides adequate tidal volume to sustain the patient. However, using this method is strongly discouraged. You cannot take proper body substance isolation precautions. The mouth-to-mask technique is preferred.

Mouth-to-mouth ventilation was studied as part of a Basic Life Support course. For more information, refer to Appendix B.

> **D.O.T. OBJECTIVE**
>
> Describe how to artificially ventilate a patient with a pocket mask.

Mouth-to-Mask Ventilation

Mouth-to-mask ventilation is a simple and effective technique of artificial ventilation. A pocket face mask with a one-way anti-reflux valve is the preferred method of performing artificial ventilation (see Fig. 7.20). Oxygen is connected to the pocket mask through an inlet valve. The mask protects you from direct contact with the patient. The one-way valve prevents exposure to the patient's exhaled air and secretions.

Mouth-to-mask ventilation may have been part of your Basic Life Support course. The procedure is summarized below (see Fig. 7.21):

1. Connect the one-way valve to the mask. Connect the oxygen tubing. Set the oxygen flow to 15 liters per minute. Make sure you are using the proper sized mask for the patient.

2. Position yourself above the patient's head.

3. Open the airway.

4. Place the apex of the mask over the bridge of the patient's nose. Lower the mask over the mouth and upper chin.

5. Seal the mask to the face using your thumbs and index fingers.

6. Inhale normally, seal your mouth around the ventilation port, and exhale for 1.5 to 2 seconds. Stop when you see the patient's chest rise.

7. Remove your mouth from the valve and allow the patient to exhale passively.

8. Continue to ventilate at least once every 5 seconds for adults or every 3 seconds for children and infants.

For smaller children and infants, you might have to turn the adult mask upside down, placing the wider portion of the mask over the bridge of the patient's nose. This allows you to obtain a more effective seal than the traditional position.

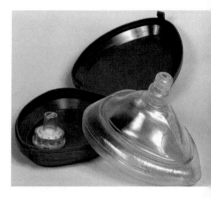

Figure 7.20 *A pocket mask with a one-way valve is an effective tool for artificial ventilation as well as a safe piece of equipment for the provider to use.*

CD-ROM Link

The video "Mouth-to-Mask Technique" in the Airway Management chapter and the Video Appendix on the MedEMT CD-ROM show the steps for using a pocket mask.

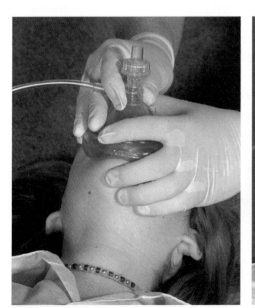 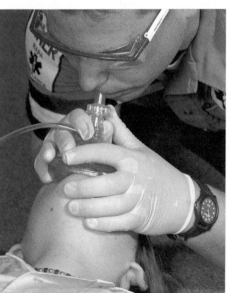

Figure 7.21 *Hold a tight seal of the pocket mask around the patient's mouth (left). Deliver slow breaths through the one-way valve (right).*

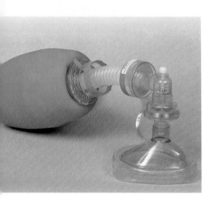

Figure 7.22 *A BVM with a reservoir for supplemental oxygen is one of the most effective ventilation devices available to the EMT-Basic.*

Bag-Valve Mask Device (BVM) | *Oxygen delivery device comprised of a self-inflating bag, face mask, one-way valve, and oxygen reservoir*

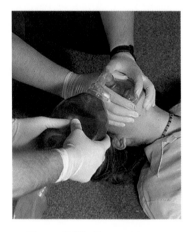

Figure 7.23 *For maximum effectiveness when performing bag-valve mask ventilation, have one person hold the seal around the face mask while another squeezes the bag.*

D.O.T. OBJECTIVES

List the parts of a bag-valve-mask system.

Describe the steps in performing the skill of artificially ventilating a patient with a bag-valve mask for one and two rescuers.

Bag-Valve Mask Ventilation

The **bag-valve mask device** (BVM) consists of a self-inflating bag with a one-way valve and an oxygen reservoir (see Fig. 7.22). This attaches to a soft, pliable mask. The BVM typically delivers less volume than mouth-to-mask ventilation. This type of ventilation is most effective when used by two EMTs. One person may have difficulty squeezing the bag while maintaining an adequate mask seal.

The bag-valve mask device has a self-refilling bag. Some bags are discarded after a single patient use. Others are easily cleaned and sterilized. For optimum results, the bag is connected to an oxygen source. Use a connecting valve that cannot be easily jammed or kinked. The fittings on the bag-valve mask are standardized 15/22 mm. The oxygen inlet and reservoir allow for a high oxygen concentration and an inlet flow of 15 liters per minute. Some devices have pop-off valves. If this type of valve is present, it must be disabled to allow for adequate ventilation. A true one-way valve prevents rebreathing the exhaled air. The BVM will perform in all environmental conditions and temperature extremes.

Bag-valve masks are available in infant, child, and adult sizes. The adult bag holds a maximum volume of about 1600 mL. Insert an oral or nasal airway before using the bag-valve mask device.

When using the BVM device, you must ventilate at a rate of at least 12 times per minute for adults and 20 times per minute for infants and children. Always evaluate the adequacy of the ventilations you are delivering. The chest should rise and fall with each ventilation. The heart rate may return to normal. You may also note an improvement in the patient's color.

Bag–Valve Mask Technique: Nontrauma Patient

Use the following procedure when two EMTs are available and trauma is not suspected (see Fig. 7.23).

EMT #1:

1. Insert the appropriate airway adjunct, if necessary or required by local protocol.

2. Select the correct mask size (adult, infant, or child).

3. Attach the mask and oxygen tubing to the bag-valve mask device. Set the oxygen flow to 15 liters per minute. Confirm that the reservoir is filling properly.

4. Position yourself behind the patient's head.

5. Open the airway using the head-tilt/chin-lift maneuver.

6. Position your thumbs over the top half of the mask. Place your index and middle fingers over the bottom half.

7. Position the top of the mask over the bridge of the nose. Lower the mask over the mouth and upper chin. If the mask has a large round cuff surrounding a ventilation port, center the port over the mouth.

8. Hold the mask securely, bringing the jaw up to the mask with your fourth and fifth fingers.

9. Maintain the mask seal and the open airway.

10. Monitor rising of the chest during each ventilation.

EMT #2:

1. Ensure that the reservoir is refilling properly and confirm that the oxygen flow is 15 liters per minute.

2. Squeeze the bag with both hands until you see the chest rise.

3. Allow the patient to exhale passively.

4. Deliver each ventilation evenly, with a duration of 1.5 to 2 seconds for adults and 1 to 1.5 seconds for children and infants.

5. Continue to ventilate at least every 5 seconds for adults and every 3 seconds for infants and children.

One-person bag-valve mask ventilation. Performing bag-valve mask ventilation with no assistance is sometimes necessary. When no trauma is suspected and you are alone, perform the bag-valve mask technique as follows (see Fig. 7.24):

1. Insert the appropriate airway adjunct, if necessary or required by local protocol.

2. Select the correct mask size (adult, infant, or child).

3. Attach the mask and oxygen tubing to the bag-valve mask device. Set the oxygen flow to 15 liters per minute. Ensure that the reservoir is refilling properly.

4. Position yourself behind the patient's head.

5. Open the airway using the head-tilt/chin-lift maneuver.

EMT Tip

An OPA or NPA may be necessary with the bag-valve mask. However, some patients who need ventilatory assistance cannot tolerate airway adjuncts.

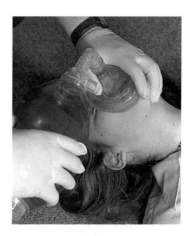

Figure 7.24 *When only one rescuer is available to ventilate a patient, a C-shaped hold on the face mask will help to seal it to the face.*

CD-ROM Link

See the video "Bag-Valve Mask" in the Airway Management chapter and the Video Appendix on the MedEMT CD-ROM for a demonstration of the techniques for using this device.

6. Position the top of the mask over the bridge of the nose. Lower the mask over the mouth and upper chin. If the mask has a large round cuff surrounding a ventilation port, center the port over the mouth.

7. Form a "C" around the ventilation port with the thumb and index finger of one hand. Place your other three fingers under the jaw to maintain the chin lift and to complete the mask seal. Hold the mask securely.

8. Using your other hand, squeeze the bag evenly to deliver each ventilation over 1.5 to 2 seconds for an adult.

9. Monitor the chest rise.

10. Allow the patient to exhale passively with each ventilation.

11. Continue to ventilate at least every 5 seconds for adults or every 3 seconds for children and infants.

> **D.O.T. OBJECTIVE**
>
> Describe the steps in performing the skill of artificially ventilating a patient with a bag-valve mask while using the jaw-thrust maneuver.

Bag–Valve Mask Technique: Trauma Patient

You must take special precautions if trauma or spinal injury is suspected. Establish and maintain in-line spinal stabilization before beginning ventilation (described in Chapter 22). Avoid any movement of the head, neck, or spine before the patient has been fully immobilized on a long backboard.

1. Insert the appropriate airway adjunct, if necessary or required by local protocol.

2. Select the correct mask size (adult, infant, or child).

3. Attach the mask and oxygen tubing to the bag-valve mask device. Set the oxygen flow to 15 liters per minute. Ensure that the reservoir is refilling properly.

4. Position yourself behind the patient's head.

5. Open the airway using the jaw-thrust maneuver.

6. Ask another EMT to manually stabilize the spine by holding the patient's head. If no assistant is present, immobilize the head by holding it between your knees and thighs.

7. Position your thumbs over the top half of the mask and your index and middle fingers over the bottom half.

8. Position the top of the mask over the bridge of the nose. Lower the mask over the mouth and upper chin. If the mask has a large round cuff surrounding a ventilation port, center the port over the mouth.

9. Hold the mask securely, bringing the jaw up to the mask with your fourth and fifth fingers. Avoid tilting the head back or moving the neck.

10. Maintain the mask seal and the open airway.

11. If present, EMT #2 squeezes the bag with both hands until the chest rises. Do this with your free hand if you are working alone.

12. Allow the patient to exhale passively.

13. Deliver each ventilation evenly with a duration of 1.5 to 2 seconds for adults and 1 to 1.5 seconds for children and infants. Continue to ventilate at least once every 5 seconds for adults and every 3 seconds for infants and children.

14. Maintain the airway and continue manual in-line spinal stabilization until the patient has been fully immobilized.

D.O.T. OBJECTIVES

Describe the signs of adequate artificial ventilation using the bag-valve mask.

Describe the signs of inadequate artificial ventilation using the bag-valve mask.

Common Problems with Bag-Valve Mask Ventilation

If the patient's chest does not rise and fall, if you have difficulty maintaining the ventilation rate, or if the pulse does not return to normal, reevaluate your technique:

- Reposition the head to ensure that the airway is opened correctly.

- Check the mask seal. Listen for air escaping under the mask. Reposition your fingers and the mask to tighten the seal.

- Check for airway obstruction. Suction the mouth or use the foreign body airway obstruction maneuver, if necessary.

- Try an alternative method of artificial ventilation, such as a mouth-to-mask or oxygen-powered ventilation device.

- If you have not done so previously, consider the use of an oral or nasal airway adjunct.

If the abdomen is distended or it enlarges during ventilation, air is entering the esophagus and stomach. Check your ventilation technique:

- For nontrauma patients, reposition the head and neck to correct an inadequate head-tilt/chin-lift maneuver.

- For trauma patients, maintain cervical spine control. Reposition the jaw to correct the jaw-thrust maneuver.

- The ventilation rate may be too fast. Ventilate at 12 breaths per minute in adults or 20 per minute in children.
- Tidal volume may be excessive. Deliver the bag volume over a 2-second interval. Wait for exhalation before ventilating again.

Flow-Restricted, Oxygen-Powered Ventilation Device

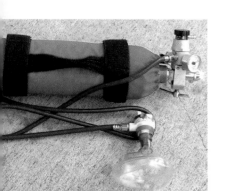

Figure 7.25 *Flow-restricted, oxygen-powered ventilation device.*

The flow-restricted, oxygen-powered ventilation device (FROPVD) was formerly called a demand-valve device (see Fig. 7.25). This device quickly provides oxygen under pressure. The force of the oxygen expands the chest and delivers oxygen to the alveoli.

A properly designed flow-restricted, oxygen-powered ventilation device delivers 100 percent oxygen. It can deliver up to 40 liters per minute in normal environmental conditions or extreme temperatures. There is a trigger next to the mask, so you can use both hands to hold the mask in position. An inspiratory pressure relief valve that opens at 60 cm of water (60 mmHg) will stop the gas flow or vent excessive flow to the atmosphere. An audible alarm will sound if the relief-valve pressure is exceeded.

Ventilation with the FROPVD can cause gastric distention. Improper use could rupture a lung. For this reason, watch out for overinflation of the chest. In addition, never use the device on children or infants.

EMT Alert

The FROPVD should never be used on a patient with COPD or emphysema because the lungs have lost their elasticity and cannot tolerate the pressure of the demand valve.

> **D.O.T. OBJECTIVE**
>
> Describe the steps in artificially ventilating a patient with a flow-restricted, oxygen-powered ventilation device.

Flow-Restricted, Oxygen–Powered Ventilation Device Technique: Nontrauma Patient

Follow this procedure in adults when no spinal injury is suspected:

1. Check the FROPVD unit for proper functioning and adequate oxygen supply. Attach the mask.
2. Open the patient's airway using the head-tilt/chin-lift maneuver.
3. Insert the correct size oral or nasal airway adjunct.
4. Position your thumbs over the top half of the mask. Place your index and middle fingers over the bottom half.
5. Position the top of the mask over the bridge of the nose. Lower the mask over the mouth and upper chin.
6. Hold the mask securely, bringing the jaw up to the mask with your fourth and fifth fingers. Ensure a tight seal.

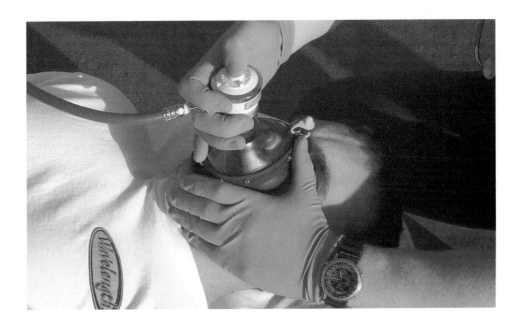

Figure 7.26 *The FROPVD has a trigger on the mask, which allows a single EMT-B to maintain the mask seal with both hands.*

7. Press the trigger until the patient's chest rises (see Fig. 7.26).

8. Release the trigger and allow passive exhalation.

9. Ventilate once every 5 seconds.

Flow-Restricted, Oxygen-Powered Ventilation Device Technique: Trauma Patient

1. Open the airway using the jaw-thrust maneuver.

2. Check the unit for proper functioning and adequate oxygen supply. Attach the mask.

3. Ask another EMT to manually stabilize the spine by holding the patient's head. If no assistant is present, immobilize the head by holding it between your knees and thighs.

4. Position your thumbs over the top half of the mask. Place your index and middle fingers over the bottom half.

5. Position the top of the mask over the bridge of the nose. Lower the mask over the mouth and upper chin.

6. Hold the mask securely, bringing the jaw up to the mask with your fourth and fifth fingers. Ensure a tight seal. Do not tilt the head or neck (see Fig. 7.27).

7. Press the trigger until the patient's chest rises.

8. Release the trigger and allow passive exhalation.

9. Ventilate once every 5 seconds.

10. If necessary, consider using an airway adjunct.

EMT Alert

Using a positive pressure ventilation device can force foreign material deep into the airway if the patient has not been suctioned first.

Figure 7.27 *Maintain spinal immobilization when using the FROPVD on a trauma patient.*

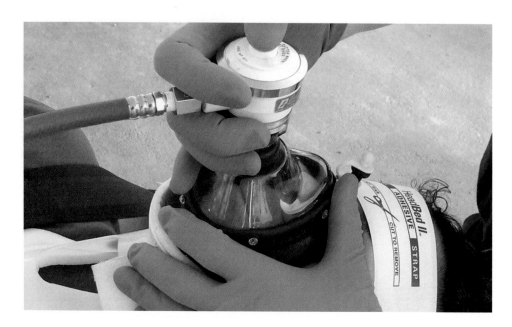

Common Problems with Flow-Restricted, Oxygen-Powered Ventilation

The flow-restricted, oxygen-powered ventilation device is subject to the same problems as the bag-valve mask. Reposition the head or jaw if the chest does not rise and fall or if the abdomen rises. Check the seal of the mask against the face. Look for an airway obstruction. Consider using a different method of ventilation, such as the pocket mask. Occasionally, the oxygen source powering the device runs out. If this occurs, use an alternative ventilation method.

> **D.O.T. OBJECTIVE**
>
> Define the components of an oxygen delivery system.

Supplemental Oxygen

The air we breathe contains a concentration of about 21 percent oxygen. Many illnesses and medical emergencies cause a decrease in the oxygen supplied to the tissues. Other conditions increase the body's demand for oxygen. This can be true even when breathing is adequate. You can improve tissue oxygenation in hypoxic patients by providing supplemental oxygen therapy. Patients who are cyanotic, cool, clammy, or short of breath need supplemental oxygen.

In contrast to assisted artificial ventilation, supplemental oxygen is usually provided at low pressure. It moves passively into the airway during normal inspiration. This delivery method is preferred for patients with good tidal volume and respiratory rates.

Oxygen is stored in cylinders as a compressed gas or liquid. It is delivered to the patient through a pressure regulator and tubing connected to a personal delivery device. In the EMS setting these commonly include the non-rebreathing mask and the nasal cannula.

Oxygen Cylinders

Oxygen cylinders come in several sizes (see Figs. 7.28 and 7.29). Each size is designated by a letter. These steel or aluminum tanks store oxygen at a pressure of 2,000 pounds per square inch (psi) when full. The pressure may vary with the temperature. Medical (USP grade) oxygen containers are often distinguished by their green or gray color. The cylinder sizes common in emergency use are:

- D cylinders, which hold 350 liters
- E cylinders, which hold 625 liters
- M cylinders, which hold 3,000 liters
- G cylinders, which hold 5,300 liters
- H cylinders, which hold 6,900 liters

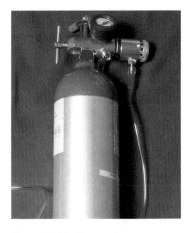

Figure 7.28 *Due to its convenient and manageable size, the D cylinder is the most common oxygen tank used on ambulances.*

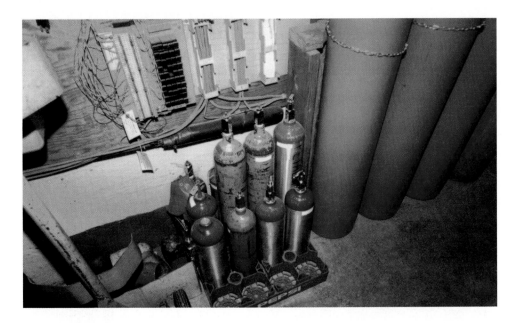

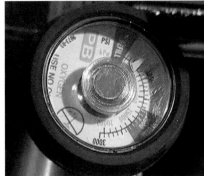

Figure 7.29 *Oxygen tanks come in several sizes for use in the home, on the ambulance, and at the station for resupply.*

Pressure Regulators

A pressure regulator controls the pressure of the cylinder contents. The regulator has a yoke that attaches over the tank valve. The regulator has a gauge that indicates the pressure in the cylinder (see Fig. 7.30). As the tank empties, the pressure changes proportionally. Pressure in a full tank of oxygen is 2,000 psi, regardless of cylinder size. Therefore, a pressure reading of 1,000 psi shows that the cylinder is half full. Most agencies consider tanks to be empty when

Figure 7.30 *A pressure regulator indicates the oxygen pressure in the tank.*

the pressure drops below 500 psi, or some other designated pressure. Agencies with only a few calls a day may require changing the tank after each call. Remove tanks from service according to your agency's protocol.

A high-pressure regulator limits the tank pressure, but has no mechanism for regulating or measuring the flow rate of the oxygen. A therapeutic regulator includes an adjustable flow meter that controls the amount of oxygen delivered to the patient (see Fig. 7.31).

Figure 7.31 *A flow meter attached to the oxygen tank controls the flow rate and quantity of oxygen delivered to the patient.*

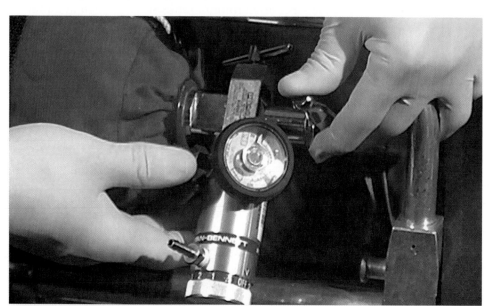

Figure 7.32 *Non-rebreather masks are used for patients who are hypoxic or short of breath.*

EMT Tip

In previous years, EMT-Basics used a variety of devices to provide oxygen. Besides the nasal cannula, simple face masks and Venturi masks were common. Be aware of differences in training and follow your local treatment protocols.

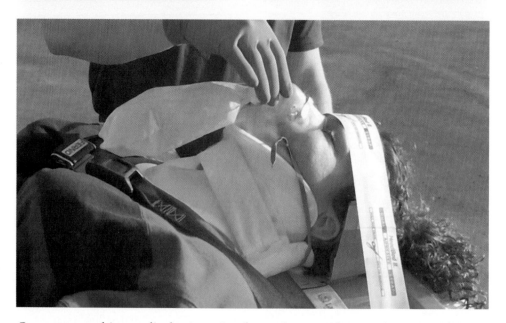

Oxygen stored in a cylinder is emitted as a dry gas. This can be irritating to the patient's mucous membranes and respiratory tract. The addition of a humidifier to the oxygen line can reduce the irritation. This is particularly important during a long transport. Dry oxygen is not harmful for short-term use, so humidifiers may not be used by your agency.

Safety Measures

Oxygen is stored under very high pressure. A punctured tank or broken valve assembly can act like a missile. An oxygen tank has enough projectile force to penetrate a concrete wall. Therefore, always handle cylinders with care. Secure the cylinder in the ambulance or horizontally on a stretcher. Avoid dropping or puncturing the tank or damaging the valve. Always face the regulator away from yourself and others.

Oxygen increases the combustibility of other materials. Therefore, do not allow smoking in an area in which oxygen is being used. Never allow oxygen delivery components to come into contact with oil, grease, petroleum-based lubricants or adhesive tape. This could cause an explosion.

When working with oxygen equipment, use BSI precautions if you are likely to contact body fluids, secretions, or mucous membranes.

> **D.O.T. OBJECTIVES**
>
> Identify a non-rebreather face mask and state the oxygen flow requirements needed for its use.
>
> Identify a nasal cannula and state the flow requirements for its use.
>
> Describe the indications for using a nasal cannula versus a non-rebreather mask.

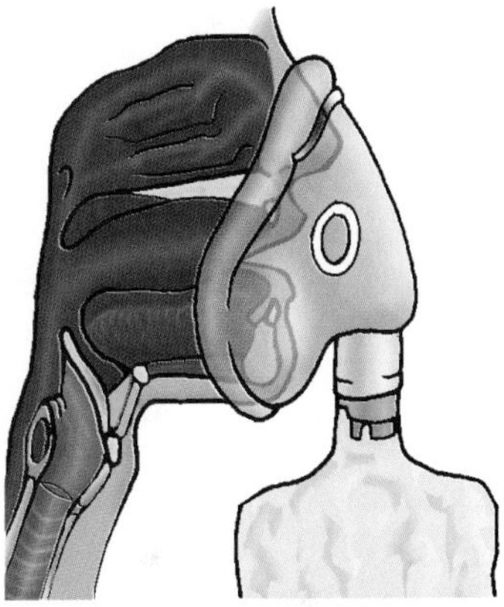

Oxygen Delivery Equipment

A variety of oxygen delivery devices is available. The two most common types are the **non-rebreather mask** and the **nasal cannula**.

The non-rebreather mask is the preferred ventilation device for prehospital care (see Fig. 7.32). The mask is attached to a reservoir bag that is filled from the oxygen cylinder. When the patient inhales, he or she draws oxygen from the bag. The oxygen mixes with a small amount of air that leaks around the edges of the mask. The result is an oxygen concentration of approximately 90 percent (see Fig. 7.33). A one-way valve prevents the patient's exhaled air from mixing with the oxygen in the reservoir. This prevents rebreathing of exhaled air. The non-rebreather mask is connected to oxygen supplied at a rate of 15 liters per minute.

The nasal cannula is an alternative method for administering oxygen (see Fig. 7.34). A cannula is used when the patient requires oxygen at 2 to 6 liters per minute. The cannula is a low-flow system with no oxygen reservoir bag. This decreases the concentration of delivered oxygen to 24 to 44 percent oxygen. Despite this limitation, cannulas are common in the prehospital setting. The

Non-Rebreather Mask | High-flow oxygen delivery device characterized by an inflatable oxygen reservoir bag and a one-way valve that prevents exhaled air from being reinhaled

Nasal Cannula (NAY-zul KAN-yuh-luh) | A tube inserted into the nose to deliver low-flow oxygen

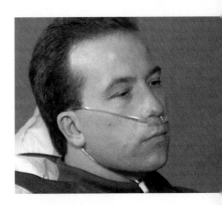

Figure 7.33 *With a correct mask seal, the non-rebreather mask delivers about 90 percent oxygen to the patient.*

Figure 7.34 *The nasal cannula provides low concentration oxygen.*

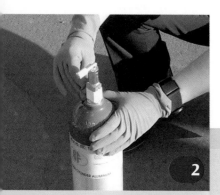

nasal cannula is used when a patient cannot tolerate a non-rebreather mask. If the patient resists the mask, try to coax him or her into accepting it. Use the cannula only when patient cannot tolerate a mask.

Procedures for Administering Oxygen

Before administering oxygen, the cylinder and regulator must be prepared (see Procedure 7.3). When a tank is empty, you must change it and reattach the regulator.

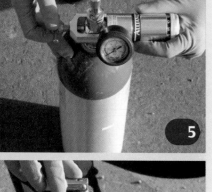

Procedure 7.3 • PREPARING AN OXYGEN CYLINDER

Personal Safety

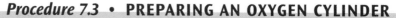

1. Identify the cylinder contents as USP (medical grade) oxygen.

2. Remove the protective seal from the tank valve.

3. Quickly open and then shut the main cylinder valve to remove dust and debris. Direct the valve away from people or objects.

4. Attach the yoke of the regulator-flow meter to the tank, aligning the pins.

5. Tighten the screw by hand.

6. Open the valve to check the pressure of the contents. Replace the tank as required by local protocol (usually below 500 psi).

7. Attach the oxygen delivery device (non-rebreather mask or nasal cannula) to the flow meter. Adjust to the proper flow rate.

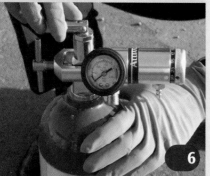

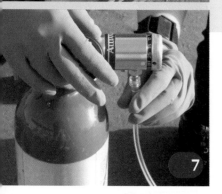

To administer high-concentration oxygen through a non-rebreather mask:

1. Explain to the patient that you will be giving oxygen through a mask. Advise him or her to breathe normally.

2. Select the correct size mask for an adult, child, or infant.

3. Open the flow meter and adjust the flow rate to 15 liters per minute.

4. Fill the reservoir bag before placing the mask on the patient.

5. Position the mask to ensure an adequate seal with the face. Adjust the elastic strap and pinch the nasal bridge piece for a snug fit.

6. Check the flow rate by watching the reservoir bag inflate. If the bag does not reinflate quickly, you may have to increase the flow of oxygen. Adjust the flow to prevent the reservoir bag from collapsing when the patient inhales. Also check for leaks or tears in the reservoir bag.

To administer low-concentration oxygen through a nasal cannula:

1. Position the two prongs of the cannula in the patient's nostrils. The curve of the prongs is designed to follow the natural curve of the nose.

2. Place the tubing over the patient's ears and secure it under the chin with the slip-loop.

3. Open the flow meter. Adjust the flow rate to between 2 and 6 liters per minute.

When oxygen delivery is no longer required:

1. Remove the oxygen delivery device from the patient.

2. Close the main cylinder valve.

3. Allow any oxygen in the regulator to run out until the pressure gauge reads zero.

4. Turn off the flow meter control.

SPECIAL CONSIDERATIONS

You will encounter patients with many special circumstances. In some situations, you must adjust your airway management and assisted artificial ventilation techniques.

Infants and Children

Proper airway and breathing management is the most important aspect of prehospital care for infants and children. The principles of emergency care are the same for children and adults. However, you must remember that infants and children have important anatomical differences. These differences require special consideration when managing the airway and providing artificial ventilation.

Anatomical Differences in Children

The airway structures in children are smaller than adults (see Table 7.4 and Fig. 4.39 in Chapter 4). They become obstructed more readily. A child's trachea is narrow and the tongue takes up proportionally more space in the pharynx. This increases the risk of airway blockage from tissue swelling. For example, epiglottitis, a rapid swelling of the epiglottis, occurs most commonly in young children.

CD-ROM Link

The "Nasal Cannula" video in the Airway Management chapter and the Video Appendix on the MedEMT CD-ROM shows the procedure for providing oxygen using a cannula.

National Registry Examination Tip

Correctly administering supplemental oxygen is a required step in some of the practical skills stations. Review the skills evaluation forms to determine when oxygen is required. Practice proper sizing, setting flow rates, and reassessing respiratory effort for each patient requiring oxygen. When using a nasal cannula, do not exceed the maximum oxygen flow of 6 LPM. Check the oxygen supply to be sure there is enough oxygen to complete a call using a high-flow delivery device. Review the basic safety precautions for working with oxygen. Be sure the oxygen cylinder is secure.

Table 7.4 • AIRWAY ANATOMY IN CHILDREN

Structure	Characteristics in Infants and Children
Head	Proportionally larger than in adults
Nose and Mouth	Nose breathers
Tongue	Proportionally larger tongue than an adult's; pharynx is easily blocked
Trachea	Smaller, narrower trachea that is easily blocked
Cricoid Cartilage	Less rigid and developed than in adults
Chest Wall	Softer and more pliable than in adults
Diaphragm	More dependent on diaphragm for breathing

Cartilage has not yet developed its full rigidity in infants and children. The trachea and cricoid cartilages are soft and flexible. Excessive flexion or hyperextension of the neck may result in airway blockage. The chest wall is soft. This causes infants and children to rely more heavily on their diaphragms for breathing. In addition, the chest wall can be easily overinflated during assisted ventilation. This can lead to lung injury.

Airway Management for Pediatric Patients

Establishing and maintaining the airway may be difficult in pediatric patients. Follow these guidelines:

- Clear any foreign body airway obstruction in infants using a combination of back blows and chest thrusts (see Figs. 7.35 and 7.36).

- When performing the head-tilt/chin-lift maneuver on infants or children with no suspected spinal injury, avoid excessive hyperextension or flexion of the neck. This could cause the trachea to collapse with complete airway

Figure 7.35 *Use back blows to clear foreign body airway obstructions in infants.*

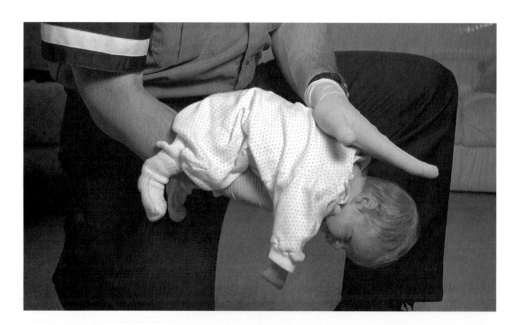

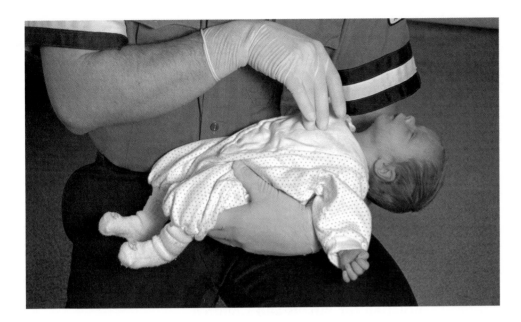

Figure 7.36 *Chest thrusts for airway obstruction and chest compressions for CPR are both performed using two fingers on the anterior chest.*

obstruction. Gently tilt an infant's head back to a "sniffing" or neutral position. Do not overextend the head. When treating small children, tip the head slightly beyond the neutral position. Use only one or two fingers to lift the chin and jaw (see Fig. 7.37). Otherwise, place your hands and perform the maneuver in the same way you would for adults.

- Insert an oral or nasal airway adjunct if you cannot maintain a clear airway by other methods.

Suctioning Infants and Children

When suctioning an infant or child, remember:

- Infants and small children may need frequent suctioning of their nasal passages with a soft catheter.
- Use a rigid tip for suctioning larger children or when the foreign objects in the airway are large or there is a continuous flow of fluids.
- Suctioning may slow the heart rate. This is particularly true if you touch the posterior portions of the airway. Take care not to touch the back of the airway with the catheter. Also avoid causing soft tissue trauma.
- Suction for no more than 5 seconds at a time.
- Carefully observe the patient for signs of deterioration during suctioning. A slow, rapid, or irregular heart rate suggests a dangerous decline in oxygen, which may be caused by excess suction or by stimulation of the airway by the catheter. If this occurs, remove the catheter immediately. Ventilate with oxygen for at least 30 seconds.

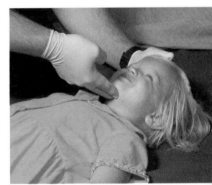

Figure 7.37 *Be sure not to hyperextend the neck of a child when opening the airway with a head-tilt/chin-lift maneuver.*

Breathing Assessment

When a pediatric patient's breathing has been compromised by illness, obstruction, or injury, the child must work hard to attain his or her normal level of oxygenation. This can cause a pediatric patient to tire rapidly and to stop breathing. When assessing an infant or child for signs and symptoms of inadequate breathing, look for:

- A respiration rate outside of the normal range (see Table 7.1)
- Shallow breathing
- Retractions above the clavicles, between the ribs, and below the rib cage
- Nasal flaring
- A seesaw breathing pattern, with the abdomen and chest moving in opposite directions

Artificial Ventilation for Infants and Children

Observe the following differences from the adult procedure:

- Ventilate children for 1 to 1.5 seconds. Adjust the rate of ventilation to once every 3 seconds. This is the equivalent of 20 times per minute.
- Provide only enough tidal volume to make the chest rise. Excessive volume readily leads to gastric distention. This condition compromises ventilation and may cause vomiting. Excessive volume could also injure the child's lungs.
- Continually assess the effectiveness of assisted ventilations. Ventilation is adequate if the chest rises and falls with each ventilation and if the heart rate returns to normal. Ventilation is inadequate if the chest does not rise and fall, if the breathing rate is too fast or slow, or if the heart rate does not return to normal.
- Use a properly sized face mask to ensure a good seal.
- Avoid using a bag-valve mask device with a pop-off valve. This could cause inadequate ventilation. If a pop-off valve is present, close it to disable it.
- Never use a flow-restricted, oxygen-powered ventilation device on children or infants.

Administering Oxygen to Infants and Children

The indications and technique for administering supplemental oxygen to pediatric patients are similar to those used for adults. Consider the following points when administering supplemental oxygen to infants and children:

- Administer high-flow oxygen by non-rebreather mask, if tolerated.
- If the patient will not tolerate having a mask fastened to the head, ask a parent or familiar caregiver to hold the mask in place. An alternative is to hold the mask 1 to 2 inches from the child's face.
- Select a mask that is the correct size for the patient's face.

List the steps in performing the actions taken when providing mouth-to-mouth and mouth-to-stoma ventilation.

Stoma or Tracheostomy Tube

A **stoma** is a surgically created opening into the body. A stoma at the base of the neck is created during a **tracheostomy**. A tracheostomy is performed for some respiratory emergencies. A permanent tracheostomy is done in other situations. A patient with a **laryngectomy** has had the larynx completely or partially removed. These patients also have a tracheostomy.

A short, plastic **tracheostomy tube** may be inserted through a stoma (see Fig. 7.38). This provides unobstructed access to the trachea. Some patients breathe entirely through the stoma or tracheostomy tube. Others breathe some air through their noses and mouths (see Fig. 7.39).

Stoma | *A surgically created opening into a body cavity*

Tracheostomy (tray-kee-AHS-tuh-mee) | *Surgical opening of the trachea*

Laryngectomy (lair-en-JEK-tuh-mee) | *Removal of the larynx*

Tracheostomy Tube | *A specialized airway device for surgical placement into a tracheal stoma; used to maintain an airway passage*

Figure 7.38 *A tracheostomy tube was placed in this patient to provide an open airway.*

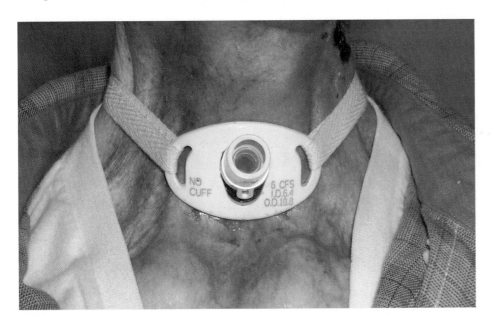

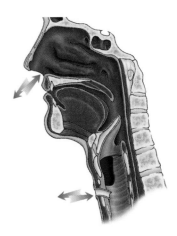

Figure 7.39 *Some patients with a tracheostomy are able to breathe partially through the mouth and nose.*

Avoid getting the stoma area wet. Keep powder from your gloves and other foreign material away from the opening. Anything that enters the stoma will be inhaled directly into the lungs.

A tracheostomy tube is easily obstructed from an accumulation of mucus. Suctioning with a soft catheter may be needed to open the airway. Air can escape through the mouth and nose while ventilating through a stoma or tracheostomy tube. If this occurs, close the mouth and pinch the nostrils to seal them off.

Figure 7.40 *Bag-valve mask ventilation of a stoma patient.*

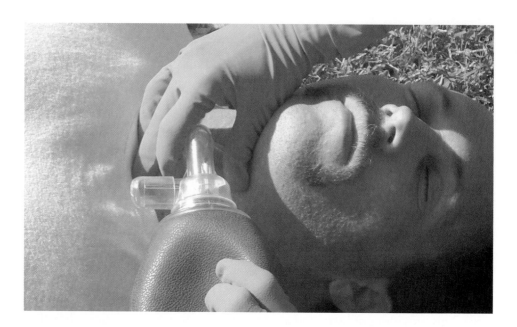

Bag-Valve Mask Ventilation: Stoma or Tracheostomy Tube

Follow this procedure for bag-valve mask ventilation of a stoma or tracheostomy tube (see Fig. 7.40):

1. Suction the stoma or tracheostomy tube with a soft catheter to remove mucus or secretions. Suction for no more than 15 seconds at a time.

2. Keep the head and neck in a neutral position.

3. The bag-valve device is designed to attach directly to a tracheostomy tube. Use an infant or pediatric mask to establish a seal around a stoma.

4. Deliver each ventilation evenly, with a duration of 1.5 to 2 seconds for adults or 1 to 1.5 seconds for children and infants. Continue to ventilate at least once every 5 seconds for adults and once every 3 seconds for infants and children.

5. Allow the patient to exhale passively following each ventilation.

6. Monitor the rising of the chest. If the chest does not rise, manually seal the mouth and nose to prevent air from escaping.

7. If you are unable to artificially ventilate through the stoma, suction with a soft catheter. Then seal the stoma and attempt to ventilate through the mouth and nose.

Facial Injuries

You have learned that the face is very vascular. Because of this, blunt injuries to the face often cause severe swelling or bleeding. This makes airway management challenging. Frequent suctioning may be necessary. Carefully insert an oral or nasal airway to help maintain respirations.

Dental Appliances

Whenever possible, leave dentures in place during ventilation. Dentures provide structure and form to the mouth. This makes sealing a mask much easier. Partial dentures, full dentures, or other dental appliances may become dislodged in an emergency. In extreme situations, they can slip into the throat. Leave dental appliances in place. Remove them if they are loose or if the airway becomes compromised.

National Registry Examination Tip

Practice the skills associated with airway management often. Be sure you understand all the proper ratios, rates, depths, and sequences. Master the skills used for infants and children. Constantly reassess your interventions. Airway position is a common cause of ventilation complications. Remember to take or verbalize infection control precautions at all times.

Chapter Seven Summary

- Airway management is a critical intervention you must master. All prehospital care depends on your ability to maintain the patient's airway. The patient will die if the airway cannot be protected or adequate ventilation is not provided. During your initial assessment, you must establish and maintain an open and clear airway for every patient.

- To ensure an open and clear airway, use the jaw-thrust or the head-tilt/chin-lift maneuver. Suction the patient as necessary. Consider placing an oropharyngeal or nasopharyngeal airway adjunct to maintain airway patency.

- If the patient's breathing rate is within normal limits and air exchange is adequate, consider giving supplemental oxygen, especially if the patient is unresponsive.

- If the breathing rate is too fast (above 24 breaths per minute) or too slow (less than 8 breaths per minute), provide high-flow supplemental oxygen. The nasal cannula is only indicated for patients who cannot tolerate a non-rebreather mask. Also consider assisting the patient's ventilation.

- If the patient's ventilation is inadequate or signs of air hunger are present, you must provide assisted artificial ventilation using the mouth-to-mask technique, bag-valve mask ventilation, or a flow-restricted, oxygen-powered ventilation device. While using these devices, be sure the patient is receiving high-flow oxygen.

- Always use BSI and standard precautions when performing airway management skills.

Key Terms Review

Review Questions

1. All cells require _____ to carry out their vital processes.
   a. Carbon dioxide
   b. Oxygen
   c. Blood
   d. Secretions

2. A patent airway is _____.
   a. Closed
   b. Narrowed
   c. Partially blocked
   d. Open

3. Which is the INCORRECT statement? In infants and children, _____ than in adults.
   a. The head is proportionally larger
   b. The tongue is proportionally larger
   c. The trachea is narrower
   d. The chest wall is firmer

4. When no spinal injury is suspected, open an adult's airway using the:
   a. Jaw-thrust maneuver
   b. Head-tilt/chin-lift maneuver
   c. Oropharyngeal airway adjunct
   d. Crossed-finger technique

5. The term aspiration refers to:
   a. Spirometer dependency
   b. Aspirin overdose
   c. Inhaling foreign matter or fluids into the lungs
   d. Suffocation due to lack of air or oxygen

6. The term bronchus refers to the:
   a. Small branch of the airway which leads to the alveoli
   b. Large airway branch connecting the lungs and trachea
   c. Branch of the trachea that connects to the oropharynx
   d. Branch of the airway connecting the bronchioles and carina

7. The term bronchiole describes a:
   a. Small branch of the airway that leads to the alveoli
   b. Large airway branch connecting the lungs and trachea
   c. Branch of the trachea that connects to the oropharynx
   d. Branch of the airway connecting the bronchioles and carina

8. When suctioning a patient:
   a. Use the same size catheter each time
   b. Start suctioning immediately upon inserting the catheter
   c. Insert the suction catheter into the throat
   d. Suction an adult for no more than 15 seconds

9. Which statement about oropharyngeal airway adjuncts is NOT true?
   a. They keep the tongue away from the back of the throat
   b. They can be used with artificial ventilation
   c. They protect the airway from aspiration
   d. They should be removed if a patient becomes responsive

10. The following statement regarding body substance isolation techniques during assisted artificial ventilation is true:
    a. Wear gloves and eyewear only if available
    b. Always use a mask and gown
    c. Use a HEPA respirator for possible exposure to tuberculosis
    d. Mouth-to-mouth ventilation is safe and convenient

11. Which of the following statements is NOT true about the non-rebreather mask:
    a. It is the preferred method of giving oxygen to pre-hospital patients
    b. It can deliver up to 90 percent oxygen
    c. It is usually connected to oxygen at 6 liters per minute.
    d. It includes an oxygen reservoir bag

Review Questions *(cont.)*

12. Which of the following statements is NOT true? A tracheostomy tube:

    a. Allows unobstructed access to the trachea
    b. May become obstructed with mucus
    c. Rarely needs suctioning
    d. May be found at the base of the neck

13. Your patient is choking on a hamburger. The patient is turning blue. What should be your first action?

    a. Call for law enforcement
    b. Apply gloves and a gown
    c. Perform the Heimlich maneuver
    d. Apply high-flow oxygen

14. With appropriate personal protective equipment already in place, you enter a safe scene where a man is unresponsive and not breathing. He is lying on his kitchen floor. What should be your first action?

    a. Head-tilt/chin-lift maneuver
    b. Jaw-thrust maneuver
    c. Begin artificial respiration
    d. Apply high-flow oxygen

15. Air travels to the lungs through a tube formed by cartilage rings. This tube is called the:

    a. Pharynx
    b. Esophagus
    c. Trachea
    d. Carina

16. The bronchi immediately divide into:

    a. The pulmonary capillaries
    b. The bronchioles
    c. The carina
    d. The alveoli

17. The alveoli are _____.

    a. Small airways
    b. Capillaries through which blood passes to exchange gases
    c. Membranes covering the lungs
    d. Microscopic, elastic air sacs where exchange of gases occurs

18. The part of the airway that can create the greatest resistance to air flow is the _____.

    a. Nasal cavity
    b. Trachea
    c. Bronchi
    d. Bronchioles

19. What occurs during normal inspiration?

    a. Intercostals and diaphragm relax
    b. Intercostals and diaphragm contract
    c. Intercostals relax and diaphragm contracts
    d. Intercostals contract and diaphragm relaxes

20. What occurs during normal expiration?

    a. Intercostals and diaphragm relax
    b. Intercostals and diaphragm contract
    c. Intercostals relax and diaphragm contracts
    d. Intercostals contract and diaphragm relaxes

21. The normal respiration rate for an adult is _____.

    a. 7 to 10 breaths per minute
    b. 12 to 20 breaths per minute
    c. 15 to 30 breaths per minute
    d. 25 to 50 breaths per minute

CASE STUDIES

Airway Management

1
You have just finished your morning equipment checkout. You are dispatched to respond to the college dorm for a patient who is having difficulty breathing. A student who looks scared and excited meets you at the door. She states that her roommate has been having breathing problems all night. When you enter the room, you see a 20-year-old woman kneeling on the floor. She looks exhausted and cyanotic about the lips. She is unable to speak in full sentences. You notice three inhalers lying on the coffee table. The roommate states that her friend has severe asthma. Last month she spent several days in the hospital for asthma complications.

A. Based on the information given, is the patient breathing adequately?

B. How will you further evaluate the adequacy of the patient's breathing?

C. You determine that the patient's respiratory rate is 38. When you listen to her chest with your stethoscope, you hear very little air movement. What is your treatment plan for this patient?

2
Bystanders report an accidental shooting. This is gang territory, so your EMS team suspects that the shooting may not be accidental. Your patient has been shot just above the right ear and is breathing irregularly. His airway is full of blood, so maintaining a patent airway is difficult. Your partner determines that the patient is pulseless.

A. What is your first concern in this situation?

B. Upon arriving at the patient's side, you realize that you did not replace the bag-valve mask used the night before. What other methods of artificial ventilation can you use to treat the patient (list in order of preference)?

C. What steps can you take to improve efforts to ventilate the patient?

D. What body substance isolation precautions should you use when you treat this patient?

3
You and your partner are assigned to standby duty during a large parade in a neighboring town. You have parked the ambulance in a visible spot and are enjoying the parade. Suddenly, you hear someone pounding on the ambulance, yelling for help. You find a father holding his 2-year-old child. He states that the child is highly allergic to bee stings and must have been stung while playing in the grass. The child is blue around the lips and fingers and is breathing very slowly.

A. What is your first step for managing this patient?

B. What special considerations should you observe as you perform the head-tilt/chin-lift maneuver on this child?

Stories from the Field
Wrap-Up

Good airway management skills are essential for providing quality emergency medical care at any level. When uninjured persons begin to vomit, they naturally lean forward or turn their heads to the side. This helps to clear the airway and prevents aspiration. In this situation, your patient is immobilized and cannot clear her airway without assistance. Immediately tilt the backboard to one side. Remove the non-rebreather mask if it restricts the free flow of vomitus. Suction the oropharynx with a large-diameter suction catheter.

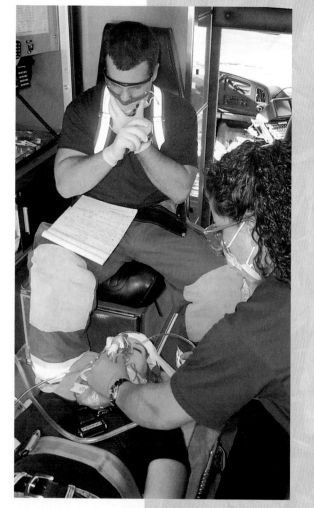

Leave the patient in the tilted position, if possible. After her airway is clear, consider placing an airway adjunct. You must rapidly assess the patient's breathing again. Assisting ventilations with a bag-valve mask device and supplemental oxygen are often necessary. If the patient's breathing is adequate, apply a new non-rebreather mask. Closely monitor the airway and breathing. Consider the patient's injuries life-threatening and transport her to the nearest appropriate facility.

D.O.T. Module 3
Patient Assessment

Chapter 8

Scene Size-Up and Initial Assessment

Stories from the Field

Your squad is dispatched to a local textile plant for a patient with an unknown medical problem. When you arrive at the scene, a security officer meets you. As you cross the plant, the guard starts to take a shortcut through a construction area. He comments, "Don't worry about the danger signs. It's safe." Kim, your partner, refuses to follow the guard unless he finds an alternate route. He reluctantly agrees and leads you around the site.

You arrive to find the patient sitting in a chair in the break area. The patient is leaning forward in the chair. He has his arms extended, holding his knees. You can see that he is in respiratory distress. Kim asks you to give him high-flow oxygen by a non-rebreather mask, and then begins her assessment. The patient's nostrils are flaring with each breath. You can see the muscles between his ribs moving as he breathes. You hear wheezing. Kim questions the patient about his medical history and the current event. He can only speak one or two words at a time. She prepares to urgently move the patient. En route to the hospital, Kim continues to question the patient about his condition. She asks you to take the vital signs frequently.

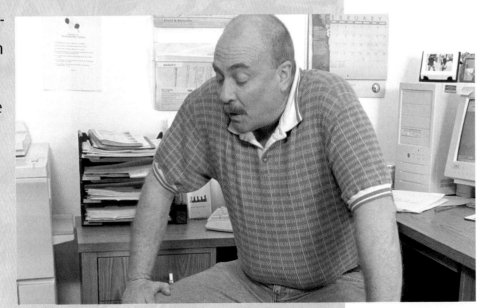

*T*his chapter presents a systematic approach from your arrival at the scene (scene size–up) through performing your initial assessment of a patient's chief complaint. During **scene size-up**, you evaluate scene safety and determine the need for additional resources. During your **initial assessment** of a patient, you will identify and treat life-threatening problems related to the patient's mental status and ABCs (airway, breathing, and circulation). This will help to establish the patient's priority for transport. Patient assessment requires different techniques for an injured patient than for someone with a medical problem. You will evaluate and provide critical interventions based on the mechanism of injury (for trauma patients) or the nature of illness (for medical patients) (see Fig. 8.1). Chapter 9 will present information on performing a focused history and physical exam after the initial assessment.

Scene Size-Up | *The process of determining scene safety, the nature of the problem, total number of patients, and need for additional resources*

Initial Assessment | *Conducted after scene size-up in order to find and manage any life-threatening conditions*

Figure 8.1 *The steps in patient assessment.*

EMT Alert

Note that critical interventions and transport may be required at any time during your assessment. Use the patient's condition as a guide.

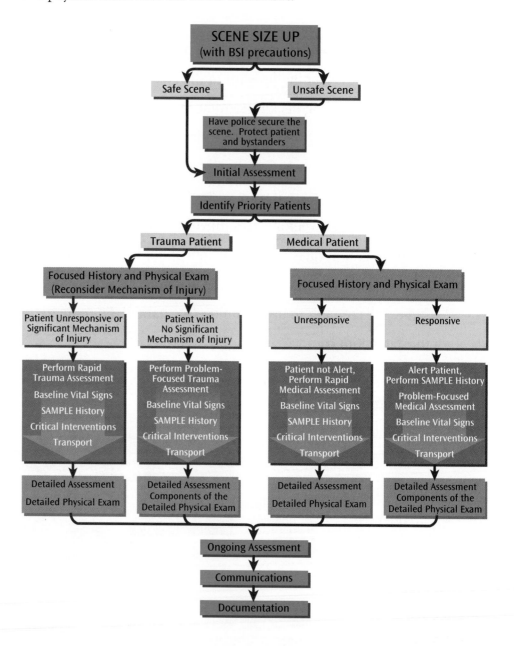

Patient assessment findings are the foundation for many patient care decisions. In mastering this skill, you will ensure consistent, safe, and competent emergency care for every patient you treat. Patient assessment is a series of procedures designed to:

• Identify the patient's chief complaint

• Identify signs and symptoms

• Guide you in setting patient priorities

• Guide your treatment decisions

• Determine the priority for patient transport

National Registry Examination Tip

Review the checkoff sheet for the National Registry's Patient Assessment and Management Practical Examination. Compare the flow with the steps in the Patient Assessment Diagram.

SCENE SIZE-UP

Scene size-up is an important first step in patient assessment (see Fig. 8.2). A complete scene size-up reduces the risk of injury to you and others at the emergency scene.

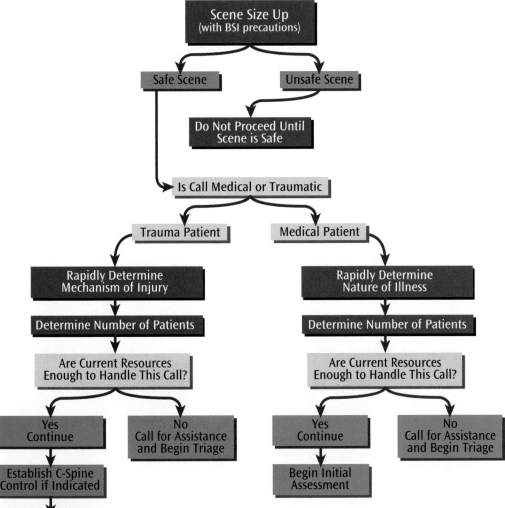

Figure 8.2 *Critical steps in scene size-up.*

Visually assess the scene before you physically approach. Dispatch may have provided some information, but you must reassess the scene upon arrival. When you arrive, you must evaluate:

• Scene safety

• The patient's chief complaint

• The mechanism of injury or the nature of illness

• The need for additional help

D.O.T. OBJECTIVES

Describe common hazards found at the scene of a trauma and a medical patient.

Recognize hazards/potential hazards.

Determine if the scene is safe to enter.

EMT Alert

Never enter a hazardous scene or attempt a hazardous rescue unless you are trained and equipped to do so.

Scene safety assessment is an essential step. Anticipating and eliminating risks ensures the well-being of those on the scene (see Fig. 8.3). Scene safety assessment protects:

• All EMS personnel

• Patient(s)

• Bystanders

You will apply many safety principles to protect yourself and all others at the scene. Safety principles include using personal protective equipment and applying BSI precautions.

Figure 8.3 *Always assess scene safety before approaching.*

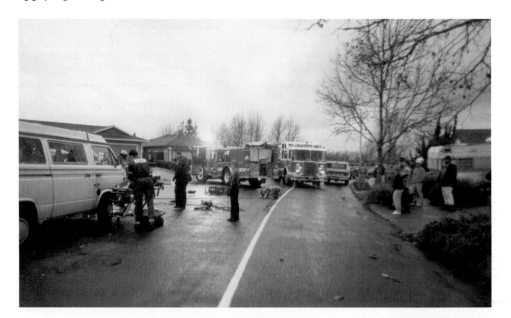

Table 8.1 • SENSORY CLUES TO AN UNSAFE SCENE

Sense	Clues
Sight	Unstable vehicles, structures, ground
	Hazardous material spills or placards
	Dark, poorly lit areas
	Presence of drug paraphernalia or gang materials
	Presence of visible or overtly displayed weapons
	Many bystanders or onlookers
Smell	Unusual or unclassifiable odors
	Smell of smoke, natural gas, propane, wires burning, drug use
Hearing	Sounds of an argument or fight
	Loud, boisterous conduct
	Gunfire or explosions
	Comments from bystanders or onlookers
Tactile	Presence of concealed weapons on patient
Intuition	If your intuition (based on your experience) tells you a scene may be unsafe, be especially alert even if no other clues are present

Personal Protection

Upon arrival at the scene of an emergency, your first priority is to assess scene safety. Determine whether the scene is safe or unsafe (see Table 8.1). Never enter an unsafe or unstable scene. This is the most important precaution you will take. You cannot help the patient if you become a patient yourself.

The following scenes may have particular hazards or concerns:

- Crash and rescue scenes
- Presence of toxic substances
- Low oxygen areas
- Unstable surfaces
- Crime scenes

Any scene may be safe initially, then become unsafe while you are caring for the patient. Continually reassess scene safety. If the scene becomes unsafe, use an emergency move to remove the patient as quickly as possible. Maintain as much spinal immobilization as you can under the circumstances. Always make sure that you have a safe route of exit. Never allow family members, suspects, onlookers, other persons, or objects to block your exit. Barroom scenes can be unpredictable and may turn violent quickly. Waiting for your eyes to adjust to the low lighting in the room may delay patient care. Work as efficiently and unobtrusively as possible.

EMT Alert

Use body substance isolation and standard precautions routinely for all patients. This includes use of gloves, gowns, eye protection, and masks, if necessary. Chapter 2 lists guidelines for prevention of transmission of bloodborne pathogens.

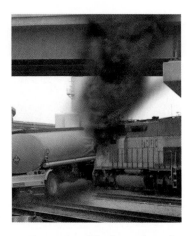

Figure 8.4 *The hazards multiply when a tanker collides with a train.*

Taking body substance isolation precautions is an essential part of scene safety. Take steps to reduce the risk of exposure to harmful substances before you approach the patient.

Crash and Rescue Scenes

When approaching the scene of a motor vehicle collision, evaluate the area for real or potential hazards to the patient, EMS responders, and the ambulance (see Figs. 8.4 and 8.5). Potential hazards include:

- Vehicle instability
- Broken utility poles, exposed or downed power lines
- Sharp or broken material
- Leaking fuel
- Hazardous material spills
- Smoke
- Fire

Traffic moving past an accident scene is one of the greatest hazards to which emergency personnel are exposed.

Figure 8.5 *Severely damaged vehicles present many potential safety hazards.*

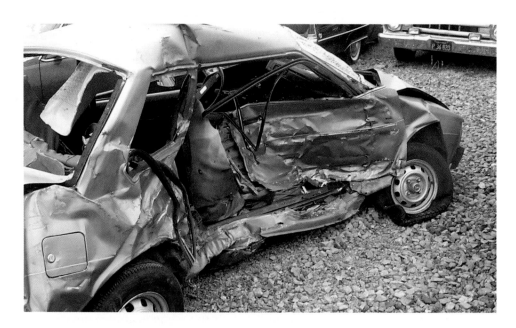

Visually assess vehicle crash scenes to identify areas in which you might lose your footing. Coolant, oil, gasoline spills, or broken glass may make walking a challenge. In addition, be careful that traffic has been safely diverted around the scene. Watch for other hazards such as downed power lines and hot metal when on scene of a motor vehicle crash.

Toxic Substances and Low-Oxygen Areas

Assess the scene for toxic substances and the possibility of low oxygen levels. These problems are possible on the scene of:

- Toxic chemical spills or leaks
- Fires
- Confined spaces

Suspect toxic substance exposure if many persons at the scene have similar respiratory symptoms. Some of these individuals may be in respiratory distress. If you suspect the presence of toxic substances, you must wear respiratory protection. Additional protective equipment may also be necessary. If you suspect hazardous materials are involved, do not enter unless you have been adequately trained and are properly equipped.

Unstable Surfaces and Slopes

Environmental hazards at some scenes may interfere with your ability to safely provide care. Hazards that may interfere with your ability to care for the patient are:

- Unstable surfaces
- Uneven terrain
- Ice
- Bodies of water

If the emergency scene is on or near a cliff or slope, take special precautions to ensure safety of the patient and your crew (see Fig. 8.6). Watch for heavy objects that may fall or move during rescue. Move the patient away from unstable or dangerously uneven ground, if this is safe. Specialized training is required for high-angle rescue. Perform this type of rescue only if you have been trained and have the necessary safety equipment and sufficient personnel.

Ice

If you are working in an area with snow and ice, take safety precautions to stabilize your footing. Apply sand, salt, or gravel to ice-coated surfaces. Try to stand on a tarp or a rug while caring for the patient. If possible, avoid walking onto frozen bodies of water. Instead, call for a specialized rescue team to remove a patient from this potentially dangerous situation. Always follow local protocols. Advanced training for emergency response and rescue in extreme weather conditions may be available in your area.

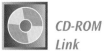

CD-ROM Link

See the "Fallen Climber" and "Climber's Descent" videos in the Authentic Emergency Scenes section of the Video Appendix on the MedEMT CD-ROM for a view of how rugged terrain affects patient care.

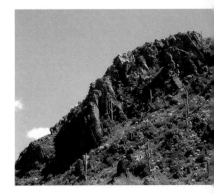

Figure 8.6 *Watch your footing at all times.*

Water

Never attempt a water rescue alone. If assisting with a water rescue, always wear a personal flotation device (PFD). Work from a position of safety and avoid entering the water. Attempt to reach the patient by throwing flotation devices or ropes. You may be able to reach the patient by extending a pole. Water rescues require special training (see Fig. 8.7). If you are not trained, call for assistance from specialized rescue teams.

After the patient has been removed from the water, you will assume care. Always assess for signs and symptoms of hypothermia (discussed fully in Chapter 17). This is a common problem requiring special treatment. It is often not recognized in warm bodies of water. Hypothermia can occur in any body of water in which the water temperature is below body temperature.

Crime Scenes

The most important step in crime scene size-up is ensuring your personal safety. Do not knowingly enter a crime scene until law enforcement personnel arrive and secure the scene. When in doubt, call law enforcement and wait. Stay away from the scene until police have verified that the scene is secure.

After scene safety, your primary responsibility is patient care. Focus on the mechanism of injury, emergency care, and transport decisions. Law enforcement will focus on the details of the crime. However, try to preserve the integrity of any evidence as much as possible (discussed further in Chapter 3).

When approaching a potential crime scene, remember that firearms may be involved. Remain outside the *killing zone*. This is an area controlled by hostile fire. The area is approximately 100 to 150 yards away and 120 degrees in front of the suspected site of firearms.

Remember the following about crime scenes:

- Never enter a crime scene until it has been secured by law enforcement
- Do not touch or move anything unless absolutely necessary for patient care
- Preserve any evidence on the victim's clothing by cutting around bullet holes, knife tears, etc.
- Preserve any bindings, gags, ropes, etc., and carefully document any movement or removal of these items
- Document all actions and surroundings to the best of your ability
- Restrict the number of EMS personnel allowed into the crime scene, and carefully record crew names
- Do not use the telephone or bathroom without explicit permission from law enforcement

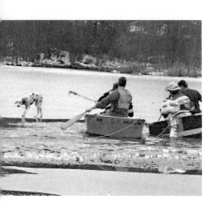

Figure 8.7 *Some specialized rescue teams use dogs for their tracking ability.*

Arrive at a crime scene quietly, initially parking a safe distance away. Do not approach until law enforcement has arrived and secured the scene. Observe the scene and approach only if you believe it is safe. A group of bystanders or onlookers in the area does not mean that a scene is safe. The group should be considered a possible threat to your safety as well. There is further discussion about gangs in the Enhanced Study section at the end of this chapter.

When approaching a patient at a crime scene, remember the following safety measures:

- Walk single-file. At night, the lead person holds a flashlight by his or her side. Approaching in this manner keeps you from being singled out as a target (see Fig. 8.8).

- Avoid standing directly in front of doors or windows, especially when knocking to gain entrance (see Fig. 8.9).

- Note possible protective barriers in case taking cover becomes necessary.

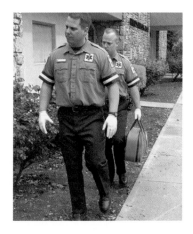

Figure 8.8 *Approach all potential crime scenes with caution.*

Figure 8.9 *Never stand in front of doors or windows.*

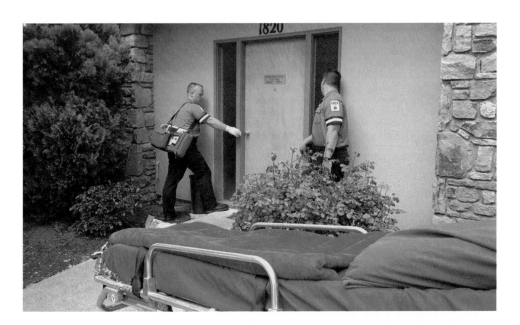

**CD-ROM
Link**

For a true picture of the risk of exposure to blood, see the "Stabbing" video in the Authentic Emergency Scenes section of the Video Appendix on the MedEMT CD-ROM.

Understanding the difference between cover and concealment is important to EMS providers in potentially hostile situations. Taking cover means situating yourself behind an object capable of withstanding a hit from a weapon. If you are behind an adequate cover, you will not be injured. Items such as a vehicle's engine block or a brick wall can be used for cover. Concealment prevents a potential assailant from seeing you. It provides almost no protection from firearms. You should not feel secure because you are sitting in the ambulance. Ambulances are not constructed to provide cover.

Protecting the Patient

Environmental factors can greatly influence the patient's comfort and safety. A heavy, fireproof blanket provides excellent protection against the most common scene hazards. Protecting the patient's privacy helps to prevent stress and embarrassment during an emergency.

Protect the patient from:

• Extremes of cold or heat

• Wet weather

• Danger from traffic or extrication equipment

• Public attention

• News media

Protecting Bystanders

Try to keep bystanders away from dangerous areas. You must also try to keep them at a safe distance so that they do not interfere with the rescue. Allow bystanders to assist if the task is not too dangerous. They can provide crowd control or help to move the patient, if needed. If you ask bystanders for assistance, explain their duties carefully.

Members of the news media may arrive at the scene of many serious incidents. Reporters listen to scanners and often arrive before patients are transported from the scene. In some states, members of the media can cross barrier tape and enter hazardous scenes at their own risk. Avoid concentrating on what the media is doing. Remain focused on providing good patient care and protecting the patient's privacy. Cover the patient's body, exposing only the area you are working on. If media representatives are in the way or interfere with patient care, request assistance from your supervisor or law enforcement.

Most agencies have a public relations or public information officer. These individuals work with the media and are trained to answer sensitive questions. Never release information about a patient or incident on your own. Refer media representatives to the designated person in your agency.

CHIEF COMPLAINT

After ensuring scene safety and taking BSI precautions, you must determine the patient's chief complaint. A medical patient has complaints, signs, or symptoms caused by an underlying illness. **Trauma** patients have complaints, signs, or symptoms caused by external forces, such as a fall or vehicle collision.

Trauma | *A serious injury to the body or a severe emotional shock*

If the chief complaint is medical, you must determine the **nature of illness**. Ask about the nature of the chief complaint by asking, "How can I help you today?" and "Why was EMS called?" Use the SAMPLE and OPQRST questions to elaborate on the patient's chief complaint. Later in the chapter, we will return to specifics of assessing a medical patient (see the section called Initial Assessment).

Nature of Illness | *The type of condition or complaint a medical patient has*

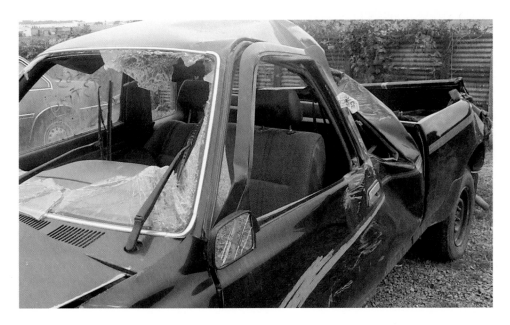

Figure 8.10 *Pickup truck involved in a rollover.*

For trauma cases, you must determine the **mechanism of injury (MOI)**. Observe the scene and ask questions about the specific forces or events that caused the injury. The mechanism of injury and forces involved will influence the type of injury sustained. Determining the mechanism of injury will provide clues to the patient's problem (see Fig. 8.10). The following section discusses the mechanism of injury and how this relates to assessing a trauma patient.

Mechanism of Injury (MOI) | *The forces involved or factors influencing an injury*

 EMT Alert

Remember that any trauma patient may have a cervical spine injury that requires spinal stabilization.

D.O.T. OBJECTIVES

Discuss common mechanisms of injury/nature of illness.

MECHANISM OF INJURY

Understanding the mechanism of injury is critical to assessing and treating the trauma patient's injuries (see Table 8.2). Hospital personnel rely heavily upon the information you provide about the scene of an accident and the mechanism of the injury. Upon arrival, note:

• The type of traumatic event, such as motor vehicle collision, fall, or gunshot wound

Table 8.2 • EVALUATING THE MECHANISM OF INJURY

Type of Trauma	Questions
Motor Vehicle Collisions	How fast was the vehicle traveling? What part of the vehicle was impacted? How extensive is the damage? Were passengers restrained? Did the airbags activate? Were passengers ejected from the vehicle? Are passengers trapped in the vehicle?
Falls	How far did the patient fall? What body part did the patient land on? What type of surface did the patient fall onto? Is the patient having head, neck, or back pain? Did the patient lose consciousness?
Penetrating Wounds	What size and type of weapon or object is causing the injury? Does the patient have any hidden wounds? Does the wound go all the way through a part of the body?

- An estimation of the energy exchanged; for example, the speed of the vehicle upon impact, distance of the fall, or size and type of weapon
- The impact of the patient with the object, such as a car, airbag, knife, bat, or bullet

This information is important in identifying hidden injuries in a trauma patient (see Fig. 8.11).

Blunt Trauma

Blunt Trauma | *Injury caused by non-penetrating forces*

Blunt trauma is a common cause of hidden injury. These injuries are caused by a force that strikes the body, but does not penetrate the skin. Blunt trauma results from many mechanisms of injury. The most common are motor vehicle collisions and falls (see Fig. 8.12). Usually, blunt trauma affects the head, cervical spine, chest, abdomen, and pelvis. Injuries commonly caused by blunt trauma are closed fractures, internal bleeding, and respiratory compromise.

Motor Vehicle Collisions

Three impacts occur in every motor vehicle collision (MVC). This may be called a motor vehicle accident (MVA) in your area (see Fig. 8.13). First, the vehicle collides with another vehicle or object. Then the occupant moves within the vehicle, colliding with the interior (dash, side posts, floorboards, etc.). The type of passenger restraint influences the extent of this impact. Restraints include lap or shoulder belts, air bags, child seats, and combinations of these. Finally, the occupant's internal organs collide with the surrounding body

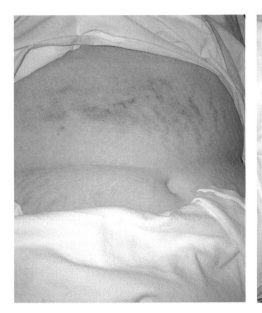

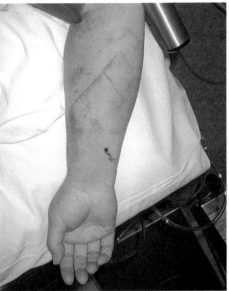

Figure 8.11 *Contusions are clues to the mechanism of injury. This patient's abdomen collided with the steering wheel (left) and his arm impacted the dashboard (right).*

framework (e.g., the heart compresses against the chest wall, or the aorta is torn within the chest cavity).

You will get an idea of the type of injuries to expect by assessing the damage inside the car. During your assessment, inspect the steering wheel and patient compartment to estimate the force of potential injuries. Lift and look beneath the air bag after the patient has been removed. Inspect the steering column, dash panel, and floorboard for clues suggesting additional injuries. Any visible deformation of the steering wheel suggests possible internal injuries.

Different types of motor vehicle collisions result in different types of injuries. For example, you may see imprints in the dashboard where the occupant's knees have hit. The head may hit the windshield, causing head trauma. An

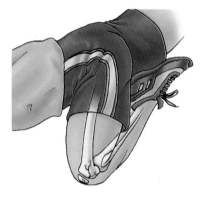

Figure 8.12 *Blunt trauma to the knee resulting in a fractured patella and femur.*

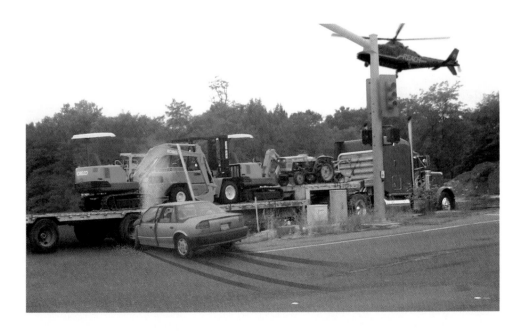

Figure 8.13 *Vehicle collisions can cause both external and internal injuries.*

CD-ROM Link

See the animations in the "Mechanism of Injury" section in Chapter 8 and the Video Appendix on the MedEMT CD-ROM. These animations depict the consequences of various vehicle accidents.

injury of this type may also cause hyperextension or compression of the cervical vertebrae. Head impact can cause a spiderweb-shaped break in the windshield. Body impact may bend the steering wheel. The Enhanced Study section at the end of this chapter goes into more detail about injuries from different types of motor vehicle collisions.

The fact that a patient was wearing a seat belt does not automatically rule out serious injuries. Seat belts, even when properly used, can cause injury to a patient's pelvis, abdomen, chest, or shoulders. Without seat belts, air bags may not provide adequate protection against injury. In some crashes, a patient can still strike the steering wheel after the bag has deflated. Air bags can also cause serious injuries, especially to children and small adults.

Motorcycle and Bicycle Accidents

Cyclists are only protected from impact by their clothing and helmets. The most common injury in cyclists is a closed head injury. (Management of head injuries is discussed in Chapter 22.) Wearing a helmet reduces the mortality rate. Several types of injuries are possible. The nature of the injury depends on:

- Speed
- Type of impact
- Nature of impact (whether a car, truck, brick wall, etc. was hit)
- How far the patient was ejected

Cyclists are usually involved in frontal or side-impact collisions. In either case, the cyclist often suffers lower extremity injuries from the initial impact. The cyclist is usually ejected upon impact. If the impact is frontal, the ejected victim may incur femur fractures from being thrown over the handlebars. After the initial impact, the cyclist may strike the car's windshield, the car's roof, or the road surface. The patient usually lands on his or her head. This results in severe head, neck, and spinal trauma. Ejected cyclists may be found several yards from the scene of the accident. If a cyclist is missing from the immediate scene, make sure a thorough search of the area is conducted.

Falls

Falls are the most common causes of injuries in the United States. The outcome of a fall can be affected by the:

- Distance fallen
- Type of surface impacted
- Part of the body that hits first

A fall of more than 10 feet for a child or 20 feet for an adult usually requires evaluation at a trauma center. If no trauma center is available, transport the patient to the community facility with the highest level of care. Follow local

EMT Tip

If a patient falls from a height greater than his or her own standing height, he or she should be evaluated at an emergency department. (Follow local protocol.)

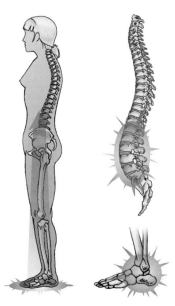

Figure 8.14 *Feet-first falls often cause injury to the heel and lumbar region.*

protocol. The patient may have serious internal injuries that are not readily apparent. A feet-first fall often causes skeletal injuries to the heel (see Fig. 8.14). The force of the impact may cause lumbar compression injuries. A head-first fall usually causes injury to the head and cervical spine.

Penetrating Trauma

Penetrating trauma occurs when the skin is broken by an object or projectile. The object could be a knife. A bullet or shrapnel are examples of projectiles. Penetrating trauma readily damages internal structures. You may be called upon to assess patients with stab or gunshot wounds. Patients with these injuries often develop internal bleeding, external bleeding, shock, and respiratory compromise. The extent of the injury depends on the type of projectile, its size, how fast it is traveling when it hits the body, and the area of the body penetrated.

Cavitation is tissue compression caused by the pressure wave of a projectile. Damage from cavitation is increased by:

- A large frontal area of the projectile at the point of impact (from a large projectile or a bullet that is designed to spread out or explode upon impact)
- High density of the tissue it enters
- Higher projectile velocity

Thus, a large bullet traveling through dense tissue at high speed will cause the most damage.

Exit wounds are usually larger than entrance wounds (see Fig. 8.15). This is due to the surface area, tissue density, and velocity through which the energy is dissipated. Look under the armpits and breasts, on the back and buttocks, and in the groin. Note all wounds on the patient. You aren't expected to classify wounds as entrance or exit wounds in your documentation.

Penetrating Trauma | *An injury caused by an object that pierces the skin or other body structure*

Cavitation | *Tissue compression and cavity formation caused by the pressure of a projectile entering the body*

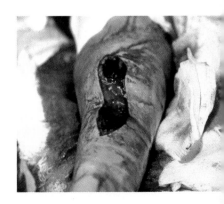

Figure 8.15 *Exit wound.*

Weapons

Weapons that cause penetrating trauma are divided into three categories, based on their initial energy or speed:

- Low-energy weapons, such as knives or other sharp objects
- Medium-energy weapons, such as handguns
- High-energy weapons, such as hunting or military rifles

Always relay information to hospital personnel about the length and type of knife used to inflict the patient's injury. A long kitchen or hunting knife causes more damage than a short pocketknife. However, the external wound may look the same. Never remove an impaled object, such as a knife, from a patient. Removing an impaled object may worsen bleeding. Exceptions to this general rule include impaled objects in the cheek and those that restrict the airway or keep the provider from performing chest compressions. Bring the knife to the emergency department if it is found outside the body. In some communities, law enforcement will transport the weapon. Management of impaled objects is discussed in Chapter 20.

Firearms are medium- and high-energy weapons (see Figs. 8.16 and 8.17). The severity of injuries is determined by the:

- Type of bullet
- Bullet caliber
- Distance fired
- Location of the shooter

If you are unfamiliar with weapons, ask a law enforcement officer about the weapon involved.

Figure 8.16 *Entrance and exit wounds caused by a medium-energy weapon.*

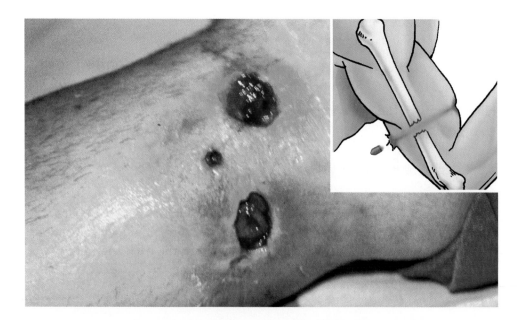

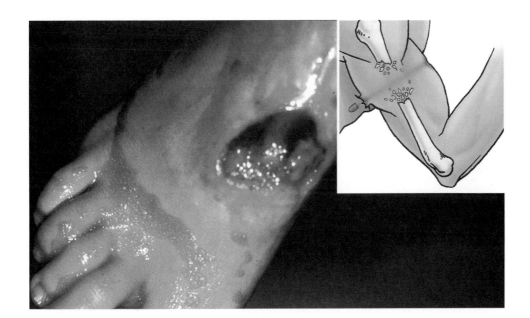

Figure 8.17 *Wound caused by a high-energy weapon.*

Figure 8.17 *Wound caused by a high-energy weapon.*

Blast Injuries

Blast injuries are caused by powerful explosions (see Fig. 8.18). There are three distinct patterns of explosive injury:

- Injuries caused by the initial pressure wave
- Injuries caused by objects becoming projectiles from the blast wave
- Injuries that occur if an individual is thrown a distance by the blast wave

A pressure wave occurs immediately after an explosion. This wave has the same effect as any other blunt trauma on the body. Internal injuries from the blast wave are usually the most severe. However, they may not be the most obvious. These injuries often affect the hollow organs, such as the ears, lungs, intestines, and stomach. The eardrum is the most vulnerable to pressure and may rupture.

The victim may also be injured by objects within the blast wave. Many soft tissue injuries occur when the body is struck by flying glass, metal, and other items. These injuries are obvious, but are usually not the most serious.

Additional injuries occur when the patient is part of the blast wave. In strong explosions, the patient may be thrown a significant distance. Head, neck, and spinal injuries are common from explosions.

Compounding Factors

Assess every trauma patient thoroughly for multiple injuries. A coexisting medical illness may have caused the injury. For example, a heart attack (myocardial infarction) could lead to a vehicle collision. Low blood sugar in a

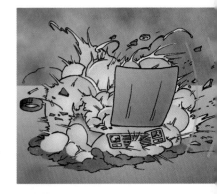

Figure 8.18 *Blast injuries can be due to the pressure wave, propelled objects, and the individual being launched.*

diabetic can cause a fall. Always consider the possibility of traumatic injury first, then look for medical causes of the accident. Be aware that preexisting medical problems can also complicate traumatic injuries.

D.O.T. OBJECTIVES

Discuss the reason for identifying the total number of patients at the scene.

Explain the reason for identifying the need for additional help or assistance.

NEED FOR ADDITIONAL HELP

EMT
Tip

The best time to call for additional help is when you arrive at the scene, before getting out of the ambulance.

The last element of your scene size-up is to count the number of patients quickly. Next, you must decide whether additional help or specialized resources are needed (see Figs. 8.19 and 8.20). You may need to request:

- Advanced life-support backup
- Aeromedical (helicopter) evacuation
- Specialized rescue teams
- Fire departments
- Law enforcement
- Hazardous materials teams

Figure 8.19 *In mass casualty incidents, helicopters are often used for patient transport.*

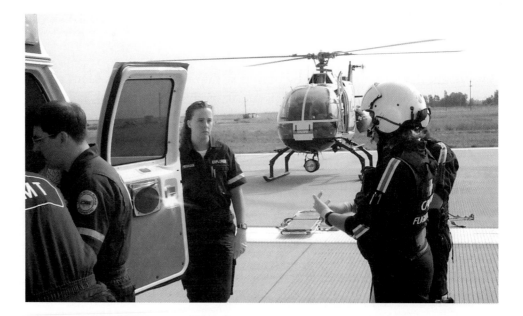

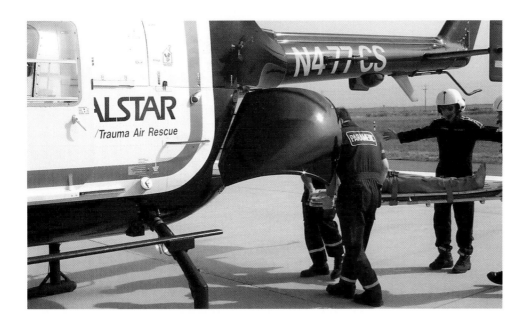

Figure 8.20 *Airlifting the patient can greatly reduce transport times to the trauma facility.*

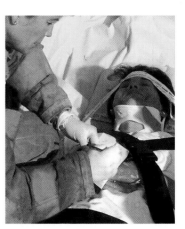

Figure 8.21 *Treatment is prioritized by writing descriptions on a triage tag.*

When the scene includes multiple casualties, follow triage protocols before beginning any extended patient care. **Triage** enables EMS responders to do the greatest amount of good for the greatest number of people in the shortest possible time. You will quickly assess all potential patients. Sort the patients into categories, based on the severity of their injuries. Prioritize each patient for treatment and transport (see Figs. 8.21 and 8.22). Triage identifies patients with life-threatening emergencies, enabling you to provide critical **interventions**. It also helps you to determine transport priorities. Triage is covered in detail in Chapter 24.

Call for additional help early in the response. The sooner you call for additional help, the sooner it will arrive.

Figure 8.22 *Treating patients at a mass casualty event.*

Triage | *The process of prioritizing patients to receive the appropriate level of care or transportation*

Interventions | *Procedures done in an effort to improve the patient's condition*

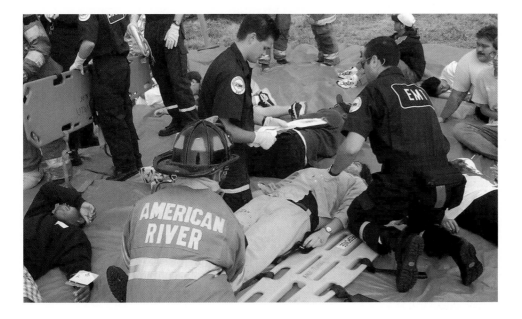

> **D.O.T. OBJECTIVE**
>
> Explain the value of performing an initial assessment.

INITIAL ASSESSMENT

The purpose of the initial assessment is to identify and treat life-threatening problems related to the ABCs (see Table 8.3). The steps of the initial assessment include:

- Form a general impression
- Assess mental status
- Assess the airway
- Assess the breathing
- Assess circulatory status
- Identify priority patients

Sometimes, you may need to begin an intervention before proceeding with the complete assessment. In Stories from the Field, during the scene size-up, you found a man obviously in respiratory distress. He was immediately placed on high-flow oxygen. Once his airway was managed, the assessment could be continued. This assessment and your earliest interventions may save a person's life or prevent serious disability.

Table 8.3 • **COMPONENTS OF THE INITIAL ASSESSMENT**

Assessment Step	Notes
Form a General Impression	
Assess the Mental Status	AVPU evaluation—Alert, Verbal, Pain, Unresponsive
Assess the Airway	Assume control of the cervical spine, if indicated Open the airway using the appropriate maneuver Ensure that the airway is free from obstruction; provide suction if needed
Assess the Breathing	If adequate, consider providing high-flow oxygen by non-rebreather mask If inadequate or absent, assist ventilation at the proper rate with supplemental oxygen
Assess the Circulation	Assess for the presence of a pulse. If pulseless, consider use of AED (see Chapter 13) Assess for and control major bleeding
Determine the Patient's Priority for Transport	

The initial assessment is presented here as a step-by-step process. When you are actually performing the initial assessment, you may perform more than one step at a time (for example, skin temperature can be checked at the same time you are taking a pulse or counting respirations). Conduct each assessment systematically, following a consistent, logical pattern. The initial assessment should be completed as quickly and efficiently as possible.

Whether a patient's chief complaint is due to illness or trauma, you will always assess the ABCs. You can establish cervical spine control, assess mental status, and assess the airway simultaneously.

D.O.T. OBJECTIVE

Summarize the reasons for forming a general impression of the patient.

Forming a General Impression

The first step in the initial assessment is to form a **general impression** of the patient. You will determine the seriousness of the patient's condition, the priority for emergency care, and the priority for transport. Your general impression is based on an immediate assessment of the environment and the patient's chief complaint.

General Impression | *The first step in initial assessment to quickly identify what is wrong and how serious it is; a time to use instinct and draw upon past experience*

You must quickly determine whether the patient has a life-threatening condition. If a life-threatening condition is found, begin treatment immediately.

The general impression will also identify:

• The mechanism of injury or nature of illness
• The patient's age and gender

You will become skilled at forming a general impression as you gain experience.

As part of the general impression, determine whether there is a potential for cervical spine injury. If you believe a potential for spinal injury exists, immobilize the spine immediately (refer to Chapter 22). Next, you will assess the patient's mental status.

D.O.T. OBJECTIVES

Discuss methods of assessing altered mental status.

Differentiate between assessing the altered mental status in the adult, child, and infant patient.

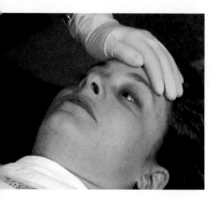

Figure 8.23 *The patient's mental status is important for determining the seriousness of his or her condition.*

AVPU | *Memory aid used to help categorize a patient's level of responsiveness: A = Alert, V = responds to Verbal stimuli, P = responds to Pain, U = Unresponsive*

CD-ROM Link

See the "AVPU" video in Chapter 8 and the Video Appendix on the MedEMT CD-ROM for a demonstration of this assessment method.

Assessing Mental Status

Assess the patient's mental status and responsiveness (see Fig. 8.23). This information is valuable in determining the seriousness of the illness or injury. Assessment of mental status will also be part of your ongoing assessment. Changes in mental status can alert you to changes in the patient's condition.

When you approach the patient, state your name, identify yourself as an EMT, and explain that you are there to help. Determine the patient's level of responsiveness using the **AVPU** method (see Table 8.4).

- Is the patient alert? A patient is alert if he or she is communicative and awake. An alert patient requires no stimulation to respond to your questions or commands. Depending on their ability to speak, alert patients may or may not be able to answer questions about who they are, where they are, what time it is, and what has happened.

- Does the patient respond to verbal stimuli? A patient is responsive to verbal stimuli if he or she responds only to verbal commands or requests. The patient offers no independent action or communication.

- Does the patient respond to painful stimuli? A patient who is not alert and does not respond to verbal commands may be responsive to painful stimuli. To determine responsiveness to painful stimuli, firmly rub the sternum, stimulate the palm of the hand or arch of the foot, or pinch the patient's neck muscles and observe for a response (see Fig. 8.24).

- Is the patient unresponsive? A patient who fails to respond to both verbal and painful stimuli is unresponsive.

You can use the AVPU method of evaluating mental status on adults, infants, and children. When evaluating a child's mental status, monitor how the child interacts with the primary caregiver. Ask the caregiver if the response or activity is normal for the child. If it is not, ask exactly how the current behavior is different from normal.

Table 8.4 • AVPU ASSESSMENT OF MENTAL STATUS

Mental Status	Indicators
Alert	The patient is alert, aware, and responsive In the case of an infant or child, he or she cries or follows eye contact
Verbal	The patient is not alert, but responds to verbal stimuli
Pain	The patient is not responsive to verbal stimuli, but responds to pain such as a pinch on the skin
Unresponsive	The patient is unresponsive to all stimuli; no gag or cough reflex

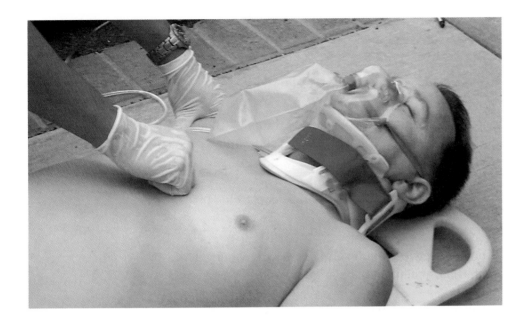

Figure 8.24 *Determining response to a painful stimulus.*

EMT Tip

The difference between a patient who is alert and one who responds to verbal stimuli can be difficult to assess. It is most important to establish a baseline response level and then watch for changes.

D.O.T. OBJECTIVES

Discuss methods of assessing the airway in the adult, child, and infant patient.

State reasons for management of cervical spine once the patient has been determined to be a trauma patient.

CD-ROM Link

The "Head-Tilt, Chin-Lift" and "Jaw-Thrust" videos in the Airway Management chapter of the MedEMT CD-ROM demonstrate these maneuvers.

Assessing and Opening the Airway

The mechanism of injury as well as the patient's age and size determine the method of opening the airway. If a responsive patient is talking or crying, you know the airway is secure. If trauma is suspected, immediately stabilize the cervical spine. For an unresponsive medical patient, use the head-tilt/chin-lift maneuver. If a trauma patient is unresponsive or if the mechanism of injury is unknown, use the jaw-thrust maneuver to open the airway. If there is obstruction, clear the airway. Once you have established that the airway is open and clear, proceed to assessing the breathing and circulation. For further information on the techniques of opening the airway, see Chapter 7.

Assessing Breathing

Place your ear and face close to the patient's mouth and nose. Look down at the chest and feel for air movement on your cheek and ear (see Fig. 8.25). Recall from Chapter 7 that anything that affects the rise and fall of the chest or rate of respirations will interfere with the patient's ability to breathe normally. Monitor breathing rate, tidal volume, and chest expansion. You must also assess changes in level of consciousness, skin signs (particularly cyanosis), and respiratory effort.

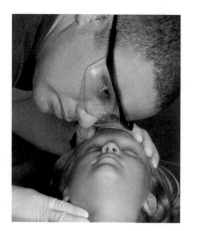

Figure 8.25 *Look, listen, and feel when assessing breathing and circulation.*

When you assess a patient's breathing, decide whether supportive measures are necessary. If a responsive patient's breathing is adequate, determine the need for oxygen therapy. Administer oxygen at 15 liters per minute through a non-rebreather mask if the rate is slow (<8 bpm) or fast (>24 bpm). If the patient is unresponsive, open and maintain the airway. Insert an airway adjunct, if the patient tolerates it. Deliver oxygen at 15 liters per minute through a non-rebreather mask if respirations are adequate. If breathing is inadequate or absent, use an adjunct, then begin supplemental oxygen immediately. Determine the need for positive pressure ventilation.

The following summarizes breathing assessment and supportive interventions:

• If breathing is adequate and the patient is responsive, oxygen may be indicated.

• All responsive patients with respiratory difficulty and breathing >24 breaths per minute or <8 breaths per minute should receive high-flow oxygen.

• If the patient is unresponsive and breathing is adequate, open and maintain the airway and provide high-flow oxygen.

- If breathing is inadequate, open and maintain the airway, assist the patient's breathing, and utilize airway adjuncts. Always apply oxygen.

- If the patient is not breathing, open and maintain the airway and ventilate using an adjunct. Always apply oxygen.

Infants and Children

When dealing with an infant or child, your assessment of breathing adequacy is extremely important. Most cardiac arrests in pediatric patients occur because of respiratory compromise. Look for an altered mental state combined with accessory muscle use and cyanosis as the key indicators of breathing inadequacy. If the pediatric patient is breathing adequately, provide supplemental oxygen by a non-rebreathing mask. If breathing is inadequate, assist ventilations while you provide supplemental oxygen. Assessment of airway and breathing for infants and children is also discussed in Chapters 7 and 23.

Assessing Circulation

Assess the circulation by determining the presence and quality of the pulses, adequacy of skin perfusion (color and temperature), and skin condition using the methods discussed in Chapter 5. In children less than 6 years old, use the capillary refill rate as an indicator of circulation. Identify and control any life-threatening bleeding.

D.O.T. OBJECTIVES

Describe the methods used to obtain a pulse.

Differentiate between obtaining a pulse in an adult, child, and infant patient.

Assess the Pulse

Assess the pulse by palpating or feeling for the radial pulse. If the pulse is weak, the patient may be in shock. Bleeding and shock are discussed in Chapter 19.

If a peripheral pulse cannot be felt, check the carotid pulse (see Fig 8.26). If the carotid pulse is absent, begin CPR and assist ventilations with supplemental oxygen. For medical patients older than 12 years in age or more than 90 pounds in weight, apply the automated external defibrillator (AED) immediately. The operation of the AED is discussed in Chapter 13.

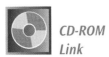

CD-ROM Link

See the "Vital Signs–Breathing" video in the Airway Management chapter of the MedEMT CD-ROM for steps in assessing breathing adequacy.

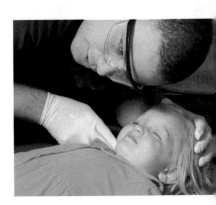

Figure 8.26 *Checking the carotid pulse.*

Figure 8.27 *Checking the brachial pulse in a child.*

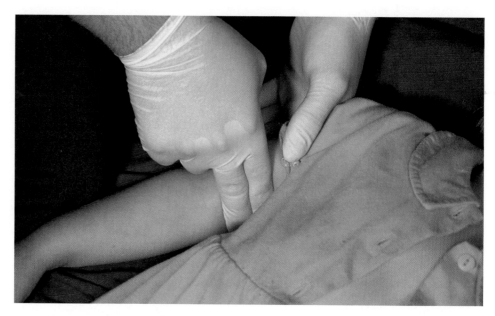

For patients who are less than 1 year old, assess the peripheral pulse at the brachial artery (see Fig. 8.27).

CD-ROM Link

The "Bleeding Control" video in Chapters 8, 19, and the Video Appendix on the MedEMT CD-ROM demonstrates the technique of applying direct pressure to control bleeding.

> **D.O.T. OBJECTIVE**
>
> Discuss the need for assessing the patient for external bleeding.

Look for Bleeding

Rapid control of major bleeding can be lifesaving. A hemorrhaging patient can lose enough blood to die in less than 2 minutes. Quickly check the patient for major bleeding. Look for blood-soaked clothing or pools of blood around the patient. Upon finding a major source of bleeding, quickly cut away the clothing in order to expose the area. Place your gloved hand over the wound and apply direct pressure. When bleeding has been controlled, apply a pressure dressing. You must control major bleeding before continuing the assessment. Bleeding control and pressure dressings are discussed in Chapter 19.

> **D.O.T. OBJECTIVES**
>
> Describe normal and abnormal findings when assessing skin color, temperature, and condition.
>
> Describe normal and abnormal findings when assessing skin capillary refill in the infant and child patient.

Assess Tissue Perfusion

The next step in checking the patient's circulation is assessing perfusion and skin color, temperature, and condition. Examine the color of the skin, lips, eyes, and nail beds. Normal skin feels warm and dry. Check capillary refill time in children under 6 years old (see Fig. 8.28). Capillary refill time greater than 2 seconds indicates inadequate perfusion. Monitor closely and check for signs of bleeding. For a review of how to assess tissue perfusion, including a discussion of abnormal findings, refer to Chapter 5.

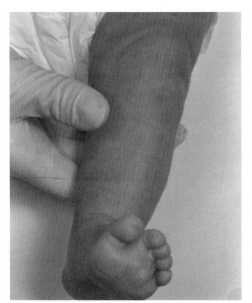
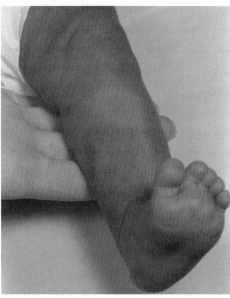

Figure 8.28 *The leg is another location for assessing capillary refill.*

D.O.T. OBJECTIVE

Explain the reason for prioritizing a patient for care and transport.

DETERMINING PATIENT PRIORITY

Once you have gathered enough information to form a general impression and have assessed the patient's ABCs, the next step is to identify priority patients. You must determine the priority of each patient for treatment and transport. You will make your decision based on your general impression, the patient's mental status, and the ABCs. Conditions that suggest a high priority for immediate transport are:

• Poor general impression

• Unresponsive patient

EMT Tip

Do not attempt to control minor bleeding or other minor injuries during the initial assessment. This may be difficult when minor wounds are actively bleeding. Only treat bleeding that is life-threatening during this part of the patient assessment.

- Responsive patient who is not following commands
- Difficulty breathing
- Shock (hypoperfusion)
- Complicated childbirth
- Chest pain with systolic BP <100
- Uncontrolled bleeding
- Severe pain

Expedite the transport of priority patients. If you decide that the patient's condition requires immediate transport, continue assessment and treatment in the ambulance. Consider calling for advanced life support assistance if available.

After your initial assessment and critical interventions, you will continue the assessment with a focused history and physical exam. The mechanism of injury (for trauma patients) or the nature of the illness (for medical patients) determines the type of physical exam. The next chapter gives information on how to perform these exams. Information from your initial assessment will guide you in deciding how to proceed with the focused history and physical exam.

Chapter Eight Summary

- A thorough, organized patient assessment is the key to providing good patient care. All care is based on assessment.

- The scene size-up is an evaluation for threats to safety and the need for additional resources. You will also determine the mechanism or nature of the injury or illness.

- Scene assessment does not stop after you approach the patient. Continuously evaluate the scene while caring for the patient. Monitor for changes that may threaten your safety or the safety of your crew, the patient, or bystanders.

- Body substance isolation measures are initiated before you approach the patient. BSI and standard precautions are an important protective measure at an emergency scene.

- The initial assessment focuses on identification and treatment of life-threatening problems related to the airway, breathing, or circulation.

- Your general impression is an important tool that, when refined by experience, will help you to manage a patient correctly. Your impression includes basic information on the mechanism of injury or illness, the patient's sex, age, and chief complaint.

- If you suspect traumatic injury, always control the cervical spine while assessing the patient's mental status and airway patency.

Key Terms Review

AVPU | *page 274*
Blunt Trauma | *page 264*
Cavitation | *page 267*
General Impression | *page 273*

Initial Assessment | *page 254*
Interventions | *page 271*
Mechanism of Injury
  (MOI) | *page 263*
Nature of Illness | *page 263*

Penetrating Trauma | *page 267*
Scene Size-Up | *page 254*
Trauma | *page 262*
Triage | *page 271*

Review Questions

1. At every scene you are responsible for the safety of many people. You generally do NOT have responsibility for which of the following responders?

   a. Law enforcement
   b. Yourself
   c. Patient
   d. Bystanders

2. You are at the scene of a house fire when you get word that there are two children trapped in a first-floor bedroom. The mother is frantic for you to rescue the children, despite your lack of firefighter training. What should you do?

   a. Await trained and equipped fire department personnel
   b. Don protective equipment and try to locate the children
   c. Order your partner to get the children while you back him up
   d. Instruct a law enforcement officer to bring the children to you

3. As you enter an office building where several patients are passed out, you smell an odd odor. You have nearly reached your first victim, but cannot determine if that patient is breathing. What should be your next action?

   a. Proceed to the patient and begin life saving treatment as necessary
   b. Quickly assess the patient and continue on to find others who are ill
   c. Proceed to the patient and notify the fire department of the odor
   d. Leave the building until fire personnel investigate the odor

4. At the scene of a bar fight, which of the following would NOT usually be considered a potential safety hazard for you and your crew?

   a. Beer bottles
   b. Large crowd
   c. Displayed weapons
   d. Patient's wife

5. You are responding to a call for a person thrown out of a raft into the river and stranded in the water. He is very near shore, and the water does not appear to be moving too fast. It will take 20 minutes for the water rescue team to reach your location. What should you do?

   a. Don a personal flotation device and swim to the patient
   b. Await arrival of the water rescue team
   c. Try to reach the patient in another raft
   d. Instruct the patient to swim toward the riverbank

6. You arrive at a residence where a woman has been held hostage. The perpetrator has been removed from the scene by police. You discover that your patient has been bound with rope around the wrists and ankles and has been gagged with duct tape. How should you treat this patient and the evidence?

   a. Leave ropes and tape in place until law enforcement can examine them
   b. Remove all bindings as quickly as possible for patient comfort
   c. Transport your patient with bindings in place for removal at hospital
   d. Carefully remove bindings, documenting their position and removal

7. Never attempt a water rescue:

   a. If you are alone
   b. If it is dark
   c. If the water appears rough
   d. Without your supervisor present

8. If you suspect significant traumatic injury in a single patient who has been injured in a motor vehicle accident, you should immediately:

   a. Start CPR
   b. Cover the patient to ensure warmth
   c. Secure the cervical spine
   d. Call for a second ambulance

9. A patient who fails to respond to both painful and verbal stimuli is considered to be:

   a. Dead
   b. Unresponsive
   c. Responsive
   d. Comatose

10. For infants, the pulse should initially be assessed at the ___ artery.

    a. Radial
    b. Carotid
    c. Femoral
    d. Brachial

11. A patient with darker skin can be assessed for skin signs in the:

    a. Ear
    b. Lower eyelid
    c. Nose
    d. Arm

12. When should an EMT-B attempt to enter a hazardous scene?

    a. When directed into the scene by a bystander
    b. When the hospital directs you into the scene
    c. When you are specially trained and equipped
    d. You should never enter a hazardous scene

13. What is the most important step in crime scene size-up?

    a. Preserving the evidence for law enforcement
    b. Ensuring your own and your partners' personal safety
    c. Documenting all of the evidence that you see
    d. Reporting all visual evidence to the hospital

14. Part of an EMT-B's job includes triaging patients at an incident with multiple patients. This means that the EMT:

    a. Loads the patients into ambulances for transportation to the hospital
    b. Completely treats each patient before establishing contact with other patients
    c. Contacts a supervisor for advice on where to transport all of the patients
    d. Rapidly assesses patients and prioritizes them for treatment and transport

15. The mnemonic AVPU is used when assessing:

    a. Blood pressure
    b. Level of shock
    c. Mental status
    d. Breathing status

CASE STUDIES

Scene Size-Up and Initial Assessment

1 The air is extremely cold. Even your gloves cannot keep out the wind and snow. You have been dispatched to respond to a man who is ill at a local homeless shelter. The staff advises you that the man has been there for three days. He has become progressively weaker each day. They finally decided to call 9-1-1. The 40-year-old male is weak, warm to the touch, and coughing constantly. He states that his cough has been getting worse since he left a shelter in San Francisco four months ago. You notice some terrible bruises on the patient's arms and feet. Two of the bruises are bleeding lightly. You also notice a distended right upper abdominal quadrant and a yellow tinge to his skin.

A. What personal and scene safety issues concern you?

B. What personal protective equipment will you use to decrease your risk of exposure to infection?

2 You are looking forward to your shift with the volunteer rescue squad. The captain mentioned that the department will be working with the police in a mock hostage situation. They want your squad to be on scene in case something goes wrong. As luck would have it, just as you finish washing the unit and are about to leave for the drill, the pager sounds. You are dispatched to the scene of a violent assault. As you arrive at the apartment complex, a sheriff's officer who is standing in a doorway hurriedly waves you up. You see blood all over the walkway. When you enter the door, you see two patients lying on the floor, covered with blood. It looks like the male shot himself beneath the chin with a large caliber gun. You can see only part of the female's upper body.

A. What is your general impression of this scene? How did you reach this impression?

B. What is triage? How does it apply to this case?

C. Has the patient suffered a significant mechanism of injury? Will this decision make a difference in the type of assessment that you will conduct? If so, how?

Stories from the Field
Wrap-Up

Accurate assessment is the key to appropriate treatment. An organized, thorough assessment of the patient's physical condition provides a picture of what is wrong with the patient. It will also reveal what is not wrong.

Kim's refusal to enter an unsafe area was a correct course of action. A thorough scene size-up is always done to ensure the safety of yourself and others. Your initial assessment is done to identify and correct problems that are an immediate threat to life. The scene size-up and initial assessment determine the type of focused history and physical exam you will perform. It also helps you to determine the patient's initial priority for transport. Asking detailed questions is important so that you don't overlook important aspects of the patient's history. Reassessing the patient's condition frequently is also very important. Your observations of changes in the patient's condition are important to the physicians at the receiving facility.

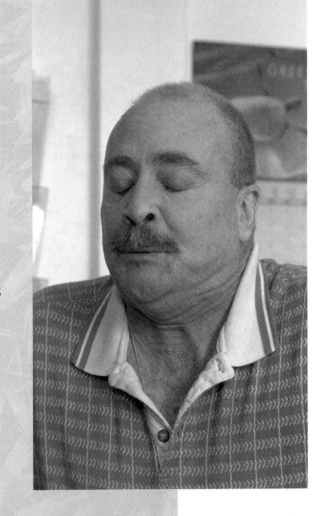

ENHANCED STUDY

Mechanism of Injury in Motor Vehicle Collisions

Recall from the discussion on mechanism of injury that three collisions occur in every motor vehicle collision (MVC): the vehicle impact, the occupant impact, and the internal organ impact. With practice and experience, you will learn to recognize the types of injuries to expect by assessing a vehicle's damaged interior. This section contains further information about mechanisms of injury in motor vehicle accidents, including information about the potential injuries a cyclist or pedestrian can sustain if involved in a collision with a motor vehicle.

Frontal Impact Collisions. In a frontal impact MVC, suspect these injuries:

- Head and cervical spine injuries (see Enhancement Fig. 8.1)

- Chest wall injuries, such as contusions and rib fractures

- Heart and lung injuries, including pneumothorax, cardiac, or pulmonary contusions

- Transection, or tearing of the aorta due to rapid deceleration of the internal organs

- Injuries to the spleen and liver

- Posterior fracture or dislocation of the ankle, knee, or hip

Enhancement Table 8.1 describes the type of injuries that may occur in a frontal impact MVC.

Side Impact MVCs. In a side impact accident, look for injuries on the side of the body nearest to the impact (see Enhancement Fig. 8.2). Notice the amount of intrusion of the vehicle frame into the passenger compartment. Suspected injuries from a side-impact MVC are:

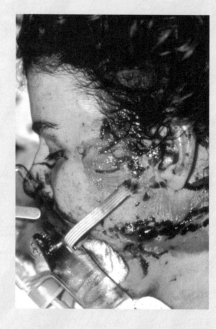

Enhancement Figure 8.1 *This patient was involved in a frontal impact collision. The facial injuries were caused by impact with the windshield.*

- Head and contralateral neck injuries

- Lateral chest wall injuries, such as contusions and rib fractures

- Pneumothorax

- Injuries to the liver or spleen, depending on the side of impact

- Fractures of the pelvis or hip

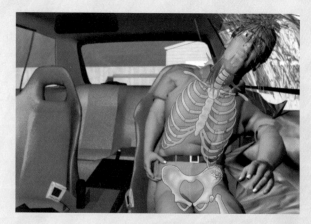

Enhancement Figure 8.2 *The door is often pushed into the passenger compartment in side impact collisions.*

Enhancement Table 8.1 • INJURIES IN FRONTAL IMPACT COLLISIONS

Type of Frontal Collision	Description	Examples of Injuries
Down-and-Under Impact	The occupant is thrown down and under the steering wheel (see Enhancement Fig. 8.3)	Ankle injuries Fractured kneecap or femur Dislocated hip joint
Up-and-Over Impact	The occupant is thrown up and over the steering wheel (see Enhancement Fig. 8.4)	Internal injuries such as heart contusions, liver and spleen damage, and internal bleeding
Combination Impact	The occupant first follows a down-and-under pathway, then continues up and over the steering wheel (see Enhancement Fig. 8.5)	A combination of the injuries listed above

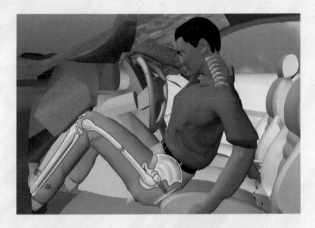

Enhancement Figure 8.3 *Down-and-under frontal impact.*

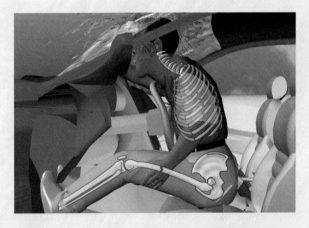

Enhancement Figure 8.5 *Combination impact.*

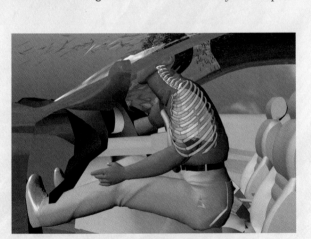

Enhancement Figure 8.4 *Up-and-over frontal impact.*

Rear Impact MVCs. In most rear impact accidents, a stopped vehicle is hit from behind. An occupant can suffer spinal injuries when the torso accelerates forward, snapping the head backward. Properly adjusted headrests prevent or minimize this type of injury. These injuries can also result from head-on, rollover, and lateral impact collisions.

Rollover or Ejection MVCs. An unrestrained occupant can sustain multiple severe injuries in a rollover crash. The vehicle may roll over many times or collide with many objects

ENHANCED STUDY

Mechanism of Injury in Motor Vehicle Collisions *(cont.)*

before coming to a stop. The person can strike anything in the vehicle, so you cannot predict the pattern of injuries.

Unrestrained occupants can be ejected through a window or convertible roof, or from a truck bed or motorcycle (see Enhancement Fig. 8.6). Ejection from a vehicle increases the severity of injuries. The risk of death also increases significantly. The patient contacts so many objects that the injury pattern is difficult to predict. The vehicle may hit the person after ejection. He or she may become trapped under the wreckage. These objects may be inside or outside the vehicle. Ejection from a vehicle also increases the risk of hypothermia and other injuries caused by environmental exposure.

Pedestrian Injuries. A pedestrian hit by a motor vehicle may sustain injuries to any part of the body. In adults, the bumper commonly hits the pelvis and legs first. Next, the person may be thrown onto the hood, striking the windshield. This can cause injuries to the torso, head, neck, and arms. Finally, the victim is often thrown to the ground, causing serious head and spine injuries.

Children are usually hit in the chest and abdomen. They are often knocked to the ground by a vehicle, and then run over. When a child is hit by a car, suspect:

- Severe crushing injuries to the chest and abdomen

- Head, neck, and spinal trauma

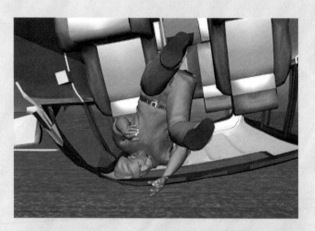

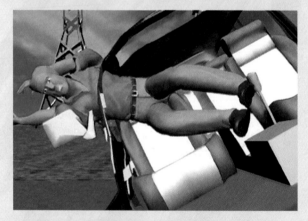

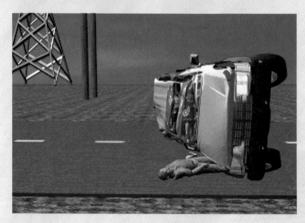

Enhancement Figure 8.6 *When a vehicle rolls over, an unrestrained occupant collides repeatedly with the interior (top). He may also be ejected from the vehicle (center) and become trapped under it (bottom).*

ENHANCED STUDY

Gangs

Many states and municipalities have specific legal definitions for gangs. For your purposes, a gang is a group that gathers or associates regularly. The primary purpose of a gang may be to engage in criminal activity.

Hundreds of gangs are active across the United States. They are found in both metropolitan areas and small towns. Both males and females belong to gangs. Do not assume that all gang members are male. Most gangs are highly organized, with a formal hierarchy. They are cohesive and very serious about their activities. Members are rarely alone. One or more gang members are usually always in the vicinity. Gang-controlled areas may have graffiti and unusual symbols painted in various locations. Some of the graffiti may have been crossed out. Rival gangs do this as a sign of disrespect or as a threat to the writer. Gang members may communicate by using a series of hand signals. Most, but not all, gangs use identifiable colors and symbols. Some wear items of their clothing in a certain way.

Personal Safety. If you suspect that you are in a gang-controlled area, call for law enforcement backup. Also call for backup if you are dispatched to a medical or trauma scene that you suspect is related to gang activity. Avoid entering the scene until police personnel advise that the scene is safe.

When working with suspected gang members:

- Be fair, but firm. Avoid giving the impression that you feel superior. As always, show respect for the individual.

- Avoid overreacting to possible gang membership.

- Whenever possible, try to deal with a gang member alone. Remove other members from the room or area. If this is not possible, consider moving the patient to the ambulance and continuing your care en route to the hospital.

- Be aware that alcohol or drug use may mask symptoms of a medical problem.

- Be aware that members may carry concealed weapons. Be on guard, and never risk your personal safety.

- The hat can be an important garment. If you are at a scene of suspected gang activity, avoid bumping or stepping on members' hats. Likewise, avoid cutting or tearing clothing whenever possible.

Chapter 9

Patient Assessment

Stories from the Field

For the last few weeks, John and Robin have been letting you take the lead on medical calls. They critique your performance and make suggestions regarding areas in which you can improve. They are still taking the lead on trauma calls. Just after noon, you are dispatched to a possible shooting. As you drive to the staging area, Robin informs you that you will take the lead on this call. You must assess the patient, make a plan for treatment, and see that it is carried out.

The location of the call is a convenience store. There is a great deal of activity when you arrive. You wait in the staging area until you are cleared to enter by law enforcement on the scene. A police officer directs you inside the store, where the clerk is lying in a pool of blood on the floor behind the cash register. The clerk is conscious and alert and complains of hip pain. After taking body substance isolation precautions, you approach the patient. She states that a man shot her with a handgun from about 10 feet away. You notice a spurt of blood coming from a wound in the patient's left hip. John hurries outside to get more equipment. Robin turns to you. What do you do first?

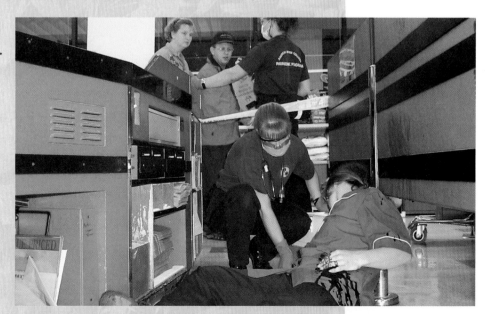

I n Chapter 8, you learned that a thorough and organized initial assessment is the key to providing effective patient care. After completing the initial assessment, immediate life-threatening problems will have been discovered and managed. Now you will continue to evaluate the patient by conducting a **focused history and physical exam** (see Fig. 8.1 in Chapter 8). This exam will enable you to discover whether any further interventions are necessary or whether rapid transport is required. This chapter describes a general plan for patient assessment. Details for many types of injury and illness are presented throughout the book. Chapters 12–18 provide specific assessment and treatment procedures for emergency medical patients. Assessment and treatment of traumatic injuries are discussed in Chapters 19–22.

If your initial assessment indicates that the patient has been injured, you must reconsider the mechanism of injury. If the mechanism of injury is significant, you will conduct a rapid trauma assessment of the entire body to identify hidden injuries. If the mechanism of injury is not significant, you will only perform components of the rapid trauma assessment related to the injured area. If your patient's chief complaint is medical in nature, you will complete a rapid medical assessment after determining the patient's mental status. If a medical patient is responsive and able to tell you what the problem is, you will perform components of the rapid medical assessment specific to the patient's chief complaint. An unconscious patient will require a full-body rapid medical assessment.

Normally, you will perform the focused history and physical exam immediately after completing the initial assessment. If there is a delay in completing the assessment, quickly reevaluate the patient's mental status, airway, breathing, and circulatory status before continuing. If you find critical injuries or if the patient begins to deteriorate during your exam, reconsider previous interventions and transport decisions. Also consider requesting support from other resources, such as:

- Advanced life support units
- Aeromedical evacuation agencies
- Other specialized resources

If you have time, a detailed physical exam is performed after the rapid assessment. This is a careful, more thorough, head-to-toe assessment. The detailed physical exam is most often performed in the ambulance while en route to the hospital. Based on the patient's chief complaint, there may be specific signs or symptoms you will look for.

FOCUSED HISTORY AND PHYSICAL EXAM: TRAUMA

If your patient's chief complaint is caused by trauma, you must first reconsider the mechanism of injury to decide how to proceed with the focused history and physical exam (see Fig. 9.1). If you determine that the mechanism of injury is significant, or if you cannot determine the mechanism of injury, conduct a complete **rapid trauma assessment**. This is a quick head-to-toe examination that will help you to identify key signs, symptoms, and additional injuries. Pay particular attention to areas related to the complaint or mechanism of injury.

Rapid Trauma Assessment | *A physical exam designed to quickly identify critical injuries and emergency interventions*

Figure 9.1 *Assessment procedure for a trauma patient.*

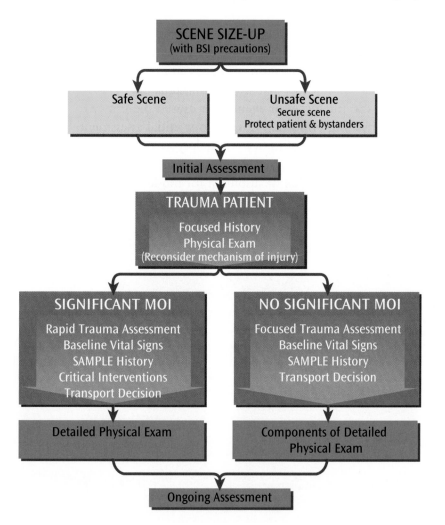

If the mechanism of injury is not significant, conduct a focused trauma assessment concentrating on the specific injury site. This is also referred to as a problem-focused history and physical exam. For example, if the patient has a laceration on the leg, complete an assessment of the injured leg. If you encounter critical findings or multiple injuries, or if the patient's condition deteriorates, proceed with a head-to-toe rapid trauma assessment.

After completing the focused history and physical exam for a trauma patient, you will obtain baseline vital signs and a SAMPLE history. You will provide interventions as needed and prepare the patient for transport.

D.O.T. OBJECTIVE

Discuss the reasons for reconsideration concerning the mechanism of injury.

Reconsidering Mechanism of Injury

During your initial assessment of a trauma patient, you considered the mechanism of injury (MOI) to help evaluate the patient's chief complaint. Now you will reconsider the mechanism of injury in more detail. Some trauma patients have critical injuries that are not immediately obvious. You will reevaluate the specific forces or events that caused the injury to be sure you did not miss anything important during your initial assessment. Reconsideration of the mechanism of injury will help you anticipate, recognize, and manage hidden injuries such as internal bleeding. Based on the mechanism of injury, maintain a high index of suspicion for hidden injuries on every trauma scene (see Fig. 9.2).

Figure 9.2 *Gunshot holes in a windshield suggest that the MOI may be significant.*

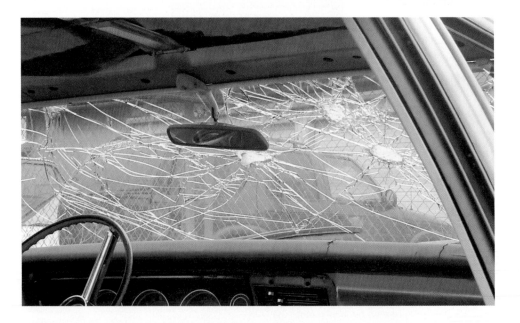

Mechanisms of injury indicating the need for a rapid trauma assessment include:

- Fall greater than 20 feet (adult)
- Diving accident
- Penetrating trauma to the head, chest, or abdomen
- Ejection from a vehicle
- Death of another passenger in the vehicle
- Vehicle rollover
- High-speed collision
- Vehicle-pedestrian collision
- Motorcycle crash
- Seat belts not worn
- Seat belts worn (buckles can cause injuries; wearing a seat belt does not preclude other injury)
- Airbags deployed (may not be effective without seat belt; patient may hit steering wheel after deflation)
- Deformities in the steering wheel (a strong indicator of potentially serious internal injuries)
- Unresponsive patient or altered mental status
- Indeterminate mechanism of injury

Examples of mechanisms of injury that are not significant are:

- Low-velocity collision in which the patient complains of neck pain
- A tennis player with an injured ankle
- A young child with a minor hot-water burn on one arm

Special Considerations

Trauma can cause serious injuries to infants, children, and the elderly in situations where a healthy adult might be less seriously injured.

Assessing the mechanism of injury in a child is very important. An infant or child may appear healthy, even with significant injuries. Infants and children may compensate very well for blood loss for a brief time, but then decompensate very quickly. You must rely on the mechanism of injury to identify the need for rapid trauma assessment and intervention. Be particularly cautious in bicycle accidents, falls greater than 10 feet, or moderate-speed vehicle collisions.

The mechanism of injury should be considered carefully when elderly patients sustain trauma. Coexisting medical conditions such as arthritis and osteoporosis (a demineralization and weakening of the bones) can make a patient more susceptible to injury (see Fig. 9.3). In an elderly patient, significant injury can result from relatively minor events.

CD-ROM Link

Review the "Mechanism of Injury" series of animations in Chapters 8, 9, and the Video Appendix on the MedEMT CD-ROM to see depictions of various vehicle collisions and the injuries predicted from each.

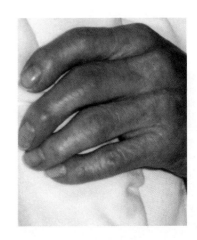

Figure 9.3 *Arthritic patients are more susceptible to bone injuries.*

EMT Tip

Complete the scene survey and initial assessment before beginning the rapid trauma assessment. Maintain in-line spinal stabilization and recheck the ABCs, if indicated.

CD-ROM Link

For a demonstration of the steps of a rapid trauma assessment, see the video "Rapid Trauma Assessment" in the Patient Assessment chapter and the Video Appendix on the MedEMT CD-ROM.

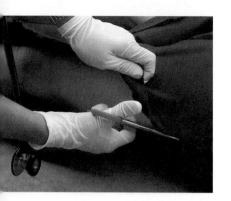

Figure 9.4 *Cut or remove clothing to expose an injured area for assessment.*

Stabilizing the Cervical Spine

While reconsidering the mechanism of injury, ensure that the cervical spine is maintained correctly. The head should be in a neutral, in-line position. Spinal immobilization is suggested in all cases with significant, unknown, or uncertain mechanisms of injury. Patients without a significant MOI should be immobilized if the chief complaint involves any potential for spinal injury. For example, immobilize the spine when a patient has head or facial injuries.

> **D.O.T. OBJECTIVES**
>
> State the reasons for performing a rapid trauma assessment.
>
> Recite examples and explain why patients should receive a rapid trauma assessment.

Rapid Trauma Assessment

The purpose of the rapid trauma assessment is to locate serious injuries and to ensure that you have not overlooked anything significant during your initial assessment. Continue with a rapid trauma assessment if you:

- Encounter a significant mechanism of injury
- Cannot clearly identify the mechanism of injury
- Detect critical injuries
- Are unsure of extent of injury

In most situations, the rapid trauma exam can be completed by one EMT-Basic. Other crew members may prepare a stretcher or immobilization equipment or obtain SAMPLE history information. To perform the rapid trauma assessment, quickly but thoroughly inspect and palpate each area of the body sequentially (see Table 9.1). Focus on finding major injuries or problems. You will not look for every minor injury at this point.

In some cases, you will need to remove some or all of the patient's clothing to properly inspect the body. It may be necessary to cut shoelaces or clothes to expose an injured body part (see Fig. 9.4). In such cases, begin by covering the patient with a blanket. Expose the body under the blanket, with minimal manipulation. When removing clothing, maintain the patient's modesty and respect. Also protect the patient from weather elements. If the patient's condition allows, perform this part of the rapid trauma assessment inside the transport vehicle.

Table 9.1 • RAPID TRAUMA ASSESSMENT

Area of Body	Assessment
Assess head	Evaluate for DCAP-BTLS
Assess neck	Evaluate for DCAP-BTLS Assess for jugular venous distention or crepitation Manually stabilize spine during assessment, then place cervical spinal immobilization collar
Assess chest	Evaluate for DCAP-BTLS Assess for paradoxical motion or crepitation Seal any open chest wounds with occlusive dressings (see Chapter 20) Determine whether breath sounds are present or absent on each side Determine whether breath sounds are equal on each side Determine whether breath sounds are normal or abnormal
Assess abdomen	Evaluate for DCAP-BTLS Note whether abdomen is firm, soft, or distended
Assess pelvis	Evaluate for DCAP-BTLS If there is no pain, compress pelvis to determine tenderness and stability
Assess extremities	Evaluate for DCAP-BTLS Evaluate distal pulses, motor function, and sensation
Assess posterior body	Roll the patient onto one side with cervical spine control Evaluate for DCAP-BTLS Place long spine board under patient, if indicated

DCAP-BTLS

DCAP-BTLS is a mnemonic used to help you to remember the signs of injury you should look for while completing a systematic survey of the patient. Use your senses of hearing, vision, smell, and touch. You will inspect and palpate the head, neck, chest, abdomen, pelvis, extremities, and posterior body, looking for:

D | Deformities

C | Contusions

A | Abrasions

P | Punctures and penetrations

B | Burns

T | Tenderness

L | Lacerations

S | Swelling

EMT
Tip

Remember that time is the enemy of a critically injured trauma patient. You must be able to complete a focused history and physical exam quickly. You do not have time to "stumble, fumble, and forget."

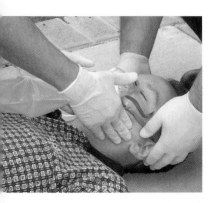

Figure 9.5 *Avoid touching deformities or depressions during a head assessment.*

Crepitation (krep-eh-TAY-shun) | *A crackling sensation felt and heard beneath the skin; caused by broken bone ends grating against each other or by subcutaneous air*

Head Assessment

Evaluate the mechanism of injury, level of consciousness, and signs of external deformity. Rapidly assess the patient's head for DCAP-BTLS (see Fig. 9.5). Avoid touching deformities or depressions if you discover any. Listen and feel for **crepitation** of the bones, a crackling feeling and sound. Crepitation, also called crepitus, is caused by the grating of bone ends against each other. Crepitation can be exaggerated due to air underneath the skin, called subcutaneous air or subcutaneous emphysema.

Ask the patient to smile or frown to assess motor function of the facial muscles. As an EMT-Basic, you cannot measure the severity of a head injury, particularly if there are internal injuries. More detailed information on treating head injuries is presented in Chapter 22.

Neck Assessment

Rapidly assess the skin, cervical spine, trachea, and jugular veins for DCAP-BTLS. Maintain cervical in-line spinal stabilization while inspecting the neck (see Fig. 9.6). Avoid compromising the cervical spine to inspect or palpate it.

Figure 9.6 *Maintain manual spinal stabilization while inspecting the neck.*

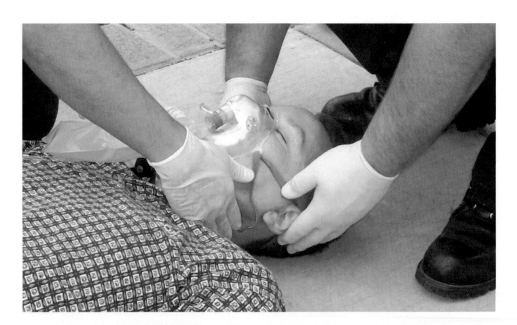

Look for a medical identification insignia. This will alert you to allergies or medical conditions that are important in the treatment of the patient.

Assess the jugular veins (see Fig. 9.7). Normal jugular veins are slightly distended in the supine position. They flatten when the patient's head is elevated more than 45 degrees. A major blood loss will result in decreased circulatory volume. This will cause the jugular veins to remain flat when the patient is in the supine position. **Jugular venous distention (JVD)** is a bulging of the jugular veins. The bulging appears over more than two-thirds of the distance from the base of the neck to the angle of the jaw. JVD suggests serious injury to the heart or chest. For example, cardiac tamponade may cause jugular venous distention upon elevation of the head. This is a serious condition (discussed further in Chapter 22) in which blood leaks into the space between the heart muscle and the membrane covering the heart.

Normally, the trachea lies at the midline position. **Tracheal deviation** is a condition in which the trachea is pushed to one side of the midline. This suggests severe injury to the chest or lungs and requires aggressive airway management. Tracheal deviation is almost always a very late sign. Do not wait until deviation occurs before you begin airway management.

Crepitation of the neck may be recognized by a puffy appearance. You will observe a crackling feel and sound on palpation. This suggests possible disruption of the bony structures and/or air under the skin and is a sign of severe neck or chest injury.

Management of the Cervical Spine. As you assess the neck, the following interventions are indicated:

- Ensure that manual, in-line immobilization is being done correctly
- Ensure that the cervical spine is adequately protected
- After evaluation of the anterior and posterior neck, apply a cervical spinal immobilization collar (CSIC). Make sure you select a collar that fits the patient properly (see Fig. 9.8). This is described fully in Chapter 22.
- Continue to maintain in-line spinal stabilization until the patient is completely immobilized on a long backboard

Chest Assessment

It may be necessary to remove clothing to expose the chest for complete assessment. Assess for chest injuries using the DCAP-BTLS mnemonic. Inspect the rib cage, clavicles, and sternum for damage or crepitation (see Fig. 9.9).

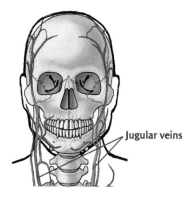

Jugular veins

Figure 9.7 *Jugular veins are located on both sides of the neck near the front.*

Jugular Venous Distention (JUG-yuh-ler VEE-nus di-STEN-shun) (JVD) | *Abnormal bulging of the jugular veins indicating injury to the heart or chest*

Tracheal Deviation (TRAY-kee-ul dee-vee-AY-shun) | *A shifting of the trachea to either side of the midline caused by the pressure of air trapped in the chest cavity*

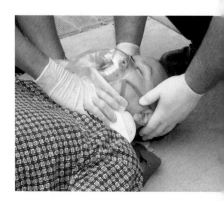

Figure 9.8 *Continue manual immobilization while applying a cervical collar.*

Figure 9.9 *Remove clothing to expose the chest area for assessment.*

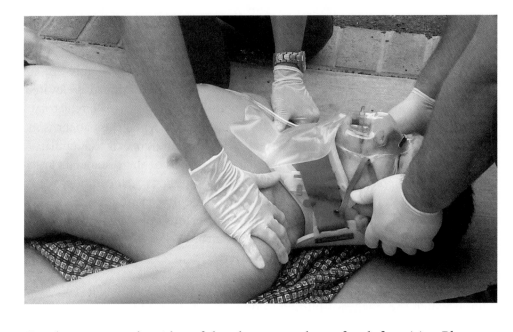

Paradoxical Motion | *Chest movement during breathing in which one section of the chest moves in the opposite direction from the rest; indicates multiple rib fractures (flail chest)*

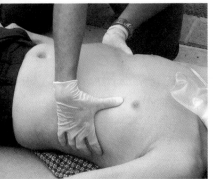

Figure 9.10 *Palpate the rib cage, clavicles, and sternum for damage or crepitation.*

Figure 9.11 *In a flail segment, several adjacent ribs are broken in more than one place. This can be detected by the paradoxical motion seen during breathing.*

Gently compress the sides of the chest to evaluate for deformities. Place your hands around the ribs. Look and feel for equal motion of the chest wall on both sides (see Fig. 9.10). Notice if one section moves differently than the rest of the chest wall. A common sign in patients with significant chest trauma is **paradoxical motion**, a sign of a flail chest. This occurs when a section of ribs is broken in two or more places (see Fig. 9.11). The damaged ribs, or flail segment, move in a direction opposite to the rest of the chest wall during respiration. As the normal part of the chest expands, the damaged area moves inward. When the uninjured part of the chest contracts, the broken ribs move outward. Paradoxical motion can contribute to inadequate respiration and, in severe cases, is considered a type of airway obstruction. It is sometimes easier to feel than to see. You should suspect other severe internal injuries if a flail segment is present.

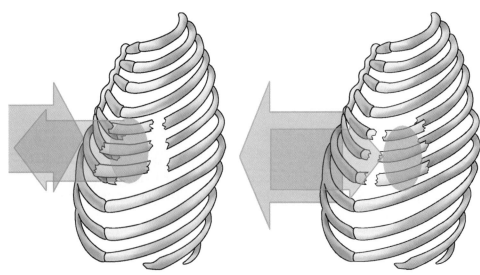

Another chest injury you will encounter is pneumothorax (pneumo = air, thorax = chest). This occurs when air is present in the chest cavity between the lung and chest wall. It may be caused by a punctured lung, blunt chest trauma, or as a complication of positive pressure ventilation. Occasionally, it is seen in chronic lung diseases such as emphysema.

Auscultate the lung sounds using a stethoscope. Listen for the presence and quality of breath sounds during inspiration and expiration. Compare the right and left sides for symmetry of breath sounds, motion, and shape.

For each lung, listen at the:

- Apex, along the midclavicular line (see Fig. 9.12)
- Base, on the midaxillary line (see Fig. 9.13)
- Midpoint of an imaginary line drawn between the apex and base (see Fig. 9.14)
- Anterior and posterior chest

When evaluating breath sounds, notice whether breath sounds are:

- Present or absent
- The same on the right and left sides
- Normal or abnormal (noisy)

If you detect a life-threatening problem during the chest evaluation, intervene immediately. Interventions are determined by the suspected nature of the problem. For example, immediately stabilize the injured area of a flail chest using your gloved hand or a bulky dressing. For all injuries, reassess breathing and reconsider assisting ventilations with supplemental oxygen.

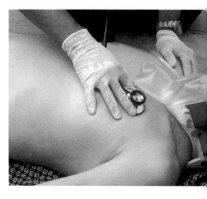

Figure 9.12 *Listen to the apex of each lung along the midclavicular line.*

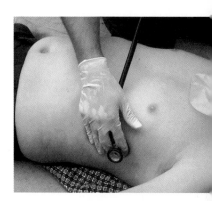

Figure 9.13 *Listen to the base of each lung at the midaxillary line.*

Figure 9.14 *Locations for listening to lung sounds (circles).*

CD-ROM Link

The "Flail Chest" animation in Chapter 9 and the Video Appendix on the MedEMT CD-ROM illustrates the signs of a flail chest.

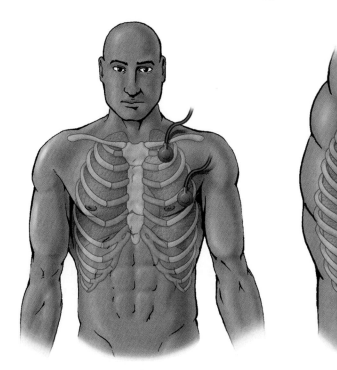

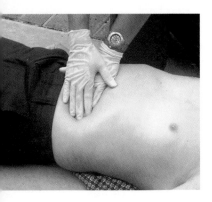

Figure 9.15 *Gently depress the surface of the abdomen about an inch.*

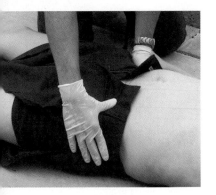

Figure 9.16 *If there is no pain or obvious injury, gently flex and compress the iliac crests with your hands.*

EMT Tip

To evaluate for a pelvic fracture, place your fist between the patient's knees. Instruct the patient to squeeze the legs together. Pain during this maneuver suggests a pelvic injury.

Abdomen Assessment

After assessing the chest, move to the abdomen. Check DCAP–BTLS signs. Palpate each of the four quadrants, using the flat surface of the fingers of one hand. Begin with the nontender quadrants. End with the quadrant of complaint or obvious injury. Gently rest your other hand over the examining hand (see Fig. 9.15). Depress the surface about an inch. Watch the patient's facial expression for evidence of tenderness. Normally, the abdomen is not painful or tender to touch. If it is injured, it may be tender or painful.

The abdomen should feel soft. It may feel swollen, firm, or distended. Distention of the abdomen can be caused by the presence of air, fluid, or blood. Swelling of the abdomen suggests internal bleeding. Look for signs and symptoms of shock if the abdomen is distended. A firm abdomen may indicate irritation, which causes muscle tension. It also suggests an infection of the abdominal lining, called peritonitis.

A pulsating mass in the abdomen suggests an injured aorta, called an aortic aneurysm. This is a life-threatening condition requiring surgical intervention. If you detect a pulsating mass, avoid pressing too hard. Note the location of the mass. Transport the patient immediately to a medical facility. The patient may need immediate surgery.

Pelvic Assessment

Expose the pelvis and evaluate for DCAP–BTLS. Protect the patient's modesty during your exam. If the patient complains of pain or if an injury is evident, do not palpate, flex, or compress the pelvis. If no pain is reported and if you cannot find an obvious injury to the pelvic girdle, continue the assessment. Place your hands around the iliac crests. Gently flex and compress the pelvis to evaluate stability (see Fig. 9.16). Gently push posteriorly to flex the pelvis. Gently push toward the midline to compress the pelvis. Assess for any signs of tenderness or motion. If the patient complains of pain or if the bones feel unstable, stop the exam immediately. Immobilize the patient. Stabilize the pelvis with a pneumatic anti-shock garment (PASG) and follow local protocol. Use of the PASG is described in Chapter 19.

Note whether the patient is incontinent (has lost control of bowel or bladder). Check for swelling in the sacral area. In male patients, check for an erection, which suggests a neurological injury.

Extremities Assessment

Next, examine the patient's arms and legs. Follow the DCAP–BTLS list. Look for angulations or abnormal positioning of the extremities. Check the skin, pulse, and the sensory and motor functions for each extremity. Look for a medical identification tag on the wrists or ankles.

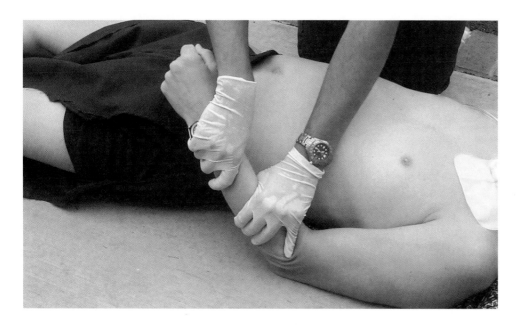

Figure 9.17 *Gently palpate the extremities for a spongy feeling when checking for edema.*

Edema (eh-DEE-muh) | *Abnormal accumulation of fluid in the tissues causing swelling*

Inspect for the presence of **edema**, or swelling. Edema, a collection of fluid in soft tissue, suggests underlying tissue injury resulting in bleeding. The area will feel spongy and form dents with pressure (see Fig. 9.17). The presence of edema may also suggest congestive heart failure or blockage of a vein in an extremity by a blood clot.

Next, palpate the distal pulses in all four extremities. Include the:

- Radial pulse (at the wrist near the base of the thumb; see Fig. 9.18)
- Dorsalis pedis pulse (on top of the foot; see Fig. 9.19)
- Posterior tibial pulse (behind the medial ankle bone)

All of the distal pulses should be strong and equal.

Lightly touch the toes and fingers. Note if the patient experiences abnormal sensation or is unresponsive to touch. Try to determine the degree of abnormality. If the patient is unresponsive, pinch his hand and watch for a response to the painful stimulus. Look for a grimace or movement of the extremity. If numbness or tingling is present, touch the distal end of the affected extremity and move up the limb. Ask the patient to indicate when sensation is normal. In spinal cord injuries, the region of abnormal sensation corresponds to the level of the injury. Assess the motor functions by asking the patient to move the toes and fingers and to squeeze your fingers.

Posterior Body Assessment

When the examination of the extremities is complete, log roll the patient onto one side. Maintain cervical spine control throughout the move and assessment (see Fig. 9.20). Examine the spine, back, buttocks, and posterior extremities. Assess for signs of injury, including DCAP-BTLS.

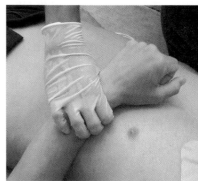

Figure 9.18 *Palpate the radial pulse at the base of the thumb.*

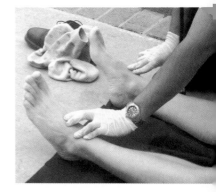

Figure 9.19 *Palpate the dorsalis pedis pulse on top of the foot.*

Figure 9.20 Maintain spinal immobilization during the posterior assessment.

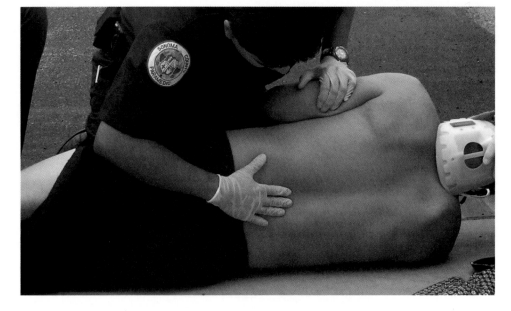

After completing the posterior assessment, place a spinal immobilization device under the patient. Carefully log roll the patient onto the long spine board. Completely immobilize the patient on the backboard (see Chapter 22).

Vital Signs and SAMPLE History

After completing the rapid trauma assessment, obtain the baseline vital signs and SAMPLE history as discussed in Chapter 5. Observe the rate and quality of respirations. Record the pulse rate and character. Assess skin color, temperature, and condition. Assess pupil response. Measure the blood pressure. If the patient is stable, continue to monitor the vital signs every 15 minutes. If the patient is not stable, assess vital signs every 5 minutes or more often, if necessary.

After taking the first set of vital signs, obtain the SAMPLE history. If the patient is responsive, take the SAMPLE history during transport. If the patient is unresponsive, ask others at the scene to give you a quick history. During transport, you will perform a more detailed physical exam and continue with ongoing assessment.

FOCUSED HISTORY AND PHYSICAL EXAM: MEDICAL

When the patient's chief complaint is medical, you will complete a focused history and physical exam based on the nature of the illness. This assessment looks at the patient's past medical history and the signs and symptoms of the present illness (see Fig. 9.21). First, you must quickly assess the patient's mental status. Use the AVPU evaluation described in Chapter 8 to determine whether the patient is responsive or unresponsive.

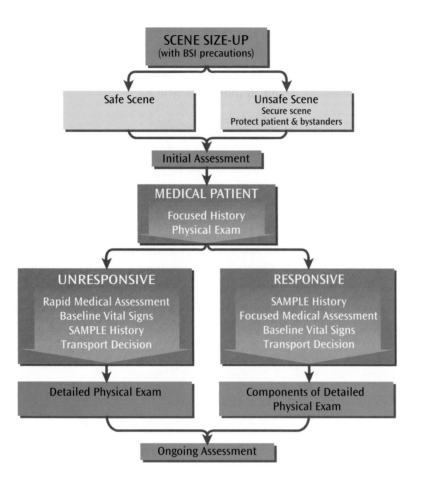

Figure 9.21 *Sequence of steps in the assessment of a medical patient.*

EMT Alert

Do not allow history-taking to delay the assessment and treatment of critical injuries or illnesses. If necessary, take a family member along in the ambulance to provide information while en route to the hospital.

A responsive patient will be able to tell you about his or her symptoms. In this case, you can generally determine the nature of the illness and conduct a physical examination specific to the problem. You will obtain:

1. History of the present illness and SAMPLE history

2. Rapid medical assessment focused on the area of chief complaint

3. Baseline vital signs

Begin by assessing the chief complaint and the associated signs or symptoms as discussed in Chapter 5. Use the OPQRST questions to assess the chief complaint. Obtain additional history using SAMPLE questions. It is important to gather this information quickly. The patient's condition may deteriorate at any time. He or she might speak and respond clearly one minute but become unresponsive the next. This is the primary reason for beginning with the focused history in responsive patients. If the patient loses consciousness, family members, friends, or bystanders can often provide you with valuable information.

Move to your physical exam after completing the history. Knowing the patient's medical history will help you to concentrate on areas that are directly related to the chief complaint. You will also have a better idea of the background of the current emergency.

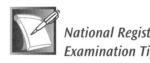

National Registry Examination Tip

Be prepared to read several different written scenarios and identify the appropriate history and physical exam questions for each case. Try to anticipate possible responses that a patient might give to these questions. Review the patient management diagram.

An unresponsive medical patient or one with altered mental status is not able to tell you what is wrong. You must first perform a physical examination to determine the nature of the illness and whether an injury has occurred in addition to the illness. For example, a patient with altered mental status could be a diabetic experiencing hypoglycemia (see Chapter 14). Or the patient could be suffering from a traumatic head injury that occurred the previous day. Your examination will guide the interventions you provide.

For an unresponsive medical patient, you will obtain:

1. A rapid medical assessment from head to toe

2. Baseline vital signs

3. A SAMPLE history (as far as family members or bystanders can provide)

Remember that an unresponsive patient may not be able to maintain his or her airway. Position the patient to protect the airway. Continually evaluate the adequacy of breathing.

Rapid Medical Assessment

Rapid Medical Assessment | A physical exam designed to quickly determine the nature and severity of an illness and identify necessary interventions

Rapid medical assessment techniques are similar to the rapid trauma assessment steps discussed previously. You will systematically examine the head, neck, chest, abdomen, pelvis, and extremities as needed. Table 9.2 summarizes important points to observe in each region.

If the patient is responsive and has a specific chief complaint, focus your rapid assessment on the area or body system involved. For an unresponsive patient, assess all of the areas. As you quickly inspect and palpate the entire body, look for physical signs associated with the patient's medical illness. Also make sure that the medical patient hasn't sustained any trauma. Use the DCAP-BTLS list to guide your evaluation. Spinal immobilization during a rapid medical assessment is not required, unless the chief complaint suggests the possibility of a spinal injury.

If at any time you discover life-threatening conditions, manage them immediately.

Table 9.2 • **RAPID MEDICAL ASSESSMENT**

Area of Body	Assessment
Assess head	Evaluate pupil response Look for drainage from ears, nose, throat
Assess neck	Assess for jugular venous distention or tracheal deviation Check for tracheostomy tube and whether suctioning is needed
Assess chest	Listen to breath sounds (present, normal or abnormal, equal)
Assess abdomen	Palpate for masses, tenderness, distention, swelling
Assess pelvis	Assess for bowel or bladder problems Evaluate whether the patient could be pregnant or have an ectopic pregnancy
Assess extremities	Assess pulses, movement, and sensation Look for medical identification bracelet Look for edema around the sacrum (suggests fluid overload or congestive heart failure)

PROVIDING EMERGENCY CARE

For every patient, the purpose of assessment is to discover conditions that require your emergency care. You will provide interventions, as authorized by medical direction and local protocols, based on your findings during the focused history and physical exam. Detailed assessment steps and interventions for specific medical and trauma situations are presented in later chapters of the book.

Remember that your major concern is always to ensure adequate breathing. Maintain an open airway, provide suction, and assist ventilations as necessary. Always provide high-flow oxygen to unconscious patients using a non-rebreather mask. Also establish and maintain in-line spinal stabilization for any suspected spinal injury. Always offer support and reassurance to responsive patients.

TRANSPORTING THE PATIENT

For a noncritical patient, prepare for transport after completing the focused history and physical exam and providing basic emergency care. In a critically ill or injured patient, rapid transport is a key to survival. Only life-threatening emergencies should be managed before transport. Work with your team to expedite rapid assessment and preparation for transport.

If spinal injury is not suspected, transport the patient in the recovery position. This position improves drainage of secretions from the mouth and helps to keep the airway open. If you observe signs of spinal injury, immobilize the cervical spine. If the nature of illness or mechanism of injury is unknown, assume that the patient is a victim of traumatic injury and proceed accordingly.

If you are maintaining the airway in a patient with spinal immobilization, turn the patient on his or her side while immobilized. After clearing the airway, you can rotate the patient back into a supine position. If the airway remains full of fluid or foreign material, ask another EMT-B to keep the backboard turned slightly to allow the material to flow out by gravity. Pay extra attention to monitoring and maintaining an airway in a patient who is immobilized.

D.O.T. OBJECTIVES

Discuss the components of the detailed physical exam.

Explain what additional care should be provided while performing the detailed physical exam.

Distinguish between the detailed physical exam that is performed on a trauma patient and the one that is performed on the medical patient.

State the areas of the body that are evaluated during the detailed physical exam.

DETAILED PHYSICAL EXAM

Detailed Physical Exam | A careful, comprehensive examination of the body performed on critical patients, usually while en route to the receiving facility

The **detailed physical exam**, or detailed assessment, is usually a head-to-toe physical examination. Its steps are similar to the rapid trauma and rapid medical exams (see Table 9.3). However, this time you will perform your evaluations slowly and methodically. The purpose of the exam is to gather additional information about a patient's injuries or signs of illness. This exam is not required for every patient. Determine whether this exam is indicated based upon the severity of the patient's injury or illness. For example, a patient with a cut finger would not need a detailed physical exam.

Complete the detailed physical exam only if conditions and time allow. It is most often performed while en route to the receiving facility. Try to conduct the detailed exam on all unresponsive patients and all trauma patients with multiple injuries or significant mechanisms of injury. In a life-threatening emergency, complete critical interventions before initiating the detailed exam.

Conduct the examination systematically for each area of the body (see Procedure 9.1 on pp. 310–11). Inspect and palpate for signs of illness or injury

Table 9.3 • DETAILED PHYSICAL EXAM

Area of Body	Assessment
Assess head	Evaluate entire skull and face for DCAP-BTLS and crepitation Evaluate ears for drainage Evaluate eyes for discoloration, unequal pupils, foreign bodies, blood in anterior chamber Evaluate nose for drainage or bleeding Evaluate mouth for loose or broken teeth or dentures, swollen or lacerated tongue, odors, discoloration, any object that could cause obstruction
Assess neck	Evaluate for DCAP-BTLS and JVD or crepitation
Assess chest	Evaluate for DCAP-BTLS and crepitation, paradoxical motion, breath sounds (present, equal, normal)
Assess abdomen	Evaluate for DCAP-BTLS and whether firm, soft, or distended
Assess pelvis	Evaluate for DCAP-BTLS and stability (gently flex and compress)
Assess extremities	Evaluate for DCAP-BTLS and distal pulses, sensation, and motor function
Assess posterior body	Evaluate for DCAP-BTLS

using DCAP–BTLS. Always attend to the patient's psychological needs during the assessment. Explain your actions and why each action is necessary. Being calm, efficient, and reassuring helps to build the patient's confidence in your ability to manage his or her care.

Reassess vital signs after the detailed physical exam if time and the patient's condition permit. If you are busy, have another member of your team complete this task. Vital signs are measured during the focused history and physical exam, after the detailed physical exam, and as part of ongoing assessment. Compare the results with baseline vital sign values and note any changes.

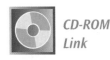

CD-ROM Link

See the "Detailed Physical Exam" video in the Patient Assessment chapter and the Video Appendix on the MedEMT CD-ROM for a demonstration of this examination.

D.O.T. OBJECTIVE

Describe the components of the ongoing assessment.

ONGOING ASSESSMENT

In order to ensure appropriate care, you must reevaluate the patient frequently. The **ongoing assessment** serves three purposes:

- To identify any missed injuries or conditions
- To detect any changes in the patient's condition
- To determine the effectiveness of interventions

Ongoing Assessment | *Frequent reevaluation of a patient after initial assessment and primary interventions; to identify changes in patient condition and ensure appropriate care*

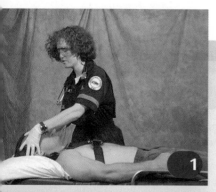

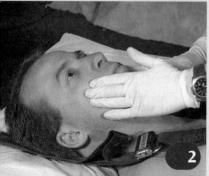

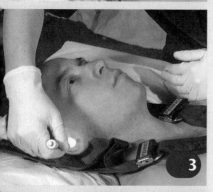

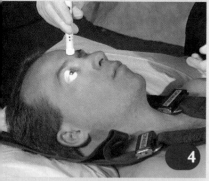

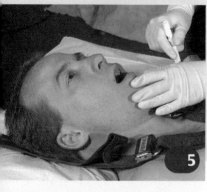

Procedure 9.1 • DETAILED PHYSICAL EXAM

 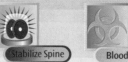

Stabilize Spine   Bloodborne   Video Appendix

1. Assess each area of the head individually during the detailed examination. Inspect and palpate the entire skull. Access may be limited by spinal stabilization or immobilization. Avoid palpating obvious deformities of the skull. Gently place your palms on the top of the patient's head, in the parietal region. Then palpate the back of head, in the occipital region. Sequentially palpate the side, or temporal region, and the frontal region. Look for the DCAP-BTLS signs of injuries. Listen and feel for crepitation of bones and look for blood on your gloves.

2. Inspect and palpate the cheekbones, forehead, and lower jaw. Assess for DCAP-BTLS. Look for signs of a possible mandibular injury or dislocation. Inability to close the mouth, misaligned teeth, and signs of an airway obstruction suggest injuries to the mandible.

3. Use a flashlight or penlight to examine the ears and nose. Some signs suggest a basilar skull injury. Look for drainage of cerebrospinal fluid or blood from the ear. You might also see Battle's sign (bruising behind the ear and mandibular joint) or raccoon eyes (bruises around the eyes). Assess the DCAP-BTLS checklist for injuries to the nose and ears.

4. Examine the eyes using a flashlight. Inspect the eyelids, pupils, sclera, and conjunctiva. Do not force the lids open. Evaluate DCAP-BTLS and look for foreign bodies in the eyes. Inspect for blood in the anterior chamber of the eye. This indicates that the patient has received a serious blow. Shine a light in each eye from the lateral side. Check for a reddish discoloration or a dependent pool of blood in the lower portion of the pupil. Look for discoloration of the sclera or conjunctiva. The sclera should be white. Yellow or red color suggests disease or injury. The conjunctiva is normally pink, but some diseases cause it to appear pale or red. Check the pupils for size and reactivity. Normal pupils are equal-sized, round, and reactive to light. Classify the pupil response as reactive (brisk), sluggish, or nonreactive (fixed). Classify the pupil size as normal, pinpointed, or dilated. Abnormal findings are most significant in an unresponsive patient.

5. Open the mouth and inspect the teeth, tongue, and mucosa with a flashlight. Use the DCAP-BTLS method. Remove loose or broken teeth or dentures that could obstruct the airway. A swollen tongue may also block the airway. Lacerations of the tongue may suggest a recent seizure. Check for mucosal discoloration or burns. Smell for unusual odors that could indicate diabetes, alcohol, or ingestion of a toxic substance.

Procedure 9.1 • Detailed Physical Exam *(cont.)*

6. Inspect and palpate the anterior neck, if it is accessible. Assess the jugular veins and trachea. Check for JVD. Listen and feel for crepitation. This indicates trauma to the airway, lungs, or esophagus. The cervical spine will already be immobilized if you suspect a spinal injury. Removing the front of the cervical collar may be necessary to thoroughly inspect and palpate the neck. Your partner must maintain in-line spinal stabilization during this part of the exam. The device may have an anterior opening or window that allows you to assess the neck without removing the collar.

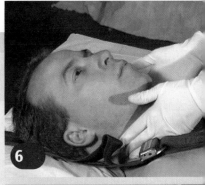

7. Inspect and palpate the chest beginning with a DCAP-BTLS assessment of the clavicles. Move sequentially to the sternum, ribs, and as much of the back as you can reach without moving the patient. Check the chest for crepitation, suggesting an air leak from a punctured lung. Reassess for chest injury and breathing difficulty, including use of accessory muscles (see Chapters 4 and 5). Observe the patient taking a deep breath. Auscultate the lungs with your stethoscope.

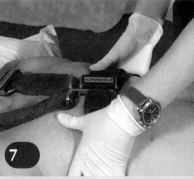

8. Inspect and palpate all four quadrants of the abdomen. The normal abdomen should feel soft, not firm or distended. Also check for DCAP-BTLS signs.

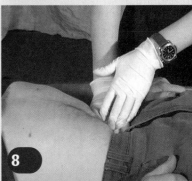

9. Inspect and palpate the pelvic girdle by placing your hands on both iliac crests. Do not palpate the pelvis if an obvious deformity is present or if the patient complains of pain. If you observe pain or motion of the normally fixed bones, suspect a serious pelvic injury. Examine the pelvis if the patient is unresponsive or has no complaints of pain in that region.

10. Inspect and palpate one extremity at a time, beginning with the lower body. Check the extremities for DCAP-BTLS signs. Palpate the distal pulses and compare the left and right pulses for equality. Use the dorsalis pedis or posterior tibial pulse in the lower extremities. In the upper extremities, use the radial pulse.

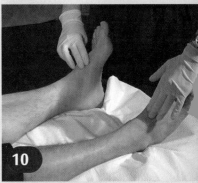

11. If a spinal injury is not suspected, log roll the patient to inspect and palpate the upper and lower back, buttocks, and posterior extremities. If a spinal injury is suspected, the patient will already be immobilized on a backboard. Carefully slide your hands under the patient and palpate for abnormalities.

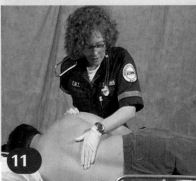

The ongoing assessment is performed on all patients while en route to the hospital (see Table 9.4). Repeat the ongoing assessment every 15 minutes if the patient is stable and at least every 5 minutes if unstable. If you discover a life-threatening problem during assessment, provide emergency care immediately.

Table 9.4 • ONGOING ASSESSMENT

Reevaluation	Assessment
Repeat initial assessment	Reassess mental status Maintain open airway Monitor breathing for rate and quality Reassess pulse for rate and quality Monitor skin color and temperature Reestablish patient priorities
Reassess vital signs	Record pulse, respiratory rate, and blood pressure
Repeat focused assessment	Reevaluate patient's complaints or injuries
Check interventions	Ensure adequacy of oxygen delivery and ventilation Ensure management of bleeding Ensure effectiveness of all interventions
Repeat ongoing assessment	Every 5 minutes for critical patients Every 15 minutes for stable patients

> **D.O.T. OBJECTIVE**
>
> Discuss the reasons for repeating the initial assessment as part of the ongoing assessment.

EMT Tip

Remember: Maintaining the airway, breathing, and circulation takes priority in all patients.

Repeating Initial Assessment

Repeat the initial assessment as though you were examining the patient for the first time, and compare your observations with your initial findings. Conditions for examining the patient may be more favorable in the ambulance, revealing additional injuries, signs, or symptoms. The patient may also become responsive and report additional history or complaints.

Identify any missed injuries or conditions and anything that requires immediate intervention. Identify changes in the patient's condition and reassess the effectiveness of interventions. Reassess the mental status of the patient. Observe for changes in speech, orientation, and level of awareness. If the patient becomes unresponsive, assess AVPU mental status.

Reassess the airway to be sure it is open and that there are no secretions or anything that could cause airway obstruction. A conscious patient who is talking comfortably has an airway that is open and clear. Next, look, listen, and feel for breathing rate and quality. If deficiencies or problems are seen, you may need to deliver supplemental oxygen or assist ventilations.

Reassess the patient's circulation. Changes in pulse rate or quality indicate improvement or deterioration of the circulatory system. Determine if the radial pulse is present, lost, or regained. Reassess the skin color, temperature, and perfusion. Monitor capillary refill in children less than 6 years old. Check sites of major bleeding for recurrence. Look for signs of shock or signs of improvement.

Once the initial assessment has been repeated, reconsider your patient priorities and adjust the emphasis of care as necessary. Immediately transport any patient with a deteriorating status or critical conditions you cannot adequately manage.

CD-ROM Link

The "Assessment in the Ambulance" video in the Authentic Emergency Scenes section of the Video Appendix on the MedEMT CD-ROM depicts an EMT monitoring a patient while en route to the hospital.

D.O.T. OBJECTIVE

Describe trending of assessment components.

Reassessing Vital Signs

Again assess and record the breathing rate and quality, pulse rate and quality, pupil response, and skin color, temperature, and condition (perfusion). Measure the blood pressure. Record the time of reassessment.

Carefully look for trends that demonstrate improvement or deterioration in the patient's condition. Always be prepared to provide interventions if the patient's condition worsens. Constantly look for subtle changes or trends in vital signs. If the systolic blood pressure drops, the difference between the systolic and diastolic pressure will decrease. The difference between the systolic and diastolic pressure readings is the pulse pressure. When measuring successive vital signs, look for changes in both pressures. Narrowing pulse pressure may suggest life-threatening traumatic injury and shock. If the systolic blood pressure is less than 100 mmHg with a pulse pressure of less than 30 mmHg, consider the possibility of severe blood loss and shock.

Repeating Focused Assessment

During transport, the patient may begin to complain about symptoms or injuries not initially disclosed. An unresponsive patient may regain consciousness and be able to provide a history. Perform a focused history and rapid physical exam that is specific to the patient's complaint or injury.

Checking Interventions

National Registry Examination Tip

Understand the purpose for the ongoing assessment and recognize the steps included in this assessment.

Reassess the appropriateness and adequacy of interventions by observing the patient's responses. Check the following interventions for effectiveness:

- Airway management, including OPAs and NPAs

- Oxygen delivery, artificial ventilation, and chest compressions; ensure that the oxygen tank isn't empty and that ventilation is adequate with good chest rise and fall

- Management of bleeding; check all dressings to ensure that bleeding is controlled

- Spinal immobilization

- Splinting

- Other interventions

Adjust emergency care as needed if there is no improvement or there is deterioration of the patient's condition. Check your equipment to verify that it is functioning properly and that it is correctly applied. If necessary, change any ineffective interventions and reassess the effects.

Chapter Nine Summary

- If the patient has suffered a traumatic injury, perform the focused history and physical exam for a trauma patient. If the mechanism of injury (MOI) is significant, complete a rapid examination of the patient from head to toe (the rapid trauma assessment). If the MOI is minor, examine only the affected area.

- For responsive medical patients, perform a medical focused history and physical exam. If the patient is unconscious, perform a thorough head-to-toe assessment (the rapid medical assessment). Carefully evaluate unconscious patients to be sure that traumatic injury is not involved.

- The detailed physical exam is often performed while en route to the hospital. The detailed exam is a careful, more thorough assessment of the patient from head to toe. Based on the patient's chief complaint, there may be specific signs or symptoms you will look for.

- While en route to the receiving facility, it is very important to perform ongoing assessments. For unstable patients, you should perform these every 5 minutes. For stable patients, reevaluate every 15 minutes. The ongoing assessment involves repeating the initial assessment, remeasuring vital signs, and checking any interventions you may have performed.

Key Terms Review

Crepitation | *page 298*
Detailed Physical Exam | *page 308*
Edema | *page 303*
Focused History and Physical Exam | *page 292*

Jugular Venous Distention (JVD) | *page 299*
Ongoing Assessment | *page 309*
Paradoxical Motion | *page 300*

Rapid Medical Assessment | *page 306*
Rapid Trauma Assessment | *page 293*
Tracheal Deviation | *page 299*

Review Questions

1. Which mnemonic will help you to further assess a patient's chief complaint?

   a. OPQRST
   b. SAMPLE
   c. CHART
   d. AVPU

2. At what point during treatment and transport of a patient from a motor vehicle accident would you perform a detailed physical exam?

   a. Upon initial contact with the patient
   b. During transport of the patient
   c. As soon as the patient is on a backboard
   d. Immediately after extrication

3. Which of the following is NOT part of the ongoing assessment?

   a. Baseline vital signs
   b. Intervention check
   c. Repeated focused assessment
   d. Repeated initial assessment

4. Paradoxical movement of the chest may suggest:

   a. Cerebral edema
   b. Flail chest
   c. Cardiac contusion
   d. Abdominal contusion

5. Distention, firmness, or rigidity of the abdomen may suggest:

   a. Internal bleeding
   b. Cardiac contusion
   c. Flail chest
   d. Head injury

6. Reevaluating the patient helps to:

   a. Detect initial problems
   b. Identify any missed injuries or conditions
   c. Detect any patient changes
   d. Detect any patient changes and identify missed injuries or conditions

7. The mnemonic OPQRST can assist the EMT-B while assessing the chief complaint. What does the letter "P" stand for in this mnemonic?

   a. Perfusion
   b. Pupil size
   c. Position
   d. Provocation

8. When assessing the patient's ears and nose, the EMT-B should look for Battle's sign. This is:

   a. Blood or clear fluid oozing from the ears
   b. Blood or clear fluid oozing from the nose
   c. Bruising behind the ears and mandibular joint
   d. A ringing sensation deep inside the ears

9. Which of the following is NOT a circumstance in which you would perform a rapid trauma assessment?

   a. When you encounter a significant mechanism of injury
   b. When you detect critical injuries or findings
   c. When you are unsure of the extent of injury
   d. When the patient has suffered an isolated extremity injury

10. In the mnemonic DCAP-BTLS, what does the B stand for?

    a. Bilateral
    b. Burns
    c. Blow by
    d. Brachial

11. A flail chest occurs when:

    a. Two or more ribs are broken in at least two places
    b. There is an open chest wound
    c. There is a sucking chest wound
    d. The diaphragm is displaced upward

12. For the purpose of assessment, the abdomen is divided into:

    a. Four quadrants
    b. Top and bottom halves
    c. Front and rear sections
    d. Central and peripheral areas

CASE STUDIES

Patient Assessment

1
The scene is remarkably quiet for a drive-by shooting in this part of town. The city police have the area surrounded with yellow tape and have covered one body. Several officers have detained a group of young men on the front lawn of a small brick house. One officer directs you to your patient, a 50-year-old female whose son was just killed. She is sitting on the porch complaining of moderate shortness of breath and mild chest pain. During your physical exam, you notice some crackling sounds when you palpate the patient's left shoulder.

A. Considering the discovery of crackling sounds together with shortness of breath, what is the most likely mechanism of injury or nature of illness?

B. When assessing lung sounds in this patient, what should you try to determine?

2
Most of the people headed out of town this holiday weekend seem to be driving responsibly. As you enter the cross-town freeway after a busy shift, you see traffic slowing. A car looks like it has just come to a stop across the second and third lanes of traffic. Several people have left their vehicles and are attempting to open the driver's door. You cannot see any signs of a traffic crash. The people assisting do not seem agitated or angry. After you safely park your vehicle, a bystander advises you that the car had been weaving across traffic and then suddenly came to a stop. The driver, an elderly female who is slumped over the steering wheel, appears unresponsive.

A. Describe the steps you will take once the scene is safe and you have gained access to the patient.

B. You are unable to find any obvious signs of injury on the patient. What other items might you look for to indicate this patient's immediate problem or medical history?

C. What medical conditions might require rapid transport?

D. When you assess the patient's sacral area and ankles, you notice significant edema. What might be the medical cause of this condition?

CASE STUDIES

Patient Assessment (cont.)

3 The weather has turned ugly. Many of the rural roads will soon be flooded. A highway patrol officer requests emergency service for a three-car crash about eight miles south of town. When you arrive on scene, two volunteers have just completed triage. They direct you to a patient who was ejected from a small pickup truck that appears to have rolled several times. He is a 16-year-old male with obvious head injuries and bilateral deformity of the lower extremities. Volunteer first responders are maintaining spinal precautions and ventilating the patient with a pocket mask.

A. Should this patient receive a rapid trauma assessment or a focused history and physical exam? Why?

B. How does the rapid trauma assessment differ from the focused history and physical exam?

C. What do the letters DCAP-BTLS stand for? Why are they important?

D. The volunteer who is working with you is providing the patient with artificial ventilation. He has only worked with the rescue squad for two months and is still unsure of his skills. As he begins another round of ventilations, he stops and reports that his ventilation is not causing the chest to rise. The patient is cyanotic around the lips and earlobes. What should you do in this situation?

E. When you begin your rapid assessment of the patient's neck, what specific things will you look for?

4 Transport times from your new response area are commonly in excess of thirty minutes. You were comfortable with the ten- or fifteen-minute transports from your previous assignment, but are still learning how to handle calls that last longer. The patient in your unit has been complaining of general weakness and dizziness. She is 73 years old and denies any significant medical history. She has been vomiting for several hours and has been unable to eat since yesterday morning. Your initial assessment and physical exam have revealed no significant problems or findings. Her baseline vital signs are normal except for blood pressure slightly lower than average.

A. What are the reasons for the ongoing assessment?

B. If the patient's condition were unstable, how often would you take vital signs? Why?

C. One step in the ongoing assessment is to check interventions. What does that step include?

Stories from the Field
Wrap-Up

The critical patient is often difficult to assess due to the drama of the call. For a new EMT-Basic, encountering a large amount of blood, a possible crime scene, and the need for quick action can lead to problems. There can be a tendency to freeze or to develop a sort of tunnel vision that causes you to miss important details. This is why assessing a patient must follow a standardized procedure. You must act quickly, yet remain focused on performing a thorough rapid trauma assessment.

In all critical situations, the EMT team must quickly take charge of the scene, perform a rapid assessment, and transport the patient. Trauma has become recognized as a disease that can only be treated adequately in the hospital. The clock is already ticking when you arrive, so you must not waste precious time on the scene. Your rapid assessment and early transport may be the difference between life and death. For a noncritical patient, rapid assessment and transport may not be as essential, but you must still follow a standardized procedure to ensure nothing is missed. Assessment is a critical skill to develop because every patient you encounter will need a competent analysis of his or her condition.

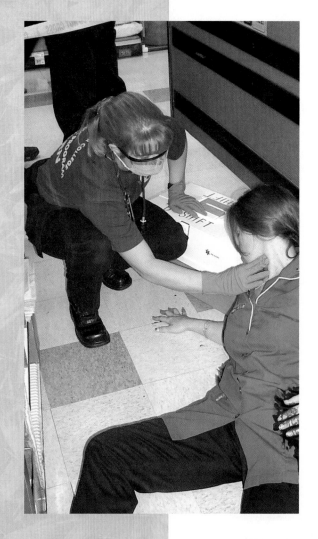

Chapter 10

Communications and Documentation

Stories from the Field

Your crew is asked to respond to a local school one Tuesday evening. The dispatcher advises you that a young girl was injured while participating in a gymnastics meet. When you arrive, you find a 12-year-old girl sitting on the bleachers. She landed incorrectly from a vault and hurt her lower left leg. Your patient appears to be very quiet and depressed. Robin's initial assessment reveals no life-threatening conditions.

The teacher hands you a copy of the parent's permission form, which includes consent for you to treat and transport the girl to the local hospital. Robin and John ask you to obtain a history and vital signs while they evaluate and splint the injured ankle. The patient's vital signs are: pulse 68, respiration 22, blood pressure 114/68, pupils equal and reactive, skin color pink, and skin condition warm and moist. Although the girl doesn't know much about her own medical history, the permission form states the following: allergies—codeine, medications—none, and past history—heart murmur since birth. Splinting the leg takes longer than usual. While en route, the patient complains that her leg hurts worse. Robin asks you to call the receiving facility and give a preliminary report.

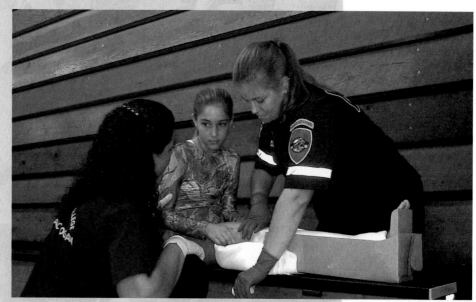

C ommunication is an essential part of prehospital care. Although your patient care centers on assessment and intervention, you also need excellent verbal and written communication skills. You will use both verbal and written methods of communication during every response. The continuum of patient care is based upon effective and efficient communication. You must be able to communicate your findings accurately to other healthcare providers. The best prehospital care will suffer at the receiving facility if the staff is not properly prepared for the patient's condition.

You must also create written records describing all aspects of your patient's emergency situation. Complete and accurate documentation helps to ensure high-quality patient care. A prehospital care report must be filled out for every patient encounter. This documents the nature and extent of your emergency medical care. It will become a permanent part of the patient's hospital record. Written communication is generally completed at the receiving facility. Well-prepared reports are important for both medical and legal purposes.

COMMUNICATIONS

You will communicate vital patient information to the appropriate people during dispatch, throughout the call, and after completion of transport (see Fig. 10.1). Three forms of verbal communication are used during a call:

- Radio communications
- Communications with staff at the receiving facility
- Interpersonal communications with the patient and others on scene

Radio Communications

Radio communication is essential in emergency medical systems. You will use radios to communicate with dispatch, medical direction, and the receiving facility (see Fig. 10.2). During a typical emergency response, radio transmissions are used when:

- EMS dispatch transmits a call to the EMS unit
- Your unit acknowledges that the call was received
- You notify dispatch that you are en route
- Dispatch contacts other agencies as necessary, such as medical direction or the local hospital
- You notify dispatch that you have arrived at the scene
- You contact medical direction to report the patient's condition or request orders

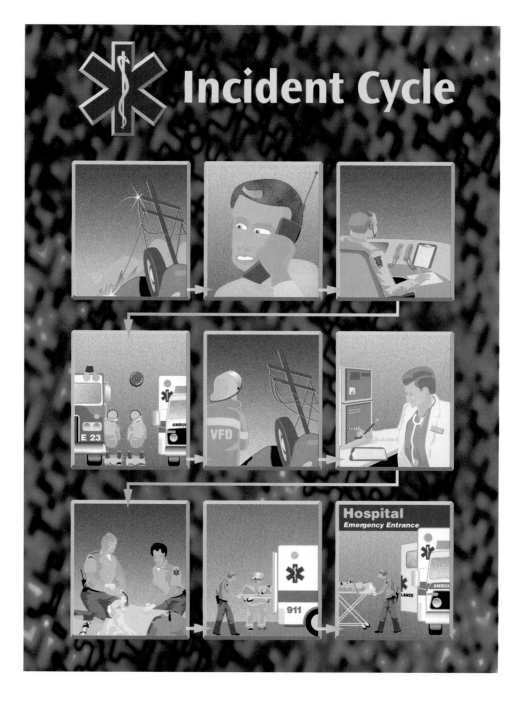

Figure 10.1 *Communications that occur during a typical incident: Someone at the scene contacts the dispatch center, which notifies EMS personnel. Medical direction is consulted as the EMTs gather information from the patient. After transport, the EMTs provide a report to hospital staff.*

- You notify dispatch that you are leaving the scene
- You contact the receiving hospital to give a patient report
- You notify dispatch of your arrival at the hospital
- You notify dispatch that you have left the hospital
- You notify dispatch of your arrival back at the station

Radio communications are regulated and monitored by the Federal Communications Commission (FCC). Specific frequencies are assigned and licensed for EMS operations. The FCC also approves the equipment that is used.

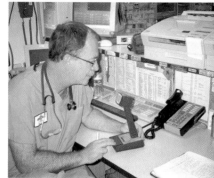

Figure 10.2 *Communication with medical direction.*

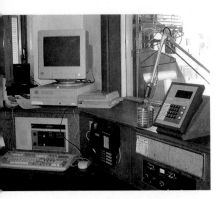

Figure 10.3 *Base stations are often located in hospitals or on mountaintops.*

Base Station | *Radio used for central dispatch operations and coordination of emergency services in an EMS communication system*

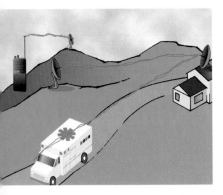

Figure 10.4 *Repeaters help communications among EMS personnel over a wide area or difficult terrain.*

Mobile Radio | *Two-way radios that are usually built into emergency vehicles*

Repeaters | *Communications devices that receive a low-power transmission and rebroadcast the signal at higher power*

Communications Equipment

Although local systems and protocols vary considerably, most prehospital care communications systems rely on common types of equipment (see Table 10.1).

- A **base station** is a radio that is located at a stationary site. This might be at a hospital or public safety agency or on a mountaintop (see Fig. 10.3). The base station is used for dispatch operations and coordination of emergency services. It has superior transmitting and receiving capabilities (80 to 150 watts).

- Mobile two-way radios are usually mounted in the vehicle. Most **mobile radios** transmit at 20 to 50 watts. They have a relatively long transmission range of 10 to 15 miles over average terrain.

- Portable radios are handheld transmitter/receivers. Their power output is 1 to 5 watts and their range is approximately 1 to 5 miles. With a portable radio, you can maintain communication while away from the ambulance.

- **Repeaters** form a system of remote receivers for communication over a wide area or difficult terrain. Repeaters receive a transmission from a low-power portable or mobile radio on one frequency. They rebroadcast the signal at higher power on another frequency (see Fig. 10.4).

- Digital radio equipment uses encoders and decoders to isolate specific frequencies for different transmissions. This allows for more efficient use of crowded broadcast frequencies.

- Cellular telephones are increasingly used in EMS communications. They are portable and can serve a wide area. They are useful in areas where a radio system is not well established. They can also be used as secondary backup in case of radio failure.

Constant maintenance of radio communications equipment is essential to assure effective delivery of emergency medical services. All emergency radio equipment should be kept clean and in good working order at all times. Batteries must be checked and replaced regularly. Your agency should have a protocol for periodic inspection and service by a qualified technician. It will also provide for backup methods in case the usual procedures do not work.

D.O.T. OBJECTIVES

List the proper methods of initiating and terminating a radio call.

Describe the attributes for increasing effectiveness and efficiency of verbal communications.

Table 10.1 • EMS COMMUNICATIONS SYSTEMS

Type of System	Range	Advantages	Disadvantages
VHF-Band Transmission	15–20 miles (mobile radio) 1–5 miles (portable radio) Signal can be increased using repeaters	Widely available Guaranteed channel access Most common system	Expensive to purchase and maintain Requires FCC license Requires line-of-sight between parties
UHF-Band Transmission	15–20 miles (mobile radio) 1–5 miles (portable radio) Signal can be increased using repeaters	Widely available Guaranteed channel access Less dependent than VHF on line-of-sight between parties	Expensive to purchase and maintain Requires FCC license
Cellular Telephone Transmission	20 miles from cell site, otherwise unlimited	Inexpensive Widely available Person being called requires no special equipment	Cell site availability becomes a problem during events Dependent on third party for channel access Calls can be overheard on scanners
Digital Transmission	3–5 miles from digital cell site, otherwise unlimited	Secure connections Excellent clarity High reliability	Not widely available Dependent on third party for channel access

Principles of Radio Communications

The following general principles should be used for all radio communications. Learn your local protocols for communicating.

- Turn on the radio and adjust the volume. If necessary, close the ambulance windows to reduce background noise.

- Use an assigned EMS frequency. Listen to the channel before beginning transmission to ensure that it is clear.

- Press the *press to talk (PTT)* button on the radio. Wait for one second before speaking. This will prevent having your first words cut off.

- Hold the microphone 2 to 3 inches from your lips as you speak. Speak clearly and slowly, in a monotone voice (see Fig. 10.5).

- Address the unit being called. Then identify your unit by name and number. For example, say "Mercy Hospital, this is Ambulance 2."

- The unit being called will signal you to begin transmission. They might reply "This is Mercy Hospital, go ahead." A response of "Stand by" means you must wait for further notice before continuing.

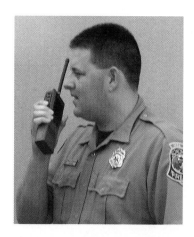

Figure 10.5 *Speak slowly and clearly when using a portable radio.*

- Keep transmissions brief. On long transmissions, stop speaking after thirty seconds and pause for a few seconds. This will allow other emergency traffic to use the frequency if necessary.

- When the transmission is finished, say "Over." Wait for confirmation that the message was received.

During your radio communications, speak in plain English. Don't use codes, except those that are standard for your department. Avoid meaningless phrases such as "Be advised." Say "Affirmative" and "Negative" instead of "Yes" and "No," which can be difficult to hear. When transmitting a number that could sound like another, state the number, then the individual digits. For example, say "Sixteen, one-six" to avoid confusion with the number sixty.

Courtesy is assumed in your transmissions. There is no need to say "Please," "Thank you," or "You're welcome." Also, say "We" instead of "I." An EMT rarely acts alone.

Radio transmissions are not private. Many people monitor radio frequencies used by public agencies, including emergency medical services. Scanners are popular. They allow the general public and media personnel to listen to your calls. Therefore:

- Do not give a patient's name over the air.

- Only give information about your assessment and the treatment rendered. Use the standard reporting format. Avoid offering any diagnosis of the patient's condition.

- Remain objective and impartial when describing patients. You could be sued for slander if you injured someone's reputation over the airwaves.

- Do not use profanity on the air. The FCC can impose substantial fines.

EMT Tip

Interference with emergency radio communications and the use of obscene or offensive language are strictly prohibited.

D.O.T. OBJECTIVE

List the correct radio procedures in the following phases of a typical call: to the scene, at the scene, to the facility, at the facility, to the station, and at the station.

Communicating with Dispatch

You will be given vital information by the dispatch center about the nature of your call (see Fig. 10.6). The dispatcher will also inform you of any coordinating agencies involved. You must keep dispatch informed of your status and location. Notify the dispatcher:

- Acknowledging that a call has been received

- When your unit is en route

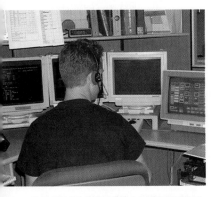

Figure 10.6 *Communication with dispatch is necessary for vital information.*

- Upon arrival at the scene
- When you leave the scene
- Upon arrival at the hospital
- When leaving the hospital for the station
- Upon arrival at the station
- At other times as required by local protocol

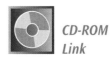

CD-ROM Link

See the "Paramedic in the Ambulance" video in Chapters 10, 24, and the Video Appendix on the MedEMT CD-ROM for an example of radio communications in the tense atmosphere while en route to the hospital.

The dispatcher will tell you the time of the communication. Enter the time into your written report. Record times using the 24-hour military system. All elements of the EMS system must use accurate and synchronized clocks. Recorded times can be important for legal reasons and for quality control. Accurate times are also necessary as you monitor changes in the patient's vital signs. Set the ambulance clock and your watch to match the dispatch center's clock.

It is customary for all dispatch calls to be recorded. The recording becomes part of the legal record.

Communicating with Medical Direction

After assessing your patient and providing emergency interventions, you may need to contact the medical direction physician. Medical direction can give you permission for administration of medications. The physician might recommend other treatments or assessment procedures that are appropriate for the patient. The medical direction physician may or may not be located at the receiving facility.

Medical direction relies on your information about the patient's condition. Your communications must be organized, clear, concise, accurate, and pertinent. To ensure that all communications are clearly understood, follow these guidelines:

- Speak slowly and clearly.
- Report accurate, concise information using the standard medical report format (discussed in the next section).
- Immediately repeat all orders for medications or procedures exactly as you heard them. Also repeat any denials of your requests.
- Ask medical direction to repeat any order that you didn't hear clearly. Then repeat it exactly as heard.
- If you do not understand an order or have any questions about it, ask for clarification. The medical director may have misunderstood part of your transmission. He or she might state orders in a way that is unfamiliar to you. Always clear up anything you are not sure about. This is better than making a potentially harmful mistake.

Communicating with the Receiving Facility

The staff at the receiving facility needs clear, concise, accurate information about the patient's condition. They must prepare their personnel and resources before your arrival. This ensures efficient continuity of care. Usually you will communicate with the receiving facility in three ways:

- By radio, while en route to the facility
- In person, when you transfer patient care to another healthcare professional
- In writing, on your patient care report (see the discussion on Documentation later in this chapter)

While en route, your radio reports to the receiving facility will follow the format of the standard medical report. You will continue your ongoing patient assessment and reassessment of vital signs during transport. Update your reports with any new information that becomes available. Include any improvement or deterioration in the patient's condition.

D.O.T. OBJECTIVE

State the proper sequence for delivery of patient information.

Standard Medical Report

When reporting patient information to medical direction and the receiving facility, you will use the standard medical report format. This ensures that critical data is presented in a concise, well-organized way. A typical standard medical report should include the following information, given in this order:

- The identity of your unit and the levels of providers who are present
- Your estimated time of arrival
- The patient's age and sex
- The chief complaint
- A brief, pertinent history of the present illness
- Information on major past illnesses
- The patient's mental status
- The baseline vital signs
- Pertinent findings from your physical exam
- A summary of emergency medical care that has been provided
- The patient's response to the emergency medical care

Communications at the Receiving Facility

After arrival at the hospital, give a verbal report to the staff. This will ensure continuity of care. Introduce the patient by name, if known. Summarize the information given over the radio in your standard medical report. Note any new or changed information. Include the following information in your verbal report:

- Chief complaint
- Any history or information that was not transmitted previously
- Additional treatment given en route
- Additional vital signs taken en route

Communicating to receiving facility staff is essential for both medical and legal reasons. Giving information to the proper healthcare professional is part of transferring patient care. You could be charged with abandonment if you failed to give a complete and accurate report of the patient's condition.

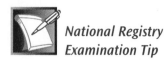

National Registry Examination Tip

Review the responsibility of the FCC for EMS communications. Briefly review the various types of communications systems used in EMS. Understand the basic components of an EMS radio report and the principles of radio communications. Be familiar with the typical progression of radio transmissions throughout a response. Note the basic skills for interpersonal communication and communication with medical direction.

Interpersonal Communications

When you enter a scene, you will communicate with the patient, family, friends, or bystanders. These individuals are often frightened, upset, angry, or confused. You must assess the situation and communicate effectively in order to establish trust and rapport.

Apply these skills for effective communication at the scene:

• Enter the scene in a calm, confident, and caring manner.

• Identify yourself and tell the patient that you are there to help.

• Ask the patient his or her name and what he or she likes to be called. With older people, use the patient's formal name, unless given permission to use the first name. Use the patient's name throughout the contact.

• Ask the patient if it is all right to provide treatment. If the patient says no, continue to question in a reassuring manner. Make sure you do not begin care until you receive consent.

• Make and keep eye contact with the patient. This shows respect and interest. However, note that direct eye contact may seem rude or be uncomfortable for people from some cultural backgrounds. Adjust your behavior accordingly.

• Position yourself at or below the patient's eye level in order to appear less intimidating. Occasionally, you may want to assume a taller stance to establish authority.

• Be aware of what your body language communicates to your patient. Do you appear open or closed, caring or impatient, respectful or annoyed?

• Speak clearly, slowly, and distinctly. Use language that the patient can understand.

• Allow the patient enough time to answer a question before asking the next one. This is especially important with young and elderly patients.

• Be honest. Listen to the patient's questions and answer as fully as possible. Explain what you are doing.

Special Circumstances

Communicating with some people requires special skills or arrangements.

Hearing-impaired individuals:

• Speak clearly with your lips visible to the person

• Use any American Sign Language (ASL) interpreters at the scene

• Use written notes

Non-English speaking individuals:

• Use any interpreters on scene

• Request an interpreter from dispatch or medical direction

Elderly individuals:

- Talk slowly and listen to each response
- Treat the person with respect
- Accommodate any visual or hearing deficit
- Do not immediately assume visual, hearing, or mental impairment

Children:

- Stay at the child's eye level and speak calmly
- Be honest
- Parents should be on scene if possible, and remain calm and confident

DOCUMENTATION

Your written reports detailing an emergency response and your prehospital care serve as important medical documents (see Fig. 10.7). They help to ensure continuity of care for your patient in the emergency department as well as later, when they may be referred to for important information. These reports also become permanent legal documents. You may be required to testify in court based on the forms you complete.

The information in your reports is often used for other purposes. It may provide an educational case study that demonstrates how to handle unusual circumstances. It may be evaluated as part of continuous EMS quality improvement, to analyze and improve various components of the system or to prevent problems from occurring. Details of a situation may provide valuable health research data. The documentation may also be used administratively, for patient billing or to compile service statistics for your agency.

A good report describes the status of the patient upon arrival at the scene, what emergency medical care was provided, and any changes in condition before arrival at the receiving facility. Documentation should include both objective and subjective information stated clearly and accurately.

Remember these sayings when filling out reports—if it isn't written down, it wasn't done, and if it wasn't done, don't write it down.

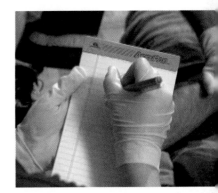

Figure 10.7 *Documentation may be used for medical, educational, legal, and informational purposes.*

D.O.T. OBJECTIVES

Explain the components of the written report and list the information that should be included on the written report.

Discuss all state and/or local record and reporting requirements.

Prehospital Care Report

Prehospital Care Report (PCR) | *Documentation of the assessment and treatment of a patient in the field*

The **prehospital care report (PCR)** is the major document that you will complete regarding your emergency care. In the PCR, you paint a picture of the patient's condition. This will assist the hospital staff in understanding what occurred before arrival at the hospital. The ongoing record of vital signs and mental status indicates whether the patient is improving or deteriorating. Your descriptions of the patient's condition on arrival, any procedures done, and the response to treatment give the emergency staff valuable information that allows for continuity of care.

Figure 10.8 *Example of a prehospital care report.*

PREHOSPITAL CARE REPORT

Dispatch

MONTH/DAY/YEAR | PATIENT CARE TRANSFERRED TO: | TIME | ☐NON TRANSPORT ☐ALS ☐BLS ☐TRANSFER | PATIENT STATUS ☐STAT ☐NONSTAT | NO OF PATIENTS ____ OF ____ | FIRE #

PATIENT'S NAME LAST FIRST | UNIT # | AMB#

PATIENT'S ADDRESS | CITY | STATE | ZIP

LOCATION OF INCIDENT | CALL RECEIVED : | ENROUTE : | AT SCENE : | TO HOSPITAL : | AT HOSPITAL :

FIRST RESPONDERS | AID GIVEN ☐O_2 ☐CPR | ☐CPR STARTED AT ____ ☐TIME WITHOUT CPR ____ ☐OTHER ____ | CODE TO 2 | 3 | CHANGED 2 | 3 | AGENCY

Patient Medical Information

AGE____ GENDER ☐M ☐F WEIGHT______ (KG LB) PVT MD LEVEL OF DISTRESS ☐MILD ☐MOD ☐SEVERE LOC 1 2 3 4

CHIEF COMPLAINT & CURRENT HISTORY ____
P
Q
R
S
T

PAST MEDICAL HX. | ALLERGIES

TIME	PULSE + EKG		BLOOD PRESSURE	RESPIRATION & BREATH SOUNDS		O_2SAT	PT. MEDICATIONS
							FIELD IMPRESSION

Breathing	Skin Color	Skin Moist/Temp	Capillary Refill	Pupils	Eye Opening	Verbal Response	Motor Response	TRAUMA SCORE
☐Normal ☐Labored ☐Shallow ☐Retractive ☐Absent	☐Normal ☐Pale ☐Flushed ☐Cyanotic ☐Other	☐Normal ☐Dry ☐Moist ☐Normal ☐Cold ☐Cool ☐Hot	☐Normal <2 Secs ☐Delayed >2 Secs ☐Absent	☐PERL ☐Pinpoint ☐Dilated ☐Reactive ☐Nonreactive ☐R>L ☐L>R Size	4☐Spontaneous 3☐To Voice 2☐To Pain 1☐None	5☐Oriented 4☐Confused 3☐Inappropriate Words 2☐Incomprehensible Sounds 1☐None	6☐Obeys Commands 5☐Localizes Pain 4☐Withdraws To Pain 3☐Flexion To Pain 2☐Extension To Pain 1☐None	TIME

	WNL	ABN		WNL	ABN	
HEAD	☐	☐	ABDOMEN	☐	☐	☐C Spine ☐SCOOP ☐K.E.D. ☐Extrication ☐Splint ☐Dressing ☐Other
NECK	☐	☐	BACK/SPINE	☐	☐	
CHEST	☐	☐	PELVIS	☐	☐	
LUNGS	☐	☐	EXTREMITIES	☐	☐	

Treatment & Response

AIRWAY MANAGEMENT ☐O_2 ____ L/M ☐SUCTION ☐ASSIST VENT ☐OPA/NPA ☐CANNULA ☐CRICO ☐MASK ☐CO2 MON | ☐NTT ☐ET ☐EOA | # ATT. | TIME | SIZE | ☐I.V. ☐I.O. SITE____ CATH. SIZE____ ☐I.V. SUCCESSFUL | ☐T.K.O. RATE____ TOT. VOL____ ☐I.V.UNSUCCESSFUL | ☐BLOOD DRAW BLOOD SUGAR____ # OF ATTEMPTS____

TIME ORDERED	TREATMENT	DOSE	TIME DONE	RESPONSE	TIME ORDERED	TREATMENT	DOSE	TIME DONE	RESPONSE

Destination

TRANSPORTED ☐YES ☐NO | CODE 2 | 3 OTHER: | ☐11-44 | ☐AMA ☐DNR | REQUESTED FACILITY | DESTINATION | ☐PT ☐FAM ☐MD ☐NEAREST FACILITY ☐OTHER:

BASE HOSPITAL CONTACT ☐YES ☐NO ☐QVH ☐SHH | ☐DISRUP. COMMUNICATION | MICN | M.D.

FIELD PERSONNEL NAMES: 1. | # 2. | # 3. | # 4. | #

RELEASE: I, THE UNDERSIGNED, HAVE BEEN ADVISED THAT MEDICAL ASSISTANCE IN MY BEHALF IS NECESSARY AND THAT REFUSAL OF SAID ASSISTANCE AND TRANSPORT MAY RESULT IN DEATH OR IMPERIL MY HEALTH. NEVERTHELESS, I REFUSE TO ACCEPT TREATMENT OR TRANSPORT AND ASSUME ALL RISKS AND CONSEQUENCES OF MY DECISION AND RELEASE THE PROVIDER OF EMS SERVICE FROM ANY LIABILITY ARISING FROM MY REFUSAL.

PATIENT'S SIGNATURE DATE WITNESSED BY

The prehospital care report should be neat and legible. It is essential that other healthcare workers are able to read and understand your report. You should also remember that this report reflects directly upon your professionalism. Patient care reports are a permanent legal document. Both the document and its information are confidential.

The traditional report form contains boxes to check or bubbles to fill in plus a written narrative section (see Fig. 10.8). Some forms are designed to be scanned by computers; be sure to fill in the boxes completely and avoid stray marks. A recent development in prehospital records is the electronic clipboard or pen-based computer. This handheld computer can recognize handwriting and convert it to electronic text.

Local and state protocols will determine where copies of the forms are distributed. Generally, you should not distribute copies of the PCR except as stated in local or state protocol or procedures.

Minimum Data Set

The U.S. Department of Transportation has established a **minimum data set** to be included in each prehospital care report (see Fig. 10.9). The required data ensures a uniform standard of care and provides a valuable tool for research and education.

Minimum Data Set | *Patient and administrative information required to be included in a prehospital care report*

The minimum data set has two components: patient information and administrative information. The information recorded should be accurate and pertinent, documenting patient care from initial contact through arrival at the receiving facility. Check with your local department for specific forms and regional reporting requirements.

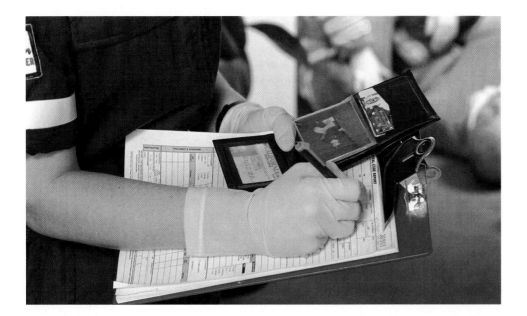

Figure 10.9 *The minimum data set must be included with every PCR.*

Patient information is gathered:

- On scene at the time of your initial contact
- After any interventions
- Upon arrival at the receiving facility

The information must include the:

- Chief complaint
- Level of consciousness and mental status (AVPU)
- Systolic blood pressure for patients older than 3 years
- Skin perfusion by capillary refill for patients under 6 years old
- Skin color and temperature
- Pulse rate
- Respiratory rate and effort

The administrative information must include the:

- Time of the incident report
- Time the unit was notified
- Time of arrival at the patient
- Time the unit left the scene
- Time of arrival at destination
- Time of transfer of care

D.O.T. OBJECTIVES

Identify the various sections of the written report.

Describe what information is required in each section of the prehospital care report and how it should be entered.

Sections of the Prehospital Care Report

A prehospital care report consists of sections for run data and patient data. It generally includes check boxes and a narrative report. There may also be sections for other state or local requirements. Whenever the PCR includes a section with check boxes, it is important to fill in the boxes completely and to avoid stray marks.

Dispatch								
MONTH/DAY/YEAR	PATIENT CARE TRANSFERRED TO: TIME		☐ NON TRANSPORT ☐ ALS ☐ BLS ☐ TRANSFER	PATIENT STATUS ☐ STAT ☐ NONSTAT	NO OF PATIENTS ___ OF ___ UNIT #		FIRE # AMB#	
PATIENT'S NAME LAST FIRST								
PATIENT'S ADDRESS		CITY			STATE		ZIP	
LOCATION OF INCIDENT		CALL RECEIVED :	ENROUTE :	AT SCENE :	TO HOSPITAL :	AT HOSPITAL :		
FIRST RESPONDERS	AID GIVEN ☐ O₂ ☐ CPR	☐ CPR STARTED AT _____ ☐ TIME WITHOUT CPR _____ ☐ OTHER _____				CODE TO 2 | 3	CHANGED 2 | 3	AGENCY

Figure 10.10 *Run data section of a prehospital care report.*

Run data (see Fig. 10.10) includes the administrative portion of the minimum data set with additional information:

- Agency name
- Date
- Run or call number
- EMS unit number
- Times
- Names and number of crew members and levels of certification

EMT Tip

Run data requires accurate and synchronized times. Be sure to check your clocks before beginning every shift.

Patient Medical Information						
AGE_____ GENDER ☐ M ☐ F WEIGHT_____ (KG LB) PVT MD LEVEL OF DISTRESS ☐ MILD ☐ MOD ☐ SEVERE LOC 1 2 3 4						
CHIEF COMPLAINT & CURRENT HISTORY _____						
P						
Q						
R						
S						
T						

PAST MEDICAL HX.					ALLERGIES	
TIME	PULSE + EKG	BLOOD PRESSURE	RESPIRATION & BREATH SOUNDS	O₂SAT	PT. MEDICATIONS	
					FIELD IMPRESSION	

Breathing	Skin Color	Skin Moist/Temp	Capillary Refill	Pupils	Eye Opening	Verbal Response	Motor Response	TRAUMA SCORE
☐ Normal ☐ Labored ☐ Shallow ☐ Retractive ☐ Absent	☐ Normal ☐ Pale ☐ Flushed ☐ Cyanotic ☐ Cold ☐ Other	☐ Normal ☐ Dry ☐ Moist ☐ Normal ☐ Cold ☐ Cool ☐ Hot	☐ Normal <2 Secs ☐ Delayed >2 Secs ☐ Absent	☐ PERL ☐ Pinpoint ☐ Dilated ☐ Reactive ☐ Nonreactive ☐ R>L ☐ L>R Size___	4☐ Spontaneous 3☐ To Voice 2☐ To Pain 1☐ None	5☐ Oriented 4☐ Confused 3☐ Inappropriate Words 2☐ Incomprehensible Sounds 1☐ None	6☐ Obeys Commands 5☐ Localizes Pain 4☐ Withdraws To Pain 3☐ Flexion To Pain 2☐ Extension To Pain 1☐ None	TIME
	WNL ABN				WNL ABN			☐ C Spine ☐ SCOOP ☐ K.E.D. ☐ Extrication ☐ Splint ☐ Dressing ☐ Other
HEAD	☐ ☐		ABDOMEN		☐ ☐			
NECK	☐ ☐		BACK/SPINE		☐ ☐			
CHEST	☐ ☐		PELVIS		☐ ☐			
LUNGS	☐ ☐		EXTREMITIES		☐ ☐			

Figure 10.11 *Patient data section of a prehospital care report.*

Patient data forms the main portion of the prehospital report. It contains information about the patient, his or her condition throughout the call, and any treatment given (see Fig. 10.11). The specific components are:

- The patient's legal name, age, sex, and date of birth
- The patient's home address
- Insurance or billing information

- Nature of the call

- Mechanism of injury or chief complaint

- The location of patient

- Any treatment administered prior to your arrival

- Signs and symptoms

- Baseline and subsequent vital signs

- SAMPLE history

- Care administered and the effects of that care

- Changes in condition

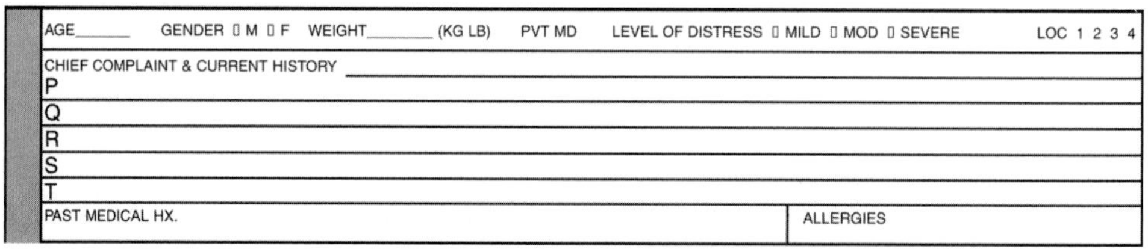

Figure 10.12 *Narrative section of a prehospital care report.*

Narrative Section. The narrative report allows you to provide a more detailed description of the patient, the chief complaint, the care provided, and responses to any interventions (see Fig. 10.12). In this section, you will describe the patient's condition for review by other medical professionals. When writing your narrative, be sure to only use medical terminology that you understand, and use terminology correctly. There is an introduction to the study of medical terminology in Appendix D.

The narrative must be accurate and complete, with pertinent information presented in a logical order. The narrative section includes:

- Type of call dispatched to

- Explanation of any delay in responding to the call (traffic, etc.)

- Description of the patient's condition upon arrival at the scene

- Chief complaint (record the patient's own words in quotes, if possible)

- SAMPLE history

- Physical assessment

- Treatment provided and patient's response to treatment

- Changes or trends in the patient's condition

- Information from the scene (surroundings, family, bystanders)

Remember these tips when writing your narrative report:

- Describe observations, don't draw conclusions.

- Include pertinent negative findings.

- Record important observations about the scene (e.g., suicide note, weapon, etc.).

- Avoid using radio codes.

- Use abbreviations only if they are standard (see Table 10.2 later in the chapter).

- When information of a sensitive nature is documented (e.g., communicable diseases), note the source of that information.

- Include any state reporting requirements.

- Be sure to spell words correctly, especially medical words. If you do not know how to spell it, find out or use another word.

- Record the time and findings of every reassessment.

EMT Tip

If you have problems with spelling, carry a pocket-sized medical dictionary.

D.O.T. OBJECTIVE

Describe the legal implications associated with the written report.

Legal Issues

The prehospital care report is a legal document. As such, issues of confidentiality and accuracy must be kept in mind.

Confidentiality. Both the PCR form itself and the information it contains are considered confidential. Do not discuss the patient with unauthorized people. Be familiar with state and local laws. As discussed in Chapter 3, there are very strict guidelines for the release of medical information. Do not violate the patient's right to privacy.

Falsification of Information. When an error in patient care occurs, do not try to cover it up. Falsification of information on the prehospital care report will lead to suspension or revocation of an EMT's certification or license in most states. It also leads to poor patient care. Other healthcare providers will be given a false impression of assessment findings or the treatment that was provided.

An error of omission involves something that should have been done or recorded, but wasn't. An error of commision occurs when an inappropriate action is taken, or when inaccurate information is recorded. In case of any error, document the actual events and what steps (if any) were taken to correct the situation. Only record vital signs that were actually taken. If a treatment such as oxygen was overlooked, do not record that the patient was given oxygen.

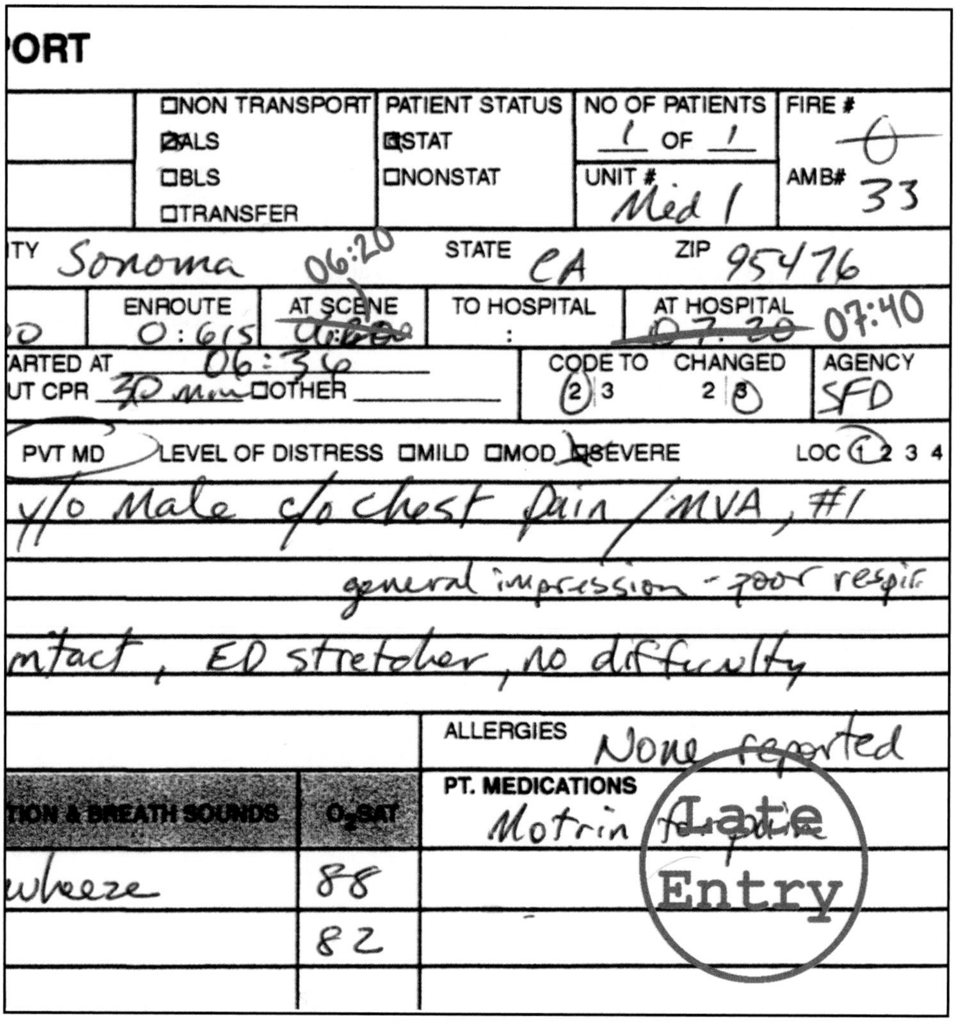

Figure 10.13 *Proper correction of errors on a prehospital care report.*

Correction of Written Errors. If you discover an error in a report as it is being written, draw a single horizontal line through the error, initial it, and write the correct information above or beside it (see Fig. 10.13). Do not try to obliterate the error. This could be interpreted as an attempt to cover up a mistake.

If you find an error after the report has been submitted, contact your supervisor or local medical direction and follow their specific directions. In some cases, you may be asked to write the correct information as described above. If information was omitted, you might add a note with the correct information, the date, and your initials. Make sure that any additional notations or changes are distributed to the all individuals who received a copy of the original PCR.

D.O.T. OBJECTIVE

Define the special considerations concerning patient refusal.

Documentation of Patient Refusal

As discussed in Chapter 3, competent adult patients have the right to refuse treatment. Before leaving the scene, however, you should:

- Try again to persuade the patient to go to a hospital.
- Inform the patient why he or she should go to the hospital, and what might happen if he or she does not.
- Ensure that the patient is able to make a rational, informed decision. If you suspect that the patient is under the influence of alcohol or other drugs, or if the patient's thinking is affected by illness or injury, consult medical direction as directed by local protocol. The physician may make a recommendation or talk directly with the patient. Advise law enforcement, if appropriate.

If the patient still refuses care:

- Document any assessment findings and emergency medical care given, then have the patient sign a Refusal of Care form (used in most departments).
- Have a law enforcement officer, family member, or bystander sign the form as a witness. If the patient will not sign the refusal form, ask a witness to sign verifying that the patient refused to sign.
- Suggest alternative methods of obtaining care, such as taking private transportation to see a doctor.
- State your willingness to return if the situation changes or the patient changes his or her mind.
- Complete the prehospital care report. Record as much of the patient assessment as possible, including physical exam and vital signs. Document all care given. Also describe the care you wanted to provide for the patient. Include a statement that you explained to the patient the possible consequences of failure to accept care, including the potential for death.

Reporting Special Incidents

There are some cases when the standard prehospital report is not used, or when additional reports are necessary.

Multiple Casualty Incidents (MCI)

On a scene where multiple patients are involved, such as a plane crash or explosion, patients must be cared for quickly. Complete documentation may not be possible. If there is not enough time to complete a prehospital care report before the next patient, you will have to fill out the report at a later time.

The local MCI plan (discussed in Chapter 24) should include a protocol for temporarily recording important medical information. This is often accomplished with a triage tag that is attached to each patient (see Fig. 10.14). The

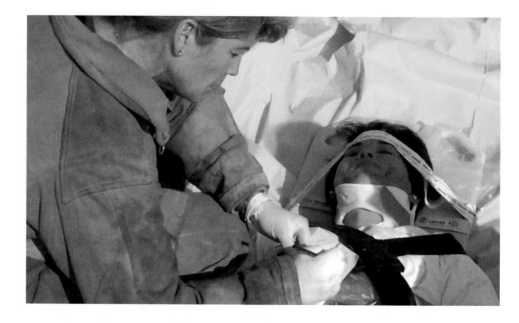

National Registry Examination Tip

You will not be asked to generate a PCR after any skill station. However, you should review the concept of standard of care, know the difference between patient data and administrative or run data, understand what belongs in each section of the standard PCR, and practice using standard medical abbreviations.

tag contains basic information about the chief complaint, vital signs, and treatment. This will stay with the patient if he or she is moved and can be used later to complete the PCR. Generally, the PCR in a multiple casualty incident will be less detailed than in simpler calls.

Special Reporting Situations

States or localities may require EMS providers to report certain events. Accurate, objective, complete documentation should be submitted to the appropriate agency in a timely manner. You or your agency should keep a copy of each report with the patient care record. Examples may include:

- Exposure to infectious disease
- Injury of EMS personnel
- Malfunction of equipment
- Use of patient restraint by EMS providers
- Suspected child, elder, or spousal abuse
- Suspected sexual assault or violent crime

COMMON MEDICAL ABBREVIATIONS

Many abbreviations are used in prehospital care reports. These abbreviations save you time when writing information. It is important that everyone understands clearly what is meant in the reports written at the scene. Therefore, a list of standard abbreviations has been created for use in these reports (see Table 10.2). Consult with your local medical director for accepted usage. The abbreviations listed in the table are common, but not universally accepted.

Table 10.2 • COMMON MEDICAL ABBREVIATIONS

Term	Abbreviation	Term	Abbreviation
After	$\bar{p}$	Milligram	mg
Alcohol	EtOH	Multiple casualty incident	MCI
As necessary	prn	Nasal cannula	NC
At	@	Nausea and vomiting	N/V
Bag-valve mask	BVM	Nitroglycerin	NTG
Before	a	No known drug allergies	NKDA
Blood pressure	BP	Obstetrics	OB
Cervical spinal immobilization device	CSID	Orally, by mouth	po
Chief complaint	CC, C/C	Oxygen	O_2
Date of birth	DOB	Patient	pt
Dead on arrival	DOA	Past medical history	PMHx
Decreased	'	Physical exam	PE
Emergency department	ED	Prior to arrival	PTA
Emergency room	ER	Prescription	Rx
Endotracheal tube	ETT	Pulse	p
Estimated time of arrival	ETA	Rule out	R/O
Every	$\bar{q}$	Shortness of breath	SOB
Every day	qd	Signs and symptoms	s/s
Four times a day	QID	Sublingual	SL
Gunshot wound	GSW	Symptoms	Sx
Hazardous materials	HAZ-MAT	Three times a day	TID
History	Hx	Transient ischemic attack	TIA
Hypertension	Htn	Treatment (also traction)	Tx
Immediately	STAT	Twice a day	BID
Increased	'	Vital signs	VS
Jugular venous distention	JVD	With	$\bar{c}$
Loss of consciousness	LOC	Without	$\bar{s}$, w/o
		Year old	y/o

Chapter Ten Summary

- Communication is an integral part of patient care. You must be able to gather and relay patient information as well as produce an accurate written report at the conclusion of each call.

- Verbal communication is an integral part of your patient care. You will communicate frequently with medical direction and dispatch, in addition to your patients.

- When communicating with a receiving facility or medical direction, you must present an accurate and concise picture of your patient. Repeat word-for-word any orders or denials you are given. Question any unclear or inappropriate order.

- Always communicate changes in your unit's status to dispatch (en route to call, arriving on scene, etc.).

- At the conclusion of the call, you will produce a written report of the patient's condition and the medical care provided. This documentation assists in the continued care of the patient and is legal evidence of the prehospital care received. These forms are often used for quality improvement, to influence patient care decisions, and for billing purposes.

- Certain situations, such as patient refusals, require careful documentation to protect you from claims of abandonment or negligence. Other situations, such as assaults, child abuse, elder abuse, domestic violence, and sexual crimes, may require you to file a report with an outside agency such as social services or law enforcement. Be familiar with local procedure.

- Patient care reports must be honest. Carefully correct any errors. If you make an error in caring for the patient, carefully document the situation and what you did to correct the problem once it was identified.

Key Terms Review

Base Station | *page 324*

Minimum Data Set | *page 333*

Mobile Radio | *page 324*

Prehospital Care Report (PCR) | *page 332*

Repeaters | *page 324*

Review Questions

1. Which of the following mechanisms for communicating with hospital personnel is the least helpful for the continued care of your patients?

   a. Patient care report
   b. Face-to-face report
   c. Pre-arrival radio report
   d. Dispatch information

2. Which of the following is NOT part of the standard medical radio report?

   a. Estimated time of arrival
   b. Patient's age and gender
   c. Patient's name and address
   d. History of the present illness

3. You are giving a radio report to the local hospital. The hospital asks for the patient's name. What should you do?

   a. Tell the hospital the patient's name
   b. Ask your partner for advice
   c. Tell the hospital you cannot give them that information
   d. Turn off the radio

4. When an EMT talks on the radio, he or she should wait for _____ second(s) before beginning a transmission.

   a. One
   b. Five
   c. Ten
   d. The EMT does not have to wait to transmit

5. To assure accuracy in record keeping, the most important aspect of the clock you use is that it be:

   a. Analog
   b. Digital
   c. Synchronous
   d. Based on military time

6. What agency is responsible for the regulation of all EMS radio traffic in the United States?

   a. Federal Emergency Management Administration
   b. Department of Defense
   c. Federal Communications Commission
   d. Department of Transportation

7. The prehospital care report is considered a(n) _____ document.

   a. Confidential
   b. Public domain
   c. Open
   d. Multi-jurisdictional

8. What is the best method to eliminate an error on a hand-written prehospital care report prior to submitting the report?

   a. Tear it up and start over
   b. Obliterate it
   c. Draw a single horizontal line through the error
   d. Staple a correction to the original

9. Who has the right to refuse treatment?

   a. All patients
   b. Competent adult patients
   c. Unconscious patients
   d. Legal citizens

10. If a patient refuses care, you should always:

    a. Call for your supervisor
    b. Document this on a patient refusal form and have the patient sign it
    c. Call for law enforcement
    d. Leave the scene immediately

11. Who is responsible for keeping a clock on all calls?

    a. Law enforcement
    b. Dispatch
    c. The base hospital
    d. The ER physician

Review Questions *(cont.)*

12. Which of the following is NOT a form of verbal communication used during a call?

    a. Radio communication
    b. Communication at the receiving facility
    c. Interpersonal communication
    d. Prehospital care report

13. What happens to the prehospital care report?

    a. It is read and discarded
    b. It becomes part of the public domain
    c. It becomes part of the patient's permanent medical record
    d. It is only sent to the local EMS agency

14. Written communications should generally be completed:

    a. At the end of the day
    b. En route to the hospital
    c. Right after the call at the receiving facility
    d. At the convenience of the EMT

15. One effective way to reduce background noise in the ambulance during radio transmissions is to:

    a. Increase the volume of the transmitter
    b. Close the windows
    c. Turn to an alternate frequency
    d. Adjust the squelch

16. An effective practice to avoid interfering with another ambulance attempting to use its radio is to:

    a. Wait 10 to 15 seconds before transmitting
    b. Announce your intention to broadcast over the air
    c. Transmit immediately
    d. Speak in specialized codes

17. To request orders to assist a patient with medication, you should contact:

    a. Your supervisor
    b. The charge nurse at the receiving facility
    c. Medical direction
    d. Any local physician

18. After receiving an order from medical direction, you should:

    a. Complete the order
    b. Repeat the order exactly as you heard it
    c. Finish your report
    d. Ask the patient about possible medication allergies

19. What does the abbreviation CC (or C/C) mean?

    a. Centimeter
    b. Chief complaint
    c. Cervical collar
    d. The diameter of the cervix

CASE STUDIES

Communications and Documentation

1 You and your partner are transporting a patient who was injured in an automobile accident. You assessed the patient and stabilized his cervical spine before transport. The patient appears to be intoxicated and is angry at the other driver. Some of his anger is directed at your partner. Before arriving at the hospital, he makes threats against both your partner and the other driver.

A. What is your best course of action?

B. Could you document in the patient care report your suspicion that the patient is intoxicated?

C. What legal protection will your patient care report give you?

2 A local reporter approaches you when you are off duty and requests information about a call you ran a week ago. You cared for a woman who was the victim of a rape. The police now have a suspect in custody. The reporter indicates that he has knowledge about the condition of the patient and the care you gave her. He only wants confirmation of certain facts about the call.

A. What should you do?

B. The reporter then produces a copy of your patient care report. He will not tell you where he obtained it. Again, he only asks you to confirm certain facts about the case. Do you answer his questions?

3 You are served with a subpoena to testify in a case in which you cared for a man who was injured in a motor vehicle accident. He has included you and your employer in a lawsuit. While on the stand, you are given a copy of your patient care report.

A. You have no memory of the call. Can you still give testimony?

Stories from the Field
Wrap-Up

To be an effective EMT, you must be able to pass along the information you have learned from your assessment. This is done verbally during your initial radio report and when you make your report to the receiving facility staff. It is put into writing in your patient care report. Information that is lost or forgotten during this process could have a negative effect on the patient's care. It could also result in legal liability for you as a healthcare professional.

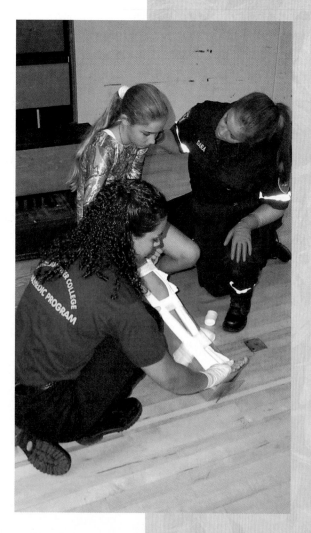

It might be unusual for an EMT-Basic student to be asked to give a preliminary report as in this scenario. However, radio reports are a skill you must master. Pre-arrival reports are essential in order to provide for continuity of your patient's care at the receiving facility. Always provide identifying information for the unit and crew, the standard medical report, and an estimated arrival time. Follow your preliminary report with an in-person report to the healthcare professional who assumes care of your patient, and leave them a copy of your legible, neatly written patient care report. Doing so will provide legal protection as well as ensuring that your patients receive the highest level of care.

D.O.T. Module 4

Medical Emergencies

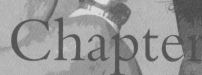

Chapter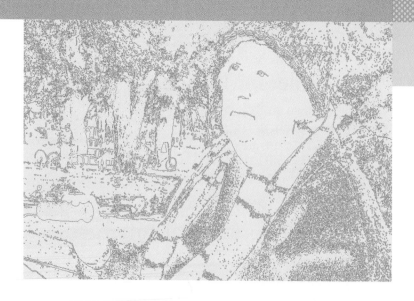

11

General
Pharmacology

Stories from the Field

You are dispatched for an ill woman found wandering in the street. The patient responds slowly to your questions. She mumbles that she was visiting a friend in the area and can't remember where she parked her car. She seems confused and puzzled by the attention. She is not dressed appropriately for the hot weather. The woman does not have identification. Although many seniors live in this neighborhood, she is not familiar to any of the bystanders. Your initial assessment shows no problems with airway, breathing, or circulation. The patient is able to follow commands and has a steady gait. She is unable to provide details about her medical history. However, she wears a medical identification necklace stating that she has a history of diabetes and is taking insulin.

Your partner finds the patient's handbag, which contains her driver's license and a small tube of oral glucose. The glucose is prescribed in the woman's name. She denies having breakfast and cannot remember when she took her last insulin injection. You notice that her responses are becoming slower and her speech a little slurred.

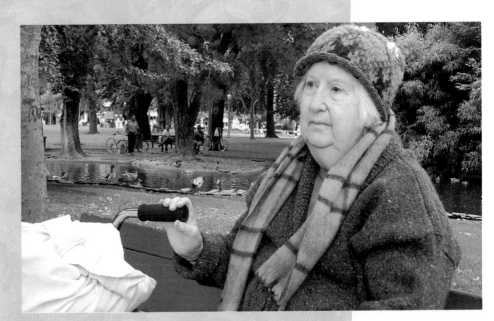

*P*rehospital medication administration can be critical in improving the outcome for many patients. You must learn and remember which prescribed medications you can administer or assist patients to self-administer. You must be able to identify when each medication is needed.

This chapter will give you a general understanding of medications. You must develop a basic knowledge of the drugs you will be administering. Specific information about individual medications is discussed in later chapters covering specific medical emergencies. EMS is a rapidly advancing field. Stay informed as changes occur regarding medication administration.

GENERAL PHARMACOLOGY

As an EMT-Basic, you can administer a few select medications to patients. You may also be directed to assist a patient in self-administering other drugs. Giving the proper medication in an emergency is critical to the well-being of the patient.

You must thoroughly understand the medications you work with in order to use them safely and correctly. You must learn the:

• Indications for use

• Contraindications

• Proper dosage

• Route of administration

• Potential side effects

Improper use of medications by emergency patients can result in serious additional injury or illness. The rules, policies, and protocols for administering medications vary widely among individual states, localities, and agencies. Always follow the guidelines provided by your instructor and medical director.

D.O.T. OBJECTIVES

Identify which medications will be carried on the unit.

State the medications carried on the unit by the generic name.

Medications Carried on the EMS Unit

Several medications are carried in the ambulance and can be administered by an EMT-B. You must have permission from medical direction before administering any drug. Permission may be in the form of a standing order in a patient care protocol. In some situations, you will receive direct, on-line orders from a medical control physician.

Medications carried on most basic ambulances are:

- Oxygen, a gas administered to supplement the oxygen in room air. It is discussed in detail in Chapter 7.

- Activated charcoal suspension (see Fig. 11.1), used in poisoning and overdose cases. It is discussed in detail in Chapter 16.

- Oral glucose gel (see Fig. 11.2), used for patients with diabetes. It is described in Chapter 14.

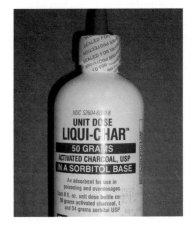

Figure 11.1 *Activated charcoal suspension.*

D.O.T. OBJECTIVES

Identify the medications with which the EMT-B may assist the patient with administering.

State the medications the EMT-B can assist the patient with by the generic name.

Medications Carried by the Patient

Some patients carry prescribed medications with them. You may be directed to help them take the drugs in an emergency. Follow your local protocol. You must have permission from medical direction in this situation. Accurate and legible documentation is important if you assist a patient to self-administer a drug.

Medications that an EMT-B may assist patients to self-administer are:

- Albuterol, isoetharine, metaproterenol, and other medications delivered by **metered dose inhalers (MDIs)**. These are described in Chapter 12, Respiratory Emergencies.

- Nitroglycerin (NTG) tablets or spray. This is discussed in Chapter 13, Cardiovascular Emergencies.

- Epinephrine for injection; described in Chapter 15, Allergic Reactions.

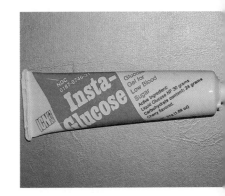

Figure 11.2 *Oral glucose.*

Metered Dose Inhaler (MDI) | *Hand-held inhalation device for delivering liquid or powdered medication in pre-measured doses*

Table 11.1 • NAMES OF DRUGS

Type of Name	Description
Generic	The official name as listed in the *U.S. Pharmacopeia (USP)*. This is given to a drug during development. Each drug has only one generic name.
Trade	The brand name given to a drug by the manufacturer for marketing purposes. A drug may have two or more trade names.

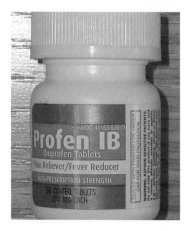

Figure 11.3 *Ibuprofen is a generic medication name.*

Generic Name | *Official, common name of a medication*

Trade Name | *Manufacturer's brand name for a medication*

EMT Tip

Drug containers or packages usually list the trade name, followed by the generic name in smaller print. The generic name is sometimes followed by the abbreviation USP.

Medication Names

All medications have more than one name. You must know the exact substance you are using. Always check the label twice before administering any medication (see Table 11.1).

The **generic name** of a drug is the name listed in the *U.S. Pharmacopeia (USP)*, a federal government publication. This book lists all drugs approved by the U.S. Food and Drug Administration. The generic name is used during drug development, before FDA approval. A generic name is usually a simple form of the compound's chemical name (see Fig. 11.3).

The **trade name** is a marketing brand name assigned by the drug manufacturer. If several different pharmaceutical companies manufacture the drug, it will have several trade names.

> **D.O.T. OBJECTIVE**
>
> Discuss the forms in which the medications may be found.

Medication Forms

Drugs come in different forms. There are many reasons for this. Having drugs available in several forms provides control over the amount of the drug in the bloodstream and targeted body systems. The form of medication influences how quickly it works, the site it affects within the body, and the stability of the drug.

The medication forms that you will administer or assist with are:

- Suspensions, such as activated charcoal or Ipecac

- Gels, such as oral glucose

- Gases, such as oxygen

- Fine powders for inhalation, such as found in metered-dose inhalers

- Compressed powders or tablets, such as nitroglycerin

- Liquids for injection, such as epinephrine

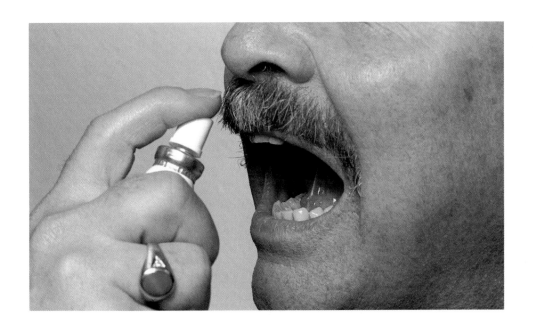

Figure 11.4 *Administering nitroglycerin spray.*

- Vaporized liquids in fixed-dose **nebulizers**, such as drugs given to treat asthma
- Sublingual sprays, such as nitroglycerin (see Fig. 11.4)

Nebulizer | *Device for administering vaporized liquid medication*

Characteristics of Medications

You must be very familiar with the characteristics of specific drugs you are authorized to administer (see Table 11.2). Always follow local protocols for administering or assisting in the administration of drugs. Read the labels and inspect each type of medication. You must know:

- **Indications** for using the drug—the specific illnesses, signs, or symptoms the drug is designed to treat. Some drugs relieve symptoms of a condition. Others treat an underlying disorder.

Indication | *A sign, symptom, or condition for which a specific medication or treatment is given*

Table 11.2 • ESSENTIAL INFORMATION ABOUT ANY DRUG

Characteristic	Description	Example
Indications	When to use a drug	Use an epinephrine auto-injector to treat a patient with a severe allergic reaction
Contraindications	When not to use a drug	Do not give nitroglycerin if the blood pressure is below 100 mmHg systolic
Action	How the drug affects the body	Metered dose inhalers dilate the bronchioles
Dosage	How much of the drug to give and when	Give one 0.4 mg nitroglycerin tablet every 5 minutes, up to a maximum of 3 tablets
Route of Administration	The method by which you administer the drug	Give an epinephrine auto-injector by injection into the lateral thigh
Side Effects	Signs or symptoms that may appear as a result of giving the drug	Patient given nitroglycerin gets a headache

Contraindication (KON-trah-in-duh-KAY-shun) | *Condition under which a specific medication or treatment should not be given*

• **Contraindications** are situations in which the drug should not be used. Administering the drug would be harmful or have no effect on the patient's condition. Never give a drug that is contraindicated.

Dosage | *Appropriate amount of a medication to administer; also dose*

• The **dosage,** or dose, is the amount of drug necessary to achieve a specific therapeutic effect. A dose that is too large can cause side effects or harm the patient. A dose that is too small may be ineffective. The correct dosage may depend on the age or weight of the patient. When you administer drugs, you must be able to differentiate adult doses from pediatric doses. The timing of medication administration is important. To reach and maintain a therapeutic effect, doses of some drugs must be given at intervals over a period of time.

Route of Administration | *Pathway by which a medication is administered: sublingual, oral ingestion, injection, inhalation, etc.*

• Each medication is given by a specific **route of administration.** The route of administration affects the length of time it takes for the drug to begin working. You will give some drugs by the sublingual route. These medications are administered by placing them under the patient's tongue. They are rapidly absorbed by the large blood vessels under the tongue. You will also give drugs by oral ingestion and inhalation. Other routes of administration include injection, topical application, and rectal suppositories.

Action | *The desired effect of a medication or treatment*

• The **action** of a medication refers to the therapeutic effect on a patient's body or systems.

Side Effect | *Unwanted effect of a medication*

• Each drug is given to achieve a beneficial effect. However, many drugs can have undesired side effects. A **side effect** is any action of the drug other than the intended one. Some side effects are common and predictable. Some are uncommon. They can be minor or serious. You must know the common side effects of the drugs you give. Be prepared to manage complications. You must reassure the patient in case of a problem.

Administration of Medications

Safe medication administration is an important responsibility.

Remember the five "rights" of medication administration:

• Right patient
• Right drug
• Right dose
• Right route
• Right time

When administering drugs to a patient, you must follow these steps:

1. Obtain permission from medical direction. This may be in the form of a standing order based on protocols or a direct on-line communication. If you are unsure about administering any drug in a specific situation, contact medical direction.

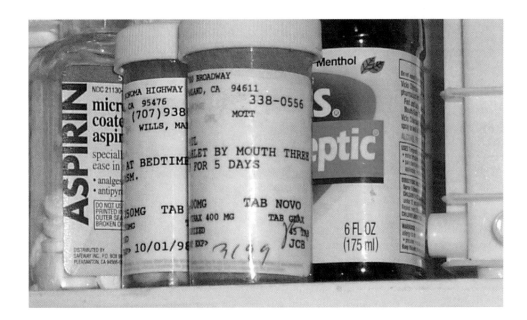

Figure 11.5 *Read the information on the label thoroughly.*

2. Select the proper medication. Read the label carefully to ensure that you are giving the correct drug (see Fig. 11.5).

3. If you will be assisting patients to self-administer their own medications, verify the prescription. Make sure that the prescription label is made out in the patient's name. Never administer a medication that is not prescribed to a patient. If the patient is unresponsive, you may be prevented from administering medications. Check your local EMS protocols.

4. Check the expiration date on the bottle or outer packaging. Never administer a drug that has expired.

5. Verify the medication form, dosage, and route of administration. Make sure that you distinguish between adult and pediatric dosages.

6. Assist the patient to self-administer the medication.

7. Document the name of the medication given, the time, dose, and route of administration.

Reassessment

You must continue to monitor the patient after administering any medication. Assess the effect of the drug on the patient's condition as part of your ongoing assessment. Repeat the vital signs. Document any improvement, deterioration, side effect, or other response to the drug.

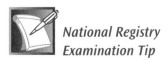

**National Registry
Examination Tip**

Review the medications that are within the scope of EMT-B practice. Be able to quickly list the indications, contraindications, and typical dosage for the drugs you can administer. Remember that your local EMS agency may allow an expanded scope of practice. In this case, you will not be tested on some drugs used by your agency.

Chapter Eleven Summary

- An EMT-Basic can administer certain medications and assist patients to self-administer others. Most EMT-B services carry oxygen, instant glucose, and activated charcoal. You may be directed to assist a patient in taking his or her own nitroglycerin, epinephrine, or prescribed inhaler. Always consult medical direction before giving these drugs.

- Some medications are known by several different names. Always read label information carefully to avoid medication errors.

- Before administering any drug, you must be familiar with the indications, contraindications, form, dose, administration, action, and side effects.

- After administering a medication, monitor the patient's response. Document improvement, deterioration, or side effects.

Key Terms Review

Action | *page 354*

Contraindication | *page 354*

Dosage | *page 354*

Generic Name | *page 352*

Indication | *page 353*

Metered Dose Inhaler
   (MDI) | *page 351*

Nebulizer | *page 353*

Route of
   Administration | *page 354*

Side Effect | *page 354*

Trade Name | *page 352*

Review Questions

1. A medication manufactured by different companies may have several _____ names.

   a. Generic
   b. Chemical
   c. Trade
   d. Common

2. An EMT-Basic might assist with administration of albuterol for what type of medical emergency?

   a. Chest pain
   b. Difficulty breathing
   c. Diabetic coma
   d. Seizure

3. Oral glucose is usually supplied in what form?

   a. Gas
   b. Suspension
   c. Gel
   d. Liquid

4. Nitroglycerin is supplied for patients in which of the following forms?

   a. Gel and powder
   b. Tablet and gel
   c. Suspension and spray
   d. Spray and tablet

5. Which of the following describes how a patient should receive a drug?

   a. Indications
   b. Route
   c. Action
   d. Side effects

6. You are dispatched to a patient who denies shortness of breath, but complains of severe chest pain. You take vitals and find: pulse 160, respiratory rate 22, and BP 90/60. The vital signs are a(n) _____ to assist him with nitroglycerin.

   a. Indication
   b. Contraindication
   c. Side effect
   d. Potential effect

7. Accurate and legible documentation is _____ important when you assist a patient in self-administering a drug.

   a. Somewhat
   b. Not
   c. Possibly
   d. Critically

8. An EMT-B must inspect the medication and label on each medication:

   a. Never
   b. Once
   c. Twice
   d. Often

9. The dosage of any specific medication is the amount that will:

   a. Help any patient
   b. Achieve a therapeutic effect
   c. Help a patient of a certain age
   d. Keep the patient from getting worse

10. The EMT-B should identify a patient's medications by locating the drug's container and verifying:

    a. The generic name
    b. The official name
    c. The brand name
    d. The trade name

11. MDI is the abbreviation for:

    a. Metered dose inhaler
    b. Multiple dose inhaler
    c. Medical dose inhaler
    d. Medical dose injector

CASE STUDIES

General Pharmacology

1

The company retreat is an annual event that everyone looks forward to all year. This year the company hired a professional catering service. They rented a private ranch in the mountains and hired live entertainment. Each member of the safety team was asked to bring gear and provide first aid, if necessary, during the three days.

The first day of the retreat went well. During lunch on the second day, Juan was eating with a group of sales staff. He began to complain of severe shortness of breath and a sore throat. Within minutes, Juan was having difficulty speaking. He complained of swollen hands and neck. He began drooling uncontrollably. Just before he lost the ability to speak, you discovered that he is allergic to crab and some other types of shellfish. He was quickly transported to a local hospital and treated for his reaction.

A. What medications can you take with you to the retreat?

B. If Juan's medication had been available, would it have been appropriate to assist him to take it once you had contacted medical direction? Would it be appropriate to assist him if it delayed transport for 2 minutes?

C. List the situations in which an EMT-B can assist a patient with a medication.

2

Tran was recently diagnosed with asthma. He is 10 years old and not quite ready to take his medication in front of his buddies. The doctor told him that his asthma could act up in cold weather. A few weeks later, he was playing touch football in cold weather. He had to stop to catch his breath. A few minutes later, he said he was not getting enough air, despite 6 straight puffs from his metered dose inhaler. Tran's breathing was becoming faster. He started walking slowly to the front office of the apartment complex, but he collapsed in front of it. You respond to a call for a child down. Your initial assessment reveals an intact airway. His breathing is inadequate. His respiratory rate is rapid, and his pulse is elevated. Tran does not respond to verbal or painful stimuli. He has an inhaler in his left hand. His friends relay the history of events.

A. What is your first priority with the patient?

B. Given the boy's obvious respiratory distress and prescribed inhaler, should you administer 2 metered doses? Justify your answer.

C. What is meant by a contraindication?

Stories from the Field
Wrap-Up

Administering drugs is a new and significant intervention for the EMT-Basic. Before administering or assisting patients with medication, you must have a thorough understanding of certain characteristics of the drug. Some drugs have multiple trade names. You must be familiar with the various drug names. You must also know how the drug is administered and its intended effect on the patient. Be able to differentiate when a drug is useful and when it is contraindicated. Knowing the route of administration and dosage is important. A dose that is too high may harm the patient. Giving a drug by the wrong route is also harmful. A dose that is too low will have no effect. Many drugs have normal and predictable side effects.

In this situation, the patient had a true medical emergency. Her altered mental status was the result of an unstable or inappropriate insulin level. After a careful assessment and consult with medical direction, you assist the woman with her oral medication. Within three minutes you notice a significant difference in her level of responsiveness. After ten minutes, she is alert and oriented and is embarrassed by the episode. As you complete the patient care record, the woman's friend arrives.

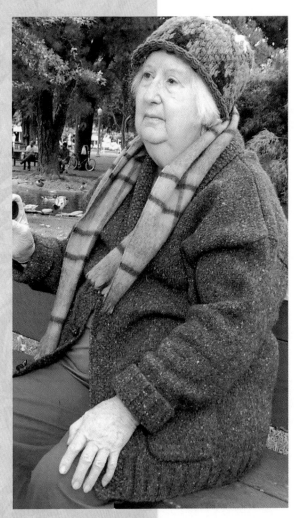

Chapter 12

Respiratory Emergencies

Stories from the Field

You are progressing well in your EMT class. Carmen and Robin ask you to become more involved in patient care. They agree to let you complete a patient assessment. Your crew is called to a large apartment complex for a patient who is having difficulty breathing. When you arrive, you find a very thin young man. He complains of severe shortness of breath. He is sitting on the edge of his bed, leaning forward. The apartment is sparsely furnished. No clues to the cause of his distress are evident as you enter the scene.

Your initial assessment reveals a 22-year-old man in obvious respiratory distress. The patient tries to talk, but can speak only one or two words at a time. If he speaks in sentences, he gasps for breath. You can understand his phrase "...hurts to breathe." The patient appears exhausted. His breathing is very rapid and shallow. The pulse is rapid. The skin is pale and cool, and the patient clutches his chest with each breath. While you are trying to obtain the OPQRST and SAMPLE histories, Robin places a non-rebreather mask with high-flow oxygen on the patient. Carmen gently nudges you and suggests you hurry things up.

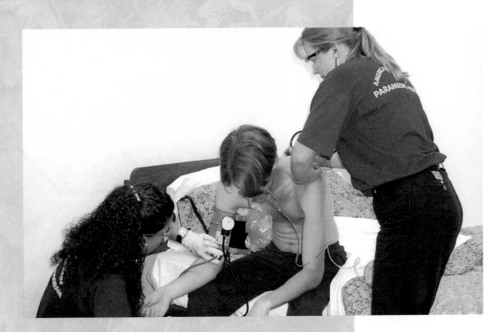

Difficulty breathing is one of the most frequent reasons for calling for emergency medical assistance. Patients and providers use many names to describe breathing problems. These include difficult or labored breathing, dyspnea, or shortness of breath (SOB). In the United States, more than 200,000 people die from respiratory emergencies each year.

Having an EMT-B present in a respiratory emergency gives the patient a real advantage. You are equipped to begin lifesaving measures quickly. Your assessment skills are vital during respiratory emergencies. You must evaluate and treat the patient for life-threatening conditions as quickly as possible. The inability to breathe is frightening for any patient. Quick administration of oxygen, assistance with a prescribed inhaler, and professional, competent help relieves anxiety. It can also save lives.

Acute Illness | *Illness with a severe, rapid onset*

Chronic Illness | *Long term illness*

An **acute illness** is a condition that develops quickly. It usually lasts a short time. A **chronic illness** is a condition that lasts a long time, perhaps for life. Many respiratory conditions are chronic illnesses. Sometimes a chronic illness will cause an acute problem. This chapter focuses on respiratory emergencies that are due to illness, rather than injury (see Fig. 12.1). Chapter 9 contains more information on evaluating and managing respiratory distress due to injury. Respiratory emergencies in infants and children are discussed further in Chapter 23.

Figure 12.1 *There are many causes of shortness of breath.*

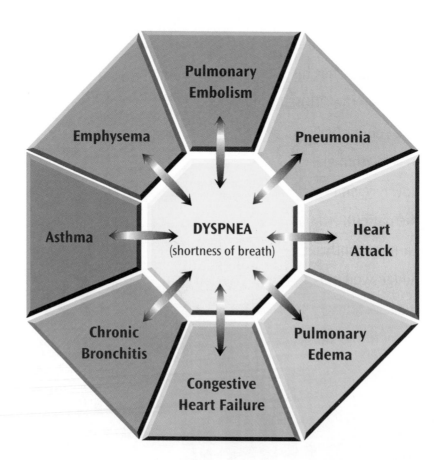

D.O.T. OBJECTIVES

List the structure and function of the respiratory system.

List signs of adequate air exchange.

National Registry Examination Tip

Review the major structures of the airway. Be able to identify each landmark quickly. Review the signs and symptoms of adequate and inadequate breathing. Be able to identify the range of normal respiratory rates in adults, children, and infants.

RESPIRATORY SYSTEM REVIEW

An EMT-B must thoroughly understand the structure and function of the respiratory system. You may want to review the detailed information in Chapters 4 and 7 before beginning this chapter. Table 12.1 summarizes the structures of the respiratory system and their functions. Table 12.2 reviews the actions of the respiratory system.

Table 12.1 • **REVIEW OF THE RESPIRATORY SYSTEM**

Structure	Function
Nose and Mouth	Warm, humidify, and clean air; mucous membranes in the nasal cavity clean and moisten air.
Pharynx	Passageway for air and food entering the body; consists of two main parts, the nasopharynx and oropharynx. The nasopharynx leads from the nasal openings. Both food and air pass through the oropharynx.
Epiglottis	Leaf-shaped, lid-like structure that covers the larynx during swallowing and prevents food and liquid from entering the respiratory tract.
Larynx	The voice box; forms the entrance to the trachea. Contains vocal cords, which produce sound. Marks the upper end of the trachea.
Trachea	Made of connective tissue, smooth muscle, and cartilage. Provides a flexible, permanent upper airway through which air enters the lungs.
Bronchi	Passageways to the lungs. The right primary bronchus divides into three secondary bronchi leading to the three lobes of the right lung. The left primary bronchus divides into two secondary bronchi feeding the left lung, which only has two lobes.
Bronchioles	Branches of the bronchi that lead to the alveoli.
Alveoli	Functional units of the lungs, where gas exchange between air and blood takes place.
Lungs	Located on either side of the thoracic cavity; protected by the ribs. Average lung volume in adults is 5 or 6 liters.
Diaphragm and Accessory Muscles	Diaphragm is a strong muscle that forms the lower border of the thoracic cavity. It expands and contracts for breathing. Accessory muscles are used during labored breathing.

Table 12.2 • **ACTIONS OF THE RESPIRATORY SYSTEM**

Action	Description
Ventilation	Breathing; the process of inhalation and exhalation. Inhalation is an active process (diaphragm and chest muscles contract); exhalation is a passive process (muscles relax).
Diffusion	Passive exchange of gases. Exchange of oxygen and carbon dioxide between the lungs and blood occurs in the alveoli. Exchange between the blood and cells occurs in the tissues.
Alveolar/Capillary Exchange	Oxygen from air passes through the alveolar membrane into the bloodstream. Carbon dioxide moves from the blood into alveoli for removal by exhalation.
Capillary/Cellular Exchange	Gas exchange between the blood and cells. Oxygen is released into cells while carbon dioxide passes into the capillaries. As oxygen-rich blood is carried past the cells, oxygen diffuses out of the capillaries while carbon dioxide diffuses in.
Oxygen Transport	Specific molecules and chemical reactions in the blood facilitate the transport and exchange of gases.
Normal Breathing	Regular, relaxed, comfortable ventilation. Accessory muscles not used, rhythm regular, breath sounds equal in both lungs, chest expansion full and equal. Normal breathing rate and depth are maintained. Adult tidal volume about 500 mL.
Inadequate Breathing	Results in reduced oxygen supply to the tissues. Signs include labored respiration, abnormal respiratory rate, inadequate tidal volume, noisy or absent breath sounds, irregular rhythm. Chest expansion may be unequal or inadequate; retractions may be present.

D.O.T. OBJECTIVES

Describe the emergency medical care of the patient with breathing difficulty.

Describe the emergency medical care of the patient with breathing distress.

Establish the relationship between airway management and the patient with breathing difficulty.

Asthma (AZ-muh) | *Reactive airway disease caused by spasmodic contraction of the bronchi; characterized by recurrent attacks of dyspnea, coughing, and wheezing*

Chronic Obstructive Pulmonary Disease (COPD) | *Generic term for emphysema, chronic bronchitis, and other obstructive airway diseases*

ASSESSMENT AND CARE OF THE RESPIRATORY PATIENT

Besides airway obstruction and injury, breathing can become compromised due to illness. For example, **asthma** is a chronic respiratory condition that can cause acute symptoms requiring an EMS response. **Chronic obstructive pulmonary disease (COPD)** includes several diseases that cause airflow obstruction. The Enhanced Study section at the end of the chapter includes background information on these respiratory diseases.

When assessing a patient in respiratory distress, be prepared to intervene immediately with supplemental oxygen or to assist with ventilations needed. Utilize appropriate BSI and standard precautions if contact with body fluids is likely. Patients with severe respiratory distress should be transported immediately and further assessment should take place while en route to the hospital.

To assess patients with nontraumatic respiratory problems, you will perform the following general steps. Details of these steps are explained in the subsequent sections.

1. Complete the scene size-up. Look for signs that the person has chronic dyspnea, including oxygen, nebulizers, metered dose inhalers (MDIs), or other supplies.

2. Complete the initial assessment. Evaluate mental status and the ABCs. Carefully assess the adequacy of breathing. Provide any necessary interventions (see Table 12.3). If supplemental ventilation is not required, place the patient on high-flow oxygen by non-rebreather mask.

3. Complete the focused history and physical exam. For responsive patients, obtain the OPQRST and SAMPLE histories. Then perform a focused physical exam of the head, neck, and chest. Obtain baseline vital signs. Consider assisting the patient with an MDI, if one is prescribed and available. Consult medical control for directions. For unresponsive patients, conduct a rapid medical assessment and obtain baseline vital signs. Try to get a history from bystanders. Begin transport early if the patient is unresponsive or in significant distress.

4. Conduct a detailed assessment while en route. Focus on assessing the head, neck, and chest. Reassess the patient continuously, depending on the severity of symptoms. Consider repeating MDI treatments, if prescribed and available, after consulting medical direction.

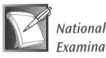

National Registry Examination Tip

Review the treatment steps for patients with each of the chronic respiratory conditions listed in this chapter. Understand the basic physiological complications behind each of the conditions. For example, you should know that asthma causes bronchoconstriction.

Table 12.3 • EMERGENCY INTERVENTIONS

Inadequate Breathing	Adequate Breathing
If the patient is conscious use MDI if prescribed with consent from medical direction	Provide oxygen at 15 LPM by non-rebreather mask
Maintain an airway	Perform focused history and physical exam
Consider ventilating with supplemental oxygen	Obtain baseline vital signs
Consider immediate transport	Transport in a position of comfort

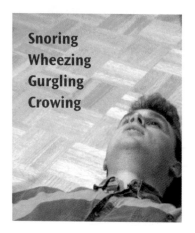

**Snoring
Wheezing
Gurgling
Crowing**

Figure 12.2 *Common signs of respiratory distress.*

Bronchoconstriction | *Narrowing of the air passageways due to contraction of the smooth muscle of the bronchi and bronchioles*

D.O.T. OBJECTIVE

State the signs and symptoms of a patient with difficulty breathing.

Signs and Symptoms of Breathing Difficulty

You must be able to differentiate between good and poor air exchange. A person in respiratory distress will show signs of inadequate ventilation or air hunger (see Fig. 12.2). Review the procedure for auscultation of lung sounds in Chapters 7 and 9. The patient assessment chapters focused on trauma patients. However, respiratory distress due to a medical condition is a frequent call that you will respond to. Always look for the following signs and symptoms of breathing difficulty:

- Dyspnea, or shortness of breath (SOB)
- A complaint of tightness in the chest
- Anxiousness, agitation, or restlessness
- Increased respiratory rate (tachypnea)
- Decreased respiratory rate (bradypnea)
- Irregular breathing rhythm
- Shallow breathing, with decreased or nearly absent breath sounds (see Fig. 12.3)
- Minimal chest movement
- Abdominal breathing
- Use of the accessory muscles
- Nasal flaring or pursed lips
- Barrel chest (a condition seen in chronic pulmonary conditions such as emphysema)
- Inability or limited ability to speak due to the effort of breathing
- Persistent cough
- Audible sounds from the upper airway and/or abnormal lung sounds upon auscultation. These may include gurgling, snoring, crowing (turbulent sounds upon inspiration), stridor, wheezing (a sign of **bronchoconstriction**), rales (now called crackles; caused by fluid in the airways), and ronchus (plural: ronchi; a low-pitched snoring sound).
- Increased pulse rate
- Skin changes such as cyanosis, pale skin, flushing or redness, or moistness

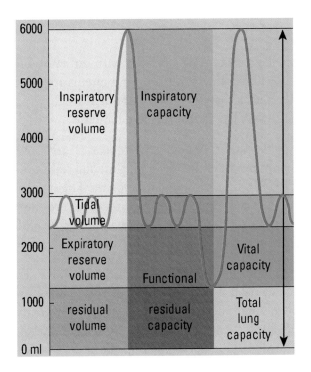

Figure 12.3 *The tidal volume is the amount of air that moves in and out of the lungs during one normal breath.*

- Altered mental status, ranging from mild to complete unresponsiveness. The effects of low oxygen and/or high carbon dioxide in the brain cause this condition.
- A patient in the **tripod position** (see Fig. 12.4). This patient will be sitting, leaning forward, supporting the upper body with hands on the knees or other surface. Sitting in this position helps to keep the airway open and maximizes respiratory effort.

Scene Size-Up

When assessing a patient with dyspnea, you must distinguish between chest trauma and a medical condition as the cause. Look for clues at the scene. Obtain information about the mechanism of injury or about the nature of illness from family and bystanders. You will usually find environmental clues to patients with a history of chronic respiratory illness. For example, the presence of an inhaler or oxygen in the home suggests a chronic respiratory problem.

For patients suffering respiratory distress caused by trauma, take any necessary spinal precautions while maintaining an open and patent airway. Rapid assessment and transport are also appropriate.

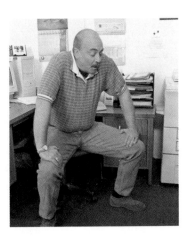

Figure 12.4 *The tripod position.*

Tripod Position | *Position that helps keep the airway open and maximizes respiratory effort: sitting, leaning forward with hands on the knees*

Initial Assessment

Conduct a rapid initial assessment of a patient with difficulty breathing. Evaluate the mental status, airway, breathing, and circulation. Look for confusion, agitation, restlessness, lethargy, or other abnormal behavior. Characterize responsiveness using the AVPU method (see Chapter 8).

Ensure that the airway is patent. The ability to speak clearly confirms an open airway. Speech also provides information about mental status. Note unusual sounds such as stridor, gurgling, crowing, or snoring. These suggest a partial upper airway obstruction (see Table 12.4). Clear and secure the airway if it is blocked. You may need to suction, use an airway adjunct, or perform the Heimlich maneuver to restore the patient's airway.

Note the rate, rhythm, and mechanics of breathing. Look for signs of inadequate breathing, such as nasal flaring, retractions, minimal chest movement, or tripod position. Quickly auscultate the lungs. Listen for abnormal sounds. Check for decreased, absent, or unequal breath sounds and poor air flow. Count the number of words the patient can speak in one breath. This often correlates to the severity of dyspnea.

If you discover that the breathing problem is due to trauma, complete the focused history and physical examination for trauma patients. Provide critical interventions, then obtain baseline vital signs and a SAMPLE history (see Chapter 9).

Table 12.4 • CHARACTERISTICS OF PARTIAL UPPER AIRWAY OBSTRUCTION

Sign	Features	Common Causes	Interventions
Gagging, gasping, coughing, or snoring	Loud, sonorous inspiration and expiration	Foreign body in airway Relaxed soft tissue partially blocking airway	Suction airway Remove foreign object Head-tilt/chin-lift or jaw-thrust maneuver
Crowing	Cawing of a crow	Spasm and narrowing of trachea	Monitor and provide oxygen
Gurgling	Moist rattling on inspiration and expiration	Blood, vomit, or liquid secretions Open chest wound	Suction immediately Cover wound with gloved hand followed by an occlusive dressing
Stridor	Harsh, high pitched sound on inspiration; "seal bark" cough	Severe upper airway swelling, allergic reaction, burns, croup, or epiglottitis	Do not insert tongue blade to examine; may cause spasm and complete obstruction Provide oxygen and transport sitting up Monitor the airway carefully

Emergency Interventions

Provide oxygen at 15 liters per minute via non-rebreather mask if adequate ventilation is present. If the patient has little or no air movement, assist ventilations with supplemental oxygen. Be sure that the airway remains open. If the patient is unable to maintain an open airway, insert the proper airway adjunct and begin artificial ventilation. Be sure to keep suction equipment nearby. For a full review of airway management techniques, see Chapter 7.

When treating patients complaining of respiratory distress, you may be faced with assisting them with their respiratory medications. In particular, you may be asked to help the patient self-administer respiratory medications via an inhaler or nebulizer (see Fig. 12.5). In these cases, medical direction should be contacted and consulted regarding the patient's complaint and condition. Always follow local protocol when assisting the delivery of medications. Never assist in the self-administration of medications that are not prescribed to the patient. Drug dosages and concentrations change for each patient even though the type of medication is similar.

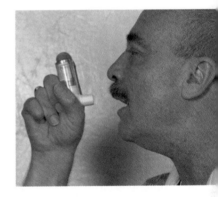

Figure 12.5 *Be available if self-medication assistance is necessary.*

Transport the patient immediately if you see evidence of:

- Airway obstruction
- Poor ventilation
- Cyanosis
- Bradycardia
- Altered mental status
- Difficulty speaking
- Severe trauma

Focused History and Physical Exam

Determining the exact cause of shortness of breath is not necessary with medical problems. However, completing a rapid physical assessment or a detailed physical exam will help you to rule out less obvious causes of the problem.

After providing emergency interventions, complete a focused history and physical exam. If the patient is responsive and stable, take a focused history.

Table 12.5 • OPQRST HISTORY: RESPIRATORY EMERGENCIES

Questions	Examples
Onset	What were you doing when the difficulty with breathing started? Was the onset sudden or gradual?
Provocation	Does anything make the breathing difficulty better or worse?
Quality	Describe the feeling of shortness of breath. If pain is present, describe it.
Radiation	Does the pain (if any) seem to radiate to other parts of the body?
Severity	Rate your breathing difficulty on a scale of 1 to 10, with 10 being the worst you can imagine or have experienced.
Time	When did the symptoms begin? Have you had this sensation before? When? How long did it last?

Conduct a focused medical assessment and measure baseline vital signs. Provide emergency care as needed, and prepare for transport. If the patient is unresponsive, perform a rapid medical exam. Measure baseline vital signs and try to obtain a history from bystanders. Transport immediately.

Focused History

Use the OPQRST questions to evaluate the chief complaint and obtain more information about the breathing problem. Adjust the questions to fit the patient's signs and symptoms (see Table 12.5). Ask about interventions: "Have you taken any medication or done anything to relieve the symptoms? If so, what? Did it help?"

The SAMPLE history questions should be phrased to gather information specifically related to patients with respiratory distress (see Table 12.6).

Rapid Medical Exam

Concentrate your examination on the body position, head, neck, chest, lungs, skin, and extremities.

Body position. Note the position and posture of the patient. The tripod position suggests significant respiratory distress. A patient in the supine position may not be experiencing severe distress. However, assess the patient carefully. He or she may have deteriorated to the point of near-exhaustion and be in need of ventilatory support.

Head. Inspect the lips and mouth for cyanosis.

Neck. Check for jugular venous distention. Inspect the trachea for deviation. Listen to the trachea for stridor. Look for retractions of the neck muscles.

National Registry Examination Tip

Be aggressive, but careful, when caring for patients in respiratory distress. Know how to manage each condition. Provide oxygen therapy for patients in distress and those with illness or injuries affecting respiratory function. Review the OPQRST questions to ask the patient in respiratory distress. Remember that he or she may have difficulty speaking. List SAMPLE questions for patients with respiratory illness.

Table 12.6 • SAMPLE HISTORY: RESPIRATORY EMERGENCIES

Questions	Examples
Signs and Symptoms	What are you feeling? Have you had any other symptoms?
Allergies	Do you have any allergies? Are you allergic to any medications? (Check for medical identification tags.)
Medications	Do you have a prescribed inhaler? When did you last use it? Do you take theophylline? Prednisone?
Pertinent Past Medical History	Do you have any other health problems? History of chronic respiratory problems or cardiac disease?
Last Oral Intake	When did you last eat or drink anything?
Events Leading to the Illness	What were you doing before you first became ill? What were the first symptoms you noticed?

Chest. Inspect for signs of trauma, chest wall movement, and retractions. Palpate for rib fractures or crepitation. These findings suggest an air leak from the lungs or bronchi. Evaluate and treat any life-threatening conditions.

Lungs. Auscultate for equal air movement and abnormal breath sounds.

Skin and Extremities. Assess skin signs, looking for color, temperature, and moisture. Check for peripheral edema and cyanosis.

Baseline Vital Signs

Measure and record the baseline vital signs (review Chapter 5). Check the circulation. Quickly feel the pulse to estimate the heart rate and strength. Look for cyanosis or edema in the extremities. Cyanosis may also be present around the lips, mouth, and nail beds. Check the skin color. If air exchange is inadequate, the skin may appear pale, flushed, or mottled. Palpate the skin temperature. Assess capillary refill time in children. Reassess every 15 minutes if the patient remains stable.

Ongoing Assessment

Continually reassess the patient. Remember that the patient may deteriorate at any time. Maintain an open airway. Establish the airway if necessary. Ensure that breathing is adequate. Provide oxygen as appropriate. If the respiratory status declines, begin assisted ventilations with supplemental oxygen. Immediately transport any critical patient.

If you are providing artificial ventilation to a patient, continuously reassess the effectiveness of ventilation. If ventilation is adequate, the chest will rise and fall with each breath. The heart rate should return to normal.

National Registry Examination Tip

Be able to assess a patient and quickly determine the level of respiratory distress. Be able to assess the patient's approximate tidal volume and respiratory rate. List the signs and symptoms of slight, moderate, and severe respiratory distress. Look for progressively increasing effort. Note the changes that occur between stages.

> **D.O.T. OBJECTIVE**
>
> State the generic name, medication forms, dose, administration, action, indications, and contraindications for the prescribed inhaler.

MEDICATIONS: PRESCRIBED INHALER

The metered dose inhaler (MDI) delivers a controlled dose of finely powdered, aerosolized medication for inhalation. Medications administered by this method go directly to the lungs, where they are rapidly absorbed. Using this route for treating a patient in respiratory distress is more effective than administering tablets or capsules. Table 12.7 summarizes the characteristics of inhaler medications. Table 12.8 lists some common MDIs you will see.

Administration

When assisting with an inhaler, follow the general principles discussed in Chapter 11. Remember the five rights of medication administration: Right patient, right drug, right dose, right route, and right time. Always consult

Table 12.7 • **METERED DOSE INHALERS**

Characteristic	Description
Names	Albuterol, isoetharine, metaproterenol, and others
Indications	Patient exhibits signs and symptoms of a respiratory emergency Patient has a physician-prescribed metered dose inhaler/handheld inhaler Specific authorization was obtained from medical direction
Contraindications	Patient is unable to use the device Medication has expired The inhaler is not prescribed for the patient Medical direction has not authorized use of the inhaler The patient has already met the maximum prescribed dose of the medication before your arrival
Actions	Cause dilation of the bronchioles or inhibit narrowing of the bronchioles by a disease process
Dosage	Varies for each patient and medication. All doses are measured in inhalations or "puffs." Medical direction will determine the appropriate dose
Route	Oral inhalation
Side Effects	Tachycardia, palpitations, tremors, nervousness, nausea, and vomiting can be side effects of most inhalers. Atrovent may cause urinary retention or glaucoma.

Table 12.8 • INHALER MEDICATIONS

Generic Name	Trade Names
Albuterol	Proventil®, Ventolin®
Bitolterol mesylate	Tornalate®
Ipratropium bromide	Atrovent®
Isoetharine	Bronkosol®, Bronkometer®
Metaproterenol	Metaprel®, Alupent®
Pirbuterol	Maxair®
Salmeterol xinafoate	Serevent®
Terbutaline	Brethaire®
Epinephrine	Primatene Mist® (nonprescription)

medical direction before assisting with this device. Various types and styles of inhalers are prescribed, so universal directions are not available. You will be assisting the patient to use the inhaler. He or she should be familiar with the specific directions for use. If the patient is mentally confused and cannot remember the directions, do not administer the drug.

Follow these guidelines when assisting patients with inhalers:

1. Obtain an order from medical direction, either on-line or off-line.
2. Check for the correct medication, patient, and route.
3. Assess the patient's mental status to learn if he or she is alert enough to use the medication.
4. Check the expiration date on the inhaler.
5. Ask whether the patient has already taken any doses of the medication. If so, how many? When was the last dose administered?
6. Ensure that the inhaler is at room temperature or warmer.
7. Read the product label carefully. Follow directions for shaking the solution. Some types require you to shake vigorously before use. Others should not be shaken.
8. Remove oxygen delivery devices.
9. Instruct the patient to exhale deeply. Seal the lips around the opening of the inhaler. Use the spacer, if available.
10. Have the patient depress the inhaler while inhaling deeply.
11. Instruct the patient to hold his or her breath for as long as comfortably possible. This provides time for the medication to be absorbed by the lungs.
12. Replace the oxygen device, if used.
13. Ask the patient to breathe normally.
14. Repeat the dose as ordered by medical direction.

National Registry Examination Tip

Review the steps for assisting a patient with the MDI. Be able to list the side effects of the medication quickly. Describe what to do if the patient has an adverse reaction. Remember to apply the principles of BSI and standard precautions. Provide ventilation assistance as needed.

EMT Tip

If you are not familiar with a certain medication, ask the patient why he or she is taking it.

Figure 12.6 *Assisting a patient with a spacing device.*

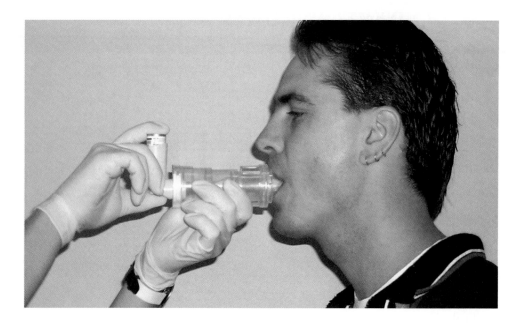

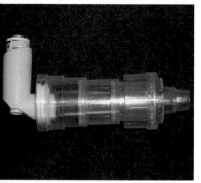

Figure 12.7 *An inhaler attached to a spacing device.*

Bronchodilator | *Drug that relaxes the smooth muscle of the bronchi and bronchioles, reversing bronchoconstriction*

Spacing Devices

The spacing device, or spacer, is a long chamber, approximately 3 ½ inches long. It attaches to the inhaler, allowing more effective delivery of medication to the bronchioles. Use a spacing device, if available. Attach the inhaler to the spacer. The patient inhales the medication slowly through the mouthpiece on the opposite end of the spacer (see Figs. 12.6 and 12.7).

Reassessment

You must reassess the patient after administering a **bronchodilator**. You should:

- Repeat the vital signs and the focused history and physical exam.

- Conduct ongoing assessments as indicated. Ask the patient if the medication relieved his or her breathing difficulty. Reassess the respiratory status. Confirm an open, patent airway. Check to see if the patient is using the accessory muscles. Auscultate the breath sounds. Note changes in skin color.

- If the first dose of medication is ineffective or minimally effective, consult with medical direction. A second dose may be ordered.

- Document your reassessment findings.

- If the patient's respiratory status deteriorates, be prepared to administer positive pressure artificial ventilation with supplemental oxygen. Transport immediately.

D.O.T. OBJECTIVE

Distinguish between the emergency medical care of the infant, child, and adult patient with breathing difficulty.

INFANTS AND CHILDREN

Respiratory failure is a leading cause of death in children. A child with **respiratory distress** can quickly deteriorate into **respiratory arrest** and eventually into cardiac arrest. Quick action is needed to block and reverse this progression.

Respiratory Failure | *When the respiratory system cannot deliver an adequate supply of oxygen to meet the body's current demand*

Table 12.9 • **PEDIATRIC RESPIRATORY DIFFERENCES**

Structure	Difference From Adults
Head	Proportionally larger than adults
Tongue	Proportionally larger; airway easily blocked
Airway	Small airway; easily blocked; natural breathing is through the nose (in infants)
Circulation	Smaller blood volume; greater risk of shock

Anatomical Differences

Remember the differences in anatomy between pediatric patients and adults (see Table 12.9). The mouth, nose, trachea, and other structures are smaller and more easily obstructed than in adults. The child's airway is at high risk for obstruction. Establishing and maintaining an airway may be more difficult. A small object can cause a serious emergency if inhaled by a child (see Fig. 12.8). A life-threatening situation will occur if the object travels to the lower airway and blocks a main bronchus.

A child's head is proportionally larger than an adult's head, so the tongue takes up more space. If the tongue swells, a blockage will occur. The child's narrow trachea is also subject to obstruction if swollen. Thus, an illness that causes swelling or obstruction anywhere in the airway will affect a child much more seriously than an adult.

Respiratory Distress | *Difficulty breathing; increased effort necessary to breathe due to impaired respiratory function*

Respiratory Arrest | *A complete lack of respiratory drive or pulmonary function*

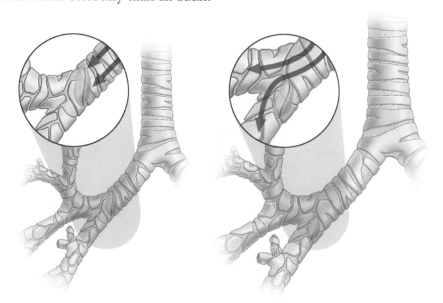

Figure 12.8 *Because a child's airway (left) is smaller than an adult's (right), a foreign object can more easily obstruct breathing.*

The cartilage in a child's trachea and chest wall is not fully developed and is less rigid. The flexible cricoid cartilage is easily damaged. The chest wall is somewhat soft, so children depend on the diaphragm for breathing. Using accessory muscles to breathe is common.

Signs and Symptoms

Retractions and use of accessory muscles are common in children with difficulty breathing. Nasal flaring and grunting are also seen. Infants may exhibit seesaw breathing. In this condition, the chest wall and abdomen move in opposite directions with each respiration. This type of breathing suggests an upper airway obstruction. The head may bob with each breath, also showing respiratory distress.

Children with bronchospasm may cough frequently, rather than wheeze. These symptoms will respond to bronchodilators.

Altered mental status in the infant or young child may be difficult to detect. One finding is an inability to recognize the parents. Cyanosis and bradycardia are both ominous, late-stage findings in infants and children, suggesting that respiratory arrest is near.

Treatment

Prompt administration of oxygen can stop or reverse the progression of respiratory distress in children. You can safely administer high concentrations of oxygen to infants and children (see Fig. 12.9). Provide humidified oxygen, if possible.

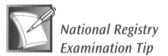

National Registry Examination Tip

Review the ranges for pediatric respiratory rates, tidal volumes, and heart rates. Recognize the reasons for changes in these vital signs. Review the treatment for pediatric patients with asthma that causes respiratory distress. Review the steps for cardiopulmonary resuscitation, artificial ventilation, and foreign body airway obstructions for infants and children.

Figure 12.9 *A parent can help to apply an oxygen mask to a child.*

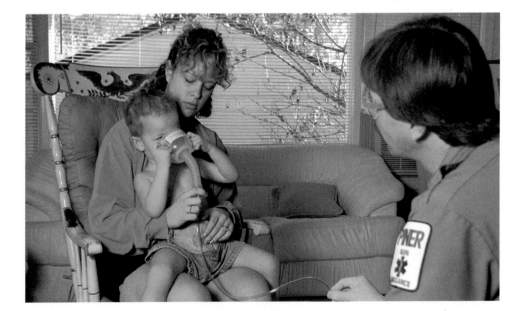

Removing a young child from the parents to apply an oxygen mask usually increases the child's anxiety and agitation. This causes respiratory distress to worsen. Unless the child is in critical condition, allow a parent to hold him or her on the lap. The parent can help by holding the mask near the child's face. Allow the parent to accompany the child in the ambulance.

If an infant or child will not tolerate a mask, be creative. Giving some oxygen to a quiet child is better than giving little or no oxygen to a panicked child. The child will be able to inhale the oxygen even though the mask is not in direct contact with the child's face (see Fig. 12.10). Place the oxygen tubing under the arm of a teddy bear or other comforting toy so the child receives blow-by oxygen (see Fig. 12.11).

Handheld inhalers are often used to treat wheezing in children. The indications and use of a metered dose inhaler are the same as they are for an adult. Delivering the correct dose may be difficult. Enlist the parent's help, if possible.

For more information about pediatric respiratory emergencies and upper airway obstruction, see Chapter 23.

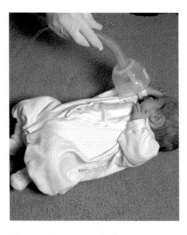

Figure 12.10 *An infant receiving blow-by oxygen.*

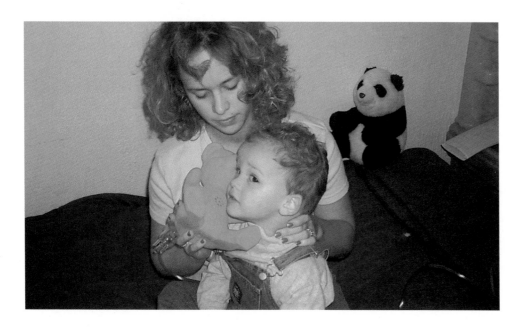

Figure 12.11 *The KidO₂™ device, distributed by BLD Medical Products.*

EMT Tip

One type of blow-by device is the KidO₂, which incorporates a friendly toy to deliver oxygen with and without medication nebulization. The KidO₂ is designed to reduce the patient's apprehension before, during, and after treatment.

Chapter Twelve Summary

- Difficulty breathing is the chief complaint in many calls. Assessing the patient's breathing is very important. Look for signs of inadequate respiration. If breathing is inadequate, begin assisting ventilation immediately. If breathing is adequate, provide high-flow oxygen by non-rebreather mask.

- Ask OPQRST questions to evaluate the patient's complaint.

- Consider assisted administration of an inhaler if the patient has one and if no contraindications exist. Always consult with medical direction before assisting with an inhaler.

- The use of handheld inhalers is a common treatment in children. Emergency care is the same as for adults. Be aware of anatomical differences in the respiratory system between children and adults. Cyanosis is a late sign of a respiratory emergency in a child.

Key Terms Review

Acute Illness │ *page 362*
Asthma │ *page 364*
Bronchoconstriction │ *page 366*
Bronchodilator │ *page 374*

Chronic Illness │ *page 362*
Chronic Obstructive Pulmonary
   Disease (COPD) │ *page 364*
Respiratory Arrest │ *page 375*

Respiratory Distress │ *page 375*
Respiratory Failure │ *page 375*
Tripod Position │ *page 367*

Review Questions

1. The exchange between oxygen and carbon dioxide takes place between the capillaries and the lung's:

   a. Secondary bronchi
   b. Trachea
   c. Alveoli
   d. Main bronchus

2. In the tissues, _____ moves into the capillaries, but in the lungs, it moves out of the capillaries into the air.

   a. Carbon dioxide
   b. Oxygen
   c. Nitrogen
   d. Hemoglobin

3. The volume of air that moves in and out of the airways in a normal breath is called the:

   a. Tidal volume
   b. Residual volume
   c. Vital capacity
   d. Expiratory reserve volume

4. If gurgling or snoring sounds are noted during the initial assessment the EMT-B should immediately:

   a. Proceed with a focused history and physical exam
   b. Properly position, clear and secure the airway
   c. Document the findings on the patient care report
   d. Auscultate for bowel sounds

5. In acute respiratory emergency cases, cyanosis is commonly seen:

   a. On the chest and abdomen
   b. On the scalp and eyes
   c. Around the lips, mouth, and nail beds
   d. Around the ankles, wrists, and knees

6. Which of the following medications may be helpful to patients with respiratory diseases?

   a. Oral glucose
   b. Nitroglycerin
   c. Bronchodilators (such as albuterol)
   d. Beta-blockers

7. Which structure is responsible for warming and cleaning air?

   a. Nose
   b. Pharynx
   c. Trachea
   d. Alveoli

8. Which structure forms the lower border of the thoracic cavity?

   a. Lungs
   b. Liver
   c. Rib cage
   d. Diaphragm

9. Which process provides the tissues with oxygen and removes carbon dioxide?

   a. Ventilation
   b. Respiration
   c. Diffusion
   d. Capillary/cellular exchange

10. The word that best describes shortness of breath is:

    a. Tachypnea
    b. Bradypnea
    c. Dyspnea
    d. Hypopnea

11. Which of the following abnormal breath sounds indicates bronchoconstriction?

    a. Crowing
    b. Gurgling
    c. Wheezing
    d. Snoring

12. What is the normal range for respiratory rate in an adult?

    a. 15 to 30 breaths per minute
    b. 12 to 20 breaths per minute
    c. 25 to 50 breaths per minute
    d. 50 to 70 breaths per minute

13. The number of words a patient can speak in one breath is a good general indicator of:

    a. Severity of dyspnea
    b. Severity of cyanosis
    c. Severity of asthma
    d. Severity of cardiac arrest

14. When an EMT-B finds a barrel chest when performing a patient assessment, the most likely cause is:

    a. Pneumonia
    b. Hypoxia
    c. Pulmonary edema
    d. Emphysema

15. What type of sound can usually be heard when listening to an asthma patient's lung sounds?

    a. Stridor
    b. Rhonchi
    c. Wheezing
    d. Crepitation

16. When comparing the adult's airway to the child's airway, which one of the following is true?

    a. The adult's airway is more likely to become obstructed
    b. The child's respiratory structures are larger and more rigid than the adult's structures
    c. The child's airway is more likely to become obstructed
    d. The adult's tongue takes up more room in the posterior pharynx

CASE STUDIES

Respiratory Emergencies

1 Recently, the air quality has been especially bad. Ozone alerts have been in effect for several days. The respiratory calls keep coming in. You arrive on the scene of another shortness of breath call. There is no response to the doorbell. You find the 31-year-old male sitting in a tripod position just outside the back door. He is unable to speak and is very anxious. His lips are slightly cyanotic, and he is gasping for air. You notice that he is using his intercostal and abdominal muscles to breathe. Family members tell you that his asthma has been especially bad recently.

A. What is your general impression of this patient?

B. What clues about the patient's position and the scene help you to develop this impression?

C. What interventions are appropriate during the initial assessment of the patient?

2 Lucinda is an active 11-year-old female. She was playing during recess when she began to complain of shortness of breath. The teacher on duty quickly sent a teacher's aide to call for help. When you arrive, you find the patient sitting in a tripod position in moderate distress. A teacher has Lucinda's emergency card, which shows a history of asthma. The card also says she uses a Ventolin metered dose inhaler. Lucinda has forgotten her medication today.

A. Why do asthma attacks commonly occur when children play outside?

B. A teacher in the school also has asthma and takes Ventolin. She offers her inhaler to Lucinda. What should you do?

3 An early morning dispatch for an automobile accident close to hospital grounds usually means someone was rushing to the emergency department. When you arrive, you notice a large sedan has crashed into several parked cars. Police officers are reaching inside the vehicle as you pull up. The driver is secured by a seat belt. Damage to the vehicle is minimal. The driver is an 80-year-old male in severe respiratory distress. He looks exhausted. The patient's respiratory rate is approximately 32 per minute. Tidal volume is diminished. The nail beds and lips are cyanotic. The patient is breathing with his lips pursed. You notice he is very thin and has a large barrel-like chest wall.

A. Do you consider this patient a medical patient or trauma patient?

B. What type of move do you suggest for this patient?

C. What are your initial interventions?

Stories from the Field
Wrap-Up

Carmen is correct in trying to speed up your assessment. The patient's sitting position and limited ability to speak are signs of severe distress. The patient may be nearing respiratory failure. Initial treatment with high-flow oxygen by a non-rebreather mask is appropriate. However, your initial assessment findings show the patient is not breathing adequately. Determining the patient's OPQRST and SAMPLE history are also important early considerations.

If the young man has a history of respiratory problems, he may have a prescribed inhaler. If so, helping him to use it before transport may be appropriate. Consult with medical direction. Otherwise, the patient's signs and symptoms suggest the need for immediate transport. You must look for other possible causes, such as recent trauma. Assisting ventilation with a bag-valve mask device or flow-restricted, oxygen-powered ventilation device is indicated if breathing remains inadequate. Insert a nasopharyngeal airway if tolerated by the patient.

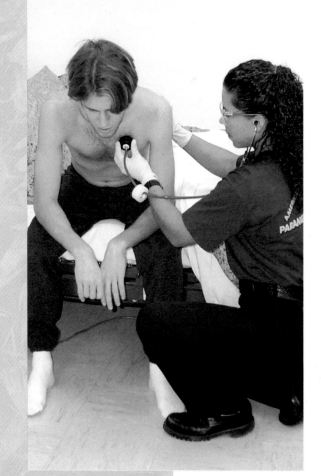

ENHANCED STUDY

Common Respiratory Diseases

As an EMT-B you will commonly care for patients with acute problems related to chronic respiratory illnesses. The conditions described in this section are chronic illnesses. You will find out about asymptomatic chronic conditions when you take the patient's history. An asymptomatic condition is one that is well controlled and is not causing the patient distress.

Oxygen concentrators are commonly used in the homes of chronic respiratory patients. An oxygen concentrator is electrically operated. It converts room air into more concentrated oxygen. However, it cannot adequately provide flow rates greater than 5 liters per minute. Patients with oxygen concentrators usually have a backup oxygen tank for use during a power failure.

Asthma. Asthma is a common chronic respiratory condition. Asthma is also called reactive airway disease. It is seen in pediatric and adult patients. An allergen such as dust or pollen, or another stimulus such as tobacco smoke or infection, causes an acute asthmatic reaction. When this occurs, the smooth muscles of the bronchioles constrict. This condition is called bronchospasm or bronchoconstriction. It obstructs the airflow, causing wheezing. The lining of the small airways swell, and mucous production increases. This leads to airway obstruction.

Signs and symptoms of an asthmatic attack are tachypnea, tachycardia, and wheezing. Retractions may be present. The patient may have some degree of hypoxia, depending on the severity of the attack. The symptoms often worsen and can become so severe that respiratory arrest occurs.

You will administer oxygen to all patients in respiratory distress. Bronchodilators such as albuterol are given to treat wheezing. The physician may prescribe steroid medications, such as prednisone, to reduce the inflammation.

Chronic Obstructive Pulmonary Disease. Chronic obstructive pulmonary disease (COPD) is a generic term. It is used to describe many chronic illnesses characterized by airflow obstruction. The two most common types of COPD are emphysema and chronic bronchitis (see Enhancement Fig. 12.1).

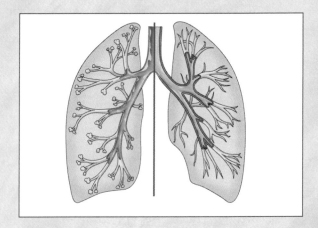

Enhancement Figure 12.1 *The effects of emphysema (left) and bronchitis (right) on the lungs.*

Emphysema. Emphysema is a chronic condition that develops over a long period of time. It often results from long-term exposure to cigarette smoke. Normally, the alveoli are like small balloons that expand and contract. Emphysema destroys the walls of the alveoli, causing them to lose elasticity and dilate (see Enhancement Fig. 12.2). Air becomes trapped in the alveoli. Because the walls have lost elasticity, they cannot push the air out. This causes poor gas exchange, resulting in low oxygen and increased carbon dioxide levels in the blood.

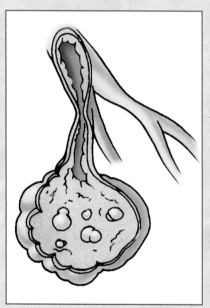

Enhancement Figure 12.2 *The air sac walls are destroyed in patients who have emphysema.*

Emphysema patients are often thin and may have a barrel chest due to trapped air. They are typically short of breath with little exertion and are tachypneic at rest. Breath sounds are chronically diminished. Rhonchi and wheezes are common. Most have a chronic cough. The condition usually worsens. Bronchodilators may help to relieve symptoms. Steroids are often necessary to control the condition.

Chronic Bronchitis. Chronic bronchitis is characterized by long-term coughing with sputum production. The bronchi are inflamed and produce excessive mucus (see Enhancement Fig. 12.3). This is often caused by infections. Airway obstruction is also present. Most patients have components of both chronic bronchitis and emphysema. Cigarette smoking is a common cause of this condition.

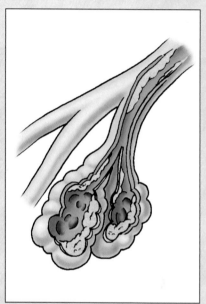

Enhancement Figure 12.3 *The bronchi are inflamed in patients who have chronic bronchitis. The swollen bronchi and secreted fluids make breathing difficult.*

A chronic, productive cough and dyspnea are common signs of chronic bronchitis. The patient may become cyanotic and tachypneic. On auscultation of the lungs, you may hear rhonchi, wheezes, and diminished breath sounds. The symptoms worsen periodically because of infection. The condition is treated with the same drugs used for emphysema. Antibiotics are used to treat the infection.

Chapter 13

Cardiovascular Emergencies

Stories from the Field

You are visiting your family during a break from your studies. An old family friend asks you to check on her husband. He recently had heart surgery and he does not look well. You tell her that you are just an EMT in training, but will be happy to talk with him. When you get inside, you find an elderly man sitting on the couch watching sports on television. He is very pale and looks sweaty. He denies chest pain. He blames his discomfort on indigestion from lunch. Your initial assessment reveals no life threatening problems. The patient is irritated by his wife's insistence that you look at him. You have a poor general impression of his condition. You really think he should be evaluated. You suggest a visit to the local emergency department. He tells you to leave him alone. You suggest calling 9-1-1 anyway, but his wife refuses to do so.

About an hour later, the woman comes running to get you again. As you approach the patient, he gasps harshly, then his breathing stops. You conduct an initial assessment and find that he is now in cardiac arrest. Relying on your Basic Life Support training, you move the patient to the floor and begin CPR. You ask his wife to call 9-1-1. You continue CPR until EMS arrives.

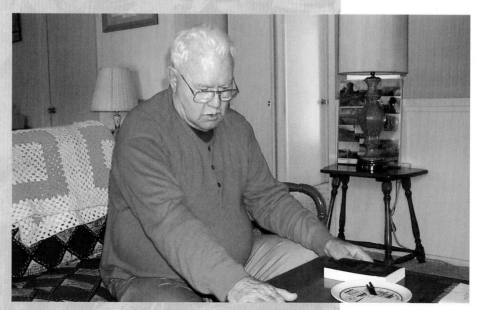

According to the National Center for Health Statistics, over 700,000 persons died in 1997 because of cardiovascular diseases. Heart disease is the leading cause of death for men above 45 years old, and for women aged 65 years and over. Unfortunately, the first sign of cardiac disease is often sudden death. As an EMT you will see many patients experiencing cardiac compromise. This condition has many causes, and the symptoms vary widely. The most common symptom is chest pain or discomfort, but some patients have no symptoms at all.

You must learn the principles and practices of emergency cardiac care. You will provide most cardiac patients with oxygen. Sometimes, you will assist a patient with nitroglycerin (NTG) administration to relieve chest pain. Occasionally, you will use either a semi-automated or a fully automated external defibrillator (AED) on an unresponsive cardiac patient. When attached to a patient, the AED records cardiac rhythm and delivers an electrical shock to the chest to restart the normal action of the heart.

D.O.T. OBJECTIVE

Describe the structure and function of the cardiovascular system.

CARDIOVASCULAR SYSTEM REVIEW

You have learned that the circulatory system transports blood to the cells, tissues, and organs of the body. Blood keeps the tissues alive by delivering oxygen, nutrients, and hormones. These substances are needed for cells to survive and function. The blood also picks up wastes produced during cellular metabolism. These waste products are carried to the kidneys, liver, lungs, and intestines for excretion. Figure 13.1 and Table 13.1 provide an overview of the structure and function of the cardiovascular system. For a full review of cardiovascular anatomy and physiology, see Chapter 4.

Inadequate Circulation

The circulatory system delivers oxygen and nutrients to the tissues and removes their waste products. Perfusion is the adequate oxygenation of body tissues. Under some conditions, the blood does not provide enough oxygen to meet the body's needs. This leads to a profound depression of vital processes. This condition is called shock or hypoperfusion. When a patient is in shock, the cells become starved for oxygen. The blood is overloaded with waste products. Eventually, the cells die. If too many cells die, the patient will die.

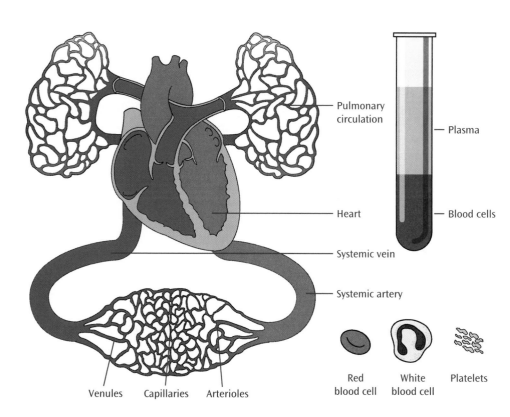

Figure 13.1 *Structures of the cardiovascular system.*

Table 13.1 • REVIEW OF THE CARDIOVASCULAR SYSTEM

Structure	Function
Heart	A muscular, four-chambered organ that functions as the cardiovascular system's pump. The upper chambers are called atria; the lower chambers are called ventricles.
Blood Vessels	Conduits for the blood. They include the arteries, arterioles, capillaries, venules, and veins. The blood vessels are able to constrict and expand, directing blood to organs that need more oxygen at any time.
Arteries	Vessels that carry blood away from the heart. The systemic arteries carry oxygenated blood to nourish the body parts.
Veins	Vessels that carry blood back to the heart. The systemic veins carry deoxygenated blood out of the tissues.
Arterioles, Capillaries, and Venules	Arterioles connect arteries to capillaries. Venules connect capillaries to veins. Capillaries allow oxygen, nutrients, and wastes to diffuse between the blood and the tissues.
Blood	Fluid consisting of plasma and cells; carries oxygen, nutrients, and waste products throughout the body.
Plasma	The fluid component of the blood that carries cells and nutrients.
Red Blood Cells	The cells that carry oxygen in the blood by means of the protein hemoglobin.
White Blood Cells	Several types of cells involved in fighting infection.
Platelets	Cell fragments necessary for blood clotting.

Shock can be caused by different conditions. For example, hypovolemic shock can occur when the volume of fluid in the body is low. This can be due to a loss of blood (known as hemorrhagic shock) or of other bodily fluids. Cardiogenic shock is caused by insufficient pumping action of the heart. Neurogenic shock occurs when blood vessels dilate excessively. Whatever the cause, shock is characterized by signs and symptoms such as:

- Anxiety or mental dullness
- Extreme thirst
- Dilated pupils
- Capillary refill time more than 2 seconds
- Nausea and vomiting
- Restlessness
- Pallor around the mouth
- Pale, cyanotic, cool clammy skin (not seen in neurogenic shock)
- Rapid but weak pulse
- Rapid and shallow breathing
- Reduction in total blood volume
- Subnormal temperature
- Low or decreasing blood pressure

Shock is discussed in more detail in Chapter 19.

CARDIAC COMPROMISE

Cardiac Compromise | *Any action or factor that reduces the functionality of the cardiac system*

Cardiac compromise is a general term used to describe difficulty with heart function. It has many potential causes. The most common and well-known cause is narrowing or blockage of the coronary arteries. These arteries supply blood and oxygen to the heart muscle. Other causes are:

- Disturbances in the heart's rhythm
- Inadequate pumping function
- Heart valve problems

More than half the Americans with heart disease will die outside the hospital, usually suddenly. Death within one hour of the onset of cardiac symptoms is called sudden cardiac death. You may be dispatched to respond to a chest pain complaint. By the time you arrive, the patient is in cardiac arrest. Or a patient you are treating for cardiac compromise may suddenly collapse. This chapter will prepare you to care for cardiac emergencies in general as well as to manage patients in cardiac arrest.

As an EMT-Basic, you will not be expected to identify different types of cardiac events. However, understanding various causes of cardiac compromise is important. Cardiac compromise is often due to underlying **coronary artery disease (CAD)**. The disease can cause a patient to incur an **acute myocardial infarction (AMI)**, commonly known as a heart attack. An AMI may lead to **ventricular fibrillation (VF)**. This is random, disorganized electrical activity of the heart that results in a life-threatening cardiac rhythm. Abnormal cardiac rhythm is called **dysrhythmia**. Arrhythmia is an older term for this activity. Ventricular fibrillation is the most common cause of sudden cardiac death. Types of cardiac compromise are discussed further in the Enhanced Studies section at the end of this chapter.

D.O.T. OBJECTIVE

Explain that not all chest pain patients result in cardiac arrest and do not need to be attached to an automated external defibrillator.

Signs and Symptoms

Patients with cardiac compromise have a variety of signs and symptoms. The most common symptom is some form of chest pain or discomfort, known as **angina pectoris**. Typically, the patient describes squeezing, crushing, tightness, burning, or aching in the chest. Some patients have no symptoms at all. Many think they are experiencing indigestion. Other common complaints are, "I think I pulled a muscle," "It's something I ate," or "I've just got gas." In addition, a patient may deny chest pain or cardiac symptoms out of fear or anxiety. Signs and symptoms of cardiac compromise include:

- Chest pain or discomfort that radiates down the arms, up to the jaw, or into the upper back
- Dyspnea, or difficulty breathing
- Pale, cool, or clammy skin
- Sudden onset of sweating (a significant finding)
- Anxiety, irritability, or feeling of impending doom
- Abnormal or irregular pulse rate
- Abnormal blood pressure
- Pain in the upper abdominal region
- Nausea or vomiting

Coronary Artery Disease (CAD) | *Condition of plaque accumulation causing narrowing within coronary artery walls; leads to decreased oxygen delivery to heart muscle*

Acute Myocardial (my-oh-KAR-de-ul) Infarction (AMI) | *Sudden cardiac muscle death or injury due to lack of oxygen; a heart attack*

Ventricular Fibrillation (ven-TRIK-yu-ler fi-bri-LAY-shun) (VF) | *Rapid, uncoordinated movements of the ventricle walls that replace the normal contraction; treated with defibrillation methods*

Dysrhythmia (dis-RITH-me-uh) | *A disturbance in heart rate and/or rhythm; formerly called arrhythmia*

Angina Pectoris (an-JI-nah pek-TOR-is) | *Severe pain and constriction about the heart; also called angina or myocardial ischemia; often treated with nitroglycerin*

It is important to realize that not all calls involving chest pain are due to cardiac compromise. Other common causes of pain are:

- Anxiety
- Lung disease
- Gastrointestinal disorders
- Musculoskeletal disorders
- Pneumonia and lung infections

D.O.T. OBJECTIVES

Describe the emergency medical care of the patient experiencing chest pain/discomfort.

Discuss the position of comfort for patients with various cardiac emergencies.

Establish the relationship between airway management and the patient with cardiac compromise.

Predict the relationship between the patient experiencing cardiovascular compromise and basic life support.

CD-ROM
Link

The Authentic Emergency Scenes section in the Video Appendix of the MedEMT CD-ROM has a video entitled "Heart Attack," which follows an emergency crew as they transport a heart attack patient to the hospital.

Automated External Defibrillator (AED) | *Defibrillation equipment designed to analyze, shock, and re-analyze cardiac dysfunction after applying electrodes to the patient*

EMERGENCY CARE: CARDIAC PATIENT

Emergency care of a patient with cardiac problems requires a rapid initial assessment and careful management. Signs, symptoms, and treatment of patients with cardiac compromise can be confusing. Most patients with chest pain do not go into cardiac arrest. Many patients experience cardiac arrest due to coronary artery disease. However, other conditions, including traumatic injury, can cause the heart to stop.

Your course of action depends largely upon whether or not there is a pulse and whether the patient is responsive or unresponsive. Environmental clues may be your only source of information about an unresponsive patient's history. Some patients will require oxygen, nitroglycerin, and transport to the hospital. Others will require more aggressive out-of-hospital treatment, including basic life support and CPR. Some patients will benefit from use of the **automated external defibrillator (AED)** (see Fig. 13.2).

You should attempt to limit a cardiac patient's anxiety. Undue stress can increase the damage to the heart muscle. Try to calm a frightened patient. If the patient asks if he or she is having a heart attack or is going to die, be careful

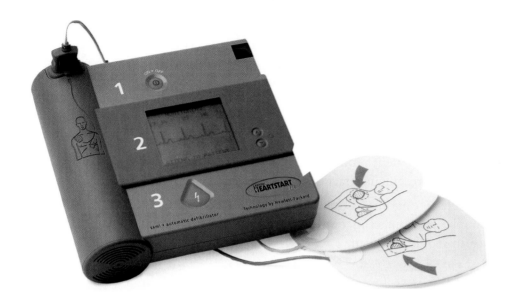

Figure 13.2 *An automated external defibrillator.**

not to offer any diagnosis. Tell the person that you are treating the signs and symptoms. Reassure him or her that advanced care will be supplied quickly.

Emergency lights and a siren may frighten some patients. However, transport delays could affect the patient's outcome. In your efforts to reduce a patient's anxiety, you must use good judgment when considering the use of your lights and siren. Weigh the risks and benefits to your patient, and decide what type of response is in his or her best interest.

Responsive Patient

Follow these guidelines for assisting a responsive patient complaining of chest pain or discomfort:

1. Complete the scene survey. Be alert for environmental clues to the patient's medical history.

2. Conduct your initial assessment. Complete a focused history and physical exam, including baseline vital signs. Look for signs and symptoms of cardiac compromise.

3. Place the patient in a position of comfort. The sitting position is often the most comfortable. Administer oxygen at 15 liters per minute via non-rebreather mask if the patient is breathing adequately. If the patient is not breathing adequately, assist ventilations and provide supplemental oxygen.

4. Conduct an OPQRST assessment and obtain a SAMPLE history. Questions to consider should include: Is the chest pain worse with exertion? Is it still present when you rest? Have you taken anything for your pain? Have you taken Viagra® or any other medications?

5. If the focused history includes cardiac complications and the patient is complaining of chest pain, ask if his or her physician has prescribed **nitroglycerin (NTG)**. Ask if the nitroglycerin is with the patient.

Nitroglycerin (NTG) | *Medication that dilates blood vessels and decreases the workload of the heart; taken sublingually by tablet or by oral spray for relief of chest pain*

*Photo courtesy of Laerdal Medical Corporation.

6. If the patient does not have any prescribed nitroglycerin, continue the focused assessment and transport immediately. If nitroglycerin has been prescribed for the patient, consider assisting the patient in taking one dose sublingually. Nitroglycerin should only be administered if the patient is complaining of chest pain, the systolic blood pressure is greater than 100 mmHg, and medical direction has been consulted. The procedure for nitroglycerin administration is described in the following section.

7. Transport the patient promptly. Conduct a detailed assessment while en route to the receiving medical facility.

8. Complete an ongoing assessment every 5 minutes. If the chest pain has not been relieved, contact medical direction to see if additional doses of nitroglycerin should be given.

D.O.T. OBJECTIVES

List the indications for the use of nitroglycerin.

State the contraindications and side effects for the use of nitroglycerin.

Nitroglycerin

Nitroglycerin (NTG) is very useful for treating chest pain related to coronary artery disease. Chest pain is caused by damage to heart tissue from lack of oxygen. Nitroglycerin relaxes the walls of the blood vessels. This decreases the heart's workload, improving oxygenation. Giving NTG often relieves chest pain. As an EMT-B, you can assist patients to self-administer nitroglycerin (see Fig. 13.3 and Table 13.2). Your skills can make a difference in the patient's outcome.

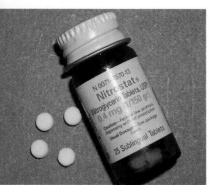

Figure 13.3 *Nitroglycerin tablets.*

Nitroglycerin Administration. In Chapter 11, general guidelines regarding the safe administration of medications were discussed. When you believe using nitroglycerin is indicated, follow these specific steps:

1. If you do not have standing orders to give nitroglycerin, contact medical direction and obtain an on-line order.

2. Remember to practice body substance isolation and standard precautions. Nitroglycerin can be absorbed through the skin. Wear gloves when handling it.

3. Complete a focused assessment, including vital signs. The patient's systolic blood pressure must be greater than 100 mmHg. Nitroglycerin dilates blood vessels and could cause a drop in blood pressure.

4. Check that the prescription label is for the correct patient, correct medication, and correct form. Always check the expiration date. Never use expired medications.

Table 13.2 • **NITROGLYCERIN**

Characteristic	Description
Names	Generic Name: Nitroglycerin Trade Names: Nitro-bid®, Nitrostat®, Nitrong®
Indications	The patient has a cardiac history and has signs or symptoms of chest pain or cardiac compromise The patient has NTG prescribed by a physician You are authorized by medical direction to administer nitroglycerin
Contraindications	Hypotension or blood pressure below 100 mmHg systolic Head injury Infants and children Patient has already met the maximum prescribed dose before you arrived Patient has taken Viagra in the last 24 hours
Actions	Relaxes blood vessels and decreases the workload of the heart
Dosage	One dose of 0.4 mg, repeated every 3 to 5 minutes if no relief was obtained, blood pressure stays above 100 mmHg, and authorized by medical control. A maximum of three doses can be given.
Forms and Route	Sublingual; tablet or spray under tongue Note: some patients may have skin patches or paste; EMS does not administer or assist with these forms
Side Effects	Hypotension Headache Pulse rate changes

5. Make sure the patient is alert. Learn the time of the last dose. Ask the patient if he or she has had side effects from the drug in the past. Make sure the patient understands the route of administration.

6. Ask the patient to lift the tongue. Tell him or her to place the tablet, or to spray one dose, under the tongue (see Fig. 13.4 and Fig. 11.4 in Chapter 11).

7. After taking the pill or spray, the patient must keep the mouth closed, without swallowing, until the medication has dissolved.

8. Record the administration and time.

9. Recheck the blood pressure within 2 minutes of NTG administration. Ask the patient if the pain has been relieved. If not, repeat the dose in 3 to 5 minutes. Contact medical direction before repeating the dose. Do not administer more than three doses.

10. Reassess vital signs and chest pain after each dose. Document your actions and findings.

Figure 13.4 *Assisting a patient to spray nitroglycerin under his tongue.*

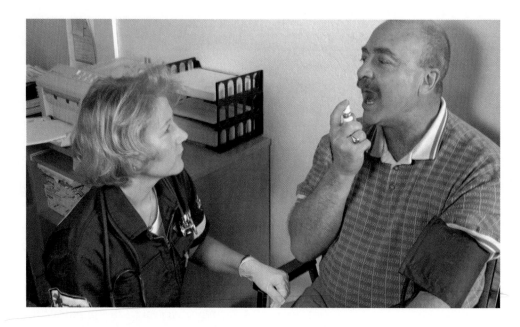

EMT Tip

Scars on the patient's chest are often a clue to previous open heart surgeries. You may also find or be told that the patient has an implanted pacemaker or defibrillator. This information should be noted on the run report. Your care will not change because of this information.

Unresponsive Patient

If a patient is unresponsive, use environmental clues to help determine whether the nature of illness is cardiovascular. Complete a scene size-up. Look for nitroglycerin nearby. Ask relatives and bystanders about a history of cardiac problems or whether the patient complained of chest pain. Consider other causes for the unresponsive state.

Conduct the initial assessment. Stop CPR, if in progress upon your arrival. Recheck the patient's airway, breathing, and circulation. If a pulse is present, transport the patient immediately. If breathing is adequate and a pulse is present, provide high-flow oxygen via non-rebreather mask and transport. If the patient is breathing inadequately or is apneic, assist ventilations using a bag-valve mask device using high-flow oxygen and transport. Continue to provide supplemental oxygen. Monitor vital signs frequently while en route. Be prepared to provide CPR or automated external defibrillation if the pulse is lost.

Pulseless Patient

A patient with no pulse is in cardiac arrest. Immediate emergency assessment and intervention are required to restore adequate perfusion of the vital tissues and prevent sudden cardiac death. If the pulse is absent, you will consider applying the AED as described in the next section.

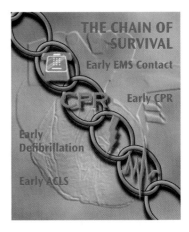

Figure 13.5 *The chain of survival.*

The Chain of Survival

The American Medical Association (AMA) and American Heart Association (AHA) are professional organizations that study diseases and make recommendations for prevention and treatment. The AMA and AHA have developed a series of critical interventions for cardiac arrest. These interventions are called the **chain of survival** (see Fig. 13.5). Each link in the chain increases the likelihood of successful resuscitation and survival. Early response and treatment are the keys to success. If a link in the chain of survival is missing, delayed, or done incorrectly, the chain will be broken. Breaking the chain can significantly reduce the patient's chance of survival.

The four links in the chain of survival are:

- Early access to the EMS system
- Early CPR
- Early **defibrillation**
- Early advanced cardiac life support (ACLS)

Strengthening the chain of survival is the key to reducing sudden cardiac death. As an EMT-Basic, you have an important role in the chain. You will implement early CPR and external defibrillation. You will also help patients to receive advanced cardiac life support care as quickly as possible. You can do this by requesting backup from an advanced life support (ALS) unit. If your area has no ALS service, you will rapidly transport the patient to a medical facility. The chain of survival is discussed further in Appendix B, Basic Life Support.

Chain of Survival | *Term used for the four interventions that provide the best chance for successful resuscitation of a patient in cardiac arrest: Early access, early CPR, early defibrillation, early ACLS*

Defibrillation | *Electrical shock or current delivered to the heart through the patient's chest wall to help the heart restore a normal rhythm*

Basic Life Support

Basic life support skills are used on cardiac patients who require life-saving interventions to maintain adequate ventilation, oxygenation, and circulatory function. These short-term life support procedures help to sustain life until more advanced staff, equipment, or interventions become available. The BLS skills you learned prior to this class are reviewed in Appendix B. As an EMT-Basic, you will usually perform two-rescuer CPR while on duty. You might perform one-rescuer CPR while your partner sets up equipment or while in transit to a medical facility. The basic skills will be enhanced by your knowledge of patient assessment, airway management techniques, lifting and moving of patients, and use of defibrillation.

> **D.O.T. OBJECTIVES**
>
> Discuss the fundamentals of early defibrillation.
>
> Explain the rationale for early defibrillation.
>
> List the indications for automated external defibrillation.

***EMT
Tip***

According to the AHA, advanced cardiac life support represents the other end of the resuscitation continuum that begins with recognition of the emergency and initiation of basic life support.

Automated External Defibrillation

The automated external defibrillator is a key link in the chain of survival. A defibrillator is used for patients experiencing ventricular fibrillation. The AED is a medical device that analyzes the patient's cardiac rhythm. It applies electrical stimulation to the heart when needed. The goal of the treatment is to reset the heart's electrical conduction system. Doing this enables the cardiac fibers to resume beating in a synchronized manner.

When a patient collapses from ventricular fibrillation, body systems begin to die. Each minute counts. Defibrillation is a very time-sensitive therapy. If applied soon after the onset of ventricular fibrillation, the chance of restoring normal heart activity is good. Successful early defibrillation also prevents lasting neurological deficits.

Automatic external defibrillation became a commonly used EMT-B skill in the late 1980s and early 1990s. Early defibrillation is now available to many patients served by EMS. This is very significant clinically. Studies have shown increased survival rates in EMS systems with early defibrillation capabilities. By combining early recognition and early 9-1-1 activation with CPR and automatic external defibrillation, EMS systems can greatly increase a patient's chance of survival. Without an EMT-B and AED that arrive together, many preventable deaths would occur. Today, AEDs are found in airplanes, stadiums, courthouses, and other public places. In many communities, members of the general public have been trained to use the AED in some situations.

Overview of Defibrillation

Two types of external defibrillators are used in EMS. The fully automated AED requires little action on your part. You apply the pads, or electrodes, to the patient's chest and turn the unit on. The AED issues a warning and delivers a shock whenever it detects ventricular fibrillation. A manual defibrillator requires the operator to analyze and interpret the heart rhythm and to administer a shock through hand-held paddles or self-adhesive pads (see Fig. 13.6).

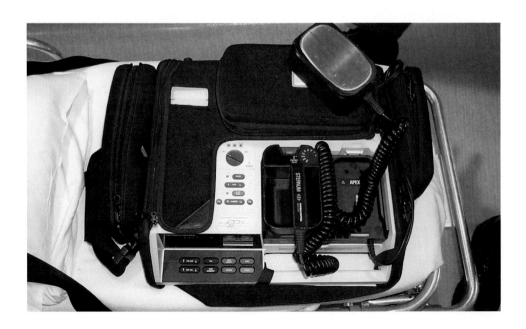

Figure 13.6 *Manual defibrillators require advanced training for operation.*

Figure 13.7 *An AED analyzes cardiac rhythms to determine if a shock is needed (left). This AED advises that no shock is needed (right).*

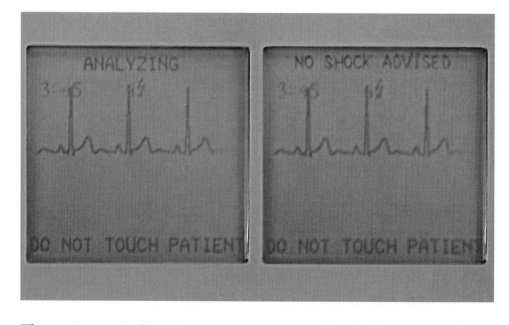

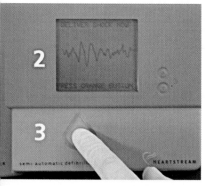

Figure 13.8 *With a semiautomated AED, you are prompted to push a button to deliver a shock.*

CD-ROM Link

The video entitled "Automated External Defibrillator" in the Cardiac Emergencies chapter and the Video Appendix on the MedEMT CD-ROM describes the purpose and procedures for using an AED.

The semi-automated AED is most commonly used in EMS. It analyzes the heart rhythm, suggests whether or not a shock is advised, then requires that the operator deliver the shock by pushing a button. First, you attach the electrodes to the patient. When you turn the unit on, it prompts you to press a button to analyze the heart rhythm (see Fig. 13.7). You are prompted to press another button to deliver a shock if the ventricular rate is above a preset rate (usually > 180 beats per minute) (see Fig. 13.8). Many AEDs are programmed to record the voices of the operators. Some machines allow the user to identify specific events during a resuscitation using push buttons. Many AEDs can download the event data to a computer for additional review and documentation.

All defibrillators check the cardiac rhythm using a computer microprocessor. This evaluates whether a shock is needed for an abnormal rhythm (tachycardia). The devices prompt both for initiation and noninitiation of electrical therapy. AED devices have very high accuracy rates for rhythm analysis and for giving the correct prompts. Correct analysis and shock delivery depends upon fully charged defibrillator batteries.

Advantages of Automated Defibillation. Using an AED has several advantages over manual defibrillation or CPR alone. Less training is required to operate an AED. Some AEDs monitor the heart rhythm continuously. To use a manual defibrillator, the operator must be proficient in rhythm recognition. After identifying the rhythm, he or she must decide if electrical therapy is needed. These skills require specialized initial training and advanced continuing education. Learning to use an AED is also easier than learning CPR, although the treatment sequence must be memorized. Both are important in the chain of survival.

Automated defibrillation is speedier than conventional defibrillation. The first shock can be delivered within one minute of arrival at the patient's side. Subsequent shocks are also delivered faster. Automated external defibrillators are designed to administer shocks in a very rapid sequence. Administering the shocks in rapid succession increases their effectiveness.

Automated defibrillation is performed remotely through adhesive electrode pads placed on the patient (see Fig. 13.9). This hands-off method is safer to administer. It also offers better electrode placement during a lengthy resuscitation and allows for the use of a larger pad. This method is often less anxiety-inducing for the operator than manual defibrillation.

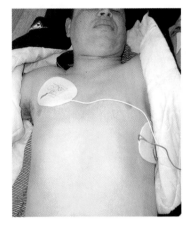

Figure 13.9 *Place the negative electrode on the right side of the upper sternum. Place the positive electrode above the ribs on the left side of the lower chest, centered on the mid-axillary line.*

D.O.T. OBJECTIVE

Discuss the need to complete the Automated Defibrillator: Operator's Shift Checklist.

AED Maintenance. Defibrillator failure is most often caused by improper equipment maintenance. Having a regular maintenance schedule for the AED is important. Dead or low batteries are the most common cause of failure (see Fig. 13.10). You must ensure proper battery maintenance and replacement to prevent this from occurring. A shift checklist for the AED, including batteries, must be completed daily. Always carry extra batteries. Follow the manufacturer's recommendations. Documentation of inspection and maintenance is important for your legal protection.

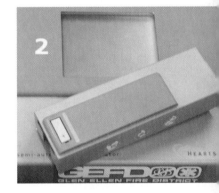

Figure 13.10 *Battery maintenance is critical for proper AED function.*

D.O.T. OBJECTIVES

List the contraindications for automated external defibrillation.

State the reasons for assuring that the patient is pulseless and apneic when using the automated external defibrillator.

Discuss the circumstances which may result in inappropriate shocks.

Discuss the special considerations for rhythm monitoring.

Explain the reason for pulses not being checked between shocks with an automated external defibrillator.

Explain the considerations for interruption of CPR, when using the automated external defibrillator.

Explain the impact of age and weight on defibrillation.

Figure 13.11 *Check for a pulse before administering a shock.*

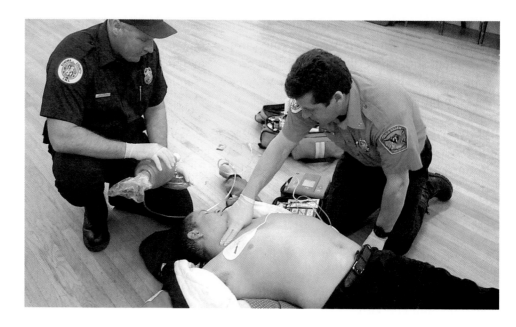

EMT Tip

Some agencies simply use the word "clear" or the phrase "clear the patient" before defibrillation. Whatever your agency advises, the intent is to ensure safety.

EMT Alert

All contact with the patient must be avoided during analysis of rhythm as well as during a shock.

Safety Considerations

An accidental shock from a defibrillator can cause serious or fatal consequences. An accidental shock may cause burns, dysrhythmias, or cardiac arrest. Inappropriate delivery of shocks is rare, but can happen because of human or mechanical error. Inappropriate shocks can result from low batteries, electrical interference, or someone touching the patient during rhythm analysis. Make sure that no one is standing or working near the patient as the shock is delivered. An inappropriate shock could also be given to a patient who is not in cardiac arrest. The AED is used only for patients who are unresponsive, without a pulse, and not breathing (see Fig. 13.11).

You must make sure the environment is safe before delivering the shock. Water and metal are both good conductors of electricity. If a patient is soaking wet, dry him or her off. Move the patient out of a wet or rainy environment. Avoid touching metal in contact with the patient, such as a metal backboard or stretcher. If any part of your body touches the patient or metal equipment, you will receive a shock. Before defibrillation, look up and down the length of the patient. Make sure that no one is in contact with him or her. A rescuer or bystander who is accidentally shocked can be seriously injured. A phrase promoted by the AMA and AHA for use before defibrillation is "I am clear, you are clear, everyone is clear." Saying this focuses your attention, and helps to remind everyone to stand back when the shock is administered.

Because no one can touch a patient while the AED is analyzing heart rhythm or delivering a shock, CPR must be discontinued at these times. This is acceptable because defibrillation is more beneficial than CPR alone. CPR can be interrupted for up to 90 seconds in cases where 3 successive shocks are necessary. Resume CPR after the shock sequence is delivered, or if the AED advises that no shock will be given.

A patient's age and weight can affect the amount of energy that arrives at the heart muscle. Use of an AED is contraindicated for patients younger than 8 years old or smaller than 55 pounds. For pediatric patients, providing an open airway and artificial ventilation are the major concerns. In larger patients, greater electrical resistance occurs because the AED shock must travel through an increased amount of tissue or a larger chest cavity. This increases the time it takes for the energy to arrive at the heart and reduces the chances of successful defibrillation.

D.O.T. OBJECTIVES

List the steps in the operation of the automated external defibrillator.

Define the function of all controls on an automated external defibrillator, and describe event documentation and defibrillator maintenance.

EMT Alert

Defibrillation comes first. Do not hook up oxygen or do anything that delays analysis of rhythm or defibrillation.

Emergency Care Using the AED

When responding to a call for a cardiac emergency, take BSI and standard precautions en route to the scene. Request assistance from ALS units, if available in your system. Upon arrival, stop CPR if it is in progress. Perform your initial assessment. Verify that the patient is unresponsive, has no pulse, and is not breathing.

Follow the steps for operation of the automated external defibrillator as described in Procedure 13.1. The machine will direct you through several cycles. These are:

- Rhythm analysis
- Shock delivery
- Reassessment of pulse and breathing
- Continued CPR

Complete the sequence as rapidly as possible. Stop only for rhythm analysis.

After defibrillation, the patient may or may not regain pulses and spontaneous respiration. Do not check for the return of a pulse until a 3-shock sequence is complete, or no shock is advised. If the patient regains a pulse at any time, stop defibrillation and immediately check the breathing. If the patient is breathing adequately, provide high-flow oxygen via non-rebreather mask (see Fig. 13.12). If the patient has inadequate breathing or remains apneic, provide ventilation with high-concentration oxygen. Transport immediately.

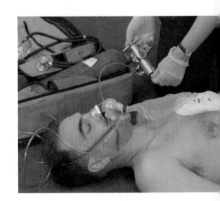
Figure 13.12 *If the patient regains a pulse, provide oxygen and assist ventilation if required.*

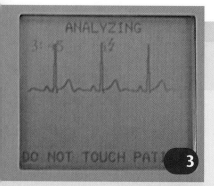

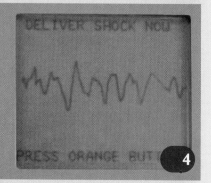

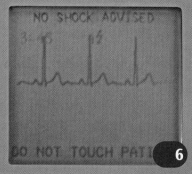

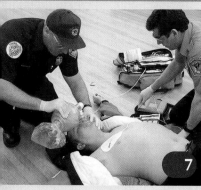

Procedure 13.1 • AUTOMATED EXTERNAL DEFIBRILLATION

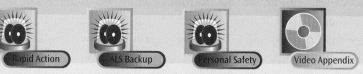

Rapid Action   ALS Backup   Personal Safety   Video Appendix

1. Stop CPR if it is in progress. Perform your initial assessment. Verify that the patient is unresponsive, has no pulse, and is not breathing.

2. One EMT-Basic resumes CPR while another sets up the AED. Attach the device to the patient and turn the power on. If the machine has a tape recorder, begin your narrative.

3. Stop CPR. Look to see that everyone is clear from the patient, and verbally warn others to stay clear. Press the ANALYZE button on the AED. The AED will analyze the heart rhythm and advise either "Shock" or "No Shock."

4. If the AED advises a shock, verify that everyone is clear of the patient, then press the SHOCK button. Immediately press ANALYZE again. If the AED again advises "Shock," verify that everyone is clear of the patient and administer a second shock. Immediately reanalyze the rhythm. If the AED advises a third shock, verify that everyone is clear. Push the SHOCK button.

5. After the third shock, check the carotid pulse. If the pulse is absent, resume CPR for one minute. Then, verbally and visually verify that everyone is clear of the patient. Repeat rhythm analysis and deliver up to 3 additional shocks. After the sixth shock, recheck the pulse. If the patient is pulseless, resume CPR and transport immediately.

6. If the AED advises you not to administer a shock after any rhythm analysis, check for a pulse. Resume CPR if the patient is pulseless. Perform 1 minute of CPR, then reassess the rhythm. If the AED advises "No Shock" again and the pulse has not returned, resume CPR for 1 minute. Reanalyze a third time. If the AED still says "No Shock," resume CPR and transport immediately.

7. If the machine advises a shock after 1 minute of CPR, deliver up to 2 sets of 3 shocks if necessary. Provide CPR for 1 minute between each set of 3 shocks.

8. Begin transport after 6 shocks have been administered, or 3 consecutive "No Shock" messages have been received, or the patient regains a pulse.

If the pulse does not return, begin transport after 6 shocks have been administered or 3 consecutive "No Shock" messages have been received (see Fig. 13.13). Additional shocks may be delivered at the scene or while en route by approval of local medical direction. In some cases, it will be more appropriate to wait for ALS backup; rely on local protocol or medical direction.

If possible, rapidly obtain an OPQRST and SAMPLE history from bystanders or family before leaving the scene. Also complete a rapid medical assessment and obtain baseline vital signs. However, do not delay transport. While en route to the closest appropriate medical facility, complete a focused history and physical exam and reassess the vital signs.

While en route, keep the electrodes attached to the patient in case cardiac arrest recurs. The AED cannot analyze cardiac rhythm in a moving vehicle. You must stop the vehicle completely if rhythm analysis or shock delivery is required. It is not safe to defibrillate in a moving ambulance.

EMT Tip

Interview bystanders and family for information about the circumstances of a cardiac arrest. Do not delay care to get the history.

AED WITH TWO OR MORE RESCUERS

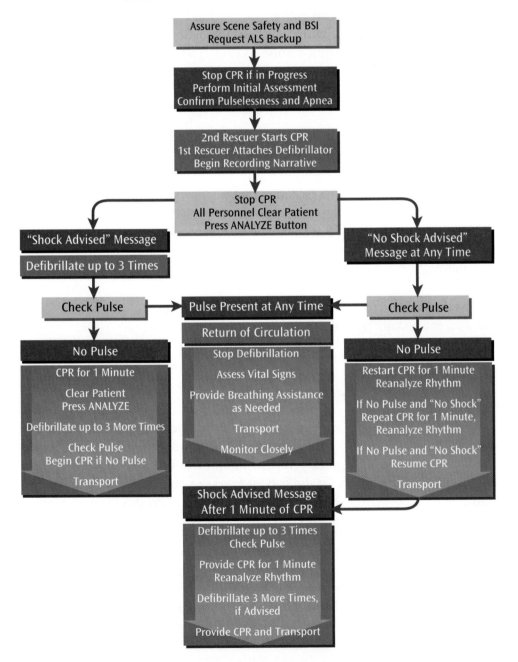

Figure 13.13 *Steps in use of the AED by two or more rescuers when caring for a pulseless patient.*

Single Rescuer AED. Since early defibrillation is the primary goal for a patient in ventricular fibrillation, there may be times when a single EMT-B must apply the AED. If you are alone, defibrillate immediately. Do not take time for initial CPR. Do not stop to activate the EMS system. Quickly complete your initial assessment to verify lack of pulse and breathing. Open the airway and give 2 breaths. This shows that airway obstruction is not causing the event. If the pulse is absent, proceed with 1 cycle of the defibrillation procedure. Continue using the AED until a pulse returns, 3 shocks have been delivered, a "No Shock" message is given, or help arrives.

Post–Resuscitation Care

After defibrillation, focus your care on supporting the airway, breathing, and circulation. If your patient remains pulseless and apneic, transport immediately and continue CPR. If the pulse returns, monitor closely for recurrence of cardiac arrest. Obtain support for the patient from personnel trained in advanced cardiac life support (ACLS) as soon as possible. You can do this through rapid dispatch of ALS crews or transport to the nearest emergency department.

Once a patient has experienced ventricular fibrillation, he or she can easily revert to this rhythm again despite multiple defibrillations. If you are en route with an unconscious patient, check the pulse every 30 seconds. If the pulse is absent and no ACLS is available, stop the vehicle and begin rhythm analysis. Deliver shocks as indicated. Do CPR if the AED is not immediately ready or if a "No Shock" message is given. Continue resuscitation according to local protocol. Follow this same procedure if a patient with chest pain loses consciousness, pulse, and breathing while en route.

If no pulse is present and a "No Shock" message is given, start or resume CPR. Continue to analyze the rhythm until you receive 3 consecutive "No Shock" messages, 6 shocks have been given, or the pulse returns. At this point, continue transport.

D.O.T. OBJECTIVES

Explain the role medical direction plays in the use of automated external defibrillation.

Explain the importance of frequent practice with the automated external defibrillation.

Discuss the goal of quality improvement in automated external defibrillation.

State the reasons why a case review should be completed following the use of an automated external defibrillator.

Discuss the components that should be included in a case review.

EMS System Requirements

For successful implementation of an AED program, the EMS delivery system should have the following in place:

- All the links in the chain of survival
- Medical direction
- Training and continuing education guidelines
- A quality improvement program

The EMS system sets training standards and equipment protocols. Medical direction is responsible for overseeing and approving AED training and usage. Before using an AED, you must receive proper training. Initial training is part of your EMT-Basic course. In addition, you must be familiar with the particular AEDs used in your EMS operational setting. After completing your training, you must be approved to use the device by state or local EMS authorities. Continuing education is an important part of skills maintenance, because you may use the defibrillator infrequently. The American Heart Association publishes training materials and continuing education information regarding AEDs. To maintain your skills, most systems require you to participate in practice drills and competency reviews every three months.

Quality improvement involves both the EMTs who operate the AED and the EMS system they work in. EMT-Basics are responsible for maintaining their skills through continuing education. The system is responsible for monitoring and improving the effectiveness of AED operation. Every use of an AED is reviewed by the medical direction physician as part of the quality improvement process. The goal of case reviews and quality improvement is to increase the survival rate for cardiac arrest patients. Each time the AED is used, the medical director or a designated representative will evaluate the:

- Timeliness of care

- Actions of the EMT-Basics

- Performance of the machine

An event can be reviewed from the written report, or from tape recordings or other memory devices that are part of the AED. The reviewer will provide feedback about the event. This helps to ensure that a high quality of care is maintained.

D.O.T. OBJECTIVES

Discuss the importance of coordinating ACLS trained providers with personnel using automated external defibrillators.

Recognize the need for medical direction or protocols to assist in the emergency medical care of the patient with chest pain.

Coordination of Personnel

Many systems dispatch both basic and advanced providers to scenes where patients complain of chest pain or shortness of breath, or where cardiac arrest is suspected. Paramedics or advanced life support personnel do not have to be present for you to use the AED. However, they should be notified of an arrest event as soon as possible. Advanced providers can place intravenous lines and administer medications. These interventions aid in the resuscitation and post-resuscitation management of the patient. They may also use an ECG to continuously monitor the patient's heart rhythm. This allows the identification of various cardiac dysrhythmias, including recurrent ventricular fibrillation. Certain conditions that increase the risk of ventricular fibrillation can be seen on the ECG. These problems can be identified and treated early by ALS personnel.

Local protocols for coordinating care are usually determined by medical direction. In most systems, ALS personnel have medical authority at the scene. Protocols should also cover the decision whether to transport a patient or await ALS arrival. These decisions may be regulated through standing orders or by on-line medical direction.

Chapter Thirteen Summary

- You will respond to many calls for "possible heart attack," or "chest pain." Some will be episodes of sudden cardiac arrest. Others may be simple indigestion. You should not attempt to learn the cause of the pain or difficulty. Treat every patient with the signs and symptoms of cardiac compromise as if the condition is life-threatening. Most chest pain patients will not become cardiac arrest patients.

- Always apply oxygen to patients with signs and symptoms of cardiac compromise. If the patient's breathing is adequate, use high-flow oxygen by non-rebreather mask. If breathing is inadequate, assist ventilations and provide supplemental oxygen.

- Ask OPQRST questions to evaluate a conscious patient's complaint. If time allows, obtain information from bystanders for an unresponsive patient.

- Consider assisting administration of nitroglycerin if a conscious patient has physician-prescribed nitroglycerin spray or tablets. Make sure no contraindications exist. Consult with medical control before assisting the patient to take this drug. Nitroglycerin dilates the coronary arteries, allowing more oxygenated blood to reach the heart muscle. This can cause a drop in blood pressure. Never administer nitroglycerin to a patient with a systolic blood pressure below 100 mmHg or to a child. Follow local protocols.

- The AED is indicated in pulseless, apneic patients who are over the age of 7 and weigh more than 55 pounds. For cardiac arrest patients less than 8 years old or 55 pounds, do CPR and transport. Never apply an AED to a patient with a pulse.

- In cardiac arrest patients, apply the AED as quickly as possible and defibrillate if indicated by the AED. Begin transport of the cardiac arrest patient after 6 shocks have been administered, 3 "No Shock Advised" messages have been received, or the patient regains a pulse.

Key Terms Review

Acute Myocardial Infarction (AMI) | *page 389*

Angina Pectoris | *page 389*

Automated External Defibrillator (AED) | *page 390*

Cardiac Compromise | *page 388*

Chain of Survival | *page 395*

Coronary Artery Disease (CAD) | *page 389*

Defibrillation | *page 395*

Dysrhythmia | *page 389*

Nitroglycerin (NTG) | *page 391*

Ventricular Fibrillation (VF) | *page 389*

Review Questions

1. The phrase used to describe a general difficulty with heart function is:

   a. Cardiac compromise
   b. Cardiac dysrhythmia
   c. Myocardial infarction
   d. Sudden cardiac death

2. All of the following are characteristics of manual defibrillation EXCEPT:

   a. Requires specialized training
   b. Operator must be skilled at rhythm recognition
   c. It is safer to administer than an AED
   d. Operator must decide if electrical therapy is needed

3. The term that describes death within one hour of the onset of cardiac symptoms is:

   a. Cardiac compromise
   b. Cardiac dysrhythmia
   c. Myocardial infarction
   d. Sudden cardiac death

4. After early CPR, the next step in the chain of survival is:

   a. Early access to the 9-1-1 system
   b. Early defibrillation
   c. Early advanced life support
   d. Early transport

5. The portion of the blood that has oxygen-carrying capacity is the:

   a. White blood cells
   b. Hemoglobin
   c. Plasma
   d. Platelets

6. After receiving an order to assist a chest pain patient with his prescription nitroglycerin, you measure his blood pressure. In order to administer nitroglycerin, the patient's blood pressure must be greater than:

   a. 80 systolic
   b. 90 diastolic
   c. 100 systolic
   d. 110 diastolic

7. You are treating a chest pain patient and have received an order to assist the patient with her prescribed nitroglycerin. When should the first nitroglycerin dose be given?

   a. As soon as you determine the chief complaint to be chest pain
   b. During transport after vital signs have been taken
   c. On scene after vital signs and the focused medical exam are complete
   d. Just before arrival at the hospital, in case she becomes hypotensive

8. Which is the most common cause of cardiac compromise?

   a. Valve problems
   b. Poor pumping function
   c. Narrowing or blockage of the coronary arteries
   d. Lack of oxygen to the thoracic veins

9. Why is nitroglycerin directly helpful in treating chest pain?

   a. It makes the patient less fearful
   b. It increases the pumping power and workload of the heart
   c. It decreases the workload of the heart
   d. It relaxes the patient

10. In order to successfully implement an AED program, the EMS system must have all of the following EXCEPT:

    a. All links in the chain of survival
    b. Training and continuing education guidelines
    c. Medical direction and quality improvement
    d. A paramedic on all AED-carrying ambulances

11. Cardiac compromise can result from:

    a. Gastrointestinal disorders
    b. Lung disease
    c. Coronary artery disease
    d. Musculoskeletal disorders

CASE STUDIES

Cardiovascular Emergencies

1 It is a Wednesday morning. You are returning to your station after a routine transport. A man standing outside his car flags you down. He tells you his 62-year-old wife is in the passenger seat and having chest pain. Your assessment reveals that she is awake and oriented. Her respiratory rate is 12 breaths per minute. The pulse is regular, with a rate of 74. Her blood pressure is 164/100. Her skin is warm and moist. Breath sounds are clear bilaterally. Your physical assessment fails to detect any other abnormalities. The patient denies shortness of breath or nausea. She tells you that she feels numbness beneath her breastbone. She uses nitroglycerin for angina. She did not take any before your arrival and wants to go to the hospital for evaluation. You have placed the patient on high-flow oxygen by non-rebreather mask. You move her to a stretcher in preparation for transport.

A. Is it necessary to learn the cause of the patient's pain to provide effective prehospital treatment?

B. Would you consider helping this patient with nitroglycerin administration? Justify your answer.

C. Medical control gives you permission to administer nitroglycerin. The patient is familiar with the medication, and administration goes without difficulty. What will you do next?

2 You are called to the home of a 58-year-old male who is complaining of chest pain. He was working in the yard when he began having chest pain and rubbing his left arm. The patient is alert and oriented. His respiratory rate is 16, pulse 76, and blood pressure 148/84. He has cool, moist skin and clear bilateral lung sounds. There is no peripheral edema or external jugular vein distention. He denies nausea, but feels slightly short of breath.

A. What questions are appropriate to help you assess the patient's signs and symptoms?

B. The patient describes the pain as a crushing sensation. He has a history of hypertension and angina. He took one of his prescribed nitroglycerin tablets before your arrival. The pain was not relieved. The patient asks you if he is having a heart attack. How do you respond to his question?

C. What interventions should you perform?

3 On an early morning call, you find a 54-year-old man sitting upright in a recliner. His skin is pale gray and he has peripheral cyanosis. The patient states that he has had chest pain, but "I am okay now." He refuses further attempts to evaluate him, becomes agitated, and asks that you leave his property. He is alert and oriented. You don't observe signs of mental problems or alcohol or drug use. As you are gathering your equipment, the patient slumps in his chair and becomes unresponsive.

A. What is your immediate course of action?

B. During rhythm analysis, the AED experiences a battery failure. There is no spare battery in the vehicle. How do you handle this situation?

Stories from the Field
Wrap-Up

Some patients experiencing a cardiac emergency will have severe signs and symptoms. Others will have no signs or symptoms at all. Understanding the EMT-B's role in recognizing and treating cardiovascular emergencies is very important. This case raises some difficult issues for you. As an EMT-Basic student, you might not feel qualified to treat the patient. If your friend called 9-1-1 as you suggested, a certified or licensed EMT-B with appropriate equipment would be able to provide more advanced emergency care.

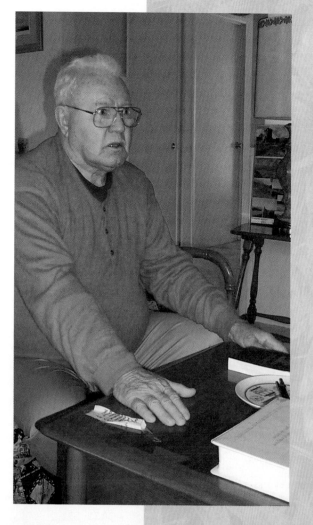

You are able to perform an initial assessment and obtain information on the husband's medical history. This information is very important for providing clues to a potential cardiac emergency. Most of the time, early transport is indicated when patients show signs and symptoms of cardiac compromise. A patient with prescribed nitroglycerin might be assisted to take a dose. However, this patient does not consent to treatment at first. When you return later, you perform CPR until EMS arrives. Once on scene, the EMTs will be able to provide supplemental oxygen and assist ventilations if necessary. They can also provide early defibrillation using an AED if the patient is in cardiac arrest.

ENHANCED STUDY

Types of Cardiac Compromise

Coronary Artery Disease. Coronary artery disease (CAD) is a condition in which the coronary arteries become narrowed. This is called stenosis. This process occurs over a long period of time. The narrowing is caused by the buildup of cholesterol-containing plaques within the arterial walls (see Enhancement Fig. 13.1). As the coronary arteries become progressively narrowed, the blood and oxygen supply to the myocardium, or the heart muscle, is reduced.

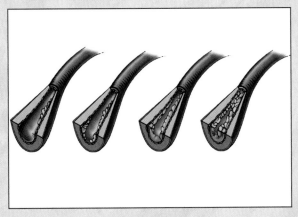

Enhancement Figure 13.1 *Atherosclerosis narrows the arteries and can deprive the heart of oxygen.*

Angina Pectoris. Angina pectoris is chest pain that develops as a result of coronary artery disease. When the myocardium does not get enough oxygen, the patient may experience chest discomfort. Angina usually appears during exertion or stress, such as walking up stairs or working outside. The pain is often described as a squeezing or tightness in the chest. The description of the pain can vary widely between patients. It may radiate into the neck, jaw, upper back, upper abdomen, shoulders, or arms. This pain is sometimes difficult to differentiate from the pain of a heart attack. The patient may have other symptoms, such as dyspnea, sweating, or nausea and vomiting.

Angina is short-lived, typically lasting less than thirty minutes. It is a chronic condition in some patients. Angina is considered stable if the patient remains pain-free at lower levels of activity or if the symptoms are reduced by nitroglycerin. Stable patients generally know how much activity will produce pain. Unstable angina occurs when chest pain develops during activities in which the patient is normally pain free, or when pain occurs with increased frequency, duration, or intensity. Rest will usually relieve angina. Nitroglycerin helps to relieve pain by dilating the coronary arteries and increasing blood flow to the heart. Supplemental oxygen also increases the oxygen to the heart muscle. This may help to relieve angina.

ENHANCED STUDY

Types of Cardiac Compromise (cont.)

Acute Myocardial Infarction. Acute myocardial infarction is the medical term for a heart attack. The term coronary may also be used. This is a shortened form of coronary artery occlusion. In this condition, the heart muscle dies from lack of oxygen.

The coronary arteries can become narrow due to coronary artery disease. The plaque may completely obstruct the blood flow. More commonly, a small blood clot forms in the artery. The obstruction plugs the narrowed artery. This blocks the flow of blood to an area of the heart. As the blockage continues, the patient experiences signs and symptoms of angina. In acute myocardial infarction, the signs and symptoms are severe and prolonged. Rest does not relieve the pain. The portion of myocardium supplied by the blocked artery will die from lack of oxygen.

Treatment for an AMI includes providing high-concentration oxygen and rapid transport to the emergency department. The patient should be placed in a position of comfort. Sitting or semi-sitting positions are usually most comfortable. Emergency lights and siren should be used carefully, because they can increase the patient's stress. However, rapid transport may improve the patient's chances for survival and recovery. You must decide, according to protocol, what is in the patient's best interest. Comfort the patient as much as possible to reduce stress and anxiety.

If available, call for advanced life support assistance. Medications are available in the emergency department that can help some AMI patients. Some advanced providers also carry these drugs. These medications, which dissolve the clot and reopen the obstructed artery, are known as thrombolytic agents. They are commonly called clot busters. By reopening the artery, clot busters can limit how much of the heart muscle dies. However, to be effective, thrombolytic agents must be given early in the course of a heart attack. Therefore, time delays cause more muscle damage. Remember this saying: Minutes equal muscle.

Congestive Heart Failure. In congestive heart failure, the heart is unable to pump effectively. As a result, fluid accumulates in the lungs and/or the extremities. The heart may not pump properly for many reasons. A previous myocardial infarction, valve disease, or other process can weaken the heart muscle. Congestive heart failure (CHF) is a chronic condition. CHF is a good example of a chronic condition that occasionally causes acute illness. When you see patients with CHF, they will probably be in acute distress because their condition has worsened.

If the right side of the heart is failing and the left side is functioning normally, fluid accumulates in the extremities and sacral area. The more severe the damage to the heart, the worse this edema will be (see Enhancement Fig. 13.2). If the left side of the heart is damaged, fluid is retained in the lungs. Patients with left heart failure experience severe respiratory distress. They may have an active cough with frothy pink sputum.

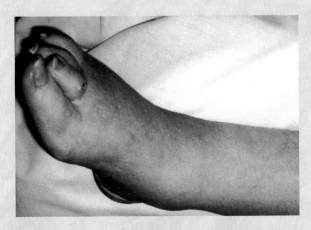

Enhancement Figure 13.2 *Edema in the lower extremities due to CHF.*

Symptoms of CHF include severe dyspnea, often coupled with angina. The patient may appear extremely short of breath. The breath sounds are often noisy because of fluid in the lungs. There may be edema of the legs due to fluid buildup.

Treatment of CHF includes the use of high-flow oxygen by non-rebreather mask. Rapid transport to the emergency department is indicated. Keeping the patient in a sitting or semi-sitting position is also important. This allows the patient to breathe more easily. Placing the patient in a supine position should be avoided unless the patient is hypotensive. The supine position increases shortness of breath. A patient in acute CHF may complain of a smothering sensation when lying down.

Ventricular Fibrillation. In a normal heart, electrical impulses transmitted through the conduction pathway cause synchronized contractions of the cardiac muscle fibers. This results in the normal cardiac rhythm. If the conduction pathway is disrupted, abnormal rhythms can occur. A myocardial infarction can cause a dysrhythmia if it damages the area of the heart that contains the electrical conduction system. Other common causes of dysrhythmias include medications, hypoxia, and electrolyte imbalances.

Ventricular fibrillation (VF) is a very serious dysrhythmia. Here, the ventricles do not contract in a synchronized fashion. This leaves the heart quivering. In this condition, the heart cannot pump blood. Patients experiencing VF are unconscious, pulseless, and apneic. If untreated, ventricular fibrillation is rapidly fatal. Use of a defibrillator can effectively reverse ventricular fibrillation by causing the cardiac cells to again beat as one unit. This is particularly true if the electrical countershock is received within minutes of arrest. Rapid application of electrical defibrillation greatly improves the patient's chance of survival.

Chapter

14

Neurological, Diabetic, and Behavioral Emergencies

Stories from the Field

When you arrive for class one evening, another student looks noticeably different. Jean is very pale and sweaty, even though the room is cool. She looks very anxious. She tells you that she is having trouble focusing on what she is doing. From casual conversations with her, you know that she is an insulin-dependent diabetic. As Kim prepares to start class, you notice that Jean looks like she is sleeping. Her head is down on the table. You bring her condition to Kim's attention.

Kim awakens Jean with little difficulty. Jean says that she does not feel well. She is concerned about her sugar level. Kim sends another student to the lounge for a candy bar and juice. The food seems to make Jean feel better. But during the break, Jean suddenly slumps to the floor in the middle of a conversation. Her airway is open, but her breathing is very shallow and rapid. You hear occasional snoring respirations. Her pulse is very rapid and weak. Kim asks another student to call 9-1-1 to request an ambulance for an unconscious person. She inserts a nasopharyngeal airway, and begins to provide ventilatory support and supplemental oxygen.

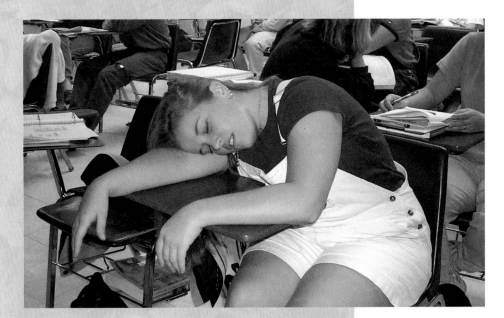

Altered mental status (AMS) is a broad term suggesting that a patient is not in a normal mental state or condition. AMS can be caused by a variety of conditions affecting brain function (see Fig.14.1). It is often due to inadequate oxygen levels in the brain. You may respond to calls involving altered mental status caused by diabetic emergencies, seizures, strokes, poisonings, infections, decreased oxygen levels, and head trauma.

Changes in mental status may cause changes in behavior. Behavior is the way a person acts in a given situation. In a behavioral emergency, the patient exhibits abnormal behavior that others consider unacceptable or intolerable.

In Chapter 8, you learned the AVPU method as a tool to assess a patient's mental status during the initial assessment. This chapter discusses altered mental status in more detail. The care of patients with diabetic or neurological emergencies is presented. You will also learn how to work with patients who are having behavioral emergencies.

Figure 14.1 *Altered mental status has many causes.*

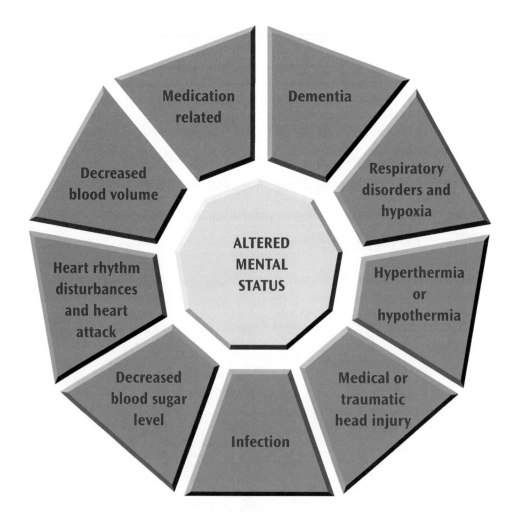

National Registry Examination Tip

Be prepared to care for patients with an altered mental status. Be aggressive when controlling the airway and providing oxygen therapy. Review and understand the conditions causing altered mental status.

ALTERED MENTAL STATUS

Altered mental status (AMS) can range from mild confusion to complete unresponsiveness. It can be due to many causes. When considered with other assessment findings, an alteration in mental status can provide clues to an underlying problem, as summarized in Table 14.1.

Maintaining an airway is especially important in patients with an altered mental state. These patients often lose the ability to protect their own airway. Patients who lose their gag reflexes are at high risk for aspiration. Be prepared to suction vomitus or secretions. Oropharyngeal or nasopharyngeal airways will help to keep the airway patent. An altered mental status suggests that the patient will need immediate transport. Without intervention, the mental status and overall condition may continue to deteriorate.

Altered Mental Status (AMS) | *Broad term indicating a change in normal thinking or clarity of thought; behavior may range from mild confusion to complete unresponsiveness*

Table 14.1 • UNDERLYING MEDICAL CONDITIONS

If You See Altered Mental Status and:	It Might Be Due to:
Bite marks on tongue; incontinence	Seizure activity
Stiffness in neck; fever	Meningitis
Traumatic injuries	Shock or head injury
Hemiparesis; facial droop	Transient ischemic attack or stroke

Information Gathering

As you approach the scene, look for clues to help explain the patient's condition. Look for signs of trauma, such as a fall or motor vehicle accident. If more than one person at the scene has an altered mental status, suspect toxic gases, and take precautions against exposure. Most of the time, the patient cannot give a reliable history. Therefore, gathering information from the scene is important. Do not delay the initial assessment or life-saving care to obtain information. You may have to gather additional information after the patient has been stabilized.

Check the patient for a medical identification tag during the focused history and physical exam. This emblem will alert you to diabetes, seizures, or other known problems causing the condition. Obtain as much information from

EMT Tip

As always, use the appropriate BSI equipment and standard precautions.

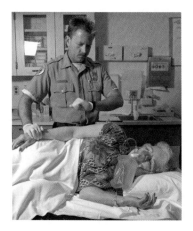

Figure 14.2 *A patient in the recovery position.*

the family or bystanders as possible. Search for prescription medications in the kitchen, bathroom, closet, and bedroom. Look on windowsills, cabinets, countertops, and nightstands. Check the refrigerator for medications such as insulin. This would suggest the patient has diabetes. Also look for empty pill bottles or signs of substance abuse.

Emergency Care: Altered Mental Status

The general procedure for treating a patient with altered mental status is:

1. Conduct a scene size-up.

2. Complete the initial assessment. If trauma is suspected, control the cervical spine. Ensure that the airway is patent. Patients with altered mental status should receive supplemental oxygen at high flow rates. If breathing is adequate, administer oxygen via non-rebreather mask. Set the flow rate at 15 liters per minute. Assist ventilations with supplemental oxygen if breathing is inadequate. Consider using a bag-valve mask device or flow-restricted, oxygen-powered ventilation device.

3. Conduct a rapid medical assessment if the patient is unconscious. If conscious, complete a focused history and physical exam. If the history or exam suggests an underlying cause for AMS, provide appropriate interventions.

4. Place the patient in the recovery position to prevent aspiration (see Fig. 14.2). If spinal injury is suspected, immobilize the patient on a long spine board prior to any movement. Tilt the board to one side as a unit if the airway needs clearing. Be careful not to compromise the cervical spine.

5. Transport. Conduct frequent ongoing assessments during transport.

> **D.O.T. OBJECTIVE**
>
> Identify the patient taking diabetic medications with altered mental status and the implications of a diabetic history.

Diabetes Mellitus (di-uh-BEE-teez muh-LEE-tus) | *A disease characterized by inadequate production or use of insulin*

Insulin | *Hormone secreted by the pancreas that regulates blood sugar levels*

Glucose | *A simple sugar that is the body's basic source of energy*

DIABETIC EMERGENCIES

Diabetes mellitus is a chronic disease caused by inadequate production or use of insulin. **Insulin** is a hormone produced in the pancreas. It enables body cells to convert **glucose** (sugar) to energy. Insulin secretion keeps the blood sugar level constant, despite meals or changes in activity. Normally, the presence of insulin allows glucose to pass into the cells (see Fig. 14.3). In a diabetic, glucose is not absorbed into the cells, so the blood sugar level rises. Elevated blood sugar is an indicator of diabetes.

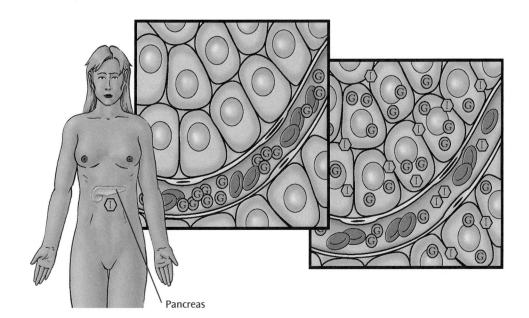

Pancreas

Figure 14.3 *Insulin (I) is produced in the pancreas (left). It helps the cells to utilize glucose (G) from the blood (right). In a diabetic, glucose cannot enter the cells (center).*

Type I diabetes is also called juvenile diabetes or insulin-dependent diabetes. It usually starts in childhood. The body does not produce enough insulin to meet daily needs. To compensate for the lack of production of insulin, the patient injects insulin or synthetic equivalents one or more times daily. Some examples are Humulin®, Novolin®, and Insulin-NPH.

Type II diabetes may be called adult onset diabetes or non-insulin-dependent diabetes, because it usually starts later in life. Adult onset diabetics do not produce enough insulin, or their bodies cannot use it correctly. This condition is usually treated with diet, exercise, and oral medications such as Diabinese®, Orinase®, DiaBeta®, Micronase®, Glynase®, and Glucotrol®. Occasionally, Type II diabetics are treated with insulin.

Signs and Symptoms of Diabetic Emergencies

In a diabetic emergency, the patient may develop altered mental status. This occurs when the blood sugar gets either too high or too low. Elevated blood sugar is called **hyperglycemia**. Low blood sugar is **hypoglycemia**. You are not expected to differentiate between hyperglycemia and hypoglycemia in the field. Most often, altered mental status in a diabetic is caused by hypoglycemia. Treating for this is appropriate, even if the exact cause is not known. This condition can cause an immediate threat to the patient's life.

Often, you will find during the SAMPLE history that the patient missed or vomited a meal after taking insulin. Or the patient may have done heavier exercise or more physical work than normal. However, don't always expect to find out why a diabetic emergency occurs. There may be no identifiable predisposing factor.

Hyperglycemia (high-per-gly-SEE-me-uh) | *Condition in which blood sugar is too high; results from inadequate insulin in the blood for glucose metabolism*

Hypoglycemia (high-po-gly-SEE-me-uh) | *Condition in which blood sugar is too low; results from too much insulin or not enough glucose in the blood*

*EMT
Alert*

If in doubt whether a patient is suffering from low blood sugar or high blood sugar, treat the patient for hypoglycemia.

When treating a diabetic emergency, airway management is extremely important. Patients with severe diabetic problems may be unable to maintain a patent airway without your intervention. You must also provide high concentrations of supplemental oxygen.

Hypoglycemia

Hypoglycemia is the most common diabetic medical emergency. It can be caused by:

- Taking too much medication (usually insulin)
- Not eating enough food
- Vomiting a meal after taking medication
- Increasing activity levels without adjusting food or medication intake

All these situations result in too much insulin, and not enough glucose in the blood. Too much insulin causes the blood sugar level to drop, resulting in hypoglycemia. This may occur with no history. The signs and symptoms are:

- Rapid onset of altered mental status
- Possible appearance of intoxication, staggering and slurred speech, or complete unresponsiveness
- Tachycardia
- Cool, clammy, pale skin
- Complaints of hunger
- Weakness, dizziness, or shakiness
- Rapid, shallow respiration
- Nervousness, excitement, anxiety, or combativeness
- Uncharacteristic behavior
- Unconsciousness
- Low blood sugar by finger stick (performed by ALS personnel)

Brain cells are very sensitive to glucose levels. If hypoglycemia lasts too long, brain cells will die. Seizures due to changes in the glucose levels in the brain are a late sign of hypoglycemia. This type of seizure is a life-threatening emergency. Seizures are discussed in more detail later in this chapter.

Oral glucose paste is given to reverse hypoglycemia. Glucose paste is rapidly absorbed by large blood vessels in the mouth. It is described fully in a later section. Follow local protocols for the amount of glucose and exact method of administration.

Hyperglycemia

Hyperglycemia occurs when the insulin in the blood is insufficient to metabolize glucose. Without insulin, blood glucose is not readily taken into the cells. It accumulates in the blood. As the blood sugar increases, glucose spills into the urine. This causes excessive urination (polyuria) and dehydration.

Eventually, the body begins to break down fat rather than glucose for its energy source. This results in a complicated metabolic process in which excess ketones and acids are produced. The process is known as diabetic ketoacidosis (DKA). As the cycle progresses, the patient may develop altered mental status. Type II diabetic patients, especially the elderly, may have some residual insulin in their systems. This results in a condition called hyperosmolar hyperglycemic nonketotic coma (HHNK). HHNK patients will demonstrate signs and symptoms similar to DKA.

Signs and symptoms of elevated blood sugar are:

- Mental confusion
- Nausea and/or vomiting
- Weakness
- Headache
- Full, bounding pulse
- Fruity smell to breath (not present in HHNK)
- Hot, dry, flushed skin
- Labored respiration
- Drowsiness
- Mental confusion
- Unconsciousness
- High blood sugar by finger stick

D.O.T. OBJECTIVES

State the steps in the emergency medical care of the patient taking diabetic medicine with an altered mental status and a history of diabetes.

Evaluate the need for medical direction in the emergency medical care of the diabetic patient.

Emergency Care: Diabetic Emergencies

When caring for a patient with altered mental status and a history of diabetes, follow these steps:

1. Conduct a scene size-up.

2. Complete an initial assessment. Evaluate the mental status using the AVPU responses. Ask about a history of diabetes. If trauma is suspected, apply spinal precautions immediately.

3. Open and manage the airway. If breathing is adequate, provide oxygen therapy. If breathing is inadequate, assist the ventilations. Position the patient on one side to prevent aspiration. Prepare to suction if necessary.

4. Complete a focused history and physical exam. Look for a medical identification tag or clues on the scene suggesting a history of diabetes. Complete a SAMPLE history and obtain a set of baseline vital signs. Find out how the episode started, its duration, whether it was continuous or intermittent, and any other symptoms. Look for evidence of trauma, seizure, or fever. Ask about the last meal, last medication dose, and any related illnesses.

5. If the patient can swallow and maintain the airway, consider administering oral glucose. Request assistance from an ALS crew that can test the blood sugar level and provide advanced care.

6. If you cannot give glucose, or if the patient's condition deteriorates, transport immediately to the closest or most appropriate medical facility. Conduct detailed and ongoing assessments en route.

National Registry Examination Tip

Recognize the most frequent signs of diabetes. Review the treatment. Always consider administering oral glucose. Remember to maintain the airway. List as many medical emergencies as possible with signs and symptoms similar to diabetic emergencies. Practice taking the history and physical exam for a diabetic patient.

> **D.O.T. OBJECTIVE**
>
> State the generic and trade names, medication forms, dose, administration, action, and contraindications for oral glucose.

Oral Glucose

Oral glucose is a concentrated sugar. It is absorbed through the mucous membranes of the mouth (see Fig. 14.4). The large blood vessels pick up the sugar, carrying it throughout the system. Oral glucose will reverse symptoms of hypoglycemia. It comes in several forms. These are gel or paste solutions (see Table 14.2). The patient must be conscious and able to swallow when you administer the solution. If the blood sugar is very low, you will not see results immediately. The patient must be evaluated by a physician after the solution is administered.

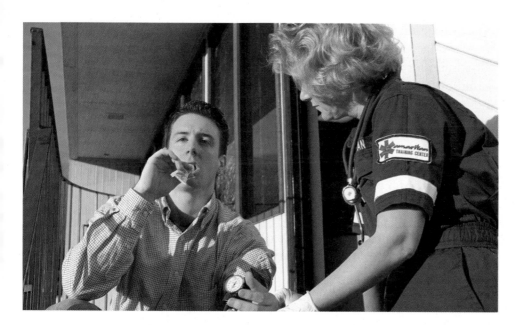

Figure 14.4 *Monitor the patient while taking oral glucose.*

Administration of Oral Glucose

1. Before giving oral glucose, complete the initial assessment. Obtain baseline vital signs and a SAMPLE history.

2. Evaluate the patient for signs and symptoms of an altered mental state.

3. Confirm that the patient has a history of medication-dependent diabetes.

4. Obtain permission from medical direction. In some systems, EMT-Bs can administer oral glucose as a standing order. Others require an on-line order. Follow your local protocols and procedures.

5. Before administering oral glucose, evaluate the level of consciousness and ability to swallow. Evaluate the patient's ability to protect his or her airway.

Table 14.2 • ORAL GLUCOSE

Characteristic	Description
Names	Generic name: Oral Glucose Trade names: Glutose®, Insta-Glucose®
Indications	Patient with altered mental status and a known history of diabetes that is normally controlled by medication
Contraindications	Unresponsive patient Patient who cannot swallow or maintain an airway
Actions	Increases blood sugar levels
Dosage	One tube
Route	Oral
Side Effects	None when given correctly May be aspirated in patients with no gag reflex

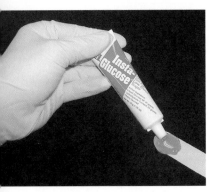

Figure 14.5 *Application of oral glucose to a tongue depressor.*

6. Place the tip of the glucose tube between the patient's cheek and gum. Slowly squeeze the contents of the tube into the mouth. The patient may also self-administer the solution. You can also apply the glucose to a tongue depressor (see Fig. 14.5). Place the tongue blade between the patient's cheek and gum.

7. Reassess the patient every 5 minutes. Intervene as needed. Oral glucose may take 20 minutes or more to improve mental status. If the patient loses consciousness or has a seizure, remove the tongue depressor or medication tube. Request that ALS personnel respond.

SEIZURES

Seizure | *Chaotic electrical activity in the brain that can lead to a momentary break in the stream of thought, muscular spasms, or a complete loss of consciousness*

Seizures are the result of a sudden, excessive electrical discharge in the brain (see Fig. 14.6). As an EMT-B, you aren't expected to identify which type of seizure a patient is having or has had, but you should be aware that not all seizures have the same signs and symptoms.

A seizure may cause the patient to lose consciousness. He or she may exhibit bizarre behavior and uncontrollable muscle activity. Seizure activity is usually brief, lasting less than 5 minutes. The following signs may or may not be seen:

• Presence of an aura prior to the seizure (unusual behavior, restlessness, or a quick change in mood)

• Involuntary crying out upon onset of the seizure

• Excess salivation

• Repetitive speech or movements

• Twitching of one area of the body or extremity

Figure 14.6 *A seizure is caused by chaotic electrical activity in the brain.*

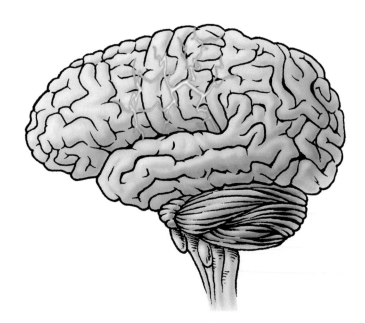

- Generalized tonic-clonic movements (tense shaking of the extremities)
- Abrupt loss of muscle tone without warning; the patient may fall
- Periods of blank staring
- Incontinence

A state of prolonged or continuous, back-to-back seizures is called **status epilepticus**. The patient remains unconscious. This is considered a life-threatening medical emergency. Untreated status epilepticus can result in brain damage or death. Rapidly transport all patients with this condition.

Active seizures are followed by a **postictal state**. This post-seizure state commonly lasts for 10 to 30 minutes. The patient will appear sleepy, confused, or unresponsive. He or she may not be able to recall the seizure events.

Causes of Seizures

Seizures suggest an underlying illness, injury, or other process affecting the brain. Chronic seizure disorders are usually controlled by medication. If a patient does not take the medication correctly, he or she will develop seizures. This is one of the most common reasons for the seizures you see in the field.

Common causes of seizure activity are:

- Epilepsy
- Noncompliance with seizure, diabetes, or other medication
- Fever
- Infection
- Hypoxia
- Hypoglycemia
- Alcohol or drug overdose or withdrawal
- Drug toxicity
- Poisoning
- Metabolic disorders and imbalances
- Congenital anomalies
- Pre-eclampsia (pregnancy-induced hypertension)
- Head injury or trauma
- Shock
- Stroke
- Tumor
- Any condition causing lack of oxygen to the brain
- Idiopathic (of unknown cause; especially in children)

Status Epilepticus (STA-tus ep-uh-LEP-ti-kus) | *A state of prolonged seizures or multiple seizures between which the patient does not regain consciousness*

Postictal (post-IK-tul) State | *A patient's condition after a seizure, during which the patient may appear sleepy, confused, or unresponsive*

 EMT Tip

Think of a seizure as a short-circuit inside the brain, causing various muscle groups to react wildly.

**EMT
Alert**

Treat all seizures as if they are life threatening.

Seizures are rarely life threatening in patients with chronic disorders. They are usually brief, and do no permanent harm. However, they may cause complications such as hypoxia and airway compromise. Treat all seizures as if they are life threatening. Immediate transport is required for:

- Patients with altered mental status (based on AVPU assessment)
- Status epilepticus
- Seizures in a diabetic or pregnant patient
- Seizures with evidence of head trauma
- Seizures while in a body of water
- Seizures in infants or children
- Patients with inadequate airway, breathing, or circulation

For these cases, perform an initial assessment, stabilize all life-threatening conditions, and transport immediately. The focused exam and additional history can be obtained while en route to the hospital.

Emergency Care for Seizures

A patient can be injured during a seizure. This is often the result of hitting or bumping into hazards in the surrounding area. The patient may also bite the tongue, causing a laceration. Follow these steps for providing emergency medical care to a patient who is having a seizure:

1. Complete a scene survey. Identify environmental hazards that could injure the patient. Protect the patient from harmful items. Do not try to restrain him or her.

2. Conduct an initial assessment. Pay particular attention to the airway and breathing. Intervene as necessary. Large amounts of saliva are often produced during a seizure. Blood may be present from airway trauma. Vomiting is also common. Do not place anything in the patient's mouth during a seizure. Consider placing a nasopharyngeal adjunct. Be prepared to suction the airway. If breathing is adequate, provide high-flow oxygen by non-rebreather mask. If breathing is inadequate, assist ventilations with high concentrations of oxygen.

3. Assess mental status by AVPU. Look for evidence of trauma as a cause for the seizure. Transport priority patients.

4. Complete a focused history and physical exam. Obtain as much information as possible from bystanders. During the SAMPLE history, address the following: What was the patient doing at the onset of the seizure? Was there an aura? Did the patient complain of headache, fever, or other signs of illness? Does

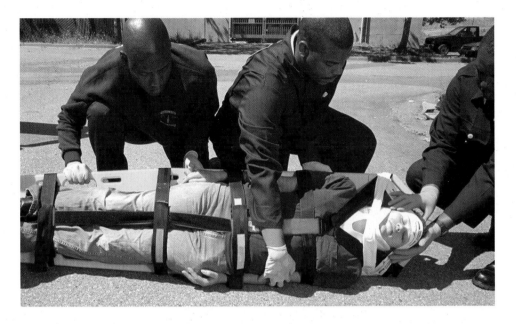

Figure 14.7 *If the airway is filled with secretions or vomit that can't be cleared by suctioning, turn the board and the patient together to clear the airway.*

the patient have a history of epilepsy or other seizure disorder? If so, when was the last seizure? What medications does he or she take for seizures? Have they been taken as prescribed? How long has the seizure lasted? Is this seizure typical in type and duration compared with previous seizures?

5. In your physical exam, note the location and extent of muscle activity (twitching, muscle spasms, stiffening). Are movements bilateral, unilateral, or spread in an orderly manner? Is the patient blinking rapidly, smacking the lips, or chewing?

6. Position the patient. If spinal trauma is not a consideration, place the patient in the recovery position with head elevated. This promotes drainage of secretions and prevents aspiration. If spinal trauma is suspected, immobilize the patient on a long backboard. Turn the board and patient as one unit if you are unable to control the airway secretions with suction devices (see Fig. 14.7).

7. Transport. The patient must be reevaluated for serious underlying conditions such as head trauma, heart conditions, or a history of stroke.

If you arrive after a seizure (postictal period), intervene as necessary after conducting your initial assessment. Keep in mind that the seizure activity can repeat without warning. Ensure that the patient's airway is patent, and that breathing and circulation are adequate. Be prepared to suction the airway. Complete a focused history and physical exam. Evaluate for injuries that may have occurred during the seizure. In the SAMPLE history, look for the same information as you would in an actively seizing patient. Transport the patient in the recovery position if there is no spinal trauma.

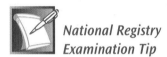

National Registry Examination Tip

Review the various causes of seizures. Review airway management and oxygen therapy for active seizures and postictal state. Recognize signs of status epilepticus. Be prepared to manage the airway aggressively and transport immediately.

SYNCOPE

Syncope (sin-KO-pee) | *Sudden onset of a temporary loss of consciousness caused by low blood pressure in the brain; fainting*

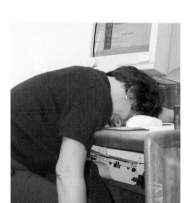

Figure 14.8 *Syncope is a sudden loss of consciousness.*

Syncope is a sudden, temporary loss of consciousness (see Fig. 14.8). It usually lasts a short time. The patient makes a complete recovery. A syncopal episode may be preceded by:

- Lightheadedness
- Visual field closing in
- Diminished hearing
- General weakness

While unconscious, the patient may have jerking of the extremities. This can be mistaken for seizure activity. Patients with syncope usually regain consciousness quickly when placed in a supine position. The patient may feel fine and not want medical attention. However, any patient with a loss of consciousness should be evaluated at a medical facility. The physician will want to rule out serious causes.

Syncope has many causes. Some are minor, such as the common fainting spell. More serious causes include:

- Abnormal heart rate (too fast or too slow)
- Hypovolemia due to dehydration or blood loss
- Inadequate vasoconstriction
- Cardiac pumping failure (valvular obstruction, tamponade, massive myocardial infarction)
- Other conditions affecting blood flow to the brain (hypoxia, anemia, ministroke, or transient ischemic attack)

Emergency Care for Syncope

1. Conduct a scene size-up. Look for environmental causes of the unconscious state.
2. Complete the initial assessment. Control the cervical spine if you suspect traumatic injury. Intervene as necessary to protect the airway, breathing, or circulation. Provide supplemental oxygen at high flow rates. Assess mental responsiveness by AVPU.
3. Complete a rapid medical assessment. Prepare for immediate transport if the patient is still unconscious. If conscious, conduct a focused history and physical exam.
4. Transport as appropriate.
5. Conduct a detailed assessment and ongoing assessments as indicated.

STROKES

A **cerebrovascular accident (CVA)** is commonly called a **stroke** or brain attack. It may also be known as a nontraumatic brain injury. A CVA is characterized by a sudden onset of loss of function. The patient may have altered mental status.

Stroke is usually caused by blockage of an artery supplying blood to one area of the brain (see Fig. 14.9). A small plaque from atherosclerosis or a blood clot blocks the artery. This is similar to the way a clot blocks a coronary artery during a heart attack. Another, less frequent cause of stroke is hemorrhaging (see Fig. 14.10). This results when a blood vessel ruptures into the brain or the space surrounding it. In either case, the brain tissue being supplied by that artery will die. This results in neurological deficit or loss of function in a corresponding area of the body.

Cerebrovascular (se-REE-bro-VAS-kyu-ler) Accident (CVA) | *Stroke or brain attack; occurs when a blood vessel in the brain becomes blocked or ruptures*

Stroke | *Common term for a cerebrovascular accident*

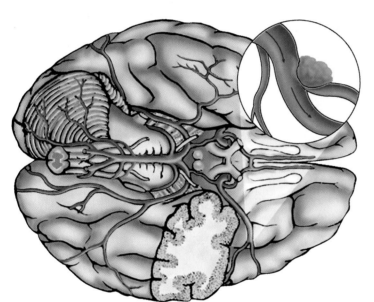

Figure 14.9 *A blood clot blocking a vessel in the brain causes a stroke.*

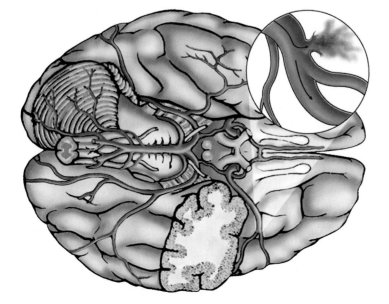

Figure 14.10 *A hemorrhagic stroke is caused by a ruptured blood vessel.*

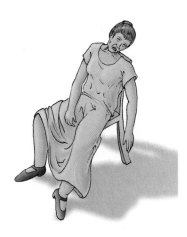

Figure 14.11 *A stroke patient may show signs of paralysis on one side of the body.*

Strokes are usually seen in elderly patients with a history of hypertension. Conditions that cause atherosclerosis, such as high cholesterol or diabetes, can also cause strokes. Occasionally, younger persons will develop stroke.

Signs and symptoms of a stroke (CVA) may include:

- Altered mental status, ranging from mild confusion to unconsciousness
- Paralysis, weakness, or disability on one side of the body, such as an arm, a leg, or one side of the face (see Fig. 14.11)
- Sensory loss on one side of the body
- Speech difficulties: slurred speech, garbled speech, unable to give the right word, unable to talk
- Unequal pupils
- Loss of vision in one eye, double vision, or other visual problems
- Severe headache
- Loss of balance or coordination
- Seizure activity
- Nausea and vomiting
- Loss of bowel or bladder control

Transient Ischemic (is-KEE-mik) Attack (TIA) | *A sudden loss of neurological functions that clears up within 24 hours; the symptoms are similar to a CVA; also called a ministroke*

A similar condition that is commonly seen during EMS responses is the **transient ischemic attack (TIA)**. This may be called a ministroke. Here, the patient has symptoms of a stroke but recovers within a short time, usually a few minutes. Occasionally, recovery can take up to 24 hours. Even if the patient recovers before transport, a physician should evaluate the condition. Patients with a history of TIA or any suggestions of TIA signs and symptoms are at high risk for having a major stroke.

Emergency Care for Strokes

Care for a stroke patient follows the general treatment guidelines for altered mental status. Avoid trying to diagnose the exact cause of altered mental status or other neurological deficit.

1. Conduct a scene size-up.
2. Complete the initial assessment. Ensure airway patency. A patient with severely depressed mental status may lose the gag reflex. This increases the risk of aspiration. Have suction ready to clear vomitus or secretions. Consider inserting an oral or nasal airway.
3. Provide oxygen and assisted artificial ventilation as needed. The brain requires high levels of oxygen during a stroke. Use 15 liters per minute via a nonrebreather mask if breathing is adequate. If breathing is inadequate, assist ventilations with a bag-valve mask and high-concentration oxygen.

4. Conduct a rapid medical assessment if the patient is unconscious. If conscious, complete a focused history and physical exam. Collect as much information as possible in the OPQRST and SAMPLE histories.

5. Position the patient. If the patient cannot protect the airway, use the recovery position to prevent aspiration. Slightly elevate the head. A responsive patient may sit up. Make sure the extremities are protected. The patient may have one or more weak or paralyzed extremities. Ensure that they are secured to prevent injury during transport.

6. Transport the patient as soon as possible. Continually reassess the patient en route. Mental status and overall condition may continue to decline. Note changes in vital signs, mental status, airway, breathing, and circulation. Provide treatment as needed. Conduct a detailed assessment and ongoing assessments as indicated during transport.

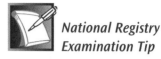

National Registry Examination Tip

Review the various causes of stroke and syncope. Be able to quickly identify the signs and symptoms of each. Review airway management steps for altered mental status. Be able to distinguish between a TIA and a stroke.

D.O.T. OBJECTIVES

Define behavioral emergencies.

Discuss the general factors that may cause an alteration in a patient's behavior.

State the various reasons for psychological crises.

BEHAVIORAL EMERGENCIES

Alterations in mental status can be closely related to abnormal behavior. A person's behavior is the manner in which he or she acts and the physical or mental activities performed. A **behavioral emergency** occurs when a patient displays behavior in a particular situation that is considered unacceptable or intolerable to the patient, family, or community.

A behavioral emergency may be related to an underlying psychological condition or mental illness. Lack of oxygen, hypoglycemia, or other physical conditions can also cause behavioral emergencies. Common factors that may alter a patient's usual behavior include:

- Medical illnesses
- Hypoglycemia
- Hypoxia or inadequate blood flow to the brain
- Infections of the spinal fluid and organic brain disorders
- Environmental conditions, such as excessive heat or cold

Behavioral Emergency | *A situation in which the patient exhibits behavior that others consider unacceptable or intolerable*

Figure 14.12 *Behavioral emergencies can be a challenge for the EMT.*

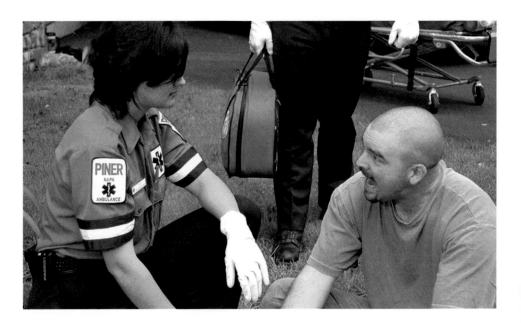

- Trauma, head injury, or significant blood loss
- Situational stresses such as money problems, loss of job, divorce, or a sudden death
- Emotional extremes, psychotic thinking, depression, or panic
- Mental illnesses such as phobias, depression, bipolar disorder, paranoia, and schizophrenia
- Mind-altering substances, including alcohol, narcotic drugs, stimulants, or psychedelic drugs

Psychological crises can result in unusual behaviors (see Fig. 14.12). These range from panic or agitation to bizarre thinking and dangerous acts. The patient may be a danger to self and others. Some psychiatric conditions that can cause a behavioral crisis are listed in Table 14.3.

Table 14.3 • PSYCHOLOGICAL CAUSES OF BEHAVIORAL CRISES

Condition	Description
Anxiety or Panic	A state of painful uneasiness about impending problems. A panic attack is an anxiety disorder. Anxiety is characterized by extreme levels of agitation, fear, and restlessness.
Phobias	Completely irrational fear of people, things, or events.
Depression	Profound feelings of discouragement, loss of control, worthlessness, helplessness, and hopelessness. Depression may be a primary factor in most suicides.
Bipolar Disorder (Manic-Depressive Disorder)	Bipolar disorders cause patients to experience widely changing moods and behaviors ranging from mania and euphoria to severe depression.
Paranoia	Behavior characterized by widely exaggerated mistrust or suspicion.
Schizophrenia	A classification or grouping that includes various mental illnesses and disorders.

Emergency Care: Behavioral Emergencies

When managing a behavioral emergency, try to determine if the patient has a behavioral problem, physical problem, or both. Never assume facts about the patient's condition. For example, diabetic emergencies can appear very similar to alcohol intoxication. Look for clues in the history or environment. This information will help you to treat the patient accurately.

Always complete an initial assessment and physical exam for patients with behavioral emergencies. Treat the underlying medical or trauma condition. Do not withhold treatment based on invalid or suspicious information.

> **D.O.T. OBJECTIVE**
>
> Discuss methods to calm behavioral emergency patients.

Methods of Calming Behavioral Emergency Patients

Few EMS workers are trained mental health professionals. However, EMT-Bs are often called upon to calm patients, family members, bystanders, and others during a crisis. Always treat behavioral emergency patients with respect and dignity. You can avoid conflict by exercising restraint and using a few proven strategies.

- Acknowledge that the person seems upset. State that you are there to help him or her.
- Tell the patient what you are doing. Try to talk him or her into cooperating with you.
- Ask questions in a calm and reassuring tone.
- Encourage the patient to talk. Ask the patient to explain what is troubling him or her.
- Avoid making quick or sudden movements.
- Involve trusted family members or friends.
- Try to eliminate or reduce any distressing stimuli.
- Be honest in your responses. Tell the patient the truth.
- Do not threaten, challenge, or argue with disturbed patients. Do not play along with or make fun of visual or auditory disturbances.
- Advise dispatch and be prepared to stay on the scene for a long time.
- Use good eye contact.
- Avoid unnecessary physical contact.
- Try to have at least two EMS providers with the patient at all times.
- Avoid the use of restraints if possible.

Begin developing a good rapport with the patient during your initial assessment. This will help to defuse and calm the situation. You may not have time to establish rapport with the patient if the situation is critical.

> **D.O.T. OBJECTIVE**
>
> Discuss the special considerations for assessing a patient with behavioral problems.

Assessing a Patient with a Behavioral Emergency

A complete and accurate scene size-up is important in behavioral emergencies. Although there is a potential for violence in all emergencies, behavioral emergencies are especially volatile. If you doubt the safety of the scene, do not enter. Wait until law enforcement personnel have declared the scene secure (see Fig. 14.13). When you enter, search for clues about living conditions, medications, and medical history. Also look for items that could be used as weapons. Make sure these items are secure.

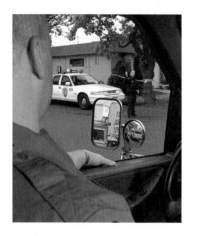

Figure 14.13 *Law enforcement must secure an unsafe scene.*

After securing and sizing up the scene, begin the initial assessment. First, identify yourself. Let the patient know you will help and will be his or her advocate. Question the patient in a calm and reassuring voice. Ask open-ended questions. For example, "How do you feel today compared to yesterday or last week? What can my crew and I do to make you feel more comfortable?" This encourages the patient to discuss feelings. Get the patient's opinion about what has happened. Even though it may be difficult at times, avoid being judgmental. Try to acknowledge the patient's feelings by listening and responding to concerns.

To show the patient that you are listening and to encourage communication, try repeating the patient's answer as a question. For example, if you ask what happened and the patient replies, "My wife just does not understand," ask him "What doesn't your wife understand?"

During your initial assessment, monitor the patient's mental status. Evaluate the following:

*EMT
Tip*

Try to get the patient to talk to you, not just at you.

- Responsiveness (AVPU)
- Appearance
- Activity level
- Clarity of speech
- Awareness of surroundings
- Orientation to time
- Awareness of others on the scene

If the initial assessment reveals any life-threatening conditions, begin treatment.

Discuss the general principles of an individual's behavior that
suggests that he is at risk for violence.

Assessing a Patient's Risk for Violence. During behavioral emergencies, watch
the patient for signs suggesting violence, hostility, or aggression. Try to find out
if the patient has a history of violence. Look at his or her eyes. The patient may
be about to strike a person or body area where the eyes are focused. Look at
the posture. Is the patient standing as if ready to bolt? Also look for:

- Clenched fists
- Swaying back and forth
- Muscle tension
- Yelling
- Verbal abuse or threats

Discuss the characteristics of an individual's behavior that
suggests that the patient is at risk for suicide.

Suicidal Patients

Suicide is any willful act designed to end one's own life. Patients who have
performed violent acts against themselves should be considered suicidal. This
is true even if the acts seem minor or insignificant. These individuals must be
evaluated by a mental health professional.

Some suicidal individuals deliberately create hostile situations with public
safety or law enforcement agencies. They may take hostages, commit a violent
crime, or intentionally begin a high-speed automobile chase. Known as "suicide by cop," this has become more common in the past decade. You must be
aware of the potential for involvement in this type of situation. Never
approach persons threatening suicide without law enforcement backup.

Assessing a Patient's Risk for Suicide. As you perform your scene size-up, look
for weapons or other objects that could cause injury. Look for signs of self-
destructive behavior (see Fig. 14.14). General risk factors for suicide are:

- Individuals over age 40 or between the ages of 10 and 18
- Single, recently widowed, or divorced individuals

*EMT
Alert*

*Be especially careful around
persons threatening to end their
lives. A person intent on suicide
may have no reservations about
taking the lives of others.*

Figure 14.14 *A wrist laceration from an attempted suicide.*

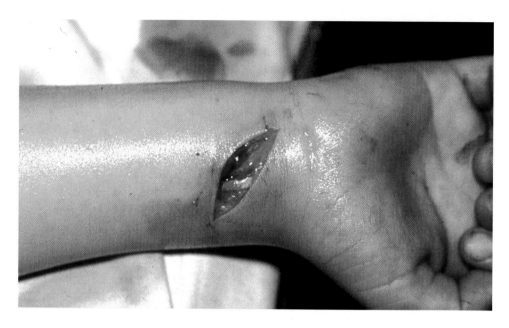

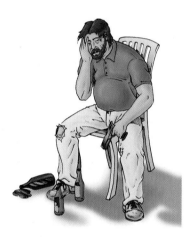

Figure 14.15 *A depressed individual with alcohol and a gun should be considered a suicide risk.*

- Persons with a history of alcoholism, substance abuse, or severe depression (see Fig. 14.15)
- Persons verbalizing a clear, lethal plan of action
- Presence of tools or materials to complete the plan of action, such as guns, ropes, or large amounts of medications
- History of self-destructive behavior
- Recent diagnosis of serious or terminal illness
- Recent loss of a significant loved one
- Recent arrest, imprisonment, or loss of job

Perform an initial assessment as usual. As you complete the assessment, consider the following questions:

- How does the patient feel?
- Is the patient thinking about hurting him/herself?
- Does the patient have suicidal tendencies?
- Is the patient a threat to self or others?
- Does the patient have an underlying medical problem?
- What interventions have been started, or what should I do now?

Emergency Care for Suicidal Patients

1. Conduct a scene size-up. Be aware of your personal safety. Never allow the patient to come between you and the escape route.
2. Complete the initial assessment. It can be very helpful to establish a rapport with a suicidal person. Perform interventions if necessary.

3. Conduct the focused history and physical exam. During the exam, try to reassure and calm the patient. If a suicide attempt involves drugs, try to find them. Bring the drug or empty container to the medical facility.

4. Complete the detailed assessment en route to medical facility if necessary.

5. Provide appropriate transport and ongoing assessment.

D.O.T. OBJECTIVE

Discuss special medical/legal considerations for managing behavioral emergencies.

Medical/Legal Considerations

You may have to make difficult decisions when managing behavioral emergencies. Legal principles can be difficult to apply to patients with behavioral emergencies. Consulting medical direction and law enforcement is a safe and effective strategy. Carefully follow your local protocols. Try to calm the patient, and get him or her to agree to treatment and transport. This can help to reduce your legal exposure.

Behavioral emergencies still require the competent patient's consent for treatment. On rare occasions, you may have to consider patients with behavioral problems or abnormal actions incompetent. Once you decide the patient cannot make competent decisions, you must secure consent for treatment. This is given by a legal guardian or law enforcement. If a legal guardian or legally responsible adult is unavailable and you believe the patient's life is at risk, you may be allowed to begin life-saving treatment based on the principle of implied consent.

An emotionally disturbed patient may resist treatment. Some patients will threaten the EMS crew, family members, mental health professionals, or bystanders. If you have reason to believe that the patient will harm self or others, consider transporting him or her anyway. You must have a firm legal foundation for caring for a patient against his or her will. Obtain consent from law enforcement or medical direction before transport. Know your local protocol regarding transporting patients with behavioral emergencies. In some areas, the police will take the patient into protective custody and then authorize treatment and transportation. For more information on patient consent, review Chapter 3.

Role of Law Enforcement and Medical Direction

Request assistance from medical direction. This reduces your legal risk when managing a behavioral emergency. Many EMS systems require contact with medical direction before restraining a patient for any reason. In some systems,

EMT Tip

Never begin treatment of a competent person against his or her will. Consult medical direction or law enforcement. In some areas, local protocol will guide your actions.

the police are simultaneously dispatched to any reported behavioral emergencies. They will ensure that the scene is safe. Officers will also assist in restraining the patient, if necessary. If a patient exhibits aggressive or combative behavior, consider the scene unsafe. Always request police assistance.

Avoiding Use of Unreasonable Force or Restraint

The safety of the EMS crew is always a primary concern. EMS personnel may use reasonable force to defend themselves against attack. Remain alert. A patient's mood can change quickly. A patient may be calm at first, then suddenly become combative or aggressive. He or she may become agitated or violent with little provocation.

Figure 14.16 *A behavioral emergency patient may become violent. Law enforcement should be on hand to ensure scene safety.*

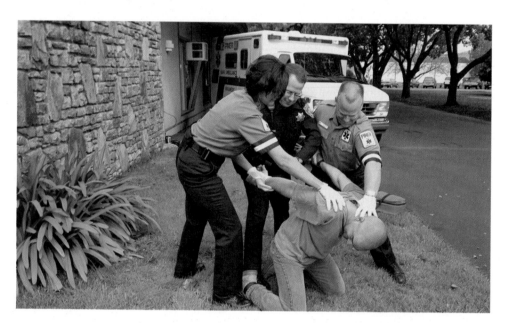

EMT Tip

Avoid acts of physical force that could injure the patient.

Force may be necessary to protect the patient or others (see Fig. 14.16). The force used to restrain or transport a patient should match the level of potential violence or harm. Excessive force increases your risk of legal challenges. Know and follow your local protocol. The amount of force that is reasonable should be determined by the following:

- Patient's size, strength, and gender
- Type of abnormal behavior
- Mental state of the patient
- Method of restraint

Protection Against False Accusations

Unfortunately, emotionally unstable patients make false accusations against EMTs. This may occur at the scene, during transport, or while at the hospital. Sexual misconduct is a common accusation. You must protect yourself against these accusations. Your best defense is to document the patient's abnormal behavior accurately and thoroughly. Include information about all phases of the response. Record all offensive or threatening comments. This demonstrates the patient's state of mind during the call. If possible, have two providers ride with the patient during transport. Preferably, one should be the same gender as the patient. Law enforcement personnel may assume this role. Third-party witnesses also help to protect you against false accusations.

Restraining Patients

The use of restraints is not desirable, but it is necessary at times (see Fig. 14.17). When restraining a patient, it is advisable to have law enforcement on the scene. Also involve medical direction in the situation.

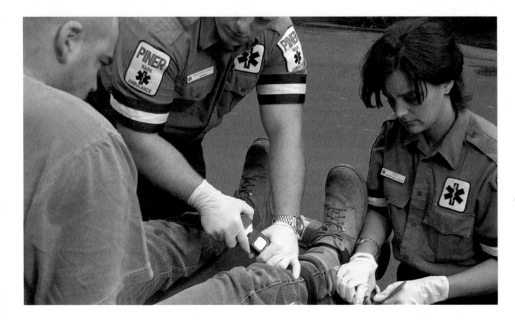

Figure 14.17 *Restraining a patient to a stretcher with ankle restraints.*

When you must restrain a patient, follow these guidelines:

- Enlist adequate help based on the patient's size, location, and aggressiveness.

- Plan your activities in advance.

- Act quickly and decisively after deciding to apply restraints. Avoid being talked out of your decision. A patient may agree to calm down to avoid restraints. Then he or she may become violent again while en route to the hospital.

- One person should continue to communicate with the patient while the others apply the restraints.

- Use the least amount of force necessary to restrain the patient.

- Include four people in the restraining plan. Each person is assigned to one of the patient's limbs. All four should approach the patient simultaneously and take control of the assigned extremities. Do not underestimate the range of motion of the arms and legs. Serious injury can result if a violent patient is improperly restrained.

Figure 14.18 *Restraining devices must be approved by medical direction.*

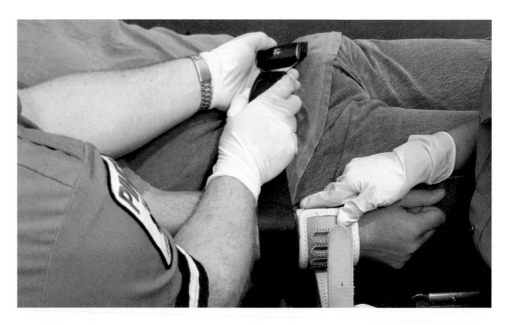

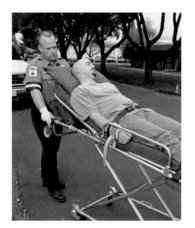

Figure 14.19 *A potentially violent patient restrained on a stretcher.*

- Secure the limbs together using restraining devices that have been approved by medical direction (see Fig. 14.18).

- In some cases, a violent patient may be placed face down on the stretcher. Continually confirm that the airway remains clear and immediately accessible. Follow local protocols.

- Secure the patient to the stretcher using multiple straps (see Fig. 14.19).

- If the patient is spitting, cover his or her face with a surgical mask.

- Reassess the patient frequently. Monitor the vital signs. Provide necessary interventions.

- Accurately and completely document the indications for use of the restraint. Record the technique used. Avoid unnecessary or unreasonable force.

Chapter Fourteen Summary

- Altered mental states have many potential causes. The most common are:

  Failure to take medications as prescribed for specific conditions, such as diabetes, seizures, or mental illness

  Alcohol abuse, drug abuse, or poisoning

  Trauma, especially in patients with head injuries

  Hypoxia due to an underlying illness

- If the patient is a known diabetic, you may not know if the problem is related to high or low blood sugar. Treat for hypoglycemia.

- Consider the administration of oral glucose for patients with an altered mental state and a history of medication- or diet-controlled diabetes. Before administering this product, assess the patient's ability to swallow and maintain the airway. Contact medical direction for permission.

- When treating patients with an altered mental status and no history of diabetes, focus on maintaining the airway. Provide supplemental oxygen and transport immediately. Be prepared to assist ventilations.

- Treat all seizure activity as potentially life threatening. If a patient is actively seizing, protect him or her from injury.

- Behavioral emergencies, like altered mental status, can have many causes. Pay close attention to scene safety in behavioral emergencies. Never allow the patient to block your exit. Many behavioral emergencies involve suicide attempts or an attempt to hurt others. Your demeanor is important when approaching and assessing the patient. Be calm and keep the patient well informed. Provide reassurance that you are there to help. Listen empathetically and acknowledge the patient's feelings.

- Know the legal procedure in your area for treating a patient against his or her will.

- Restrain patients only as a last resort. Use the least amount of physical force possible. Never restrain a patient unless there are adequate resources to conduct the task without endangering yourself, your crew, or the patient.

Key Terms Review

Altered Mental Status (AMS) | *page 417*
Behavioral Emergency | *page 431*
Cerebrovascular Accident (CVA) | *page 429*
Diabetes Mellitus | *page 418*

Glucose | *page 418*
Hyperglycemia | *page 419*
Hypoglycemia | *page 419*
Insulin | *page 418*
Postictal State | *page 425*
Seizure | *page 424*

Status Epilepticus | *page 425*
Stroke | *page 429*
Syncope | *page 428*
Transient Ischemic Attack (TIA) | *page 430*

Review Questions

1. Levels of glucose in the blood will increase when:

   a. There is a lack of insulin

   b. The patient has been fasting

   c. There is an excess of insulin

   d. The patient has taken insulin without eating

2. Diabetes mellitus is:

   a. A lack or absence of glucose in the blood

   b. An excess of glucose in the blood

   c. An excess of insulin in the blood

   d. A lack or absence of insulin in the blood

3. The breakdown of fats as an alternative energy source to sugar produces _____.

   a. Hypoxia

   b. Hyperkalemia

   c. Ketoacidosis

   d. Ketoalkalosis

4. All of the following may be causes of hypoglycemia, EXCEPT:

   a. Excessive blood sugar

   b. Too much insulin taken

   c. Insufficient food intake

   d. Excessive exercise

5. All of the following are typical signs and symptoms of hypoglycemia, EXCEPT:

   a. Unusual behavior

   b. A slow onset of symptoms (over hours or days)

   c. Rapid or normal pulse with normal blood pressure

   d. Pale, cool, sweaty skin

6. If you are not sure whether your patient is hyperglycemic or hypoglycemic, you should:

   a. Encourage the patient to take fluids

   b. Give the patient sugar

   c. Have the patient take his or her insulin

   d. Measure the patient's blood glucose level

7. All of the following are considered proper treatment for a seizing patient, EXCEPT:

   a. Try to force something between the patient's teeth

   b. Protect the patient from injury

   c. Protect the airway

   d. Transport all first-time seizures

8. A serious medical condition in which brain damage or death may occur as a result of back-to-back seizures is called _____.

   a. Tonic-clonic movement

   b. Generalized seizure

   c. Status epilepticus

   d. Postictal state

9. CVAs are commonly caused by _____.

   a. Interruption of the brain's blood supply

   b. Seizure

   c. Heart failure

   d. Low glucose levels in the brain

10. All of the following are major risk factors for a CVA, EXCEPT:

    a. Hypertension

    b. Atherosclerosis

    c. Advanced age

    d. Low serum cholesterol

11. The first treatment for an unconscious patient following a suspected stroke is to:

    a. Obtain vital signs

    b. Administer glucose paste

    c. Place the patient on one side

    d. Secure a patent airway

12. Upon arrival at the scene of a behavioral emergency, which is the correct sequence of events?

    a. Focused history and physical exam, scene size-up, initial assessment

    b. Scene size-up, initial assessment, focused history and physical exam

    c. Initial assessment, focused history and physical exam, scene size-up

    d. Scene size-up, focused history and physical exam, patient assessment

13. Oral glucose is generally given to diabetic patients because:

    a. Hyperglycemia may be a life-threatening emergency

    b. Hypoglycemia may be a life-threatening emergency

    c. Altered mental status is always a life-threatening emergency

    d. Altered mental status is never a life-threatening emergency

14. Which cells are extremely sensitive to glucose levels?

    a. Brain

    b. Liver

    c. Lung

    d. Spleen

15. You and your partner come upon an unconscious patient. Family members tell you that the patient is a diabetic who has been working outside all day chopping wood. Your partner suggests that you administer oral glucose. Administering oral glucose to this patient is:

    a. Indicated

    b. Possibly indicated

    c. Contraindicated

    d. Indicated only after speaking with medical direction

16. All seizures in adults should be treated as if they are:

    a. Life threatening

    b. Mild

    c. Recurring

    d. Traumatic

CASE STUDIES

Neurological, Diabetic, and Behavioral Emergencies

1 Your unit is on standby duty during a big football game at the university. You see a crowd gathering nearby. A young man has collapsed by the restroom. His brother says that he has a sugar problem but he cannot remember any details. You reach for your radio and advise your partner to respond. According to bystanders, the patient hit his head when he fell. A deep laceration on the forehead is bleeding profusely. The patient will only respond to a painful stimulus. You hear snoring respirations. The patient's pulse is weak and rapid.

A. What immediate intervention is necessary?

B. Is airway intervention required?

C. What can you do to provide definitive care for this patient?

D. What is diabetes? How does Type I diabetes differ from Type II?

2 Dispatch requests an emergency response on Highway 20. You are to meet a school bus parked on the shoulder. A young girl is having a seizure. All the other children are off the bus when you arrive. As you enter the bus, the driver is holding a child's head. You see the child having tonic–clonic movements. The bus driver states that the patient has been seizing continuously for 13 to 15 minutes.

A. Does this represent a life-threatening emergency?

B. Name the medical condition or circumstance of this patient.

C. What is your course of treatment for this patient?

3 A funeral for a fellow firefighter is never a happy occasion. The weather spiked to 90 degrees and the humidity is 100 percent. Your crew was asked to provide medical services for an estimated five thousand attendees. During the funeral procession, you are dispatched for a man down along the route. When you arrive, an elderly man is sitting under a tree. Bystanders are cooling and fanning him. His skin is very warm to the touch. He refuses additional services. Bystanders claim that the man was standing in the sun for 50 minutes. Suddenly, he had a syncopal episode. They state that the man started to fall against someone else. He dropped to his knees, then to his back. The woman next to him says that he did not hit his head. She tells you that several others helped him to the ground. They estimate he was unresponsive for a few seconds. The man is alert and well oriented. He denies any medical problems and has no pain. He strongly refuses transport or additional assessment.

A. What might have caused the patient's symptoms?

B. What medical care can be given to the patient in the scenario above?

C. List some causes of syncope.

D. Describe a syncopal episode in your own words.

Stories from the Field
Wrap-Up

An altered mental state has many potential causes. Diabetic emergencies are some of the most common nontraumatic causes. Diabetic patients must maintain careful control of their diets and medications to keep their blood sugar normal. Knowing Jean's medical history is essential to determining the nature of her condition. In this case, you might suspect hypoglycemia. The rapid onset of symptoms and rapid deterioration of Jean's mental state are important clues. So are her breathing and pulse. If you cannot decide whether a diabetic with an altered mental state has high or low blood sugar, treat for hypoglycemia. If not treated rapidly, hypoglycemia will become life threatening.

Kim's first priority is maintaining Jean's airway and breathing. She cannot administer oral glucose since Jean is unconscious. Kim will reassess the patient frequently. If her mental status does not improve or declines, EMS will repeat the initial assessment when they arrive and transport her immediately.

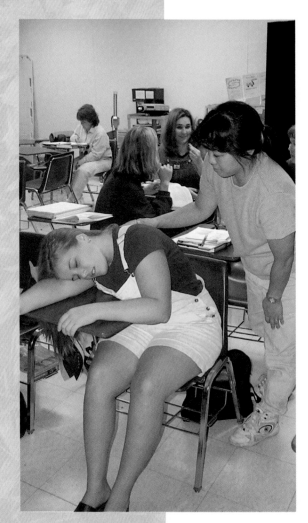

Chapter *15*

Allergic Reactions

Stories from the Field

You are attending your niece's soccer game on a Sunday afternoon. Suddenly, one of the players begins yelling and swinging her arms wildly. She runs toward the team bench. A teammate helps her to sit down and asks the girl what is wrong. The teammate calls out for help from anyone who knows first aid. You step in and identify yourself as an EMT-B student. Several bees have stung the player. Her friend states that the patient is allergic to bees.

As you approach the patient, the scene appears safe. There are no bees in the area. You observe that the patient is flushed. She is alert and oriented, although she appears anxious and very scared. Her airway is open. Her breathing is shallow and rapid. Even without a stethoscope, you can hear wheezing with each breath. The pulse is rapid. Her skin is cool and very damp. There are many bright-red, raised patches all over her body. Your general impression of the patient is very poor. You ask another teammate to call 9-1-1. While waiting for the ambulance, you continue your assessment. You attempt to calm and reassure the patient.

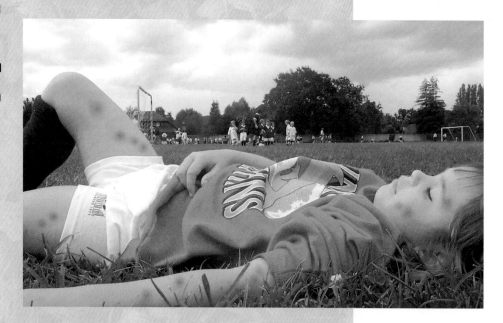

Allergies are a very common and increasing health problem in the United States. As many as 50 million persons suffer from allergies. Common allergy-related conditions you may see include asthma, hay fever, and rashes. Allergic reactions range from mild to severe. Mild allergic reactions generally affect only one area of the body. These localized reactions are seen in the tissue immediately exposed to a toxin. Mild reactions are characterized by a slow onset and minor symptoms. Some allergies, such as mild hay fever, may not require treatment. Others can interfere with day-to-day activities and diminish the quality of life (see Fig. 15.1).

Figure 15.1 *An allergic reaction.*

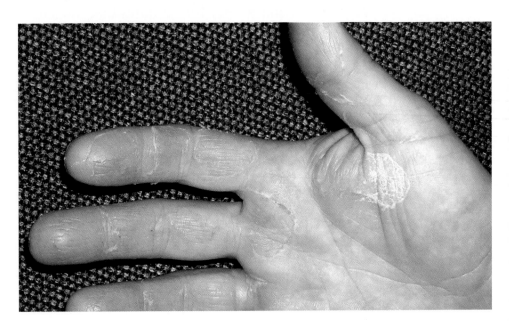

A severe allergic reaction acts on several organ systems simultaneously. It has a sudden onset with major symptoms that affect the airway, breathing, and circulation. A severe allergic reaction is called anaphylactic shock. This condition can cause death within a few minutes. For an EMT-B, recognizing a systemic allergic reaction is critical to providing early life-saving interventions. Prehospital treatment is quite different than for a local reaction. Identifying early signs and symptoms of a severe allergic reaction will improve the patient's chance of survival.

ALLERGIC REACTIONS

The immune system is part of the circulatory system. It helps to protect the body from foreign substances that might be damaging, such as viruses, bacteria, and toxins. Substances that the body recognizes as foreign are called **antigens**. Antigens enter the body through the skin, gastrointestinal tract, and respiratory system. When an antigen enters the body, the immune system produces

Antigen | *A foreign substance that enters the body and causes an immune response*

an **antibody** to that substance. Antibodies protect the person if he or she is exposed to the same substance again. The next time it is found in the body, antibodies will quickly identify it and attack. This **immune response** involves a host of complex chemical reactions that result in destruction of the invader.

Most people's immune systems function properly. However, in some conditions, the body does not react normally to harmful substances. For example, the immune system in a person with AIDS cannot distinguish between harmful and harmless substances. In other patients, the immune response becomes too aggressive. When exposed to a harmless substance, the immune system attempts to destroy it.

An allergy is a condition in which a person is very sensitive to a certain substance that is harmless to most people. Exposure to the substance triggers an **allergic reaction**, which is an exaggerated immune response. An antigen that causes an allergic reaction is called an **allergen**. Most allergens enter the body by being inhaled or swallowed, or through contact with the skin. The body's response to an allergen can be unpleasant. Most allergic reactions are mild. They produce uncomfortable symptoms, such as a runny nose or itching, watery eyes. In severe cases, allergic reactions produce life-threatening symptoms. An allergic reaction can develop within seconds. It may also be delayed for several hours. As a rule, if the reaction develops quickly, it will be more severe.

An allergic reaction involves many body systems. However, special immune system cells that act on foreign invaders are located in certain tissues. Allergy symptoms are most prominent in the:

- Skin
- Eyes
- Stomach lining
- Nose
- Sinuses
- Throat
- Lungs

Anyone can experience an allergic reaction. Age, gender, race, or socioeconomic factors do not influence allergies. People with no history of allergies can develop serious reactions. The exact mechanism of allergies is not understood. However, there appears to be a hereditary link. In susceptible people, hormones, stress, and environmental irritants such as smoke or perfume may play a role. Sometimes, an allergic reaction will recur after many years of remission.

If a patient experiences signs and symptoms of an allergy, a physician can conduct tests to try to learn what allergens are causing it. This information

Antibody | *A protein produced by the immune system that combines with a specific antigen and helps to destroy it*

Immune Response | *A series of reactions that are the body's defense mechanism against invading viruses, bacteria, and toxins*

Allergic Reaction | *An exaggerated immune response to a substance that is normally harmless*

Allergen | *An antigen that causes an allergic reaction, such as dust, mold, or pollen*

is sometimes used to prepare preventive allergy shots for a patient. These are injected over a period of time. If successful, the intensity of the allergic reaction gradually decreases. Patients may use other prescription medications to treat known allergies. The most effective way of preventing an allergic reaction is to avoid the things that trigger it.

A severe allergic reaction affects many parts of the body at once. This is known as **anaphylactic shock** or **anaphylaxis**. The effects on the airway, lungs, blood vessels, and heart are dramatic. It can rapidly result in death. Your ability to recognize and manage a severe allergic reaction may be the only thing standing between the patient and imminent death.

Anaphylactic (an-eh-feh-LAK-tik) **Shock** | *Severe allergic reaction in which blood vessels dilate rapidly, causing a drop in blood pressure and respiratory distress*

Anaphylaxis | *Another name for anaphylactic shock*

Causes of Allergic Reactions

Hundreds of everyday substances can trigger an allergic reaction (see Table 15.1). Substances that commonly cause allergic reactions are:

- Insect bites and stings—bees, wasps, yellow jackets, hornets, and some spiders. These can cause severe, rapid allergic reactions (see Fig. 15.2). Fire ant bites can also cause anaphylaxis. Some insect bites may damage local tissue or affect the nervous system without causing an allergic response. These conditions are discussed further in Chapter 17, Environmental Emergencies.

- Food—peanuts and other nuts, eggs, milk, chocolate, cottonseed oil, grains, beans, fruit, and shellfish. Reactions to food allergies generally occur more slowly than those caused by insect stings. Reactions to peanuts and shellfish are exceptions. These develop rapidly and are severe.

- Food preservatives—sulfites.

- Plants—poison ivy, plant pollen, and ragweed. Contact allergies usually cause local signs and symptoms. Although anaphylactic reactions are possible, they are less likely in plant allergies.

- Medications—antibiotics (especially penicillin), local anesthetics, aspirin, seizure medications, muscle relaxants, nonsteroidal anti-inflammatory agents, vitamins, insulin, and tetanus and diphtheria vaccines. Medicines produce both mild and severe reactions. Injected drugs are much riskier than oral medications. Chemicals injected during some x-ray studies can cause anaphylaxis. Injected medications and chemicals are a frequent cause of anaphylaxis in hospitals.

- Animals—feathers, animal dander.

- Household—molds, household dust (dust mites).

- Chemicals—soap, makeup, cleansers, industrial chemicals, glue, fertilizer, chemical fumes, latex.

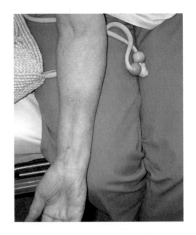

Figure 15.2 *The painful results of a bee sting.*

EMT Tip

A bee stinger must be removed carefully. Squeezing the site will force more venom into the skin. This is described fully in Chapter 17.

Latex Allergies. Allergies to natural rubber latex have become common. The exact mechanism is unknown, but some characteristics of latex cause reactions in many people. This can be a cause of anaphylaxis. Latex has become popular

Table 15.1 • COMMON CAUSES OF ALLERGIC REACTIONS

Type	Examples	Routes of Exposure
Insect Bites	Wasps, hornets, fire ants, spiders	Injection
Foods	Nuts, eggs, shellfish, berries, milk, sulfite preservatives	Ingestion
Plants	Pollens, plants, molds, and grasses	Inhalation or direct contact
Medications	Antibiotics, vitamins, aspirin, seizure medications, nonsteroidal anti-inflammatory drugs	Ingestion or injection
Other	Chemicals, animals, dust mites, latex	Inhalation or direct contact

for everyday use in a variety of products. It has many benefits. It keeps its shape and does not tear easily.

Latex allergies were almost unheard of a decade ago. They now affect up to 10 percent of all healthcare workers in the United States. This is probably due to the large increase in the use of latex products in health care. Latex gloves have been used for years to prevent infection. They effectively block the transmission of bacteria and viruses. Bandages, blood pressure cuffs, catheters, feeding tubes, IV injection ports, and rubber stoppers also contain latex. Latex allergies occur among the general public, as well. Latex is found in many common products. These include baby bottle nipples, balloons, toys, condoms, diaphragms, and rubber bands. Some patients are exposed to latex during surgery or medical procedures. Surgical gloves contact the inside of the body, which is particularly sensitive.

Most people get a rash 10 to 30 hours after contact with latex. Healthcare workers may notice an itchy, swollen rash on their hands after removing gloves. Some people experience immediate, extreme reactions. Critical reactions include asthma-like symptoms and life-threatening airway blockage. The best way to prevent reactions is to avoid contact with latex. Whenever possible, use latex-free products and equipment. Besides protecting yourself, remember that patients may also have latex allergies.

EMT Tip

As a precaution, find out if you are allergic to natural rubber latex.

D.O.T. OBJECTIVES

Recognize the patient experiencing an allergic reaction.

Establish the relationship between the patient with an allergic reaction and airway management.

Describe the mechanisms of allergic response and the implications for airway management.

Signs and Symptoms of Allergic Reactions

Hives | Raised, red blotches associated with allergic reactions

EMT Tip

Allergic reactions and anaphylaxis have many causes. Be able to recognize whether a patient is in respiratory distress or has hypotension.

You must be able to recognize early signs and symptoms of an allergic reaction. These reactions may be mild, moderate, or severe. Hay fever is an example of a mild reaction. The appearance of **hives** is a moderate reaction. Difficulty breathing, swelling of the tongue, and any altered level of consciousness are signs of a severe reaction. Table 15.2 describes signs and symptoms of allergic reactions.

A patient may not know or suspect he or she has an allergy. Some people will deny having allergies because they have never been diagnosed. A patient may complain of itching. Upon questioning, you find that the itching began after use of a new lotion or detergent. Patients may not make the connection between an allergen and a medical problem. For example, after eating shrimp, a person might get violently sick and have swelling of the hands and feet. The patient might think this is a bout of food poisoning, when it is really due to a shellfish allergy. Predicting the exact course of an allergic reaction is difficult. Sometimes you will find the patient in severe respiratory distress. You may also assist patients who have become hypotensive after a bee sting (see Fig. 15.3). Remember that severe reactions can occur rapidly and are critical.

Table 15.2 • SIGNS AND SYMPTOMS OF AN ALLERGIC REACTION

Body System	Signs	Symptoms
Skin	Hives Swelling of face, neck, hands, feet, and/or tongue Flushed or red skin Pale, clammy skin Cyanosis	Warm, tingling feeling in the face, mouth, chest, feet, and hands Itching
Respiratory	Cough Rapid breathing Labored breathing Noisy breathing: hoarseness, stridor, crowing, and/or wheezing	Lump or tickle in the throat Tightness in throat and chest Difficulty breathing Difficulty swallowing
Cardiovascular	Increased heart rate Decreased blood pressure Weak or absent pulse	Pounding or racing heart
Generalized	Itchy, watery eyes Headache Runny nose	General weakness
Mental Status	Restlessness Disorientation Seizures Unresponsiveness Decreasing mental status	Not feeling well Anxiety Sense of impending doom

Table 15.3 • SIGNS AND SYMPTOMS OF ANAPHYLACTIC SHOCK

Body System	Signs	Symptoms
Skin	Pale, clammy skin Cyanosis	Itching
Respiratory	Labored breathing Noisy breathing: hoarseness, stridor, crowing, wheezing Respiratory compromise	Tightness in the throat and chest Difficulty breathing
Cardiovascular	Increased heart rate Decreased blood pressure/hypotension Weak or absent pulse	Pounding or racing heart
Mental Status	Decreasing mental status Unresponsiveness	Not feeling well

Signs and Symptoms of Anaphylactic Shock

Assessment findings that suggest shock or respiratory distress signify anaphylactic shock. Table 15.3 lists signs and symptoms of an anaphylactic reaction. Anaphylaxis may appear mild initially, but can worsen rapidly. There can be swelling in the upper airway, which causes obstruction and reduces airflow to the lungs. Swelling and constriction of the air passages within the lungs causes respiratory compromise and hypoxia. Dilation and leakage of blood vessels can cause a dangerous drop in blood pressure (hypotension). If you suspect anaphylaxis, transport the patient immediately. Complete the focused history and physical exam while en route to the hospital.

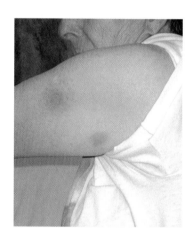

Figure 15.3 *Redness, itching, and swelling associated with an allergic reaction on the skin.*

D.O.T. OBJECTIVES

Describe the emergency medical care of the patient with an allergic reaction.

Evaluate the need for medical direction in the emergency medical care of the patient with an allergic reaction.

Differentiate between the general category of those patients having an allergic reaction and those patients having an allergic reaction and requiring immediate medical care, including immediate use of epinephrine auto-injector.

EMT Tip

Secretions may be copious and thick. Be prepared to suction. Have sterile water available to clear the suction tubing. When assisting ventilation, compressing the BVM may be difficult. This is because of airway obstruction caused by broncho-spasm (narrowing of the airway pathways).

EMERGENCY CARE: ALLERGIC REACTIONS

Follow these steps for a suspected allergic reaction:

1. During scene size-up, look for swarming bees or other unsafe conditions. Determine the number of patients. Calling for additional support or ALS backup may be necessary. Always use body substance isolation and standard precautions. Keep in mind that all body fluids are potentially infectious.

2. Complete the initial assessment. Your ability to distinguish between a mild and a severe allergic reaction may save a patient's life. Assess mental status by AVPU. If the patient is unresponsive, get as much information from bystanders as possible.

3. Maintain a patent airway. Suction secretions. Suspect a severe reaction if there is swelling inside the mouth. The uvula and soft palate may be swollen. The tongue may become so swollen that it blocks the airway. Airway adjuncts are of limited value because the airway is usually obstructed at the larynx. Instead, a bag-valve mask may be needed to force air past the swollen tissues. Positioning the patient can help to make breathing or ventilation easier.

4. If the patient is having dyspnea, is showing signs of respiratory distress, or is obviously in anaphylactic shock, administer high-concentration oxygen. Provide 15 liters per minute by non-rebreather mask. Assist ventilations with a bag-valve mask and 15 liters per minute of oxygen. A flow-restricted, oxygen-powered ventilation device may also be used. Assist respiration if necessary.

5. Evaluate the circulatory system. Ensure that the patient has a pulse. Assess perfusion by checking the skin color, temperature, and condition. Look for signs of shock, especially pale, cool, or moist skin along with a rapid pulse.

6. Conduct a focused history and physical exam. You will need SAMPLE history information immediately. This will tell you whether the patient has a history of allergic reactions. Table 15.4 lists some examples of SAMPLE questions to

Figure 15.4 *Epinephrine auto-injectors.*

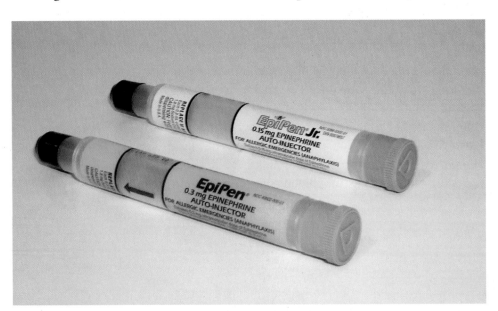

Table 15.4 • SAMPLE HISTORY: ALLERGIC REACTIONS

Category	Questions to Ask
Signs and Symptoms	Was the onset gradual or sudden? Are you feeling better or worse?
Allergies	Do you have any known allergies to food, drugs, insects, or plants? Have you had an allergic reaction before? If so, to what? How severe was it?
Medications	Have you taken any prescription or non-prescription medications recently? Have you taken any illicit drugs? Have you taken any medications to relieve your current symptoms? Do you have a prescribed epinephrine auto-injector? Do you have an anaphylaxis kit, such as Ana-Kit®?
Pertinent Past Medical History	Have you ever had an allergic reaction in the past? If so, how serious was the reaction? Do you have any other significant conditions, such as respiratory or cardiac problems?
Last Oral Intake	When did you last eat or drink anything? What/how much did you eat or drink?
Events Leading to the Injury or Illness	What were you doing before the symptoms began? Were you exercising? Were you exposed to any potential allergen? Have you been bitten or stung recently? If so, by what? Are you using any new cosmetics, soaps, clothing?

ask if you suspect an allergic reaction. Check for a medical identification tag. Find out if the patient has a prescribed auto–injector (see Fig. 15.4). Quickly obtain baseline vital signs. Look for a rapid pulse rate, rapid respiratory rate, and low blood pressure. These are signs of shock.

7. Do not delay care to ask detailed questions. Intervene if signs of respiratory distress, hypotension, or shock are present. Consider administering epinephrine as described in the following section.

8. If the reaction is severe and no preloaded epinephrine is available, transport immediately. Advise medical control of the details. Place the patient in a position of comfort. If there is hypotension, use the Trendelenburg position. If the patient is in respiratory distress, a sitting position may be preferred. Calm the patient and provide continual reassurance. Maintain warmth. Loosen tight clothing.

9. Assess the response to interventions. If the patient does not improve, transport immediately. Look for signs of deterioration, such as decreasing mental status, increasing breathing difficulty, or decreasing blood pressure. Be prepared to initiate CPR and AED if the patient becomes pulseless.

0. Rapidly transport the patient to the hospital if the patient has signs and symptoms of an anaphylactic reaction but has no prescribed auto-injector, if he or she fails to improve after administration of the auto-injector, or if the patient is or becomes unresponsive. Complete a detailed physical exam while en route to the hospital. Conduct ongoing assessments every 5 minutes.

EMT Tip

ALS personnel can provide additional therapy. Advanced airway management, IVs, and medications may be needed to reverse the effects of an allergic reaction. If available in your area, request ALS assistance early for serious allergic reactions.

EMT Tip

Epinephrine can resolve airway compromise. Medical direction may delay endotracheal intubation (see Appendix A, Advanced Airway Management) until the medication has been given.

Epinephrine | *Hormone secreted in response to stress; causes tachycardia and vasoconstriction; used as an injected medication to relieve severe allergic reactions*

Adrenaline | *Another name for epinephrine*

D.O.T. OBJECTIVE

State the generic and trade names, medication forms, dose, administration, actions, and contraindications for the epinephrine auto-injector.

Epinephrine

Epinephrine is also called **adrenaline**. Epinephrine is a naturally occurring catecholamine. It acts directly on the sympathetic nervous system. Epinephrine quickly helps to block an allergic response. It can relieve the symptoms of allergic reactions within minutes. It is easily administered using an auto-injector pen (see Fig 15.5). Table 15.5 has information on the epinephrine auto-injector.

Epinephrine dilates the bronchioles, relieving wheezing and making breathing easier. It also constricts blood vessels. This improves blood pressure and decreases tissue swelling. The patient notices improvement in seconds to minutes. The drug response is short-lived, however, lasting only about 10 to 20 minutes. You may have to contact medical direction during transport for permission to administer a second dose.

Table 15.5 • EPINEPHRINE AUTO-INJECTOR

Characteristic	Description
Names	Generic Name: Epinephrine auto-injector Trade Names: EpiPen®, EpiPen Jr.®
Indications	The patient shows signs and symptoms of a severe allergic reaction A physician has prescribed the medication for this patient Medical direction has authorized use for this patient
Contraindications	There are no contraindications for use in a life-threatening situation
Actions	Widens the respiratory passages and narrows the blood vessels, which reduce swelling
Dosage	Adult auto-injector delivers a single dose of 0.3 mg of epinephrine Pediatric device delivers 0.15 mg of epinephrine A second dose may be administered after approval by medical direction
Forms and Route	Liquid delivered by an automatic injectable needle and syringe system Note: epinephrine is also available in other forms, including those for manual injection and inhalation
Side Effects	Increased heart rate, pallor, dizziness, chest pain, headache, nausea and vomiting, excitability and anxiousness

Epinephrine Administration

To assist a patient with an auto-injector:

1. Obtain an order from medical direction, either on-line or off-line.

2. Check the auto-injector. Be sure that the prescription is written for the patient experiencing the allergic reaction. Check that the medication has not expired. Look at the liquid to make sure it is not discolored and does not contain any particulate matter. You may not always be able to see the medication.

3. Remove the safety cap from the auto-injector. Wipe the patient's thigh with an alcohol wipe, if available.

4. Place the tip of the auto-injector against the lateral portion of the patient's thigh. Center it midway between the waist and knee.

5. Push the pen firmly against the thigh until the spring-loaded injector activates.

6. Hold the injector in place until the medication is dispensed, or for at least 10 seconds.

7. Record the time, dose, and action of the epinephrine.

8. Dispose of the auto-injector in a puncture-resistant biohazard container. Handle the auto-injector carefully. The needle may protrude from the end, increasing your risk of injury.

9. Reassess the patient after 2 minutes for the effects of the medication. Report your findings to medical direction. Contact medical direction if the patient's condition deteriorates after the first dose. If symptoms do not improve, you may be approved to administer a second dose if the patient has a second auto-injector available.

Reassessment. Transport the patient soon after assisting with the administration of epinephrine. Complete any remaining assessments or treatments while en route to the hospital. Reassess the patient's airway, breathing, and circulatory status continuously. Recheck the vital signs every 5 minutes. Look for these signs of deterioration:

- Decreasing mental status
- Increasing breathing difficulty
- Decreasing blood pressure

If the patient worsens, contact medical direction. Request permission to administer an additional dose of epinephrine, if available. Some patients carry more than one injector, especially if they have a history of serious reactions. Initiate CPR and AED if the patient becomes pulseless.

If the patient's condition improves, provide supportive care:

- Give high-flow oxygen via non-rebreather mask
- Treat for shock (see Chapter 19)

EMT Tip

Remember, if the onset of symptoms is rapid after exposure to an allergen, the reaction will be more severe. If a reaction occurs within minutes of exposure, be prepared to treat a serious reaction.

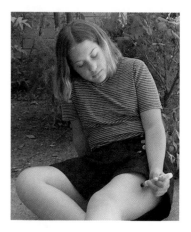

Figure 15.5 *A patient administering epinephrine from an auto-injector.*

EMT Tip

If necessary, you can inject the medication through clothing. This procedure is safe, and speeds administration.

Chapter Fifteen Summary

- Allergic reactions are exaggerated immune responses to common substances. Insect bites and stings, food (nuts, shellfish), plants, and medicines (penicillin, sulfa drugs) are among the most common causes.

- If the signs and symptoms of an allergic reaction develop rapidly, the nature of the reaction will be more severe.

- Patients with anaphylaxis may have or rapidly develop airway and respiratory compromise and/or shock.

- Patients with a known history of severe reactions often carry a physician-prescribed epinephrine auto-injector. Consider assisting with administration of the drug rapidly if signs and symptoms of shock or respiratory distress develop. Consult medical direction before administering epinephrine.

- Immediately transport a patient with symptoms and a history of serious reactions who does not have a prescribed epinephrine auto-injector.

- There are no contraindications for epinephrine in a life-threatening situation.

Key Terms Review

Adrenaline | page 456

Allergen | page 449

Allergic Reaction | page 449

Anaphylactic Shock | page 450

Anaphylaxis | page 450

Antibody | page 449

Antigen | page 448

Epinephrine | page 456

Hives | page 452

Immune Response | page 449

Review Questions

1. A substance that can cause an exaggerated immune response in some individuals is called:

   a. Antibody

   b. Allergen

   c. Pathogen

   d. Immunoglobin

2. Mary is experiencing an allergic reaction to the walnuts in her chocolate chip cookie. By what method was she probably exposed to the walnuts?

   a. Ingestion

   b. Inhalation

   c. Absorption

   d. Injection

3. What is the first thing you should do to treat an unconscious patient suffering from a severe allergic reaction?

   a. Establish and maintain a patent airway

   b. Call medical direction for guidance

   c. Administer epinephrine

   d. Administer high-flow oxygen

4. You approach a patient with classic signs of an allergic reaction. His wife says he has never had any allergies before. What is your conclusion?

   a. The patient is not having an allergic reaction

   b. The wife is wrong

   c. The patient is probably having an allergic reaction

   d. The cause is unclear

5. Pale, clammy skin, chest tightness, difficulty breathing, increased heart rate, decreased blood pressure, and unresponsiveness are signs and symptoms of which medical emergency?

   a. Anaphylaxis
   b. Arteriosclerosis
   c. Allergic reaction
   d. Aneurysm

6. For a patient with severe anaphylaxis, when should you obtain the focused history and physical exam?

   a. At the scene
   b. Within 15 minutes
   c. En route to the hospital
   d. Within 5 minutes

7. Anaphylaxis is a reaction involving the body's _____ system.

   a. Immune
   b. Respiratory
   c. Cardiovascular
   d. Skeletal

8. In general, the faster an anaphylactic reaction occurs, the _____ the effects will be.

   a. More severe
   b. Better
   c. Less
   d. Less significant

9. Bob is suffering from an allergic reaction to a bee sting. His vital signs are BP 100/50, HR 130, and RR 6. He has an altered mental status, hives, and wheezing. What is your primary concern about Bob's condition?

   a. Severe hypotension
   b. Respiratory arrest
   c. Seizure
   d. Secondary bee stings

10. Severe allergic reactions are also known as:

    a. Allergens
    b. Anaphylactic shock
    c. Antibodies
    d. Viruses

11. Involving ALS providers early in anaphylaxis reactions is important because ALS providers:

    a. Are able to diagnose anaphylaxis
    b. Know more than EMTs
    c. Can administer additional medications and treatment
    d. Can get a better history of the patient

12. After administration of epinephrine, your patient complains of the following side effects. Which of the following is probably NOT related to the administration of epinephrine?

    a. Tachycardia
    b. Chest pain
    c. Tingling in extremities
    d. Dizziness

13. You are treating a 30-year-old man who ate shellfish. He is wheezing and complaining of weakness and difficulty breathing. He has swelling and hives about his body. What sign indicates that this patient is having an anaphylactic reaction and not a simple allergic reaction?

    a. Systemic edema
    b. Weakness
    c. Respiratory distress
    d. Hypotension

14. Which of the following is NOT important for administering epinephrine to an anaphylaxis patient?

    a. Patient shows signs and symptoms of an allergic reaction
    b. Patient requests that you help to administer a prescribed EpiPen
    c. A physician has prescribed epinephrine for this patient
    d. Medical direction has authorized use for this patient

15. Which of the following can cause an allergic reaction?

    a. Lack of sleep
    b. Stress
    c. The flu
    d. Fumes

CASE STUDIES

Allergic Reactions

1

You have been dispatched to assist a 21-year-old male. He suddenly passed out in the car on the way home from the dentist. According to his wife, the patient has an abscessed tooth. He was given an oral antibiotic less than 30 minutes ago. The patient is awake, but very apprehensive. His respirations are 28 per minute. The pulse is weak and thready, with a rate of 118. The blood pressure is 90/74. His skin is flushed and sweaty. You learn the patient has a history of allergies to various medications. His physician has prescribed an EpiPen. You contact medical direction, and they authorize you to assist him with the device.

A. What type of response is this patient exhibiting?

B. What treatment is indicated based on your assessment?

C. Your patient fails to respond to the first dose of epinephrine. He continues to exhibit signs and symptoms of a serious reaction. Are there any additional options for the treatment of the patient with epinephrine?

2

You are called to the home of a 25-year-old female who is complaining of itching. She has a rash covering both legs. Her face is swollen, and the skin is flushed. She is well oriented. The vital signs are RR 12, pulse 90, and BP 116/82. The lungs are clear bilaterally. The patient has numerous minor allergies. She states that she has never had a severe allergic reaction. She tells you that she is wearing jeans just washed in a new brand of detergent.

A. Is this patient having a critical or life-threatening allergic reaction? Justify your answer.

B. When would you consider the use of an epinephrine auto-injector in this patient?

C. Why is the patient's statement regarding her jeans and detergent significant?

3

A couple drives up to the fire station. They just left a restaurant, where the 40-year-old female suddenly began itching all over and complaining of shortness of breath. She is extremely apprehensive. She has RR 27, pulse 100, and BP 100/72. Auscultation of the chest reveals bilateral wheezing. You observe flushed skin and edema about her face. Her eyes are especially swollen. She is complaining of abdominal cramps. You learn that she is allergic to shellfish. She does not have a prescription for epinephrine. Another firefighter gives you his personal EpiPen for her to use.

A. Is the use of an epinephrine auto-injector indicated for this patient? Why?

B. How will you treat this patient?

Stories from the Field
Wrap-Up

Your initial assessment is typical for a patient with a severe allergic reaction. Early recognition of a critical allergic reaction is essential to providing good care. A history of allergic reactions along with difficulty breathing, rapid pulse, rapid breathing, and hives suggest that the reaction may become life threatening. The rapid onset of these critical signs and symptoms is important. As a rule, the more quickly a reaction begins, the more serious it may be.

Before the ambulance arrives, calmly reassure the patient. Provide first aid. Place her in a position of comfort. Be prepared to assist ventilations or perform CPR if necessary. If allowed by protocol, carefully scrape away the bee stingers using a stiff edge. Provide high-flow oxygen by a non-rebreather mask as soon as possible. Complete a SAMPLE history. Ask if the patient has a physician-prescribed epinephrine auto-injector. Consider assisting with its administration. Follow local protocol and medical direction. Begin transport as soon as possible. Remember the potential for airway compromise.

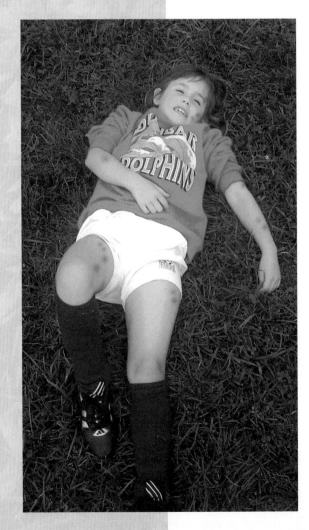

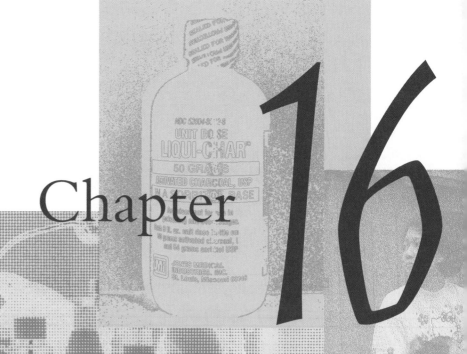

Chapter 16

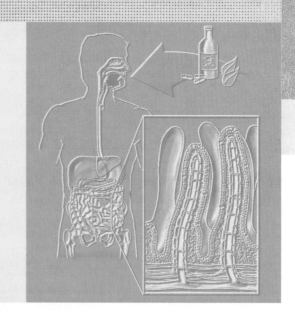

Poisoning
and Overdose

Stories from the Field

Your station receives a call for a child who has been poisoned. You respond to a small apartment complex. A young woman is sitting on a bench outside the maintenance shed with a child on her lap. She identifies herself as the boy's mother. The 4-year-old appears pale and he is drooling. His mother talked with the family doctor, who told her to call 9-1-1. The apartment manager tells you that she has been putting fertilizer, grass seed, and weed killers on the complex grounds today. The shed, which is normally locked, was left open for a few minutes. The manager returned and found the boy sitting inside. The child had opened several pint bottles. She is not sure which ones were opened previously.

The child responds to verbal stimuli. He is not crying. The inside of his mouth is very red and irritated. The boy speaks with some difficulty due to pain. His radial pulse is 140 and thready. The airway is patent and his breathing appears normal. His respiratory rate is 20. The child's skin is cold and moist.

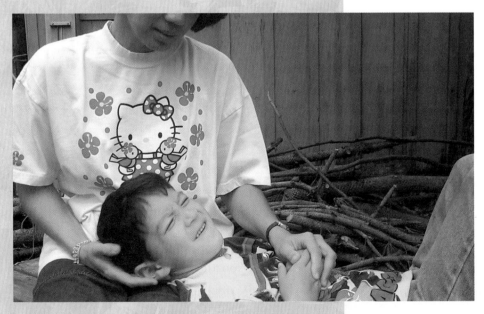

*P*oisoning due to a drug overdose or exposure to a toxic substance is a major nontraumatic cause of death in the United States. Many adults overdose on medications, either accidentally or deliberately. Thousands of children are accidentally poisoned each year. Most poisons are common household products (see Fig. 16.1). EMS providers respond to countless calls for:

• Toddlers who ingest cleaning solutions stored under the kitchen sink

• Drug abusers who are found unconscious

• Depressed teenagers who purposely take an overdose of pills

• Buildings where an unusual odor is making everyone dizzy

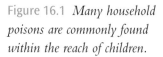

Figure 16.1 *Many household poisons are commonly found within the reach of children.*

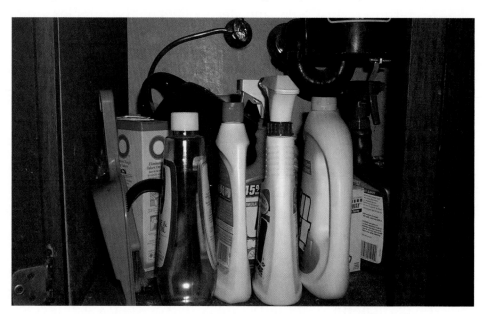

Scene size-up and the SAMPLE history are critical to recognizing a suspected poisoning. With early and appropriate prehospital care, most patients survive and recover. Prehospital treatment for ingested poisons and overdoses often includes administration of activated charcoal.

POISONING AND OVERDOSE

In 1995, poison control centers across the country responded to more than two million calls. Most of these involved accidental ingestion or exposure to toxic material. Seven hundred fatalities were reported. More than 90 percent of the reported exposures occurred in the home. These involved common drugs and household products such as aspirin, barbiturates, insecticides, and cosmetics. More than half of the poisonings occurred in children, making this the fourth most common cause of death in this age group.

There are many causes of poisoning. Preschool children are very curious. They will put any accessible household product or unsecured medication into their mouths. Some adolescents experiment with mind-altering drugs or attempt suicide. Poisoning in adults often results from an intentional drug overdose. In addition, the number of work-related toxic exposure emergencies is increasing. Elderly people may take many medications that can interact dangerously. Drug abusers also mix drugs, and they may inject drugs of unknown strength. Snakes, insects, spiders, and jellyfish can cause poisoning through injection of venom.

D.O.T. OBJECTIVE

List various ways that poisons enter the body.

Characteristics of Poisons

A **poison** is a substance that enters the body and causes illness. It can damage internal structures and interfere with body functions. There are many different kinds of poisons. Poisonous substances can be mineral, vegetable, or animal. They are found as solids, liquids, and gases. Different types of poisons have different effects on the body. It is important to understand some basic properties so that your prehospital care is effective.

Poison | *A food, plant, chemical, or drug that has an adverse effect on the body*

Poisons and toxic substances can enter the body in various ways. These routes of entry are:

• Ingestion (through the mouth)

• Inhalation (breathing)

• Injection (across the skin)

• Contact with or absorption through the skin

Depending on the route of entry, a poison may cause damage to various body systems and require different types of treatment.

Some poisons affect the body immediately, while others act more slowly. Symptoms that develop quickly suggest a serious case of poisoning. Most drugs or toxic chemicals produce symptoms within four hours. The presence of food in the stomach may delay onset of the symptoms. Some poisons cause local effects, such as a rash on the skin. Others affect entire body systems. Poisonings that affect the internal organs or central nervous system can be life threatening.

Most substances, including household products and medications, can be lethal if taken in sufficient quantity. Certain poisons, such as cyanide, are so toxic that even a small amount is harmful. Others, such as pesticide sprays, are cumulative poisons. They require long-term exposure before affecting a person's health. Poisons can also be carcinogenic, causing cancer to develop years after the exposure.

Initial Assessment

Toxin | *A substance that is poisonous to cells or tissues*

When arriving at the scene of a suspected poisoning or overdose, pay attention to scene safety. The same **toxin** may present a danger to you and your crew. Remember the possibility of poisoning if you respond to a multiple casualty incident where trauma is not involved. When several patients complain of similar medical symptoms, suspect some form of poison in the food, air, or water. If you suspect an overdose or illicit drug use, ensure that it is safe to enter the scene. Plan to withdraw if the patient becomes violent or combative. Do not reenter until law enforcement or additional help arrives. Others at the scene may also be under the influence of drugs or alcohol. Approach scenes of this nature with extreme caution.

EMT Tip

If the airway is unstable due to swelling or irritation from a toxic exposure, endotracheal intubation may be useful. See Appendix A, which discusses advanced airway management. Check local protocol.

Form your general impression of the patient. How ill does he or she appear? Is the patient awake, disoriented, or unconscious? Try to determine the route of entry of the poison during your initial assessment. For all types of poisoning, assess the patient's airway, breathing, circulation, and mental status. Be prepared to provide critical interventions.

1. Open the airway using the head-tilt/chin-lift or jaw-thrust maneuver.

2. Consider use of an oropharyngeal or a nasopharyngeal airway adjunct. Suction as needed.

3. If breathing is shallow or absent, assist ventilations with a bag-valve mask and supplemental oxygen. You may also use the FROPVD.

4. If breathing is adequate but the patient is not fully alert (as assessed by AVPU), provide 100 percent oxygen via non-rebreather mask.

5. Assess the circulation based on the pulse and the skin color, temperature, and condition. Look for signs of shock, such as tachycardia and hypotension.

6. Intervene in life-threatening problems as they are identified. A patient's condition may deteriorate quickly, so continually reassess him or her.

7. Evaluate the patient for transport priority.

Complete a focused history and physical examination and SAMPLE history. Check baseline vital signs. Examine any areas affected by the poison. If the patient is unresponsive, complete a rapid medical assessment. Try to obtain the following information in order to determine which treatments to use:

- What substance was involved?
- How long ago was the exposure?
- How much of the substance was involved?
- Was the substance taken all at once or over a period of time?
- Has anyone tried to treat the poisoning? If so, what was done? Has anyone tried to induce vomiting or given an **antidote**?
- Is the patient experiencing any effects from the poisoning? If so, what? The most common effects of poisoning are nausea and vomiting.

Medical Direction and Poison Control. It can be helpful for patient care to know information about a specific poison. Poison control centers maintain current information about many chemical compounds and their effects on the body. They provide advice on treating overdoses and poisonings. Local protocols may direct you to contact the poison control center directly for assistance. In some areas, EMS responders contact medical direction for information about poisoning. If you suspect a poisoning or overdose, do not delay transport to obtain this information. While en route, notify the receiving facility of the patient's history and condition. This is important so that appropriate treatment can begin immediately upon arrival.

INGESTED POISONS

Ingested poisons are toxic substances that enter the body through swallowing. This is the most common route of poisoning. These poisons are absorbed through the stomach or intestinal linings, where they enter the bloodstream (see Fig. 16.2). Some ingested poisons injure the gastrointestinal tract as they pass through each organ. Others affect specific organs and tissues. Some affect the entire body.

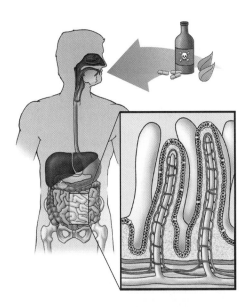

EMT Tip

Try to get the correct spelling of the poison. Many products have similar names.

Antidote | An agent that blocks or reverses the effect of a poison

Ingested Poison | A liquid or solid toxic substance that is swallowed

Figure 16.2 *Ingested poisons enter the bloodstream through the capillaries in the intestinal lining.*

EMT Tip

A patient who has overdosed may be temporarily mentally incompetent. Be very cautious if he or she refuses treatment. The person may not be capable of making a rational decision.

Most drug overdoses are ingested. Unintentional overdoses may occur when people take prescription drugs improperly. Occasionally, prescriptions are mixed with other drugs, such as alcohol. An overdose may also be due to attempted suicide. For example, physicians frequently prescribe barbiturates as sedatives. These drugs are a common source of both accidental and intentional overdose. The situation can be serious if barbiturates interact with some other drugs, including alcohol. Patients with acute barbiturate overdose may become agitated or nauseated. They may fall into a deep sleep, with shallow breathing. Over time, breathing becomes more shallow. This may be followed by unconsciousness, respiratory arrest, heart failure, and death.

> **D.O.T. OBJECTIVE**
>
> List signs/symptoms associated with poisoning.

Assessment of Ingestion Poisonings

For a suspected case of ingested poison or overdose, look for open containers, empty pill bottles, chewed-up plants, evidence of violence, or a suicide note. Try to find out what substance was taken. This will help medical direction to determine whether activated charcoal is indicated. If it is, knowing the patient's weight is helpful for calculating the dosage. Table 16.1 lists some commonly ingested poisons.

If possible, estimate the amount ingested. Parents may describe amounts in swallows. For young children, estimate a swallow to be about one teaspoonful, or 5 milliliters. In this chapter's Story from the Field, several empty pint bottles of weed killer and fertilizer were found. In this case, you may be able to compare the amount left in a bottle with the last known quantity.

Table 16.1 • **COMMONLY INGESTED POISONS**

Substance	Examples
Prescription Medications	Antidepressants, cardiac medications, sedatives
Nonprescripton Medications	Aspirin, vitamins with iron, cold medications, pain relievers
Alcohols	Alcoholic beverages, rubbing alcohol, grain alcohol
Other	Household cleaning supplies, automotive supplies, insecticides, mothballs, toiletries, plants, contaminated food

Signs and Symptoms of Ingestion Poisoning

Some common signs and symptoms of ingested poisons are:

- Nausea
- Vomiting
- Diarrhea
- Abdominal pain
- History of ingestion
- Chemical burns around the mouth
- Unusual breath odors
- Altered mental status
- Respiratory distress
- Altered heart rate
- Altered blood pressure
- Abdominal tenderness

EMT Tip

A patient who is using illicit drugs such as cocaine or amphetamines may experience medical problems such as a heart attack or stroke.

D.O.T. OBJECTIVES

Describe the steps in the emergency medical care for the patient with suspected poisoning.

Discuss the emergency medical care for the patient with possible overdose.

Emergency Medical Care: Ingested Poison

Follow these steps for the emergency medical treatment of a patient who has ingested a toxic substance or overdosed on drugs:

1. Complete the scene size-up. Perform an initial assessment.

2. Manage the airway and breathing. Suction excess secretions and remove any material from the patient's mouth, such as pills, tablets, or fragments. Remove larger particles with a gloved hand. Place the patient in the recovery position. Provide oxygen and assisted artificial ventilation, if necessary. Avoid mouth-to-mouth ventilation, because the poisonous substance may be on the lips, in the airway, or in the vomitus.

3. Complete a focused history and physical examination and obtain the SAMPLE history. Check baseline vital signs. Examine affected areas such as the mouth. If the patient is unresponsive, complete a rapid medical assessment.

4. Consult medical direction. You may be instructed to administer activated charcoal (discussed in the following section).

5. Complete a detailed assessment while en route to the receiving facility.

6. Continue ongoing assessments. Monitor the airway and breathing carefully. Reassess every 5 minutes in critical patients, every 15 minutes in others.

7. Whenever possible, bring the container of a suspected poison to the hospital. Carrying the container may not be appropriate if the substance is toxic. If safe, remove the label and note the original volume of the container. Estimate the amount remaining. If you are certain that the item is not hazardous, bring the container to the hospital. Check with poison control or medical direction to ensure this is safe. Allow the hospital time to prepare for your arrival.

D.O.T. OBJECTIVE

State the generic and trade names, indications, contra-indications, medication form, dose, administration, actions, side effects, and reassessment strategies for activated charcoal.

Activated Charcoal

Activated Charcoal | *Substance that hinders the absorption of ingested poisons and enhances their elimination from the body, preventing further damage*

Activated charcoal is the preferred treatment for ingested poison (see Fig. 16.3 and Table 16.2). Charcoal binds to poison so it cannot be absorbed. After binding, charcoal promotes elimination of the poison from the body. This reduces the risk of additional injury. Activated charcoal can absorb many times its weight in chemicals. It is most effective if given shortly after ingestion.

To administer activated charcoal, do the following:

1. If required, consult with medical direction. Obtain an order to administer charcoal and the correct dosage.

2. Shake the container to mix the charcoal thoroughly in the water. If it is too thick to shake, remove the cap. Stir until it is well mixed.

3. Activated charcoal looks like black mud. You may need to persuade the patient to drink it. Offering it through a straw from an opaque container will disguise the appearance.

4. If the charcoal suspension settles, shake the bottle. Offer it to the patient again.

5. Record the dose, the time of administration, and the patient's response.

6. Dispose of the charcoal container and equipment correctly.

7. Be prepared for vomiting after administering activated charcoal. If the patient vomits after drinking it, contact medical direction for an order to repeat the dose.

8. Transport the patient sitting up or in the recovery position to prevent aspiration. Have suction available. Reassess vital signs and mental status frequently. Monitor for signs of deterioration.

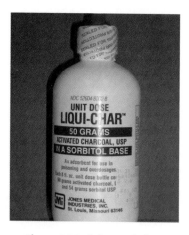

Figure 16.3 *Most ambulances are stocked with activated charcoal.*

Table 16.2 • ACTIVATED CHARCOAL

Characteristic	Description
Names	Generic Name: Activated charcoal, USP Trade Names: SuperChar™, InstaChar™, Actidose™, LiquiChar™
Indications	The patient shows signs and symptoms of an ingested poison Medical direction has authorized use for this patient
Contraindications	The patient has an altered mental status The patient has swallowed strong alkalis, acids, or caustics The patient is unable to swallow
Actions	Binds to certain chemicals and poisons and prevents them from being absorbed into the body
Dosage	Generally 1 gram per kilogram of body weight. Typical adult dose is 25–50 g; child dose is 12.5–25g. Note: different brands may bind different amounts of poison per gram. Consult medical direction for correct brand and dosage.
Form and Route	Black powder to be suspended in water and given orally. Frequently available in a plastic bottle containing 12.5 g activated charcoal in water.
Side Effects	Nausea and vomiting Black stools

INHALED POISONS

Inhaled poisons are introduced into the body through respiration. They can be in the form of gases, fumes, vapors, droplets, and sprays. These vapors and fumes are quickly absorbed into the bloodstream (see Fig. 16.4). Some gases irritate the pulmonary passages. This causes extensive edema and destroys tissue. Some inhaled poisons interfere with life-sustaining processes. For example, they may prevent red blood cells from transporting oxygen. Others interfere with the ability to use oxygen.

Inhaled Poison | *A toxic substance such as a gas, fumes, vapor, or spray that is breathed in*

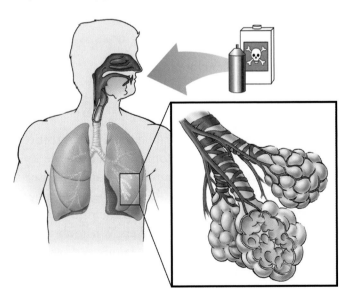

Figure 16.4 *Inhaled poisons enter the bloodstream through the capillaries in the linings of the lungs.*

Suspect the presence of toxins in any oxygen-depleted atmosphere. Some inhaled poisons are colorless or odorless so you will not be able to see or smell the substances. Some poisons, such as natural gas, have color or odor added so they can be detected readily. Common inhaled poisons include:

- Carbon monoxide
- Chlorine gas
- Freon
- Sulfur dioxide
- Ammonia
- Methylene chloride
- Hydrogen sulfide
- Hydrogen cyanide
- Nitrous oxide

EMT Alert

If toxic fumes are suspected, park your vehicle uphill and upwind of the site. To enter a site with hazardous materials, you must be specially trained and have appropriate protective equipment.

Fires are a major source of inhalation poisoning. Inhaled poisons may be used as a weapon by terrorists. Common scenes of inhalation poisoning are:

- Spills, leaks, or fires involving vehicles carrying chemicals
- Confined spaces, such as sewers, wells, and silos
- Buildings on fire
- Gases in mining, oil drilling, and similar industries

Carbon monoxide (CO) is one of the most common poisonous gases. It is an odorless, tasteless gas produced by incomplete combustion. It combines with hemoglobin much more readily than oxygen. Therefore, the blood carries less and less oxygen to the body tissues. This results in cellular hypoxia. Overexposure can be fatal. Carbon monoxide poisoning may be seen in:

- Failed heating or ventilation systems in homes or other buildings
- Inadequately ventilated areas where kerosene space heaters are used
- Cars with faulty exhaust systems
- Vehicles that are left running in enclosed spaces

Assessment of Inhalation Poisonings

Enter the scene cautiously. Note any unusual odors. Wear protective gear in the presence of known chemical hazards. Call for additional emergency services, such as the HAZ-MAT team. Count the number of patients. Suspect a toxic substance if more than one person is unconscious at the same time. For example, a family may be overcome by carbon monoxide in their home. In rural areas, toxic fumes in a silo may overcome several workers. Whatever the situation, do not become a victim. You must rely on dispatch, family, and bystanders to provide clues to events leading to your arrival and the nature of the emergency.

During the initial assessment, observe the patient's airway and breathing. Determine the patient's priority for transport. During the focused history and physical examination, obtain a SAMPLE history. Include the following questions:

- Was the patient in a confined or low-oxygen space during the toxic exposure?
- Does the patient have a history that might suggest a suicide attempt?

Signs and Symptoms of Inhalation Poisoning

The signs and symptoms of inhaled poisons are:

- History of inhalation of toxic substance
- Cough
- Difficulty breathing
- Hoarseness
- Shortness of breath
- Wheezing
- Nausea or vomiting
- Singed nasal hair
- Headache
- Cyanosis
- Chest pain
- Abnormal respiratory rate
- Dizziness
- Confusion
- Seizures
- Altered mental status
- Unresponsiveness
- Cherry red color

The signs and symptoms of carbon monoxide poisoning are:

- Headache
- Dizziness
- Yawning
- Fainting
- Weakness
- Bright, cherry red color (a late sign of significant exposure)
- Lips and ear lobes appear bluish
- Nausea and/or vomiting

Emergency Medical Care: Inhaled Poison

Follow these steps for the emergency medical treatment of a patient who has inhaled a toxic substance:

1. Complete the scene size-up. Have trained rescuers remove the patient from the source of exposure to fresh air and a safe location as quickly as possible. Minimizing exposure and absorption will improve the patient's chances for survival.

2. Complete an initial assessment. Maintain the airway. Provide oxygen and assisted artificial ventilation, if necessary.

3. Complete a focused history and physical examination and SAMPLE history. Check baseline vital signs. Examine affected areas such as the nose and mouth. If the patient is unresponsive, complete a rapid medical assessment.

4. Even if the patient is without symptoms, encourage him or her to be transported to the hospital for evaluation. Bring any containers, bottles, or labels of poisonous agents to the receiving facility. Complete a detailed assessment while en route.

5. Continue ongoing assessment. Monitor the airway and breathing carefully. Reassess every 5 minutes in critical patients, every 15 minutes in others.

Injected Poison | *A toxic substance that enters the body through a puncture in the skin; injection may be by needle, animal bite, or insect sting*

INJECTED POISONINGS

Injected poisons enter the body through punctures in the skin. This can occur from needle injections, animal bites, and insect stings. When injected directly into the bloodstream, a poison takes effect very quickly (see Fig. 16.5).

Figure 16.5 *Injected poisons may enter the bloodstream directly through a puncture into a blood vessel.*

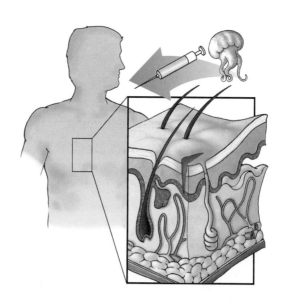

Assessment of Injection Poisonings

If the patient is outdoors, look for sources of a bite or sting during the scene size-up. Poisonous bites and stings are discussed further in Chapter 17. Also recall that an allergic reaction to a nonpoisonous insect bite or drug may cause anaphylactic shock (review Chapter 15). If you suspect illicit drug use or overdose, look for syringes and other drug paraphernalia. As you gather the history, ask:

- Has the patient been bitten by anything, especially a snake or marine animal?
- Does the patient have a history of illicit drug use?
- How much time has lapsed since the injection and the onset of symptoms?
- Is the patient allergic to any insects?

Signs and Symptoms of Injection Poisoning

The signs and symptoms of injected poisoning are:

- Weakness
- Dizziness
- Chills
- Fever
- Nausea
- Vomiting
- High or low blood pressure
- Abnormal pupillary response
- Needle marks
- Rapid or shallow respiration rate
- Skin reaction at the injection site
- Breathing difficulty

Emergency Medical Care: Injected Poison

Follow these steps for the emergency medical treatment of a patient who has injected a toxic substance:

1. Complete the scene size-up. Complete an initial assessment.
2. Maintain the airway. Suction as needed. Place the patient in the recovery position. Provide oxygen and assisted artificial ventilation, if necessary.
3. Complete a focused history and physical examination and SAMPLE history. Obtain baseline vital signs. Examine affected areas. If the patient is unresponsive, complete a rapid medical assessment. Collect any containers or bottles and bring to the receiving facility.

4. Complete a detailed assessment, usually while en route to the receiving facility.

5. Continue ongoing assessments. Monitor the airway and breathing carefully. Reassess every 5 minutes in critical patients, every 15 minutes in others.

ABSORBED AND CONTACT POISONS

Absorbed Poison | *A toxic substance taken into the body across unbroken skin or mucous membranes*

Absorbed poisons enter the bloodstream through the skin (see Fig. 16.6). They can be absorbed directly across intact skin or through a cut or scrape. They may affect the entire body or target certain organs. Substances from poisonous plants in the environment can be absorbed. Gases, fumes, mists, and liquids may also be absorbed.

Figure 16.6 *Absorbed poisons enter the bloodstream through capillaries in the skin. Contact poisons may only cause local irritation.*

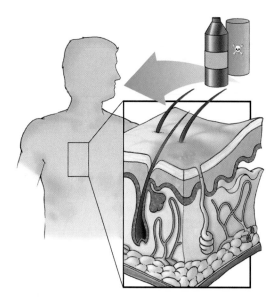

Contact poisons are usually corrosive or caustic chemicals. They cause poisoning or irritation of the skin upon contact. Localized poisons cause irritation and inflammation. This gradually worsens after exposure. Underlying tissues may also be affected.

Assessment of Absorption Poisonings

During scene size-up, note any open containers of liquid or powder. Wear protective gear and avoid contact with the suspected poison. If the call involves a potential hazardous exposure and you are not trained in managing hazardous materials or do not have the necessary equipment, request immediate assistance from the local HAZ-MAT team.

Signs and Symptoms of Absorption Poisoning

The signs and symptoms of absorbed or contact poisonings are:

- History of exposure
- Liquid or powder on patient's skin
- Burns
- Itching
- Irritation
- Redness

Emergency Medical Care: Absorbed Poison

Follow these steps for the emergency medical treatment of a patient who has been poisoned through skin absorption or contact:

1. Complete the scene size-up. The patient should be removed from a contaminated area as soon as possible by professional rescuers.

2. If the patient is contaminated and protocol allows, decontaminate him or her before beginning care. **Decontamination** ensures that others are not accidentally exposed to the toxic agent. Remove contaminated clothing and jewelry. If the substance is a dry powder, brush it off the patient. Then flush the skin with clean water. If the toxic substance is a liquid, begin flushing the affected area with clean water. Continue flushing with water for at least 20 minutes while you assess the patient. For eye splashes, irrigate the affected eye with clean water for at least 20 minutes. Whenever an affected area requires irrigation, continue irrigation while en route to the hospital, if possible.

   Decontamination | *The removal or cleansing of dangerous chemicals and other dangerous or infectious materials*

3. Complete an initial assessment. Maintain the airway. Provide oxygen and assisted artificial ventilation, if necessary.

4. Complete a focused history and physical examination and SAMPLE history. Check baseline vital signs. Examine affected areas. If the patient is unresponsive, complete a rapid medical assessment.

5. Complete a detailed assessment while en route to the receiving facility.

6. Continue ongoing assessments. Monitor airway and breathing carefully. Reassess every 5 minutes in critical patients, every 15 minutes in others.

Chapter Sixteen Summary

- Poisons may enter the body by ingestion, inhalation, absorption, or injection. Poisoning is common in young children.

- Your safety is always a top priority. Never expose yourself to toxic or poisonous substances in an attempt to rescue the patient. Before transporting any potentially hazardous substance, verify that doing so is safe.

- Always record the name of the suspected poison, if known. Record the route of exposure, the quantity of poison that entered the body, the time period in which the exposure occurred, and any interventions done before you arrived.

- Contact medical direction or poison control early so that poison-specific treatment can begin as soon as possible.

- Activated charcoal can be administered in cases of ingested poison. Activated charcoal binds to certain poisons. This prevents the body from absorbing them. Knowing the patient's weight is important to determine the dosage of activated charcoal. Never administer activated charcoal to patients with an altered mental status, those who have ingested strong alkalis or acids, or patients who are unable to swallow.

Key Terms Review

Absorbed Poison | *page 476*
Activated Charcoal | *page 470*
Antidote | *page 467*

Decontamination | *page 477*
Ingested Poison | *page 467*
Inhaled Poison | *page 471*

Injected Poison | *page 474*
Poison | *page 465*
Toxin | *page 466*

Review Questions

1. The first thing to do when arriving at the scene of an inhalation poisoning is:

   a. Provide high-flow oxygen by non-breather mask
   b. Allow trained rescuers to remove patient from the toxic environment
   c. Obtain a SAMPLE history
   d. Check for a pulse

2. The most important step in any poisoning is:

   a. Bringing the substance to the hospital with you
   b. Ensuring scene safety
   c. Maintaing the airway
   d. Administering activated charcoal

3. All of the following are common signs and symptoms of an ingested poison, EXCEPT:

   a. Vomiting
   b. Abdominal pain
   c. Burns on the back
   d. Altered mental status

4. The most common route for poisons to enter the body is:

   a. Inhalation
   b. Injection
   c. Ingestion
   d. Absorption

5. You are treating a patient who was attacked by a jellyfish. Her leg is swollen and the skin is red with blisters. How did the toxin enter her body?

   a. Ingestion
   b. Inhalation
   c. Absorption
   d. Injection

6. You respond to a 22-year-old male patient who is found on the floor in a supine position. Bystanders state that he took many "ludes" and drank a lot of "Crow." Your first step in treating this patient is:

   a. Check the patient's pupils
   b. Look for evidence of drug ingestion
   c. Clear and maintain an airway
   d. Administer activated charcoal

7. The first step in the management of an absorption poisoning is:

   a. Remove the patient from the contaminated area
   b. Irrigate the skin with water
   c. Protect yourself from exposure
   d. Brush the substance off the skin as rapidly as possible

8. You are called to a residence for a patient in respiratory distress. You find a group of teenagers in the garage. They state that they were getting high from spray paint cans. Your patient has paint on his face and hand. How did the toxin probably enter his body?

   a. Ingestion
   b. Inhalation
   c. Absorption
   d. Injection

9. You are ordered to administer activated charcoal at a dose of 1 gram per kilogram to a patient who has ingested an overdose of Valium. Your patient weighs 120 pounds. What is the proper dose to administer?

   a. 55 grams
   b. 55 milligrams
   c. 25 grams
   d. 25 milligrams

10. Activated charcoal is most effective if given:

    a. Within 24 hours of ingestion
    b. Within 12 hours of ingestion
    c. Over a 48-hour period
    d. Within 1 hour of ingestion

11. You are called to a residence for a 15-year-old male who has taken a large number of barbiturates. He was drinking alcohol for several hours. There is a strong alcohol smell on his breath. He staggers up to greet you. He says he is not certain how many pills he took. Your partner suggests that you administer activated charcoal. You decide that:

    a. Activated charcoal is indicated for this patient
    b. Activated charcoal is indicated, but patients under 18 cannot have charcoal so you cannot administer the drug
    c. You need to know the exact dose of the barbiturates ingested in order to use charcoal
    d. Charcoal is contraindicated for this patient because of his altered mental status

12. What ensures that a patient does not expose caregivers to a hazardous material?

    a. Recognition
    b. Preparation
    c. Decontamination
    d. Isolation

13. When can an EMT bring a suspected poison's container to the hospital with the patient?

    a. When the patient gives permission to transport the container
    b. When the substance has been identified by law enforcement
    c. When the medical director has issued a protocol for transportation
    d. When you are absolutely certain the substance does not present a hazard

CASE STUDIES

Poisoning and Overdose

1

You are called to the home of a 35-year-old, 160-pound female. She was overcome by fumes while cleaning the basement. She is awake and oriented. Her skin is flushed. Her respirations are 14, her pulse is bounding at 100 beats per minute, and her blood pressure is 140/64. The lungs are clear bilaterally. She has a history of allergies and asthma.

A. What is your first concern at this emergency scene?

B. What route(s) of exposure did the patient experience?

C. What should your treatment of the patient include, once a safe environment for care has been established?

2

You are dispatched to an apartment complex in the afternoon. The landlord observed a resident lying supine on the apartment floor through the patio window. The door is locked when you arrive. You can see a young man who appears to be unconscious. The landlord tells you that he lives alone. Concerned about scene safety, you notify law enforcement and await their arrival. When the officer arrives, you enter and find a brief suicide note. Several empty bottles of prescription sleeping pills are on the floor. Your initial assessment reveals a patient who is breathing at 4 to 6 respirations per minute.

A. What are your treatment priorities?

B. Should you consider the use of activated charcoal in this patient? Why or why not?

3

You are dispatched to a housing development in a rural part of your service area. The caller states that a small child has swallowed medication. Upon your arrival, you find a frantic mother carrying her 6-year-old daughter. The child is awake and oriented. Your initial assessment reveals no life-threatening injuries. The mother hands you a package of over-the-counter laxatives. She tells you that the child has taken at least five of them. The focused history and physical examination reveals no acute illness or injury. The child has no significant past medical history. Baseline vitals show a pulse of 90, a respiratory rate of 22, and blood pressure of 102/60. Her pupils are equal and reactive. The skin is pink, cool, and dry. The child tells you that she thought the medication was candy.

A. What is the route of exposure in this case?

B. How will you treat this patient?

C. After beginning the administration of activated charcoal, the child begins to vomit. Her respiratory rate slows dramatically. What should you do?

Stories from the Field
Wrap-Up

Rapid intervention and transport, with assistance from medical direction and poison control, are key to preventing deaths from overdose and poisoning. This child's pulse is thready and his skin signs are poor. His mouth is irritated, so the tissues might swell and compromise his airway. The child should be transported immediately. Obtain a complete history and try to identify the ingested substances with some certainty.

The chemicals in the shed are common and not usually hazardous if stored correctly. Therefore, bringing the containers with you to the hospital is appropriate. Follow local protocol. Notify medical direction of the patient's history and current condition. This allows time for them to contact poison control before your arrival. The use of activated charcoal is contraindicated in this patient.

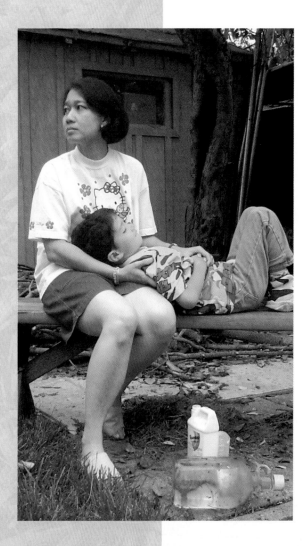

Chapter 17

Environmental Emergencies

Stories from the Field

Your shift at the fire department is scheduled on an unusually cool spring day. Although the weather has been beautiful for a week, it has been rainy and cool for the last 24 hours. You are dispatched to an unknown medical emergency in an alley behind a local bar. Because of the location and the nature of the call, law enforcement has also been dispatched. A police officer advises that the scene is safe. He states the patient is a middle-aged male who is breathing, but does not respond to questions.

The police officer escorts you to the patient. You find him sitting in the alley, leaning against a wall. You detect a strong odor of alcohol as you approach. During your assessment, the patient barely responds to painful stimuli. His airway is open. His breathing is slow and shallow. His pulse is 56. His skin is pale and cold to touch. You find no evidence of traumatic injury. Bystanders and bar patrons tell you that the patient frequently sleeps in the alley. No one knows his identity or medical history. He was last seen leaving the bar early the evening before.

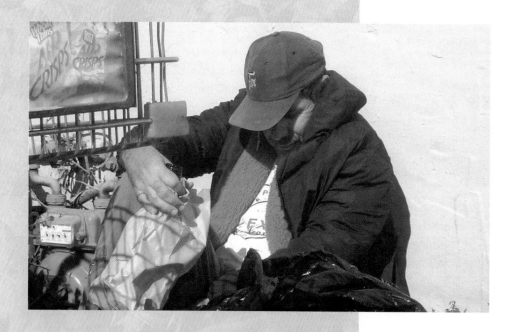

*E*nvironmental emergencies are illnesses and injuries that result from exposure to various conditions found outdoors. Some of the emergencies EMT-Basics may respond to include:

- The effects of exposure to heat or cold
- Water emergencies (drowning or near drowning)
- Bites or stings from insects or wildlife

Figure 17.1 *In the mountains, patients are subject to cold injuries, bites, and stings.*

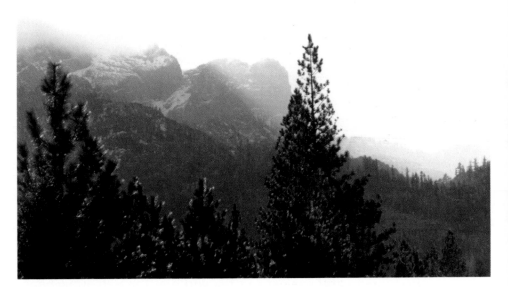

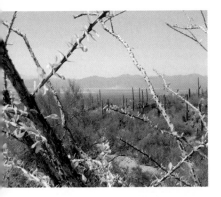

Figure 17.2 *Water emergencies, marine animal bites, and hypothermia are seen in coastal regions.*

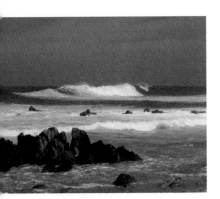

Figure 17.3 *Desert regions can cause heat emergencies, bites, and stings.*

Nature presents a multitude of environments that require emergency responses. These vary according to geographical locations. Locations range from mountains to oceans to deserts—and everywhere in between (see Figs. 17.1, 17.2, and 17.3). The type of environmental emergencies you will deal with depends upon where you practice. The climate affects the incidences of cold- and heat-related emergencies. Localized cold injuries like frostbite can range from superficial to deep. Generalized hypothermia involves the entire body and may cause death. You may also be called upon to assess and manage cases of hyperthermia. If you work in a coastal region or near bodies of water, you will probably see more near drownings and other water sport emergencies than you would in mountainous or desert regions. Marine animal bites and stings may be more common outside urban areas. However, you might be called to manage and treat insect stings almost anywhere in the country. Become familiar with the type of environmental emergencies you can expect in your area.

D.O.T. OBJECTIVE

Describe the various ways that the body loses heat.

EXPOSURE TO COLD OR HEAT

The human body can tolerate only slight changes in its core temperature. It quickly attempts to compensate for excessive heat loss or gain. Temperature regulation is an effective mechanism under most conditions. However, body temperature can be changed by environmental conditions. Medical problems combined with environmental causes can cause heat- or cold-related illnesses. Body temperature becomes an EMS concern when a person's core temperature rises or falls outside the normal range.

Hypothermia is a state in which body temperature is too low. It occurs when more heat is lost than the body can gain or produce. **Hyperthermia** is a condition in which the body temperature is too high. It occurs when excessive heat overwhelms the body's protective mechanisms so they cannot cool the person. Both conditions can cause serious health problems. The severity of a heat- or cold-related emergency is influenced by:

Hypothermia | *Abnormally low core body temperature*

Hyperthermia | *Abnormally high core body temperature*

• The exposure time

• The environment in which the exposure occurred

• Various preexisting conditions

• Post-rescue management procedures

Heat is produced by the normal metabolic processes of the body, such as muscle contraction. The body has several protective mechanisms for removing the heat to maintain its core temperature. One of these is the process of breathing. Upon inhalation, air in the lungs is replaced with cold air from the environment. The body warms this air. This cycle of exhaling warm air, then inhaling and warming colder air leads to loss of body heat. Understanding how body heat is lost will help you to prevent further heat loss in an ill or injured patient. There are four basic mechanisms for transferring heat. They are:

Conduction | *Transfer of heat from a warmer object in contact with a colder object*

Convection | *Transfer of heat from a warm object to cooler air moving past its surface*

• **Conduction**

• **Convection**

• **Evaporation**

Evaporation | *The process of converting a liquid to a gas in which heat is lost*

• **Radiation**

Table 17.1 describes how these mechanisms remove heat from the body.

Radiation | *Heat released by an object into the surrounding air as waves of infrared radiation*

Table 17.1 • HEAT LOSS FROM THE BODY

Mechanism	Description	Example
Conduction	The loss of heat that occurs when the body contacts a colder object	A person who is lying on cold ground or submerged in water
Convection	Similar to conduction, but occurs due to air that moves across the surface of the body	A person who is exposed to strong, cold wind for a long period of time
Evaporation	Body heat provides the energy required to convert water on the surface of the body from a liquid to a gas	Water evaporating from the skin when a person is wet or sweating
Radiation	Body heat that is released into the air as infrared radiation; similar to the heat given off by a lightbulb	A person who has been in freezing temperatures without a coat
Breathing	Cool air that is inhaled becomes warmed by the body, then is exhaled	Breathing cold air for a long time while outdoors on a winter day

Patient Assessment

If you suspect a patient has a temperature-related emergency, you must assess the severity of the exposure and the health risk. You do this during your focused history and physical exam. Besides the standard SAMPLE history questions, ask:

- What was the source of the exposure? Was the temperature more extreme than the individual could tolerate?

- In what environment was the patient found? Was the patient immersed in snow or water?

- Is the patient conscious? How long has he or she been unconscious? Is the mental status changing? Unconsciousness is usually a grave sign, requiring immediate care and transport.

- Is the effect of the exposure localized or general (systemic)?

- How well was the patient protected against the exposure? Does he or she have injuries or illnesses that could aggravate the effects of exposure?

- Was anything done to treat the patient's condition before you arrived?

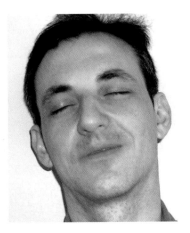

Figure 17.4 *Generalized hypothermia.*

COLD-RELATED EMERGENCIES

A person exposed to a cold environment may develop generalized hypothermia (see Fig. 17.4). Generalized hypothermia involves the entire body. Direct exposure of body tissues to extreme cold can also cause localized injuries. These injuries commonly occur on the face, ears, and extremities. You must quickly recognize the stages of hypothermia and provide prompt, appropriate care.

Cold-related emergencies are often seen among certain groups of people. For example, hunters, sailors, skiers, climbers, swimmers, and military personnel are at high risk of cold-related emergencies. Their activities often take place in cold, remote wilderness settings. If a cold-related emergency occurs, these geographical locations can cause a delay in obtaining emergency care. However, the greatest number of cold-related emergencies occurs in urban settings. Urban hypothermia is a major problem in some cities, like Chicago and New York. These cases often involve elderly persons who are homebound or people without adequate shelter.

Generalized Hypothermia

The likelihood of a person developing hypothermia and the severity of his or her condition can be influenced by predisposing factors. These are related to the patient's age and health and the environmental conditions.

Environmental Conditions

The severity of hypothermia is affected by the **ambient temperature**, the **wind chill**, and the patient's clothing. The head is the greatest area of heat loss in the body. Being outside in cold weather without a hat quickly lowers body temperature by convection. Conduction reduces body heat more effectively than convection. Therefore, a body immersed in water loses heat 25 times more rapidly than in air. A person who has been immersed in water is far more likely to suffer from hypothermia (see Fig. 17.5).

Ambient Temperature | The air temperature surrounding the patient

Wind Chill | The combined cooling effect of wind speed and ambient temperature

Suspect hypothermia whenever you believe a patient has been exposed to the cold. Common situations include:

- Obvious prolonged exposure to cold weather
- Someone who has been outdoors in low temperatures without a hat
- Immersion in water
- Cold exposure after a motor vehicle accident
- Someone in a home with little or no heat, particularly if elderly

Patient's Age

Age is a predisposing factor for hypothermia. Older persons have a much lower percentage of body fat and muscle mass than younger adults have. Because body fat and muscle are natural insulators, their risk of hypothermia is greater. The lower amount of muscle mass decreases their ability to stay warm.

The very young also have proportionally less body fat and muscle mass than adults. In addition, children have more body surface compared with their weight. The extra surface area means a child is not well protected from the effects of cold. Children too young to dress themselves cannot put on extra clothing when exposed to cold, compounding the problem.

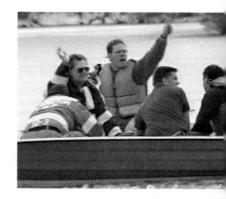

Figure 17.5 *Time is critical once rescuers retrieve a patient submerged in cold water. Urgent signals to onshore rescuers alert them to prepare for immediate transport.*

Medical Conditions

Certain factors can exaggerate the severity of hypothermia. These include:

- Underlying illnesses and chronic medical problems
- Overdose or poisoning
- Severe trauma
- Intoxication or ingestion of large quantities of alcohol
- Outdoors resuscitation attempts

With some medical conditions, the body cannot produce enough heat. For example, shock or poisoning can cause hypothermia. Following are descriptions of illnesses and injuries that can predispose a patient to hypothermia. These conditions aggravate the effects of environmental exposure.

Shock. If perfusion is inadequate, delivery of nutrients and oxygen to the tissues is reduced. This interferes with cell functions. Patients in shock cannot generate heat internally, so they develop hypothermia quickly.

Generalized Infection. Infection causes surface blood vessels to enlarge abnormally. When this happens, heat from the body's core is lost to the environment. Infection may also cause fever, which can lead to hyperthermia.

Diabetes or Hypoglycemia. Hypoglycemia, or low blood sugar, occurs in diabetics. Without sufficient fuel, shivering may be inadequate for producing heat. This exaggerates the effects of hypothermia.

Drugs and Poisons. Drugs and poisons accelerate the effects of hypothermia. These substances interfere with the body's ability to manage cold. Some drugs slow the heartbeat. This reduces the amount of warm blood circulating in the body. Other drugs and poisons short-circuit the thermoregulatory center. They interfere with the body's ability to regulate temperature. Drugs and poisons that dilate blood vessels speed the loss of body heat. Drugs may also alter the mental status. A patient may not realize that he or she is being exposed to extreme cold. He or she may lack the judgment to seek shelter.

Head Injuries. The thermoregulatory center in the brain senses and controls temperature. Head injuries can damage this part of the brain.

Spinal Cord Injuries. The nervous system controls dilation of the walls of blood vessels. Spinal cord injuries can injure the area that controls blood vessels. The blood quickly dissipates heat to the environment through radiation and convection.

Burns. Burns are soft tissue injuries that strip away the body's insulation. The epidermis and dermis help to retain heat. The fluid loss and evaporation that occur after major burns can contribute to hypothermia.

D.O.T. OBJECTIVE

List the signs and symptoms of exposure to cold.

Signs and Symptoms of Hypothermia

Generalized hypothermia begins with moderate signs and symptoms. If the body temperature remains low, the condition becomes more serious and will lead to death. Table 17.2 summarizes the signs and symptoms of hypothermia at early and late stages.

Table 17.2 • SIGNS AND SYMPTOMS OF HYPOTHERMIA

Characteristic	Early Stages	Late Stages
Blood Pressure	Normal	Hypotension
Mental Status	Normal	Altered; deteriorates as hypothermia worsens
Pupils	Normal and reactive	Sluggish; later becoming fixed and dilated
Breathing	Rapid	Slow, shallow
Pulse	Rapid	Slow and irregular
Skin	Red Shivering	Pale, cyanotic, or white May be stiff and waxy in severe cases

Patients with generalized cold emergencies are usually cool to the touch. The core temperature provides an indication of the severity of the condition. To evaluate the patient's core temperature without a thermometer, place the back of your hand against the skin of the abdomen or chest. First explain to the patient what you are going to do and why.

Decreasing mental status or poor motor function suggests severe hypothermia. Some effects you may observe are:

• Lack of motor coordination. Evaluate by asking the patient to touch his or her nose with the tip of the index finger.

• An inability or reduced ability to feel you touching a part of the body.

• Dizziness, slurred speech, or abnormal gait. These suggest that the cold has affected the central nervous system and brain.

• Temporary disruption of memory. Ask the patient who he or she is, the location, and the date or time.

- Mood changes. The patient may be combative or refuse treatment. Remember that this behavior is a sign of decreased perfusion. It has nothing to do with your professionalism or treatment.

- Poor judgment. Some patients may even remove their clothing and return to the cold environment.

- Reduced ability to communicate.

A patient with hypothermia may have stiff, rigid posture or muscular rigidity. He or she may complain of joint or muscle stiffness. The patient may be shivering. Shivering is a natural body mechanism for generating heat. The process involves repetitive contraction and relaxation of muscles. As hypothermia progresses, shivering will stop. Do not be fooled if a hypothermic patient stops shivering. This suggests a decline in his or her condition, not an improvement. Closely monitor the patient's level of responsiveness and airway.

Breathing patterns change in each stage of hypothermia. In early stages, breathing may be rapid. This indicates a mild or moderate condition. In later, more severe stages, breathing becomes shallow, slow, or absent. Assess respiration carefully in hypothermic patients. Initially, you may think that a patient is not breathing. But after careful monitoring, you might discover that the patient is actually breathing very slowly. Respiration will also be very shallow.

In early stages, the patient's pulse will be regular, but rapid. Later, the pulse becomes barely palpable and is very slow or absent. The rhythm is often irregular. The blood pressure may be low or absent because of reduced cardiac output. The pupils may respond very slowly or not at all when stimulated with light.

Skin color varies according to the severity of hypothermia. When the body first becomes cold, surface blood vessels dilate. This increases blood flow to the skin to rewarm it. The skin looks pink to deep red. With more severe hypothermia, cardiac output decreases and the body attempts to shunt blood away from the skin. The blood is needed to nourish critical areas, such as the heart, brain, and vital organs. As a result, the skin appears pale. As cold exposure continues, the patient's skin may appear cyanotic. This is a grave sign. The amount of oxygen carried by the blood may only be two-thirds of normal.

As body temperature continues to drop, superficial tissues begin to freeze. At this point, the tissues feel stiff and hard to the touch. The skin may be white in color and have a waxy appearance. In severe cases, you may feel ice crystals in the tissues on palpation.

EMT Tip

If you work in an area in which hypothermia is common, your vehicle should be equipped with a system to warm the supplemental oxygen supply.

D.O.T. OBJECTIVE

Explain the steps in providing emergency medical care to a patient exposed to cold.

Emergency Care for Hypothermia

Besides the usual emergency care procedures, a hypothermic patient must be removed from the cold environment. You will begin steps to warm him or her. The patient should be transported to a facility that can provide internal rewarming procedures. Make sure to follow your local protocols.

1. Conduct a scene size-up. Remove the patient from the environment. Protect him or her from further heat loss. Carefully remove any wet clothing. Gently but thoroughly dry the patient. Wrap in a warm blanket. Make sure to cover the head.

2. Do not allow the patient to walk or move about. Be gentle. In severe hypothermia, rough handling or activity can cause cardiac arrest. Do not allow the patient to eat or drink stimulants, including coffee, tea, or hot chocolate. Some stimulants cause vasodilation, increasing heat loss.

3. Complete your initial assessment. Assess the airway carefully. Suction if necessary. Provide high-flow supplemental oxygen via a non-rebreather mask. Warm and humidify the oxygen, if possible. Assist with ventilations if breathing is inadequate. Use a bag-valve mask or a flow-restricted, oxygen-powered ventilation device.

4. Check carefully for the presence of breathing and pulse. Take your time. Both may be slow, weak, and difficult to detect in patients with severe hypothermia. A common expression used by emergency responders is, "A hypothermia patient is not dead until he or she is warm and dead." A patient who appears to be dead may recover after rewarming and resuscitation. Before beginning CPR on a hypothermic patient, check the pulse for 30 to 45 seconds to be sure life support is required.

5. Complete the focused history and physical exam. Obtain the SAMPLE history.

6. Begin emergency interventions. Be sure the patient's body and head are wrapped in warm blankets. Turn up the heat in the patient compartment of the ambulance. Avoid massaging or rubbing frozen extremities.

7. If the patient is alert and responds appropriately, begin active rewarming. Apply heat packs to the groin, axillary, and cervical regions. These areas have large blood vessels close to the skin surface. Heat will be absorbed and quickly transferred to the inside of the body. Chemical hot packs may be hot enough to burn the patient's skin (see Fig. 17.6). Wrap them with fabric such as a towel.

8. If the patient is unresponsive or responds inappropriately, continue with passive rewarming. Cover the patient and warm the ambulance to prevent further heat loss.

9. Complete a detailed assessment while en route to the receiving facility. Conduct ongoing assessments according to the patient's condition.

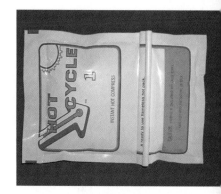

Figure 17.6 *Chemical hot pack.*

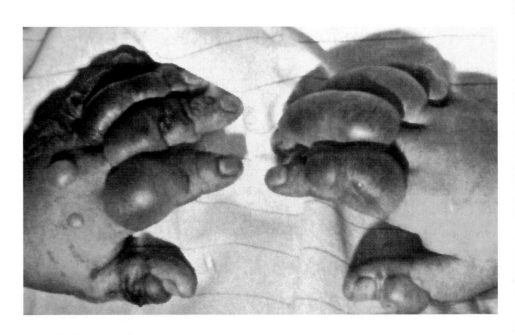

Local Cold Injuries

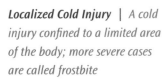

Localized Cold Injury | *A cold injury confined to a limited area of the body; more severe cases are called frostbite*

Localized cold injuries are common in areas of the body that are directly exposed to the cold. The ears, nose, face, hands, and feet are especially vulnerable.

Local cold injuries usually have a clear boundary defining the injured area. With an early or superficial injury, you may observe blanching of the skin. To check for blanching, press the skin in the affected area. Blanching is present if the skin does not return to its normal color when you release the pressure. The skin feels soft when palpated. The patient may complain of a loss of feeling in the injured area. During rewarming, the patient will report a tingling sensation.

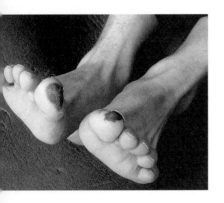

Figure 17.8 *Gangrenous tips of the toes.*

In late or deep injury, the skin will have a white, waxy, almost transparent appearance. It feels firm on palpation. In extreme cases, you will feel ice in the tissues. Swelling and blisters may be present. If tissues are thawed or partially thawed, the skin may appear flushed. The flushed area may appear purple and white. Some areas may look mottled and cyanotic. Late or deep tissue injury due to cold exposure is known as frostbite. Frostbite can lead to obstruction or loss of the blood supply. This causes death of the local tissues in a condition called gangrene. Gangrenous areas appear black (see Figs. 17.7 and 17.8).

Emergency Care for Local Cold Injuries

Follow these steps to care for a patient with a localized cold injury:

1. Complete a scene size-up. Remove the patient from the environment to prevent further heat loss. Do not reexpose injured areas to the cold. Remove wet clothing as well as any clothing that restricts circulation. If clothing is frozen

to the skin, do not try to remove it. Also remove rings, earrings, watches, and jewelry. You can expect edema when the area begins to rewarm. Jewelry will restrict circulation when swelling begins.

2. Protect the area from further injury. The patient may lose local sensation. Loss of sensation greatly increases the risk of further injury. He or she will not feel pain, heat, or cold if the area becomes further injured. Excessive heat from chemical hot packs will not be felt. Avoid rough handling. Do not allow the patient to use the injured extremity or part.

3. Complete the initial assessment. Assess the airway carefully. Suction if necessary. Provide high-flow supplemental oxygen via a non-rebreather mask. Warm and humidify the oxygen. Check carefully for the presence of breathing and pulse. Check the pulse for 30 to 45 seconds before beginning CPR.

4. Complete your focused history and physical exam. Obtain the SAMPLE history.

5. Avoid massaging or rubbing frozen extremities. If blisters have formed on the skin, avoid breaking them. Splint and cover the injured extremity. Use a dry sterile dressing and roller gauze. Medical direction or your local treatment protocols will describe further care.

6. Transport the patient to a facility equipped to provide rewarming procedures. Complete a detailed assessment while en route to the receiving facility. Conduct ongoing assessments according to the patient's condition.

Active Rewarming. If your transport time is extremely long or if transport will be delayed, you may be permitted to rapidly rewarm a localized cold injury. You will immerse the affected part in a warm water bath.

1. The temperature of the water bath should be approximately 104° F. Stir the water constantly. Monitor water temperature closely. Maintain a constant water temperature. Do not allow the bath to cool. Placing a chemical hot pack in the water will help to keep it warm.

2. Immerse the extremity in the bath. The patient will complain of severe pain during this process. Continue the rewarming until the part feels soft, and color and sensation return.

3. Gently pat the area dry. Cover it with dry sterile dressings. If the hand or foot is injured, place dressings between each finger and toe.

4. Protect from refreezing.

HEAT-RELATED EMERGENCIES

Hyperthermia occurs when the body generates more heat than it can dissipate. Heat-related problems can range from very minor to life-threatening. Like hypothermia, predisposing factors such as the patient's health and environmental

EMT Alert

Active rewarming is a potentially dangerous process. Active rewarming of a hypothermic patient with an altered mental state can cause lethal heart rhythms.

conditions can increase the severity of the condition. Heat emergencies may occur anytime. They are not limited to the hot months of the year.

Hyperthermia is usually the result of environmental exposure to high levels of heat, humidity, or a combination of the two. If the ambient temperature is high, the body cannot release heat as effectively as it does in lower temperatures. Also, as the relative humidity rises, the body's ability to eliminate heat by sweat evaporation diminishes. If the relative humidity exceeds 75 percent, sweating becomes ineffective.

Exercise and activity intensify heat-related injuries. The human body can lose more than a liter of fluid an hour during exercise. Most of this fluid is lost through perspiration, although some is lost through evaporation from the lungs. When body fluids are lost, vital electrolytes such as sodium, chloride, and potassium are excreted. This causes a potentially dangerous imbalance of fluids within the body.

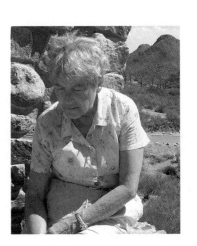

Figure 17.9 *Elderly patients are at greater risk for hyperthermia than younger adults.*

Age is a risk factor for heat-related illness. Many elderly persons have difficulty regulating their body temperatures (see Fig. 17.9). Some may not recognize the symptoms of a heat-related illness. Elderly people may not be able to readily escape a hot environment. They may also experience effects due to medications used to treat chronic illnesses. These risk factors can intensify the effects of a hot environment for an older person.

Newborns and infants may also have extreme responses to heat. Thermoregulatory mechanisms are not fully developed in children. In addition, young children are not able to remove their clothing to cool off.

High fever or serious infections are common causes of medically induced hyperthermia. Many chronic illnesses or medical conditions amplify or accelerate negative responses to heat. Examples of these conditions are:

- Heart disease
- Diabetes
- Obesity
- Fever
- Dehydration
- Fatigue
- Many drugs and medications

D.O.T. OBJECTIVE

List the signs and symptoms of exposure to heat.

Signs and Symptoms of Hyperthermia

Signs and symptoms of heat emergencies are often deceptive. In early or mild stages, the signs and symptoms are usually very subtle (see Fig. 17.10). Consequently, many EMS systems promote aggressive treatment for all heat emergencies. When caring for victims of heat-related illness, always err on the side of caution. Be aggressive in cooling a patient you suspect of suffering from hyperthermia. Heat-related emergencies are often life threatening.

Muscle cramps are a common symptom of excessive heat exposure. In early hyperthermia, the skin may be moist and pale. It feels normal or cool to the touch. This occurs because of normal body defenses. However, these are also signs of shock. Although the patient is not in imminent danger, the thermoregulatory system may have broken down. Signs and symptoms that indicate deterioration of body temperature regulation are:

- Weakness

- Exhaustion

- Dizziness

- Fainting

- Rapid heart rate

- Altered mental status

- Unresponsiveness

Skin that is very hot to the touch usually signifies a serious medical emergency. Hot skin may be dry or moist. Moist hot skin is usually caused by sweat that has not completely evaporated. If the skin feels very hot, the patient is in imminent danger. The outcome may be death or brain damage.

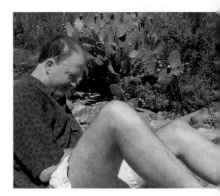

Figure 17.10 *A patient with heatstroke may have muscle cramps, weakness, and altered mental status.*

D.O.T. OBJECTIVE

Explain the steps in providing emergency care to a patient exposed to heat.

Emergency Care for Hyperthermia

Emergency care depends on the patient's skin signs and level of responsiveness.

1. Conduct a scene size-up. Remove the patient from the source of heat. Place him or her in a cool environment, such as the back of an air-conditioned ambulance.

2. Complete the initial assessment. Evaluate the airway, breathing adequacy, and circulation. Intervene immediately in life-threatening situations. Administer high-flow oxygen by non-rebreather mask or provide assisted artificial ventilations.

3. Complete a focused history and physical exam. If the patient is unresponsive, complete a rapid medical assessment.

4. If the skin is hot to touch, the situation is critical. It may feel dry or moist. Act quickly and aggressively. You must cool the patient immediately. Move him or her to the coolest environment possible. Remove all clothing quickly. Try to do this in a private area to protect the patient's dignity. Apply cool packs to the neck, groin, and armpits. Keep the skin wet to increase heat loss by evaporation. Apply water with a sponge or towel. Fan the wet patient aggressively. Transport immediately. Delays can be life threatening. Position the patient in the Trendelenburg or recovery position.

EMT Alert

Water-related emergencies are very dangerous due to the risks involved to both the rescuer and the victim.

5. If the patient is responsive, has moist, pale, skin with a normal to cool temperature, and is not nauseated, encourage fluids. Make sure that the gag reflex is intact. Offer water or a specially balanced electrolyte solution, if permitted by local protocol. Cool the patient by fanning. Position the patient in the Trendelenburg position.

6. If the patient is unresponsive, has an altered mental status, or is vomiting, position in the recovery position. This reduces the risk of aspiration. Never give the patient anything to eat or drink.

7. Conduct a detailed assessment while en route to the receiving facility. Complete ongoing assessments according to the patient's condition.

D.O.T. OBJECTIVES

Recognize the signs and symptoms of water-related emergencies.

Describe the complications of near drowning.

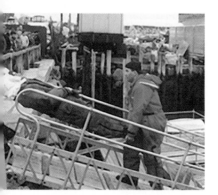

Figure 17.11 *Water rescues require specialized training and equipment.*

WATER-RELATED EMERGENCIES

Water sports and aquatic activities have grown in popularity over the past decade. As a result, the incidence of aquatic emergencies has increased. As you learn to assess and manage these situations correctly, keep in mind that water-related emergencies occur in dangerous environments. Your safety is always your primary concern. Floods, rough surf, and deep water are hazardous to rescuers. Never attempt a water rescue unless you are specially trained and have the necessary safety equipment (see Fig. 17.11). Call for backup from trained rescuers (see Fig. 17.12). Always wear a Coast Guard approved personal flotation device (PFD) when you are in or near the water (see Fig. 17.13).

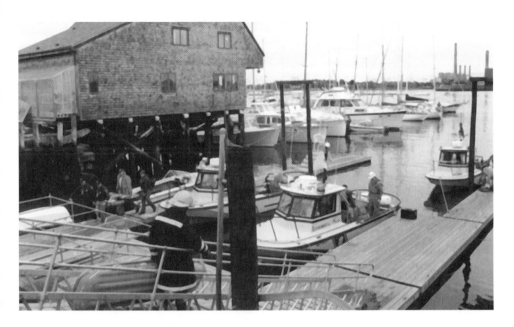

Figure 17.12 *The U.S. Coast Guard is often involved in water rescues.*

Near-Drowning Incidents

Drowning | *Death resulting from suffocation or cardiac arrest while submerged in water*

Drowning and **near drowning** are the most common aquatic emergencies that you will encounter. More than 4,500 people die annually from drowning. Many thousands more survive near-drowning incidents. A near drowning is an immersion situation. By definition, a near-drowning patient survives for at least 24 hours following the episode.

Near Drowning | *An immersion situation from which the patient is resuscitated and survives for at least 24 hours*

Drowning is a major cause of accidental death in young children. Drownings can occur in bathtubs, spas, irrigation canals, recreational facilities, and back-yard pools. Pediatric patients can even drown in a bucket. Because of the relative size and weight of their heads, they can become stuck upside down in the bucket and be unable to right themselves.

Emergency care for a near-drowning patient is described in Procedure 17.1. Always assume the possibility of spinal injury. This is especially true if the patient was involved in a diving accident or if the mechanism of injury is unknown. Maintain a neutral in-line position during removal from the water. Immobilize the patient on a long spine board as soon as possible.

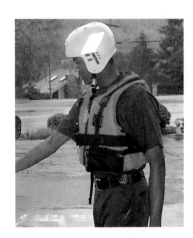

Figure 17.13 *A vest-type personal flotation device (PFD).*

A common complication with near-drowning patients is gastric distention during resuscitation. Swallowed water enlarges the stomach and pushes the diaphragm up. This prevents the lungs from expanding fully on ventilation. Place the patient in the recovery position. Set up the suction unit so it is readily available. Then apply firm pressure over the epigastric region with the palm of your hand. The patient will vomit water and gastric contents. Suction the patient as needed. Resume artificial ventilation.

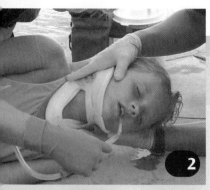

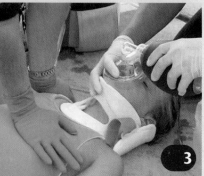

Procedure 17.1 • **EMERGENCY CARE FOR A NEAR DROWNING**

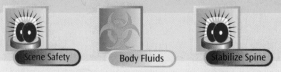

Scene Safety   Body Fluids   Stabilize Spine

1. Conduct a scene size-up. Be alert for scene hazards.

2. Complete the initial assessment. Clear the airway. This is essential for resuscitation. If necessary, immobilize the cervical spine. Place the patient in the recovery position to drain vomitus, water, and secretions. Suction as needed.

3. Treat an immersion patient like any other cardiac arrest (see Chapter 13). Administer high-flow oxygen by non-rebreather mask. Assist ventilations if necessary. Suspect gastric distention if you have difficulty ventilating the patient. Always begin CPR on a pulseless, nonbreathing patient who has been submerged in cold water.

4. Complete the focused history and physical exam. If the patient is unresponsive, complete a rapid medical assessment. For all other patients, assess and treat based on the patient's complaints. Monitor the airway and breathing closely. Respiratory failure is common in water-related emergencies.

5. Complete a detailed assessment while en route to the receiving facility. Conduct ongoing assessments according to the patient's condition.

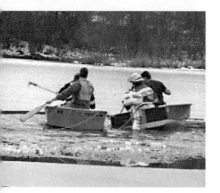

Figure 17.14 *When a victim is rescued from icy water, you must treat for severe hypothermia as well as drowning.*

When managing a near-drowning episode in which the water temperature is below 70° F, consider the length of time of immersion (see Fig. 17.14). In a cold-water immersion, the body's protective mechanisms slow the vital functions and shunt blood to critical organs. This can make the pulse and breathing difficult to detect. Always attempt resuscitation. Many patients have been successfully resuscitated after extended cold-water immersion. These episodes have been widely publicized. Follow your local protocols when caring for drowning and near-drowning patients.

When a drowning victim sinks below the water surface for the final time, he or she will attempt to hold the breath for as long as possible. However, this time is short because of previous exertion. No accurate data are available to indicate how long humans might hold their breath. Based on reports from resuscitated survivors, 15 seconds is probably the maximum.

BITES AND STINGS

You will manage many bite- and sting-related emergencies. The most common are stings from bees, wasps, or hornets. Your primary concern with these injuries is to determine whether the patient is allergic to the exposure (see Chapter 15). Calls for snake, scorpion, or marine life emergencies are less common in most areas, but can be quite serious (see Figs. 17.15 and 17.16). Some patients may suffer allergic reactions and possible anaphylaxis from marine bites or stings, as with stings from bees or wasps.

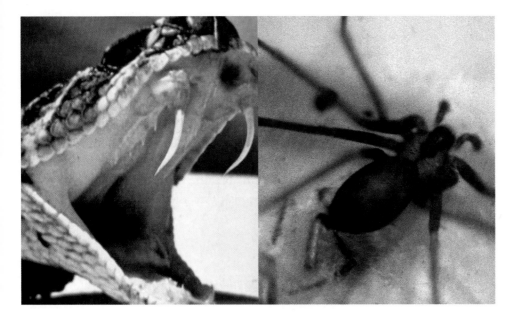

Figure 17.15 *Rattlesnakes and brown recluse spiders inject venom when they bite a victim.*

Always remember scene safety when bites or stings are suspected. Forgetting your personal safety can be a very painful lesson.

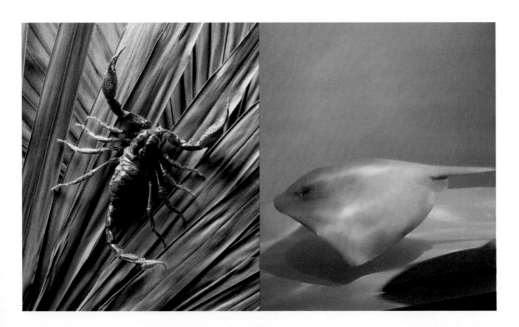

Figure 17.16 *Scorpions and stingrays deliver venom through their stingers.*

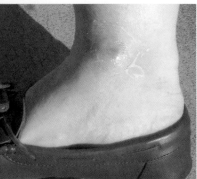

Figure 17.17 *Brown recluse spider bite.*

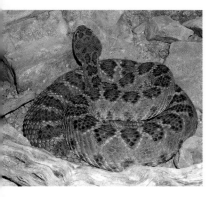

Figure 17.18 *The fangs of a rattlesnake deliver poisonous venom.*

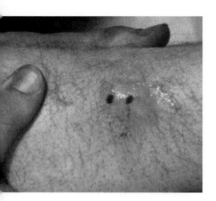

Figure 17.19 *Marks left by the two fangs of a snake.*

Signs and Symptoms of Bites and Stings

Insect bites can cause damage to tissues or affect the nervous system. For example, a brown recluse spider bite causes damage to the skin immediately surrounding the bite. The black widow spider bite, on the other hand, quickly interferes with the normal function of the nervous system. Becoming an expert in the many different types of bites and stings is not necessary. However, you must remember some common signs, symptoms, and treatments.

You usually learn about the nature of the emergency from the patient. He or she gives you a history of a bite or sting. The most common signs and symptoms are pain, redness, and swelling at the injection site (see Fig. 17.17). The patient may complain of weakness, dizziness, chills, fever, or nausea and vomiting. Inspect the skin for bite marks or the presence of a stinger (see Figs. 17.18 and 17.19). As time goes on, the venom causes more serious damage (see Fig. 17.20).

Note complaints of numbness or tingling around the patient's mouth and nose. Observe the breathing closely. Certain types of stings are neurotoxic. These will impair the patient's ability to breathe. If the airway closes, death will ensue. Focus on the patient's ability to breathe and keeping the airway open. Monitor the patient carefully for signs of an allergic reaction.

> **D.O.T. OBJECTIVE**
>
> Discuss the emergency medical care of bites and stings.

Emergency Care for Bites and Stings

These are the general steps in emergency care for bites and stings.

1. Conduct the scene size-up. Look for the source of the bite or sting. Move the patient from the area, if necessary.

2. Complete an initial assessment. Carefully assess the airway, breathing, and circulation. Use the information and skills that you learned in the airway management and respiratory emergency chapters. Be alert for signs of an allergic reaction.

3. Complete a focused history and physical exam. Keep the patient calm and quiet. Reassure the patient.

4. Position the area of injection slightly below heart level. This will slow circulation of the venom to the rest of the body. Remove bracelets, rings, watch, and other jewelry from the extremity, in case of swelling. If swelling has started, using a ring cutter may be necessary.

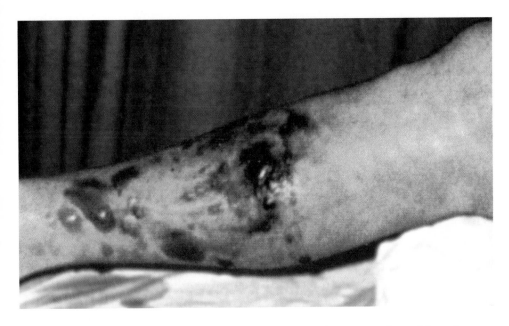

Figure 17.20 *A venomous snake bite can lead to severe complications.*

5. When treating snake bites or marine life injuries, do not apply cold packs or ice packs. For marine life injuries, applying non-scalding hot water is appropriate. Some protocols recommend rinsing the bite or sting with alcohol or vinegar.

6. Contact medical direction to determine whether to apply a constricting band for a snake bite. A band reduces blood return to the heart. It is not a tourniquet. If you are instructed to do so, apply constricting bands above and below the bite. The bands should be loose enough to slide a finger under. Periodically check the pulse below the bite.

7. Try to transport the patient to a receiving facility that has appropriate antivenom medications. Complete a detailed assessment while en route. Continue ongoing assessments. Monitor the airway and breathing carefully. Reassess every 5 minutes in unstable patients, every 15 minutes in others.

8. Observe for the development of an allergic reaction. If your protocols permit, consider treatment of the allergic response as discussed in Chapter 15.

In the case of a bee sting, you will remove the stinger from the skin. Recent research suggests that after a bee sting, the venomous sacs continue to contract and inject venom. Quick removal of the stinger and sacs is important. Follow local protocol. Examine the sting site. Look for the stinger and venom sac. If found, avoid grasping the stinger between your fingers. Do not use a hemostat, tweezers, or other grasping device. Squeezing the sac will force more venom into the skin. Instead, scrape away the protruding sac. Use a flat-bladed object, such as a tongue depressor. You can also use the edge of a credit card by sliding the card flat against the skin. Next, remove the stinger with tweezers. Wash the area gently to remove any adhering venom or toxin. Apply ice or cold packs to the sting site. This slows the spread of venom and eases the pain.

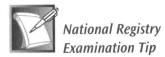

National Registry Examination Tip

Review the treatment standards for temperature-related emergencies, water emergencies, and bites and stings. Treat environmental emergencies aggressively. Remember to assess for and treat early signs of shock.

EMT Tip

Wasp stingers do not have an attached venom sac.

Chapter Seventeen Summary

- Certain factors can predispose a patient to a temperature-related emergency, including:

  Climate (high temperature, high humidity, cold temperature, immersion in water)

  Age (very old and young people are more susceptible to temperature)

  Medical conditions (trauma, dehydration, obesity, fever, fatigue, diabetes, alcoholism)

  Drugs, medications, or poisons

- Removing the patient from the environment is important when managing heat and cold emergencies.

- Generalized hypothermia involves the entire body. Actively rewarm the patient if he or she is alert and responsive. If the patient has an altered mental status, rewarm passively with warm blankets only.

- Localized cold injuries are common on the face, ears, and extremities. Blanching of the skin indicates early or superficial injury. White, waxy skin indicates late or deep injury (frostbite).

- Patients with signs and symptoms of a heat emergency should be immediately moved to a cool environment. Treatment is based primarily on the patient's skin condition and level of consciousness. Consider patients with hot skin as having a life-threatening condition.

- Always consider personal and crew safety a top priority in water-related emergencies. Never attempt a water rescue unless properly trained and equipped. Suspect spinal injury if diving is involved, or if the cause is unknown. Always attempt resuscitation on cold-water drowning victims. Follow local protocols.

- Bites and stings are common environmental emergencies involving injected poisons. Evaluate the patient carefully for signs and symptoms of an allergic reaction. Do not apply cold to snakebites or marine bites or stings. Position the injection site slightly below the patient's heart. Consult with medical direction for additional treatment instructions.

Key Terms Review

Review Questions

1. Convection refers to:

   a. Air movement within the respiratory system

   b. Normal heat transfer due to respiration

   c. Direct transfer of heat through contact with another object

   d. Transfer of heat due to air movement on the body surface

2. Vasoconstriction, shivering, confusion, lowered pulse and blood pressure, and unconsciousness can indicate various stages of:

   a. Hyperthermia

   b. Frostbite

   c. Hypothermia

   d. Cold exhaustion

3. Treatment of a hypothermic patient with altered mental status includes all of the following EXCEPT:

   a. Monitor and stabilize vital functions

   b. Active rewarming techniques

   c. Rapid transport to medical facility

   d. Prevention of further heat loss

4. You are not able to adequately ventilate a near-drowning victim due to gastric distention. What should you do?

   a. Switch to positive-pressure ventilation

   b. Insert a nasogastric tube

   c. Place pressure on the abdomen

   d. Suction the oropharynx

5. You respond to a pulseless, nonbreathing patient who was submerged in cold water for 45 minutes. You should:

   a. Assume the patient is dead and terminate care

   b. Begin resuscitation efforts immediately

   c. Call the patient's private physician for advice

   d. Ask your partner for suggestions

6. In comparison to adults, shivering is _____ effective in infants, children, and the elderly.

   a. Equally

   b. More

   c. Less

   d. Significantly more

7. If the mechanism of a water-related emergency is unknown, you should suspect possible:

   a. Cardiac injury

   b. Respiratory injury

   c. Spinal injury

   d. Localized cold injury

8. How should you treat a patient with a bee sting?

   a. Sprinkle MSG on the sting site

   b. Scrape the stinger off of the skin

   c. Remove the stinger using tweezers or forceps

   d. Gently pluck the stinger free with your fingers

9. Which signs would be inconsistent with a hypothermic patient's physical exam?

   a. Cold and stiff skin

   b. Slow, irregular pulse

   c. Hypertension

   d. Altered mental status

10. A person submerged in water loses heat _____ times as rapidly as a person in air.

    a. 2

    b. 10

    c. 25

    d. 100

11. Most cold-related emergencies occur:

    a. In rural settings

    b. In suburban settings

    c. In high-risk wilderness settings

    d. In urban settings

12. Heat lost from contact with a colder object is called:

    a. Conduction

    b. Evaporation

    c. Radiation

    d. Convection

13. Cooling of the body below normal temperature is:

    a. Systemic frostbite

    b. Exposure

    c. Hypotension

    d. Hypothermia

CASE STUDIES

Environmental Emergencies

1 You have been working as a park ranger for a little more than a month. During this time you have treated only minor cuts and bruises. Today, dispatch advises of a hiking accident on the north side of the park. When you arrive at the emergency call station, three young males are waiting. They are not properly dressed for cold nights. One is on a makeshift stretcher. You learn that they were out camping for a few days. The young man on the stretcher fell on some loose rocks, injuring both ankles. He responds slowly. His skin is cold to touch. His friends state that they walked all night to keep warm and to get help.

A. As you assess the severity of injury from exposure in this patient, list the types of questions you might ask.

B. Describe your treatment of the patient's ankle injuries.

2 The beach patrol has always been respected for its rescue efforts. You have only been with the unit for a few months. You and your partner are cruising the beach in all-terrain vehicles. You notice a surfer waving his arms up and down. You meet the patient as he exits the surf. He complains of severe pain just above his right calf. You observe a small, one-inch laceration.

A. Describe the treatment for a patient with a marine animal sting or bite.

3 The air show has been a major event for almost twenty years. Thousands gather at the local airstrip to watch supersonic and antique airplanes. Your department has provided standby medical services for the last few years. The only problem with the show has been the schedule. It is always held on one of the warmest weekends of the year. While you glance out over the large crowd, someone runs up to the ambulance. You see an elderly male lying on the pavement. A family member states that the patient has been at the show all day. He was walking around for several hours. He had no sun protection and started complaining of severe muscle cramps about 30 minutes ago. They tried to get him to sit in the shade, but he passed out. They quickly picked him up and carried him to your nearby ambulance. The patient is hot to the touch. He responds only to painful stimuli.

A. Given the above information, what should your first actions be?

B. When completing the SAMPLE history, what contributing history should you look for?

C. How will you treat this patient?

Stories from the Field
Wrap-Up

The patient's altered level of responsiveness could be caused by many factors. The history given by bystanders suggests that environmental exposure has contributed to the patient's problem. The generalized cold emergency could have been aggravated by conditions such as his age, drug or alcohol intoxication, or a possible history of chronic illness.

Your first actions must focus on the man's airway. Take spinal precautions if necessary. Provide supplemental oxygen or assisted ventilations. Move the patient from the alley to the ambulance. Handle him carefully. If he is hypothermic, rough movements may cause cardiac arrest. Remove any wet clothing and cover him with warm, dry blankets. Cover his head. Complete the focused history and physical exam and detailed assessment. Evaluate for any other potential causes of his altered mental status. Increase the heat in the patient compartment of the ambulance. Transport rapidly but carefully. Reassess the airway and breathing frequently. Be prepared to assist ventilations and provide CPR if necessary.

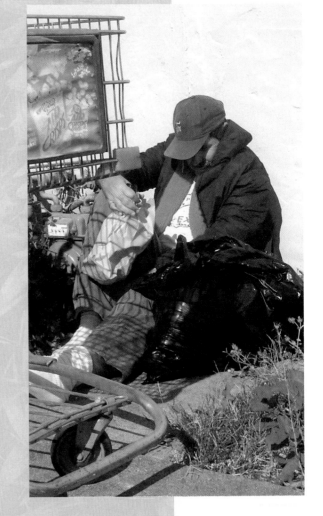

Chapter *18*

Obstetrics and Gynecology

Stories from the Field

You are working with Carmen on an early morning rotation. You are dispatched to a woman in labor. You respond to a suburban area approximately ten minutes from the hospital. When you arrive, a 24-year-old pregnant female is lying supine in bed. Her husband tells you that the baby is not due for another six weeks. As you enter the room, the young woman calls to you for help. She is in moderate distress. Her airway is open. Respirations are rapid and shallow. Her pulse is 104 and regular. When Carmen attempts to ask about the current circumstances and past medical history, the patient becomes uncooperative. She says, "Don't waste time, just help me!"

This is the patient's fourth pregnancy. She has had two children. She has seen an obstetrician regularly during this pregnancy. She has been having episodes of false labor since her twenty-fifth week. This time, regular contractions began about 30 minutes before she called EMS. The contractions are increasing in strength and duration. The husband tells you that the patient lost her plug during an episode of preterm labor. Her water broke just before you arrived. The patient is complaining of pain, but denies feeling the urge to push.

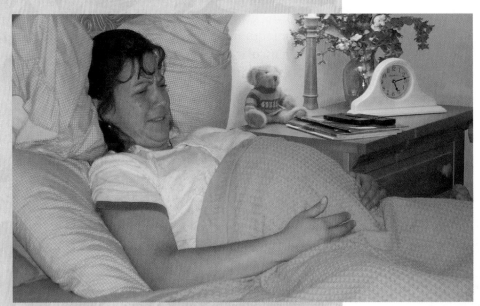

*S*ometimes childbirth occurs in the prehospital setting. Because this happens infrequently, caring for an anxious mother and newborn infant can be quite stressful. You will feel more confident in this situation if you have studied and practiced childbirth procedures. Labor and delivery are usually normal and uncomplicated. Competent, caring EMS personnel decrease everyone's stress during these situations. A relaxed atmosphere leads to better emergency care for the mother and child.

Besides prehospital childbirth, you may care for patients with obstetrical or gynecological emergencies. **Obstetrics** is the medical specialty involving care of women during pregnancy and childbirth. During pregnancy, you might respond to various predelivery emergencies. Occasionally, a prehospital delivery may involve abnormal circumstances. **Gynecology** is concerned with conditions of the female genital tract. Nonpregnant women can require care for gynecological trauma or medical conditions. Although obstetrical and gynecological emergencies are uncommon, they are private situations. Your professionalism, understanding of the condition, and patient support will enhance safe and effective care.

> ### D.O.T. OBJECTIVE
>
> Identify the following structures: uterus, vagina, fetus, placenta, umbilical cord, amniotic sac, perineum.

Obstetrics (ob-STET-rics) | *The medical specialty concerned with the care of women during pregnancy and childbirth*

Gynecology | *The medical specialty concerned with conditions of the female reproductive organs*

Uterus | *Female reproductive organ in which menstruation and fetal development occur; also womb*

Fetus | *Developing, unborn offspring in the uterus; called an embryo for the first eight weeks after conception*

Placenta | *Organ that enables the exchange of nutrients, oxygen, and metabolic wastes between the maternal and fetal circulatory systems*

Amniotic (am-nee-OT-ik) Sac | *Sac which holds the fetus suspended in amniotic fluid; also called "bag of waters"*

Umbilical (um-BILL-ik-ul) Cord | *Structure that connects the fetus to the placenta; contains arteries and veins responsible for the exchange of materials between fetal and maternal circulations*

ANATOMY AND PHYSIOLOGY OF PREGNANCY

The mother's **uterus** is the organ in which the **fetus** or developing unborn baby grows (see Figs. 18.1 and 18.2). The walls of the uterus consist of smooth muscle fibers. These stretch as the fetus grows. The walls are thick and muscular. They are responsible for the contractions during labor that lead to expulsion of the fetus. The uterus also holds the **placenta**, a complex vascular organ. The placenta exchanges nutrients and oxygen from the mother's blood supply for waste products and carbon dioxide from the fetal blood.

Attached to the placenta is the **amniotic sac**, or bag of waters. The developing fetus grows within this sac, surrounded by a protective cushion of amniotic fluid (see Fig. 18.3). The fetus is attached to the **umbilical cord**. The cord is an extension of the placenta through which nourishment and waste products pass. The umbilical cord is the fetus' lifeline to the mother. If blood flow to the umbilical cord is reduced or cut off, injury or death of the fetus can occur.

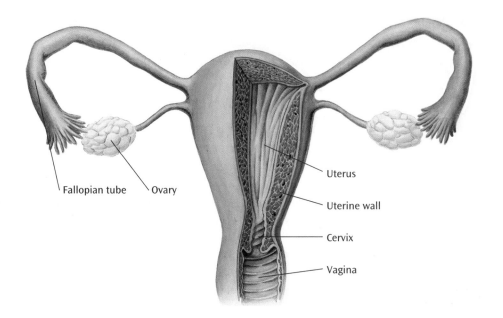

Figure 18.1 *Female reproductive structures.*

Fallopian tube — Ovary

Uterus

Uterine wall

Cervix

Vagina

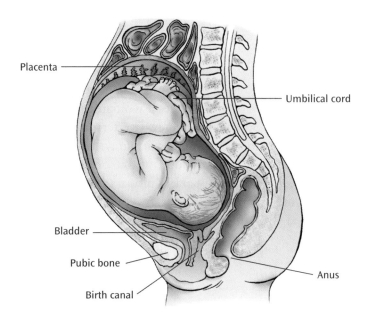

Figure 18.2 *Fetus in a normal position within the uterus.*

Placenta

Umbilical cord

Bladder

Pubic bone

Birth canal

Anus

Vagina | *Female genital structure; the lower portion of the birth canal*

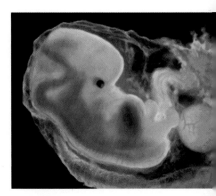

Figure 18.3 *Developing embryo within the amniotic sac.*

The birth canal consists of the cervix and the **vagina**. The cervix forms the upper portion of the birth canal. It is the lowest part of the uterus and is also called the neck of the uterus. The cervical opening is sealed with a mucous plug during pregnancy. The mucus prevents pathogens from entering the uterus, thus preventing infection. The vagina is the lower portion of the birth canal. It is lined with a soft mucous membrane. The vagina stretches wide during delivery, permitting the fetus to pass through.

Perineum (pair-eh-NEE-em) | *The area of skin between the vagina and anus in females and between the scrotum and anus in males*

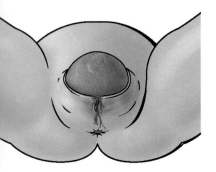

Figure 18.4 *Perineal laceration.*

Miscarriage | *Delivery of an embryo or fetus prior to viability; spontaneous abortion*

Abortion | *Delivery of the products of conception early in a pregnancy; may be spontaneous or medically induced*

The **perineum** is the outer skin of the mother's pelvic floor, posterior to the vagina and anterior to the anus. The perineum often tears during delivery because it does not stretch readily. This injury is called a perineal laceration (see Fig. 18.4).

A full-term pregnancy lasts approximately 40 weeks or 9 months. Knowing how far along a woman is in her pregnancy is important. This helps you to anticipate and prepare for complications. Ask the woman if she knows her due date or by how many months she is pregnant. If she does not, you can calculate the estimated due date. Most women do not know exactly when they conceived. Therefore, the due date is estimated from the first day of the last menstrual period. Subtract 3 months from this date, then add 7 days.

The term of a pregnancy is divided into 3-month stages. Each 3-month period is known as a trimester. A normal pregnancy passes through the first, second, and third trimesters. Normal full-term deliveries occur during the last weeks of the third trimester. The stage of development at which a fetus may be able to survive on its own is called viability. A **miscarriage** is the delivery of the products of conception prior to viability. Miscarriages are most common in the first and early second trimesters, before a fetus can survive on its own. A miscarriage is a spontaneous **abortion**. An abortion may also be deliberately induced by a physician.

Specific terminology is used to indicate the pregnancy history of a woman. Gravida (G) states the number of pregnancies a woman has had, despite the outcomes. This includes the present pregnancy. The term used to describe a woman who is pregnant for the first time is primigravida. Para (P) refers to the number of pregnancies that have produced viable offspring. A woman who has had one childbirth is called a primipara. Multipara is the term for a woman who has had two or more viable pregnancies. A woman who was pregnant four times and delivered two children would be described as G4 and P2.

> **D.O.T. OBJECTIVE**
>
> State indications of an imminent delivery.

Labor

Labor | *Physical processes of childbirth; begins with uterine contractions and leads to delivery of the fetus and the placenta*

Labor is a process that begins with the first uterine contraction. It concludes with delivery of the placenta. During this process, the smooth muscle of the uterus contracts rhythmically and forcefully. The muscular movement pushes the fetus through the vagina to the outside. Labor and delivery are broken into three or four defined stages.

Labor may begin with rupture of the amniotic sac. This appears as a warm trickle or gush of clear, straw-colored, or green-tinged fluid from the vagina.

It may be described by the mother as her water having broken. Initially, the mother may feel a tightening or cramping pain in the lower abdomen or lower back. This may signal the onset of contractions, which begins the first stage of labor.

The first stage of labor lasts until the cervix is completely dilated at approximately 10 cm wide. During this stage, the woman may pass a cluster of blood-tinged mucus called **show** or bloody show. This is due to loss of the protective mucous plug that occurs when the cervix begins to open. The first stage of labor can be difficult for the mother (see Fig. 18.5). This is particularly true for a first-time mother who has not attended childbirth preparation classes. As the fetal head descends farther into the pelvis, the pressure and force of the contractions increase. The pain is very intense. This can lead to feelings of anxiety and loss of control.

During the transition phase between the first and second stages of labor, the pain intensifies. During this stage, the fetus descends through the dilated cervix and vagina. As the fetus descends and presses against the perineum, the mother will develop an involuntary urge to push or bear down. The woman may feel nauseated. She may vomit. The second stage of labor begins when she has an irresistible urge to push. She will not be able to control this urge. The woman may mistake the pressure of the descending fetus as the need to have a bowel movement.

As the fetus descends, it reaches the end of the birth canal. Its **presenting part** presses against the perineum. The presenting part is the part of the fetus that comes out first. The infant presses on the vaginal opening, causing it to bulge and stretch wide open. Because the presenting part is usually the head, this is called **crowning** (see Fig. 18.6). Crowning signals that delivery is imminent and inevitable. Delivery of the newborn completes the second stage of labor.

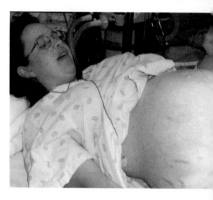

Figure 18.5 *Pregnant patient in labor.*

Show | *Discharge of small amount of blood-tinged mucus from the vagina at the onset of labor; also bloody show*

Presenting Part | *The part of a newborn that comes out of the birth canal first*

Crowning | *The stage of delivery in which the head of the fetus is first visible as it stretches the vaginal opening*

Figure 18.6 *The vaginal opening stretches as crowning occurs.*

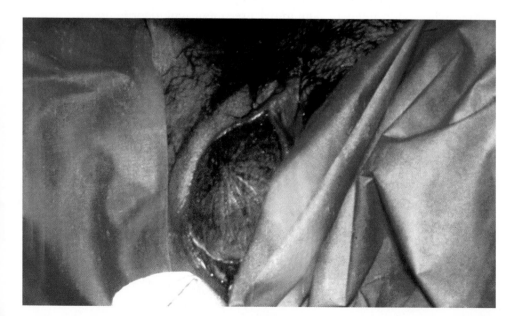

The first stage of labor usually lasts between 6 and 18 hours for a woman having her first baby. Successive labors are usually shorter. The first stage in a multipara may last from 2 to 10 hours. The second stage lasts between 30 minutes and 3 hours in a primipara. It can be as short as 5 to 30 minutes in a multipara.

The third stage of labor begins after the birth of the infant. It ends with the delivery of the placenta. This is usually within 30 minutes of birth. The placenta should deliver on its own.

The time interval between contractions during labor is called the frequency. It is measured from the beginning of one contraction to the beginning of the next. The length of each contraction is its duration. Labor is well established when contractions are 3 to 5 minutes apart or closer. During the second stage of labor, contractions are usually closer together, about every 1 to 3 minutes. The frequency and duration of contractions should be noted. In true labor, the contractions increase in frequency, strength, and duration. In a false labor, contractions are irregular. They are typically 3 to 20 minutes or more apart. They usually subside if the patient rests in bed.

OBSTETRICAL AND GYNECOLOGICAL EMERGENCIES

When responding to an obstetrical or gynecological emergency, scene size-up is critical. You must first determine whether the patient is pregnant. Not all women know that they are pregnant. Suspect the possibility of pregnancy in any woman of childbearing age, especially if the chief complaint involves abdominal pain. Look for an enlarged abdomen. Most women do not exhibit external signs of pregnancy until about the twentieth week.

Complete your initial assessment and provide interventions as you would for a patient who is not pregnant. The initial assessment will identify life-threatening problems. Determine the mother's mental status using AVPU. Her airway, breathing, and circulation are your primary concern. The mother's life always takes precedence over that of the unborn child. The fetus is dependent on the mother's blood supply. Adequate maternal oxygenation and circulation are critical. The best chance for the fetus' survival lies with survival of the mother.

Focused History and Physical Exam

To complete a focused history and physical exam for an obstetrical or gynecological patient, first obtain the SAMPLE history. Be sure to respect the confidentiality and privacy of the patient when asking questions. Ask the following focused history questions:

• Are you or could you be pregnant?

• When was your last menstrual period? Was it normal?

- Have you missed a menstrual period?

- Have you had any symptoms of pregnancy, such as breast tenderness, increased fatigue, nausea, or vomiting?

If the patient is experiencing pain or discomfort, ask the OPQRST questions:

Onset—When did the pain begin? If you are having intermittent cramps or contractions, how close together are they?

Provocation—Did the pain start gradually or suddenly? Is the pain related to sexual intercourse? Is pain present only with contractions, or does it persist between contractions?

Quality—Describe the quality of the pain. Is it dull, crampy, sharp, etc.? Can you point to the pain with one finger?

Radiation—Does the pain radiate?

Severity—How intense is the pain? If the patient is in labor, does she feel the need to have a bowel movement? Does she feel a need to push?

Time—How long have you had the pain?

For a pregnant patient, ask the following questions:

- How long have you been pregnant? Do you know your due date?

- How many pregnancies have you had, including miscarriages and abortions?

- How many children have you had?

- Have you had any prenatal care?

Ask about problems with the current or previous pregnancies:

- Has your physician expressed any concerns about the delivery or the baby?

- Did you have any complications with previous pregnancies? Were any of your children delivered by Caesarean section?

- Have you had any medical problems before or during your pregnancy?

- Have you had any unusual discharge or leakage of fluid? Was it bloody, watery, or smelly? In what amount?

Determine whether delivery is imminent by asking:

- Are you having contractions or pain?

- What is the frequency and duration of the present contractions? Exactly what time did they begin?

- When did your bag of waters rupture?

- Is the pressure in the vaginal area increasing? Do you feel an urge to push? Do you feel as if you are having a bowel movement?

- How long were previous labors?

EMT Tip

When giving a radio report about a pregnant woman, begin by stating her age. Then give her gravida and para status followed by how many weeks pregnant she is. For example, "The patient is a 23-year-old G3, P1 female who is 39 weeks pregnant and in labor." Follow local protocol.

EMT
Tip

A pregnant woman's normal vital signs are usually different than her vital signs when she is not pregnant. Her blood pressure may be lower or her pulse may be faster when she is pregnant.

To remember the most important questions to ask an obstetrical patient, use the mnemonic CCLUE:

C | Contractions (presence, frequency, duration)

C | Complications (preterm deliveries, C-sections)

L | Leaking (bloody show, vaginal bleeding, rupture of membranes)

U | Urge (urge to use the bathroom, urge to push)

E | Expected delivery date

Next, complete a physical assessment including baseline vital signs. Determine whether the patient is bleeding or passing any tissue. Observe for edema of the feet, hands, and/or face. Palpate the abdomen gently. Does it feel very hard? Observe whether crowning is occurring. A rock-hard abdomen and bulging of the perineum indicate that delivery is imminent.

D.O.T. OBJECTIVES

Identify predelivery emergencies.

Differentiate the emergency medical care provided to a patient with a predelivery emergency from a normal delivery.

PREDELIVERY EMERGENCIES

You may be called to a scene where a pregnant woman is complaining of complications prior to labor or delivery. During predelivery emergencies, the same principles of emergency care apply as for a nonpregnant patient. Consider these events predelivery emergencies:

- Vaginal bleeding, either with or without pain, especially late in the pregnancy
- Suspected miscarriage
- Seizures during pregnancy
- Trauma

These conditions require specific medical care. Start with the scene size-up, initial assessment, baseline vital signs, mental status, SAMPLE history, and focused history and physical exam. Remember that the best way to save the life of the fetus is to save the mother.

Vaginal Bleeding

Vaginal bleeding may occur anytime during pregnancy, with or without pain. It appears as fresh, bright red blood. This is not normal. Do not confuse vaginal bleeding with show, the blood-tinged mucus that is normal before labor. If you observe bleeding, place a sanitary pad over the vaginal opening (see Fig. 18.7). Do not attempt to pack the vagina. Save any passed tissue and soaked pads in a plastic bag. Transport the patient to the hospital together with the bag. In all cases of vaginal bleeding, give the patient supplemental oxygen by non-rebreather mask. Monitor for early signs of shock.

Vaginal bleeding late in pregnancy and not associated with an imminent delivery is treated as a potentially life-threatening emergency. This condition may endanger the lives of the mother and fetus. One cause of bleeding is abruptio placenta, which occurs when the placenta separates from the uterine wall before the fetus is ready to deliver. Bleeding may be concealed or heavy. Abdominal pain is typically present. Another condition is placenta previa, which occurs when the placenta blocks the cervix. This prevents the fetus from entering the birth canal. With both abruptio placenta and placenta previa, emergency surgical delivery is needed to save both lives. Apply external pads and transport immediately.

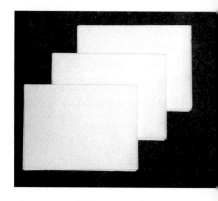

Figure 18.7 *Use external sanitary pads when vaginal bleeding is present.*

Miscarriage

A miscarriage is delivery of an embryo or fetus before it has reached viability. A fetus is usually viable after 26 to 28 weeks of pregnancy. Deliveries occurring after 28 weeks but before 38 weeks are called preterm, because the fetus is considered viable. Most miscarriages occur before the twentieth week. Preterm deliveries are most dangerous during the second and early part of the third trimesters. The fetus may have significant difficulty with survival if delivered during this stage of development.

The signs and symptoms of a miscarriage are:

• Cramp-like lower abdominal pain

• Moderate to severe vaginal bleeding

• Passage of large blood clots or tissue

• Dizziness or faintness

If you believe a patient is having a miscarriage, place sanitary pads over the vaginal opening. Collect used pads and any tissue passed in a biohazard bag. Transport the bag with the patient to the hospital. Do not try to determine the viability of the fetus. The mother may grieve over the threatened loss of the pregnancy. Be supportive. Avoid minimizing the loss. However, do not show false sympathy.

EMT Tip

Many hospitals have staff members who are specially trained to assist patients during and after a miscarriage. Encourage patients to seek support from these persons.

Ectopic Pregnancy

An ectopic pregnancy is one in which the embryo is implanted outside the uterus. Most ectopic pregnancies occur in the fallopian tubes (see Fig. 18.8). As the embryo grows and enlarges, it stretches the tube. This causes lower abdominal pain. The fallopian tube may eventually rupture. A ruptured tube can cause life-threatening internal hemorrhage.

Figure 18.8 *Embryo implanted in a fallopian tube.*

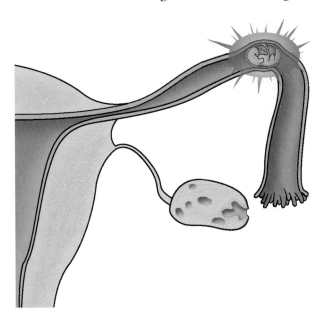

The signs and symptoms of an ectopic pregnancy are:

- Severe lower abdominal pain in early pregnancy
- Vaginal bleeding
- Shock

If bleeding is present in a suspected ectopic pregnancy, place external pads over the vaginal opening. Assess for signs of shock and manage accordingly (see Chapter 19).

Seizures

Preeclampsia is a condition of pregnancy in which the blood pressure increases. The patient's reflexes become jittery and excessive. This condition was formerly called toxemia of pregnancy.

The signs and symptoms of preeclampsia are:

- Diastolic BP above 90 mmHg
- Headache, confusion, seeing spots, or blurry vision
- Extreme edema of the face and/or extremities
- Right upper quadrant abdominal pain

***EMT
Tip***

The blood pressure in a pregnant patient should be lower than in a nonpregnant adult. A mildly elevated blood pressure in a pregnant woman suggests preeclampsia.

In severe preeclampsia, seizures may occur. Seizures in this situation suggest a life-threatening condition called eclampsia. It commonly occurs when the blood pressure rises to 160/110 or higher. In this condition, maternal mortality may be as much as 15 percent, and fetal mortality may be as high as 25 percent.

For suspected preeclampsia, transport the patient on her left side to optimize circulation to the fetus. This position also helps to lower the blood pressure. If the patient has a seizure, treat her as discussed in Chapter 14. Provide a low-stimulus environment. Avoid bright lights or noise. Provide oxygen at 15 liters per minute via non-rebreather mask and transport.

Supine Hypotensive Syndrome

Pregnant patients may develop a condition known as **supine hypotensive syndrome.** In this condition, the weight of the fetus compresses the mother's inferior vena cava. This restricts the return of blood to the maternal heart. The blood vessel compression results in a drop in maternal blood pressure. This is dangerous to both the mother and the fetus. Positioning the patient on her left side will relieve pressure on the blood vessels.

Supine Hypotensive Syndrome | Maternal hypotension caused when the mother is lying on her back and the weight of the fetus compresses her inferior vena cava

Trauma During Pregnancy

Pregnant women can sustain trauma. The uterus and amniotic fluid generally cushion the fetus from mild, blunt trauma. More severe trauma may injure the fetus as well as the mother's uterus, spleen, and liver (see Fig. 18.9). Treat trauma in a pregnant patient as you would in any other patient. Provide high-flow oxygen via non-rebreather mask. Assess baseline vital signs. Treat the patient's signs and symptoms. Treat for shock if indicated.

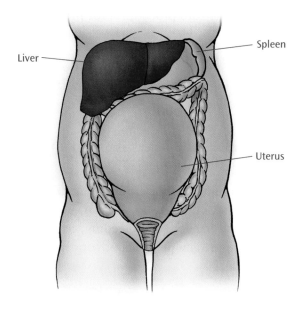

Liver

Spleen

Uterus

Figure 18.9 Because of its enlarged size and higher location, a pregnant woman's uterus is susceptible to severe abdominal trauma.

Transport the patient on her left side, if possible (see Fig. 6.27 in Chapter 6). This helps to avoid supine hypotensive syndrome. If the patient is on a backboard, place blankets under the right side of the board. This tilts her body toward her left side and slightly displaces the fetus off the major blood vessels of the abdomen (see Fig. 18.10).

Figure 18.10 *A towel wedged under the mother's right side shifts the fetus off major blood vessels (right).*

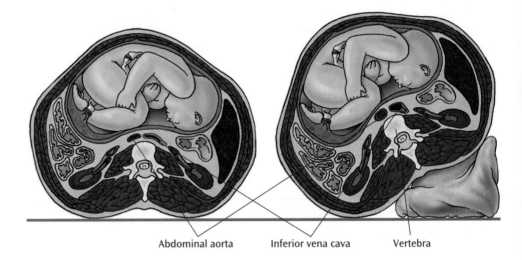

Abdominal aorta   Inferior vena cava   Vertebra

If a pregnant woman is killed in an accident, prompt initiation of CPR may save the life of a viable fetus. Follow your local protocols. If you begin CPR, continue it during transport. Immediately notify the receiving hospital. They will prepare for surgical delivery upon your arrival.

Emergency Care for Predelivery Emergencies

Follow the usual emergency care procedures for predelivery emergencies.

1. Complete a scene size-up.
2. Complete the initial assessment. Administer high-flow oxygen by non-rebreather mask if breathing is adequate. Assist ventilations with supplemental oxygen if breathing is inadequate. This helps to ensure adequate oxygenation of the fetus as well as the mother.
3. Complete a focused history and physical exam. Ask OB-specific history questions besides SAMPLE and OPQRST.
4. Provide special care for individual conditions as described in the previous sections. Treat for signs and symptoms of shock, if indicated. In cases of suspected miscarriage or late-term vaginal bleeding, cover the vaginal opening with external pads. Transport any products of conception and soiled pads in a plastic bag to the hospital.

5. Transport patients with predelivery emergencies rapidly to the closest appropriate medical facility. Follow local protocols. Complete a detailed examination while en route. If seizures are present, transport the patient on her left side in a low-stimulus environment. Use red lights and siren responsibly. Keep the patient compartment lights low.

6. Complete ongoing assessments every 5 minutes.

NORMAL DELIVERY

If you are called for a patient in labor, perform an initial assessment and focused history and physical exam. It is always best to transport an expectant mother to the hospital for delivery. However, be prepared because delivery might begin while en route. If your initial or ongoing assessment indicates that delivery is imminent, you will assist the mother with a prehospital delivery. Inform medical direction that delivery is in progress. Reassure the mother that you are ready to assist. Follow local protocols.

The procedures for assisting with a delivery are discussed in the following sections. They are summarized in Procedure 18.1. You will begin by taking BSI precautions and positioning the mother. During a normal delivery, the baby's head will emerge from the birth canal, followed by the shoulders and the rest of the body. You will then cut the umbilical cord and care for the mother and newborn. The placenta will deliver later. Birth is a normal physiologic process. It does not normally require emergency medical care. Complications that may occur during childbirth are discussed later in the chapter.

Follow these general precautions during delivery:

- Do not touch the mother's vaginal area except during delivery. Be sure your partner is present.

- Do not allow the mother to go to the bathroom. She may mistake the pressure of impending delivery for the need to have a bowel movement. Reassure her that this feeling is normal.

- Do not hold the mother's legs together. This will not delay the delivery.

- Recognize your own limitations. If the fetus has not delivered within 10 minutes of crowning, contact medical direction and prepare for transport.

EMT Alert

Out-of-hospital births involve a lot of blood and amniotic fluid. Take BSI and standard precautions in all cases of possible prehospital childbirth. Use gloves, eye protection, face shield, and gown. Handle blood- and fluid-soaked pads and linens carefully. Discard these items in the proper containers.

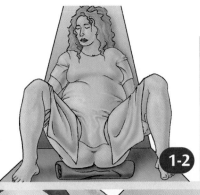

Procedure 18.1 • DELIVERY PROCEDURES

Body Fluids

Video Appendix

1. Position the mother on her back with knees up and thighs spread apart. Elevate her buttocks and prop up her back.

2. Create a sterile field around the vaginal opening. Use sterile towels or paper barriers. Place a barrier under the buttocks and thighs to receive the delivering baby. Place the OB kit within reach, but away from the birth canal.

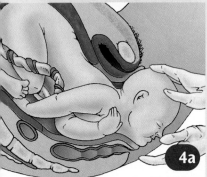

3. Assist the head to deliver as crowning occurs. If the amniotic sac is still intact, puncture it using a sterile clamp or your gloved fingers. Push the torn membrane away from the infant's head and mouth when they appear.

4. Apply gentle counter pressure as the head emerges. Place the cupped, outstretched fingers of your right hand across the top of the head. It will fit against your inner palm. Be sure to place your fingers on the bony areas of the skull. Apply gentle force with the palm of your right hand against the top of the head. Apply enough pressure to force the head to deliver in a plane parallel to the floor. Place a towel over your left hand while supporting the perineum.

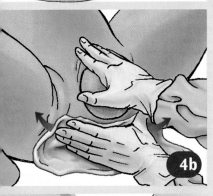

5. Determine the position of the umbilical cord as the head delivers. Feel behind the head and along the neck with your right index finger. If the cord is wrapped around the neck, try to hook it with two fingers. Slip it over the newborn's head. If it is too tight, place two clamps on the cord an inch apart. Cut between them very carefully with the OB scalpel and unwrap the cord from around the neck.

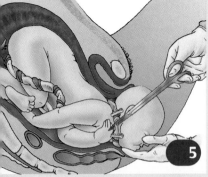

6. After the head delivers, it will probably face the mother's knee. Suction the airway while supporting the head. Use the bulb syringe to clear the airway. Compress the bulb, inserting the tip into the infant's mouth. Release the bulb to suction mucus and amniotic fluid into the syringe. Discharge the syringe contents. Suction the mouth and each nostril two or three times. Avoid contact with the back of the mouth.

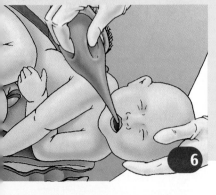

7. When assisting with delivery of the shoulders, continue to support the newborn's head. Gently cradle the skull with both hands. Cover each ear with your palm, with your fingers pointing toward the face. As the mother pushes, apply very gentle downward traction on the head, lowering it slightly. After the anterior shoulder passes below the pubic bone, raise the head upward slightly for the posterior shoulder. Be sure not to pull on the neck.

Procedure 18.1 • Delivery Procedures *(cont.)*

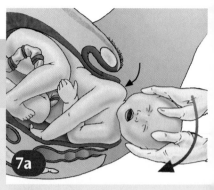

7a

8. As the rest of the body emerges, support the torso with both hands. Grasp the feet with one hand as they deliver. Support the neck and head with the other hand. Hold the slippery newborn carefully. Have someone record the time of delivery.

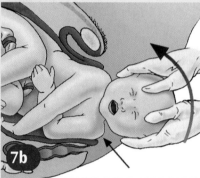

7b

9. Stabilize the newborn. Clear blood and mucus from the mouth, nose, and airway. Dry and warm the infant well. Position on its side with head lowered. Keep the infant level with the mother's vagina. Monitor the infant. Attach a temporary identification band.

0. Cut the umbilical cord when it stops pulsating. Place a clamp on the cord about three inches (four fingers' width) away from the infant's abdomen. Or tie the cord with umbilical tape. Place a second clamp about two inches closer to the placenta. Cut between the clamps with sterile scissors or the OB scalpel.

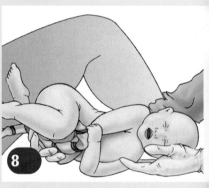

8

1. Watch for signs that the placenta is ready to deliver. Do not pull on the umbilical cord to accelerate delivery of the placenta. After it has delivered, wrap it in a towel and place it in a biohazard bag for transport to the hospital.

2. Care for the mother. Cover the vaginal opening with one or two external pads. If you notice perineal lacerations, apply firm pressure with sterile gauze for a few minutes. Lower her legs and help her to hold them together. Monitor for any signs of shock.

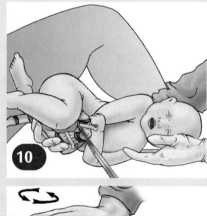

10

3. Stimulate the uterus to contract. Allow the infant to breastfeed. Place your hand on the mother's lower abdomen above the pubis, with your fingers fully extended. Feel for the top of the uterus, called the fundus. Gently massage the uterus using a kneading or circular motion.

4. Transport the mother, infant, and placenta as soon as possible. Continue your ongoing assessments while en route. If vaginal bleeding seems excessive, provide oxygen to the mother and contact medical direction.

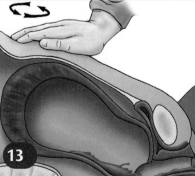

13

Identify and explain the use of the contents of an obstetrics kit.

Equipment and Supplies

A sterile obstetrics kit contains some basic supplies for assisting the mother during delivery (see Fig. 18.11). It also contains items for the initial care of the newborn. Table 18.1 lists the contents of an obstetrics kit.

Figure 18.11 *Typical items in an obstetrics kit.*

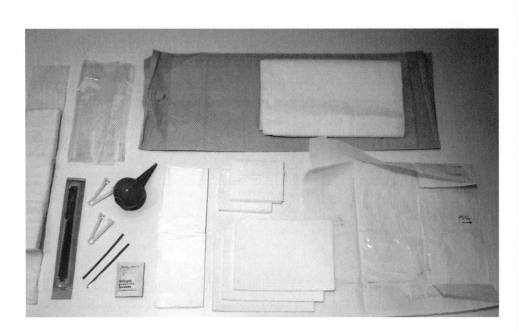

Table 18.1 • CONTENTS OF AN OBSTETRICS KIT

Item	Use
Surgical Scissors	To cut the umbilical cord
Hemostats or Cord Clamps	For clamping the umbilical cord
Sterilized Umbilical Cord Tape	To tie the cord instead of clamping
Bulb Syringe	For suctioning the newborn's mouth and nostrils
Sterile Towels or Barrier Drapes	For draping the mother
Five or More Gauze Sponges	For wiping and drying the newborn
Sterile Gloves	For protection from infection
Receiving Blanket	For wrapping the newborn and keeping it warm
External Sanitary Pads	For absorbing blood and other fluids
Large Plastic Bag	For transport of tissues and used supplies

D.O.T. OBJECTIVES

State the steps in the predelivery preparation of the mother.

Establish the relationship between body substance isolation and childbirth.

Pre-Delivery Care

Observe BSI and standard precautions. Personal protective equipment should include gloves, mask, gown, and eye protection.

While preserving the patient's privacy, remove her clothing and underclothes from the waist down. Have her lie down on her back. Position her to make the most room for the delivery. Draw the knees up, with thighs spread as far apart as possible. Elevate her buttocks with blankets or pillows. If possible, elevate the head of the stretcher to an angle of about 30 degrees. This helps the mother use the effects of gravity when she pushes, making expulsion easier. You can also prop her back with pillows.

Use sterile towels, sheets, or paper barriers to create a sterile field around the vaginal opening. Place one barrier under the patient's buttocks. Unfold it toward the feet to use as a sterile platform for the delivering baby. Place a sterile barrier over the abdomen. Drape another across the inner thighs. If time permits, tape a barrier over the back window of the ambulance to ensure the patient's privacy.

D.O.T. OBJECTIVES

State the steps to assist in the delivery.

Describe care of the baby as the head appears.

Delivery

With crowning, the perineum bulges and the fetal scalp becomes visible. The vaginal opening will stretch wide as the head delivers. This looks similar to a head pushing through a turtleneck sweater (see Fig. 18.12). Sometimes the head emerges suddenly in an explosive delivery. This doesn't give the perineum enough time to stretch properly and increases the likelihood of a perineal laceration. In addition, it can cause injury to the newborn's cranium. The delivering head also has a tendency to extend upward toward the ceiling as it delivers.

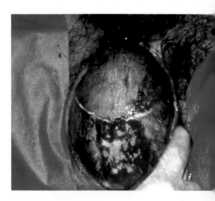

Figure 18.12 *Fetal head pushing through the vaginal opening.*

**EMT
Tip**

Remember that newborns are covered with amniotic fluid and mucous membranes. This makes them very slippery and difficult to hold. Although it sounds obvious, be careful not to drop the baby.

This increases the diameter that is passing through the perineum. In order to avoid injury to the mother or newborn, apply gentle counterpressure to the head with your right hand. This will help it to deliver slowly and keep it flexed toward the floor. Your fingers should be on the bony areas of the skull. Avoid pressing on the face or the fontanelles. Support the perineum with your left hand. The skin will be slippery from amniotic fluid.

As the head emerges, support it. The amniotic membrane should have broken before crowning, but occasionally it is still intact. If it is present as the head passes out of the birth canal, puncture it. Keep the membrane from obstructing the infant's head and mouth.

Figure 18.13 *Head facing the mother's knee after delivery.*

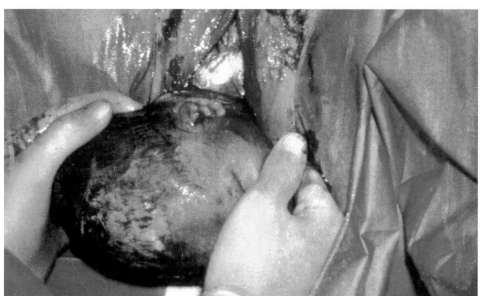

After the head delivers, it usually turns 90 degrees and faces the mother's knee (see Fig. 18.13). Feel behind it and along the neck with your right index finger. Determine whether a loop of umbilical cord is wrapped around the neck. This is called a nuchal cord. If you feel the cord, you must free it before delivering the rest of the body. Be very careful if you encounter a nuchal cord while in a moving ambulance. Consider stopping the ambulance momentarily before cutting the cord.

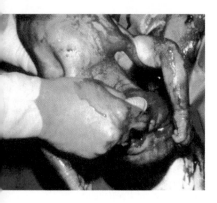

Figure 18.14 *Suctioning the infant's mouth.*

At this point, use the bulb syringe to clear the infant's airway. Suction the mouth two or three times (see Fig. 18.14). Repeat for each nostril. Avoid contact with the back of the mouth, because this can slow the heartbeat.

You may need to assist with delivery of the shoulders. As the mother pushes during a contraction, apply gentle downward traction on the newborn's head, lowering it slightly. This helps the anterior shoulder to pass under the pubic

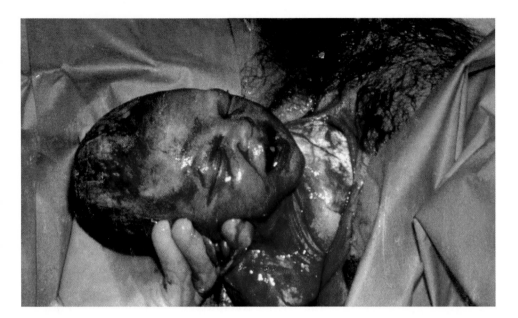

Figure 18.15 *Gently raise the head as the posterior shoulder emerges.*

bone. After the curve of the anterior shoulder becomes visible, raise the head upward slightly. This enables the posterior shoulder (the one closest to the mother's rectum) to pass through the perineum (see Fig. 18.15). Be careful when raising and lowering the head. Do not pull on the neck, because this could cause nerve damage.

Once the shoulders have delivered, the rest of the body will slip out easily (see Fig. 18.16). A gush of amniotic fluid may follow the infant. Support the feet with one hand and the neck and head with the other hand (see Fig. 18.17). The infant will be slippery. Be careful not to drop it. Never hold an infant upside down by the feet.

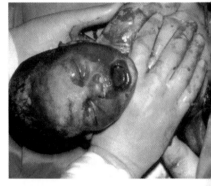

Figure 18.16 *Support the torso with both hands as it delivers.*

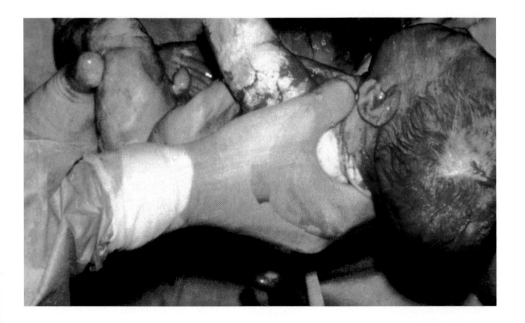

Figure 18.17 *Grasp the newborn securely.*

D.O.T. OBJECTIVES

Describe how and when to cut the umbilical cord.

Discuss the steps in the delivery of the placenta.

List the steps in the emergency medical care of the mother post-delivery.

Post-Delivery Care

After delivery, you will provide care for the newborn and the mother. First, stabilize the infant. Wipe blood and mucus away from the mouth and nose with sterile gauze. Use the bulb syringe to continue suctioning the mouth and nares until the airway is clear.

Newborns lose heat quickly. This causes their vital signs to become unstable. Dry the infant well. Drying also provides stimulation that encourages breathing. Wrap in a warm blanket, taking care to cover the head. Place the newborn close to the mother's chest to keep warm. Discard wet linens according to agency policy. Place the infant on its back or side, with the head slightly lower than the trunk. This promotes drainage of secretions. Avoid hyperextension of the neck. Keep the infant at the level of the mother's vagina until the umbilical cord is cut.

Ask your partner to assess the newborn and complete its initial care. These procedures are described later in the chapter. Attach a temporary identification band to the newborn as soon as possible. List the mother's name, the infant's gender, and the date and time of delivery. This will help to avoid confusion in case the mother and child are separated after arrival at the hospital.

If allowed by local protocol, cut the umbilical cord after it stops pulsating. Clamp the cord in two places and cut between them with sterile scissors. Leave three to four inches of the cord attached to the infant. This is a convenient intravenous site for hospital personnel to use if necessary.

The placenta will usually deliver by itself within 30 minutes after birth (see Figs. 18.18 and 18.19). Watch for signs that this is beginning. As the placenta separates from the uterus, blood may gush from the vagina. The segment of umbilical cord that is attached to the placenta may appear to lengthen. The mother may feel cramping and an urge to bear down. After the placenta delivers, bring it to the hospital with the patient. It will be evaluated later for clues about the health of the newborn.

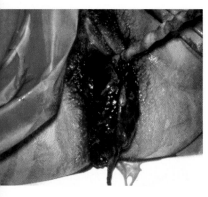

Figure 18.18 *Delivery of the placenta usually occurs within 30 minutes of birth.*

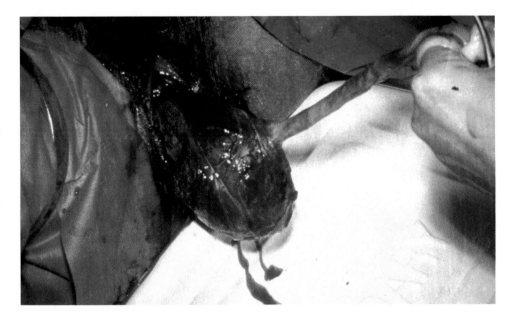

Figure 18.19 *Do not try to speed delivery of the placenta.*

Gently wipe blood away from the mother's perineum. Apply pressure to any perineal lacerations. Place a sanitary pad over the vaginal opening. Lower the mother's legs, helping her to hold them together. Transport the mother and the newborn as soon as soon as practical after delivery. Bring the placenta, if it has delivered. Do not delay transport to await delivery of the placenta. It may deliver while en route or at the receiving facility.

The normal volume of blood loss during and after delivery is approximately 500 mL. This loss will not have an adverse effect on the mother's health. You may need to reassure the mother if she is concerned about the amount of blood. Observe the mother for early signs of shock, even if blood loss does not appear excessive.

Stimulate the uterus to contract after delivery by massaging the uterus and by allowing the newborn to breastfeed. This slows the bleeding and decreases the amount of blood loss. As the uterine size is reduced, it will feel more firm and ball-shaped. Uterine massage can be very painful to the patient. Use enough pressure to knead the tissue, but not enough to cause unnecessary discomfort.

If vaginal bleeding continues, provide oxygen to the mother. Check your massage technique, and transport immediately. Continue your ongoing assessment and uterine massage while en route. If you suspect hypoperfusion, begin treatment and transport immediately. Provide supplemental oxygen. Contact medical direction. If necessary, request ALS backup.

EMT Tip

Transporting the mother and newborn in the same emergency vehicle is best. If complications occur, request additional personnel to the scene to assist. If extended resuscitation is required for either patient, separate transport units may be necessary.

ABNORMAL DELIVERIES

Emergency childbirth can involve abnormal delivery situations. Among the most common are:

- Prolapsed cord
- Shoulder dystocia
- Breech birth
- Limb presentations
- Meconium
- Multiple births
- Premature births

During any delivery, constantly reassess the condition of both patients. An abnormal delivery may not become obvious until the presenting part is visible. If you believe a delivery is abnormal, prepare to transport as soon as possible.

> **D.O.T. OBJECTIVE**
>
> Describe the procedures for the following abnormal deliveries: prolapsed cord, breech birth, limb presentation.

Prolapsed Umbilical Cord

Prolapsed Cord | Presentation of the umbilical cord before the infant's head at delivery; may cause fetal death due to constriction of blood flow through the cord

If the fetus is not positioned well into the birth canal when the amniotic sac ruptures, the umbilical cord can slip into the vagina in front of the head. This condition is called a **prolapsed cord** (see Fig. 18.20). This is a serious emergency that threatens the life of the fetus. The umbilical cord becomes pinched between the fetal head and the mother's pelvis so that the infant's blood and oxygen supply are cut off.

You will detect a prolapsed cord as it visibly protrudes from the vagina. Follow these emergency care steps:

1. Provide high-flow oxygen to the mother.
2. Position the mother on her knees with the pelvis elevated and head lowered in a knee-chest position. This uses gravity to help decrease pressure in the birth canal. In a moving ambulance, the left-lateral position may be more practical. Lower the head or raise the buttocks.
3. Insert a sterile, gloved hand into the vagina. Push the presenting part up and away from the cord. Do not attempt to push the cord back inside. Follow local protocols.

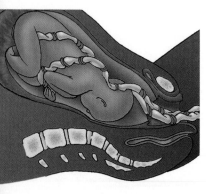

Figure 18.20 *A prolapsed umbilical cord.*

4. Wrap the cord with a damp, sterile towel to keep it moist.

5. Rapidly transport the patient.

Shoulder Dystocia

Occasionally, the fetal shoulder becomes wedged under the mother's pubic bone after the head delivers. This is called shoulder dystocia (see Fig. 18.21). The infant's body cannot continue down the birth canal because the shoulder width is too great. This can cause injury to the infant, including nerve damage or clavicle fracture. Irreversible brain damage may occur if delivery is delayed beyond 3 minutes. Death can result if delivery is prolonged beyond 6 minutes.

Shoulder dystocia cannot be detected until after the head delivers. Follow these emergency care steps:

1 Have your partner support the delivering head and monitor the delivery. Someone should call out the time every 30 seconds.

2. Help the mother to bring her thighs close to her abdomen. Keep the knees as wide apart as possible. This is the McRobert's position. It maximizes the room in the bony pelvis and facilitates delivery of the shoulder.

3. Apply pressure above the pubic bone. This helps to dislodge the shoulder. Do not apply pressure to the top of the uterus. This could cause the shoulder to become more severely wedged into the pelvis, making the condition worse.

4. Attempt to deliver the shoulder again. Keep the mother in the McRobert's position and maintain suprapubic pressure. Apply gentle traction on the head while the mother pushes forcefully. Never pull on the head or neck. This could cause permanent nerve damage.

5. Transport immediately. Be prepared to resuscitate the infant.

EMT Tip

A prolapsed cord is more common in preterm deliveries. This happens because the fetal head is small. The cord slips in front of the head easily. Prolapsed cord is also common in breech delivery. Because of the shape of the fetus' buttocks, the cord may slip past, entering the vagina.

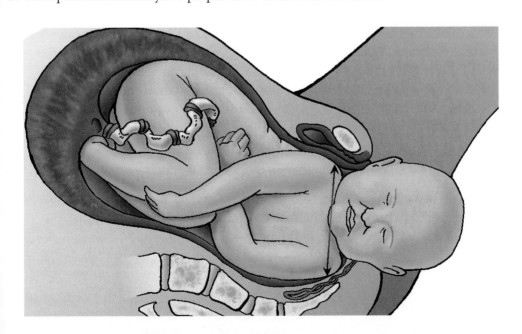

Figure 18.21 *Shoulder dystocia can lead to brain damage or death of the newborn.*

Breech Birth

A **breech presentation** occurs when the fetus' buttocks or lower extremities are the first part to deliver (see Fig. 18.22). Breech deliveries are difficult. During a breech birth, the newborn is at great risk for delivery trauma or oxygen deprivation from a prolapsed cord.

You may not know an infant is breech until the presenting part is crowning. Follow these emergency care steps:

1. Provide rapid transport immediately upon recognition.

2. Place the mother on high-flow oxygen by non-rebreather mask.

3. Instruct the mother to pant during the contractions and to stop pushing.

4. Place the mother in a knee-chest position, with head lowered and pelvis elevated. During transport, use the left-lateral position with the head lowered.

5. If delivery is imminent, you may have to deliver the infant in a breech position. Try not to attempt delivery without contact and consultation with medical direction.

6. Deliver the buttocks through the vaginal opening. If the feet are above the buttocks and delivery of the body seems delayed, you may have to free the legs. Follow local protocol.

7. Once the legs are out, deliver the infant as far as the umbilicus. Wrap the infant with a warm towel and support the body. Gently pull down a loop of the umbilical cord to decrease tension on the cord during the rest of the delivery.

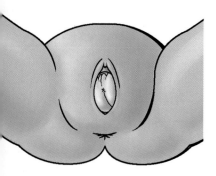

Figure 18.22 *A breech presentation with the buttocks as the presenting part.*

8. Grasp the infant at the hipbones and pull down. This helps to deliver the body as far as the upper back. Gently rotate the body so that the shoulders are vertical. Assist delivery of the shoulders, one at a time.

9. After delivering the shoulders, rotate the infant to a face-down position, supporting the trunk. While your partner applies suprapubic pressure, lower the body. This enables the back of the head to slip under the pubic bone. After the skull has emerged, continue suprapubic pressure while you gently raise the baby up and out of the birth canal. You may need to hook your finger inside of the baby's mouth to keep the head bent forward.

Limb Presentation

A **limb presentation** occurs when one of the extremities is the presenting part (see Fig. 18.23). This is often the foot of a fetus in breech presentation. You cannot manage this condition in the field.

You may first observe a limb presentation when crowning begins. A foot or arm will suddenly protrude from the birth canal. Follow these emergency care steps:

1. Begin rapid transport as soon as you recognize the condition.

2. Provide the mother with high-flow oxygen by non-rebreather mask.

3. Instruct the mother to pant through the contractions and to resist pushing.

4. Place the mother in a knee-chest position, with head lowered and pelvis elevated. Or use the left-lateral, head-down position. This may help to delay delivery.

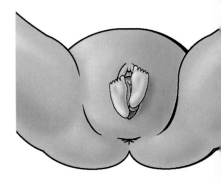

Figure 18.23 *A limb presentation with the feet as the presenting parts.*

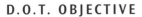

D.O.T. OBJECTIVE

Describe the special considerations of meconium.

Meconium

Meconium is fetal bowel material that passes into the amniotic fluid. This causes the colorless or straw-colored fluid to turn greenish or brownish-yellow. If an infant inhales meconium, pulmonary inflammation and pneumonia can develop. This type of pneumonia is called meconium aspiration. Meconium can vary from a thin, green-tinged fluid to a thick, pea soup consistency. If the fluid is not clear, this may be a sign of fetal distress.

Meconium (meh-KO-ne-um) | *Dark green fetal waste material that passes into the amniotic fluid; if inhaled, it will cause fetal distress*

Follow these emergency care steps:

1. Do not stimulate the infant to breathe until you have suctioned the oropharynx.

2. Suction the mouth, then the nose, after the head delivers. Quickly remove meconium from the airway. Clear as much meconium as possible. After delivery of the body, suction the airway again before the infant takes its first breath. Do not waste time.

3. Maintain the airway.

4. Transport as soon as possible. The infant may require resuscitation. Notify the receiving facility that meconium was present. Report whether you were able to suction any from the airway.

D.O.T. OBJECTIVE

Differentiate the special considerations for multiple births.

Multiple Births

Multiple births have become common because of the increased use of fertility drugs. A mother may or may not be aware of multiple fetuses. Premature delivery is a common complication of multiple births.

Follow these emergency care steps:

1. Follow the general procedures for a normal prehospital delivery. Contact medical direction. Call for additional assistance immediately upon recognition of a multiple-birth situation.

2. Be prepared for a preterm birth. Be prepared for more than one newborn resuscitation.

3. The second infant is breech in a third of all multiple births. Follow the guidelines for breech delivery.

4. If the second infant has not delivered within 10 minutes after the first birth, transport the mother and infant immediately.

D.O.T. OBJECTIVE

Describe special considerations of a premature baby.

Premature Birth

An infant born before the 38th week of development is premature. Premature infants have a low weight. They are usually small and thin, with red, wrinkled skin. Scalp hair is very fine and fuzzy looking, if present at all. The infant will not have creases on the soles of the feet, like a full-term newborn.

The earlier the birth, the greater the chance that the infant will require resuscitation. Follow these emergency care steps:

1. Resuscitation is usually needed. Follow the usual guidelines for newborn resuscitation (described in the following section). Supplemental oxygen by blow-by and artificial ventilation may be necessary.

2. A premature newborn is at great risk for hypothermia. Avoid heat loss by drying the infant quickly and thoroughly. Keep it wrapped in warmed blankets. Place the child close to the mother's skin. Heat the vehicle during transport.

3. Constantly monitor the newborn's ABCs.

NEWBORN ASSESSMENT AND RESUSCITATION

The first moments of a newborn's life are crucial (see Fig. 18.24). Your initial assessment enables you to quickly identify the need for resuscitation. Immediately after drying, positioning, and suctioning, evaluate the infant's breathing, heart rate, and color.

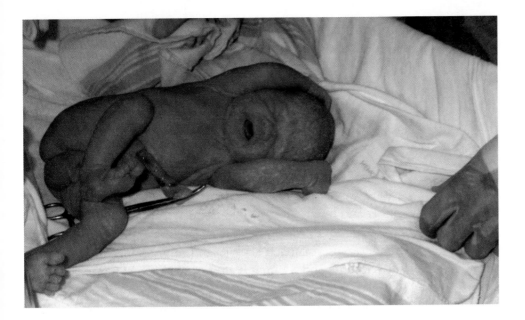

Figure 18.24 *After you have stabilized the newborn, assess its airway, breathing, and circulation.*

Assessment

Adequate oxygenation depends on a good breathing effort. If the newborn is not breathing initially, provide immediate stimulation. This may be done by slapping or flicking the sole of the foot or by rubbing the back. The rate and depth of breathing should increase in the first few seconds after stimulation. Determine whether the infant is showing good breathing effort. If the infant is still not breathing or is gasping, begin assisted artificial ventilations.

Next, monitor the heart rate. Adequate circulation to the brain and other vital organs depends upon the heart rate. Normal breathing may not provide enough oxygen to maintain the heart rate above 100 beats per minute. If the heart rate is below 100, provide artificial ventilations. Begin chest compressions and artificial ventilation immediately if the heart rate is less than 60.

As the newborn's breathing and heart rate improve, the skin or mucous membranes will begin to turn pink. Sometimes the trunk will appear blue in color, even though the infant appears to be doing well. This is a sign of inadequate tissue oxygenation. If present in a newborn with good breathing effort and heart rate, administer oxygen at 10 to 15 liters per minute. Hold the oxygen tubing as close to the newborn's face as possible (see Fig. 18.25).

Figure 18.25 *If the newborn shows cyanosis, hold the oxygen tubing and mask as close to the face as possible.*

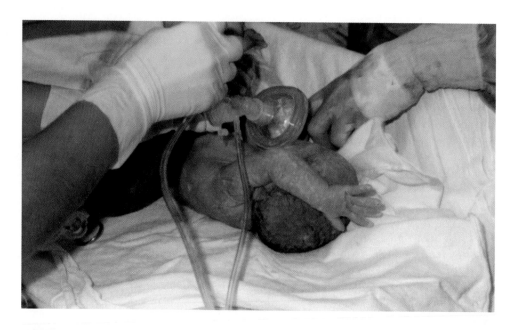

APGAR Score

APGAR Score | *Method for assessing newborns based on five ratings: Appearance, Pulse, Grimace, Activity, and Respiration*

If the breathing effort and heart rate are adequate, measure the **APGAR score.** APGAR is an acronym used to remember the steps for assessing a newborn. It stands for appearance, pulse, grimace, activity, and respiration. APGAR is usually recorded at 1 minute and 5 minutes after birth. Each component of the score is assessed separately (see Figs. 18.26 and 18.27). A numeric value is assigned to each finding (see Table 18.2). Normal findings are assigned a value of 2.

If the initial breathing effort is poor, begin resuscitation immediately. Do not delay resuscitation to calculate the APGAR score.

Figure 18.26 *Assessing the infant's skin color.*

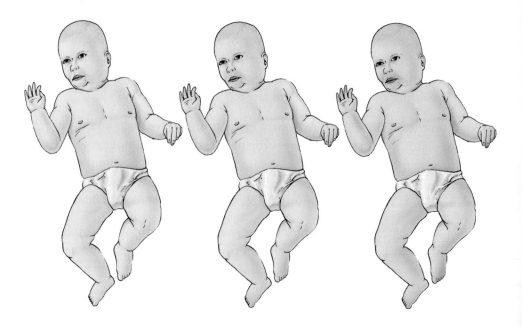

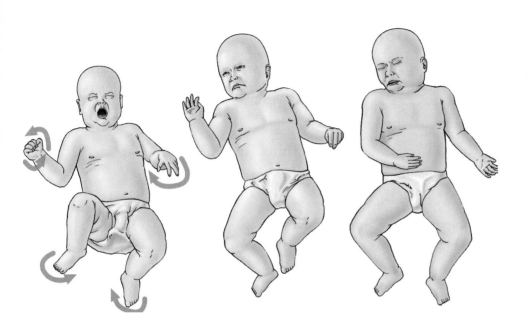

Figure 18.27 *Grimace is assessed by the reflexes displayed upon stimulation with a nasal or oral suction catheter.*

Table 18.2 • **NEWBORN ASSESSMENT (APGAR SCORE)**

Characteristic	Score=0	Score=1	Score=2
Appearance (Color)	Central cyanosis	Pink body, blue hands and feet (peripheral cyanosis)	Pink all over
Pulse	Absent	Less than 100 bpm	More than 100 bpm
Grimace (Reflex Irritability)	No response	Mild grimace or reflexes only upon stimulation	Vigorous and crying
Activity (Muscle Tone)	Limp	Some flexion upon stimulation	Active; good motion in extremities
Respiration (Breathing Effort)	Absent	Slow, irregular, ineffective	Crying, rhythmic, effective

D.O.T. OBJECTIVE

Summarize neonatal resuscitation procedures.

Resuscitation

While most infants do not require resuscitation, some delivery emergencies make the need for resuscitation more likely. You must anticipate the need for resuscitation and be prepared before delivery. Risk factors that indicate possible newborn resuscitation are:

• Maternal diabetes (also called gestational diabetes)

• Maternal hypertension

• Maternal drug use

• Meconium-stained amniotic fluid

• Multiple births

• Overdue delivery

• Premature delivery

• Prolapsed umbilical cord

• Trauma

• Vaginal bleeding

The American Heart Association and the American Academy of Pediatrics have established guidelines for resuscitation of newborns immediately after birth. An inverted pyramid is used to illustrate the relative frequencies and priorities of supportive measures (see Fig. 18.28). The items at the top of the pyramid occur most frequently. Frequency decreases toward the bottom.

Figure 18.28 *Relative frequencies and priorities of supportive measures for the resuscitation of newborns.*

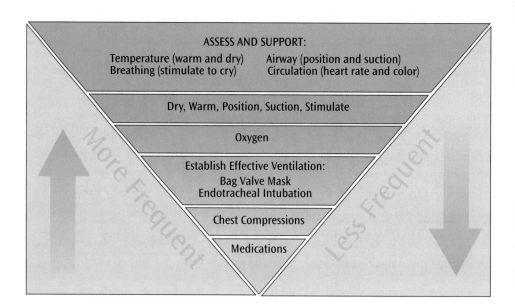

After birth, the need for resuscitation is based on your evaluation of the breathing effort, heart rate, and skin color. Usually, the newborn infant responds to the initial stimulation efforts. These are clearing the airway, drying, and stimulation. If the respiratory effort is inadequate, repeat these steps. Provide supplemental oxygen. Reevaluate respiration. If breathing is still inadequate, repeat all previous steps. Next, provide assisted ventilation. Repeat these steps during transport until the infant responds to treatment.

Provide assisted artificial ventilation with a bag-valve mask and 100 percent oxygen if the heart rate is less than 100 beats per minute, or if the infant's breathing effort is:

- Shallow

- Slow

- Gasping or absent

The mask must cover the tip of the chin, mouth, and nose. Avoid pressure on the eyes. With an airtight seal, the infant's chest will rise when you squeeze the bag. Provide enough pressure for the chest to rise normally. If the chest rises to its maximum height, the lungs are overinflated. This may cause a pneumothorax. Ventilate at a rate of 60 per minute (one per second) for 30 seconds. After 30 seconds, reassess the infant's breathing rate and effort. Continue to ventilate and reassess as necessary. Assisted ventilation may be discontinued when breathing is spontaneous and the heart rate remains above 100.

Chest compression techniques for a newborn are reviewed in Appendix B.

D.O.T. OBJECTIVE

Discuss the emergency medical care of a patient with a gynecological emergency.

GYNECOLOGICAL EMERGENCIES

The medical conditions discussed so far have been obstetrical emergencies encountered during pregnancy or childbirth. Gynecological emergencies involve the external female genitalia and the internal reproductive organs of a nonpregnant woman.

Vaginal Bleeding

Many gynecological emergencies include vaginal bleeding. Bleeding is usually caused by an abnormal menstrual period, trauma, or miscarriage. Some women are not aware they were pregnant when a miscarriage occurs. The scene size-up, initial assessment, and focused history and physical exam are similar to other medical or trauma cases. Always observe BSI and standard precautions.

Maintain an adequate airway and watch for signs of hypoperfusion. Follow these emergency care steps:

1. Complete a scene size-up.

2. Complete the initial assessment. Administer high-flow oxygen by non-rebreather mask if breathing is adequate. If inadequate, assist ventilations with a bag-valve mask and supplemental oxygen. For severe external vaginal bleeding, control hemorrhage with external pads and direct pressure.

3. Complete a focused history and physical exam. Treat for signs and symptoms of shock, if indicated.

4. Complete a detailed examination while en route to the hospital.

5. Continue ongoing assessments every 5 minutes if the patient is unstable, every 15 minutes if stable.

Gynecological Trauma

The internal female reproductive organs are generally well protected from injury. Their location deep within the pelvic cavity provides protection. The external female genitalia can sustain trauma from straddle injuries, sexual assault, or other causes. If you observe bleeding, treat as for other soft tissue injuries (see Chapter 20). Never pack the vagina with dressings to control bleeding. Reassess every 5 minutes if the patient is unstable and every 15 minutes if stable.

Provide the following emergency care in cases of genital trauma:

1. Complete a scene size-up.

2. Complete the initial assessment. Administer high-flow oxygen by non-rebreather mask if breathing is adequate. Assist ventilations with a bag-valve mask and supplemental oxygen if breathing is inadequate. Control hemorrhage with external pads. Do not pack the vagina.

3. Complete a focused history and physical exam. Treat for signs and symptoms of shock, if indicated.

4. Transport and complete a detailed examination while en route to the receiving facility.

5. Complete ongoing assessments every 5 minutes if unstable and every 15 minutes if stable.

Sexual Assault

After a possible sexual assault, the victim may be traumatized psychologically and physically. Respect the patient's need for safety and privacy. Cover her with a blanket or sheet after quickly assessing for other potentially life-threatening injuries. Examine the genitals only if profuse bleeding is present. Avoid giving details over the radio that could be overheard on commercial scanners.

Avoid passing judgment on the patient's situation. Recognize that she might respond better to a caregiver of the same gender. Do not withhold care for life-threatening injuries, however, if an EMT-B of the same gender is not available. Criminal assault situations require ongoing assessment and management of injuries. Provide psychological care as needed.

Preserving evidence is especially important in cases of alleged sexual assault. Follow local procedures for crime scene preservation. Advise the victim to avoid:

- Bathing
- Voiding or defecating
- Douching
- Washing hands
- Brushing teeth or rinsing mouth
- Cleaning wounds

EMT Tip

The general considerations and procedures in this section also apply to the sexual assault of a male patient. Also follow the usual guidelines for soft tissue trauma as described in Chapter 20.

These activities could destroy potential evidence that must be preserved until a medical exam is done in the emergency department. Observe local requirements and protocols for reporting cases of alleged sexual assault. Carefully document physical injuries and any pertinent statements made by the patient.

Follow these emergency care steps:

1. Complete a scene size-up. Request assistance from a same-gender EMT-B, if available.

2. Complete the initial assessment. Administer high-flow oxygen by non-rebreather mask if breathing is adequate. If inadequate, assist ventilations with a bag-valve mask and supplemental oxygen. Control hemorrhage with external pads. Do not pack the vagina.

3. Complete a focused history and physical exam. Treat for signs and symptoms of shock, if indicated. Ask history questions in a nonjudgmental manner. Examine genitals only if profuse bleeding is present. Discourage the patient from bathing, voiding, douching, or cleaning wounds. Protect and preserve the crime scene.

4. Transport the patient and complete a detailed assessment while en route to the receiving facility.

5. Complete ongoing assessments every 5 minutes if the patient is unstable, every 15 minutes if stable.

6. Follow local procedures for reporting sexual assault to the proper authorities.

Chapter Eighteen Summary

- Childbirth is a natural event. It is not normally a medical emergency. In an obstetrical emergency, remember that the best way to save the life of the infant is to save the life of the mother.

- Predelivery emergencies include miscarriage, vaginal bleeding, seizures, and trauma. Manage vaginal bleeding and suspected miscarriages with external pads. Treat for shock based on the patient's signs and symptoms. Bring any fetal tissues passed to the hospital. Treatment for a pregnant victim of trauma is the same as for other trauma patients.

- If delivery is imminent and crowning is present, prepare for immediate delivery. However, recognizing your own limitations is important. Transport the patient immediately if any difficulty arises, even if delivery may occur during transport.

- After delivery, dry, warm, suction, and stimulate the infant. Complete the APGAR scoring 1 minute and 5 minutes after delivery, if possible. Some infants will require resuscitation, especially if premature.

- Meconium is a dark green or brown substance that causes fetal distress during labor. It can obstruct the airway of a newborn. If present, suction the airway before stimulating the infant to breathe. Maintain the airway and transport as soon as possible.

- Abnormal deliveries can endanger the life of the fetus and mother if not managed correctly. If any part other than the infant's head presents with crowning, begin rapid transport immediately. Place the mother in the head–down, pelvis–up position. In the ambulance this may be accomplished using the left-lateral, head–down position. For a prolapsed umbilical cord, insert a sterile, gloved hand into the vagina. Gently press the fetus up to remove pressure on the cord. Follow local protocols.

- In an alleged sexual assault, try to have an EMT-B who is the same gender as the patient provide care. Remember that sexual assaults often cause tremendous psychological injury. Be calm, professional, and compassionate. Be aware of reporting requirements for criminal assault. Limit your exam to life-threatening concerns. Discourage the patient from bathing, voiding, or changing clothes.

Key Terms Review

Review Questions

1. The term amniotic sac refers to:

   a. Microscopic sacs in the uterine walls

   b. Sacs of the lungs where exchange of oxygen occurs

   c. Membranous, fluid-filled sac surrounding the fetus

   d. A complex, vascular organ that provides fetal nutrition and oxygen

2. The _____ provides nutrients and oxygen for the developing baby.

   a. Amniotic sac

   b. Fallopian tube

   c. Placenta

   d. Amniotic fluid

3. Blood is exchanged between the fetus and the placenta through the:

   a. Fallopian tube

   b. Uterine capillaries

   c. Placental blood vessels

   d. Umbilical cord

4. Labor pains are caused by:

   a. Contraction of the uterus

   b. Dilation of the cervix

   c. Growth of the fetus

   d. Loss of amniotic fluid

5. In a normal pregnancy, the developing fetus grows within the:

   a. Birth canal

   b. Fallopian tube

   c. Ovary

   d. Uterus

6. An infant born before the _____ week of pregnancy is considered premature.

   a. 40th

   b. 38th

   c. 35th

   d. 26th

7. In a birth with a limb presentation, the mother should be encouraged to _____ during the contractions.

   a. Breathe deeply

   b. Hold her breath

   c. Push hard

   d. Resist pushing

8. The knee-chest position is helpful in certain deliveries because it:

   a. Allows the pelvis to open to its widest dimension

   b. Slows delivery of the baby

   c. Keeps the mother from pushing

   d. Prevents perineal lacerations

9. The neck of the uterus is called the:

   a. Cervix

   b. Vagina

   c. Placenta

   d. Birth canal

10. The area between the anus and vagina that is commonly torn during childbirth is called the:

    a. Peritoneum

    b. Pleura

    c. Perineum

    d. Pericardium

Review Questions *(cont.)*

11. The pulse rate in a healthy newborn is:

    a. 80

    b. Over 100

    c. Unstable for the first 5 minutes

    d. Absent until the infant is dried

12. Which of the following signs and symptoms indicates that delivery is imminent?

    a. Bulging perineum

    b. Intense contractions

    c. Amniotic sac breaks

    d. Today is the due date

13. Which of the following personal protective items is NOT necessary for assisting with childbirth?

    a. Gloves

    b. Goggles

    c. Surgical cap

    d. Gown

14. Which of the following describes correct ventilation of a newborn using a bag-valve mask?

    a. The infant's chest should not rise when you squeeze the bag

    b. The infant's chest should rise slightly when you squeeze the bag

    c. The infant's arms should move actively

    d. Ventilate at a rate of 120 per minute

15. You are treating a pregnant patient who is seizing. Her husband states that she has been treated for high blood pressure and headaches during the pregnancy. She has no history of seizures. You suspect:

    a. Severe preeclampsia

    b. Epilepsy

    c. Hypertensive crisis

    d. Diabetic ketoacidosis

CASE STUDIES

Obstetrics and Gynecology

1 You are transporting a 33-year-old female in the third trimester of her first pregnancy. She has had a normal pregnancy. She is currently free of pain. Her contractions are 6 minutes apart and regular. She is having bloody show. There is no bleeding or discharge from the vagina. She is sitting in Fowler's position on the stretcher. Baseline vital signs are pulse 80, respirations 18, and blood pressure 128/72. The patient suddenly becomes sweaty and pale. She complains of lightheadedness. The vital signs are now pulse 110, respirations 26, and blood pressure 90/50.

A. What immediate action should you take?

B. What is the most likely cause of the sudden drop in blood pressure?

2 You are dispatched to an unknown emergency at a local hotel. Upon your arrival, you find several police officers standing around a partially clothed female sitting on the bed. An officer explains that the woman was raped.

A. What is your first priority after completing the initial assessment?

B. What type of physical exam should be done?

Stories from the Field
Wrap-Up

Obstetrical cases can be very stressful for EMS providers. In these situations, two or more patients are at risk. In addition, EMT-Bs infrequently care for obstetrical patients. Remember that childbirth is a natural event. Normal childbirth is not a true medical emergency.

In this case, a true emergency may exist. The patient has a history of premature labor. She is progressing toward a premature delivery. Premature infants are at risk for many medical problems. They may require extensive resuscitation due to incomplete development or stress during delivery. Transport the mother immediately to the closest appropriate facility. Try to avoid a field delivery. After completing the initial assessment, give the mother high-flow oxygen by non-rebreather mask. Increasing the mother's oxygen level increases the fetus' oxygen level. Place the patient in a position of comfort. Watch for signs of supine hypotensive syndrome. If seen, position the patient on her left side. Begin treating for shock. Performing a delivery while en route is better than delaying transport. Be prepared to resuscitate the infant. Notify the receiving facility so that they can prepare for your arrival.

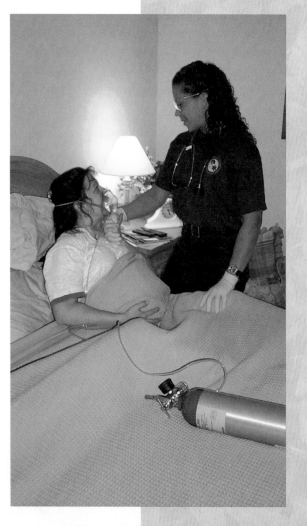

D.O.T. Module *Trauma* 5

Chapter 19

Bleeding and Shock

Stories from the Field

One Friday afternoon, you and Mark respond to an accident at a private residence. When you arrive, a woman leads you to a parking lot. She explains that her son cut his arm severely while working on her truck. As you approach, you see that the patient has his arm wrapped in a towel. A large amount of blood is visible on the driveway and the towel. The man starts to move towards you, but passes out. Mark braces him and eases him to the ground. He tells you to administer high-flow oxygen while he begins the assessment.

After a few moments, the patient begins to respond to verbal stimuli. Initial assessment reveals a large open wound to the right arm. The bone is exposed but intact. Bleeding is moderate right now. Mark controls it using a large dressing. The patient has no other obvious injuries. The SAMPLE history reveals a healthy 26-year-old male with no significant past history, no medications, and no allergies. Vital signs are respiration 24, pulse 120, and blood pressure 80/58. The skin is cool and moist. His pupils are equal and reactive. By the time Mark completes the rapid trauma assessment, the patient's dressing is soaked. Blood is running down his arm.

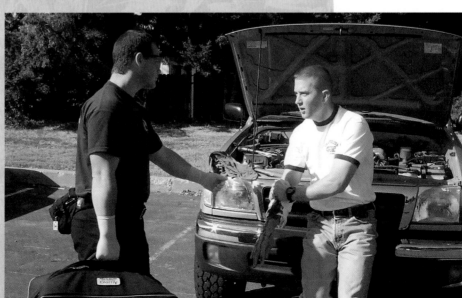

*E*xternal bleeding is a common sign of soft tissue injury. Bleeding occurs from many types of traumatic injuries. Although external bleeding is often the most obvious result of trauma, it may not be the most life threatening. Manage bleeding only after ensuring that a trauma patient's airway is patent and breathing is adequate. Bleeding can also occur internally. Internal bleeding is common from blunt trauma injuries.

Uncontrolled bleeding can cause inadequate perfusion of body tissues. This condition is commonly called hypoperfusion, or shock. You must learn to recognize the signs and symptoms of shock. This is particularly true for patients with significant external bleeding or suspected internal bleeding. After you have identified a patient who is suffering from shock, position and transport rapidly.

D.O.T. OBJECTIVE

List the structure and function of the circulatory system.

CIRCULATORY SYSTEM REVIEW

As a review from Chapter 4, remember that the circulatory system has three major components that must function adequately. First, the heart functions as a pump. The left side receives oxygenated blood from the lungs and pumps it to the body. The right side receives oxygen-poor blood from the body and distributes it to the lungs. Second, the arteries, veins, and capillaries serve as connecting tubing. Systemic arteries deliver oxygenated blood from the heart to the body under high pressure. Systemic veins deliver oxygen-poor blood from the cells back to the heart at a much lower pressure. The capillaries surround the cells and connect the smallest arterial and venous structures. The last component is the fluid, or blood. Blood carries the oxygen and nutrients needed for the cells. Blood also removes waste products from the cells for removal from the body.

A failure in any portion of the cardiovascular system will result in eventual failure of the entire system. When the system works correctly, oxygen and nutrients are delivered to the cells. Waste products are removed. Perfusion is adequate. Perfusion is the adequate circulation of blood through an organ structure. Shock (hypoperfusion) results from inadequate perfusion and oxygenation of the tissues and organs. Uncontrolled or excessive bleeding is one cause of shock. If not properly managed, shock will lead to cell and organ malfunction and eventually to death.

EXTERNAL BLEEDING

External bleeding is bleeding you can see. It may result from blunt or penetrating trauma. External bleeding occurs because of an injury to arteries, veins, or capillaries. When you care for patients with external bleeding, you must quickly determine whether the bleeding is minor or severe.

Severity of Blood Loss

The body's natural response to blood loss is to control bleeding through vasoconstriction and clotting. However, a serious injury or preexisting diseases can prevent effective clotting. Significant blood loss due to uncontrolled bleeding will lead to shock (see Fig. 19.1).

EMT Alert

You must routinely apply body substance isolation (BSI) and standard precautions (SP) when working around blood. Use eye protection, gloves, gown, and a face mask. Wash your hands thoroughly following each run.

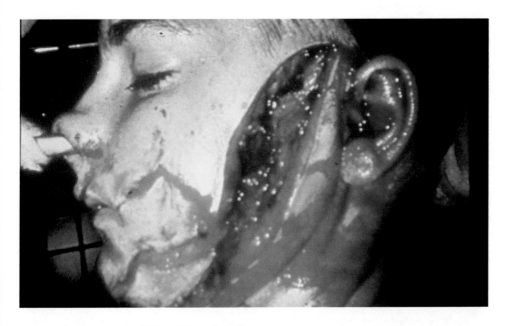

Figure 19.1 *Uncontrolled bleeding will lead to shock.*

Assess the severity of blood loss based on your general impression and an informed estimate. Also evaluate the patient's signs and symptoms. The average adult male has 5 to 6 liters (5000 to 6000 mL) of circulating blood. Most adult females have slightly less blood volume. The sudden loss of 1000 mL of blood in an adult, or 500 mL in a child, is considered serious. A 1-year-old child has about 800 mL of blood. In an infant, loss of 150 mL is significant, because this is approximately 20 percent of the circulating blood volume. Blood loss is also considered to be serious whenever a patient exhibits signs and symptoms of shock.

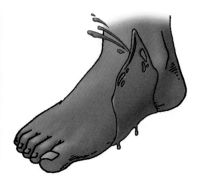

Figure 19.2 *Arterial bleeding.*

D.O.T. OBJECTIVE

Differentiate between arterial, venous, and capillary bleeding.

Types of Bleeding

Besides identifying the severity of external bleeding, you must be able to identify the source of bleeding. Bleeding may be arterial, venous, or capillary.

When an artery is cut, bright red, oxygen-rich blood spurts from the wound (see Fig. 19.2). The pumping force of the heart causes the surging action. The spurts generally coincide with the pulse. Blood pressure drops as blood is lost. When blood pressure decreases, the force of the spurting declines. Arterial bleeding is hardest to control because of the higher pressures on the arterial side of the circulatory system.

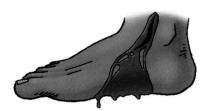

Figure 19.3 *Venous bleeding.*

When blood is lost from a vein, a steady stream of dark, oxygen-poor blood flows continuously from the wound (see Fig. 19.3). Venous bleeding can be profuse, especially if a large vein is injured. This bleeding is usually easier to control than an arterial bleed, because of lower pressure in the veins.

Capillary bleeding is usually caused by an abrasion, or scraping off of the top layers of skin. In this type of wound, dark red blood slowly oozes from the damaged capillary bed (see Fig. 19.4). This bleeding often clots spontaneously.

Figure 19.4 *Capillary bleeding.*

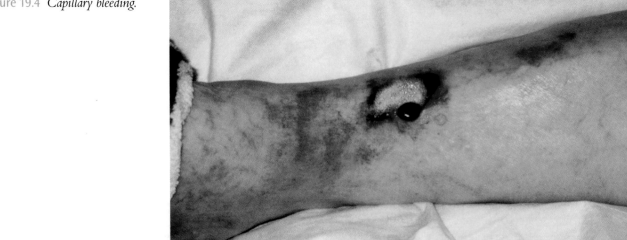

CD-ROM
Link

*Three animations in Chapter 19
and the Video Appendix on the
MedEMT CD-ROM illustrate the
differences among arterial,
venous, and capillary bleeding.*

Emergency Care for External Bleeding

The following steps outline the emergency medical care for a trauma patient
with external bleeding.

1. Conduct a scene size-up.

2. Complete the initial assessment. Manage the airway and breathing. This takes
   precedence over all other care. Provide oxygen to help to maintain adequate
   perfusion as blood volume is lost. If the breathing is adequate, use 15 LPM via
   a non-rebreather mask. If breathing is inadequate, use positive pressure ventilation with supplemental oxygen. Take cervical spine precautions, if necessary.

3. Assess circulation and control any severe or life-threatening bleeding. Follow
   the procedures outlined in the next section.

4. Conduct a rapid trauma assessment. Control any other external bleeding.

5. Complete a detailed physical examination while en route to the receiving facility.

6. Complete ongoing assessments as indicated by the patient's condition.

Bleeding Control

Controlling severe external bleeding can be lifesaving. This must be done
quickly as part of the initial assessment. To control external bleeding, you will
apply a series of methods until you find the one that works. Start with the
simplest and fastest method and work your way down the list. Methods used
to control bleeding, in order of preference, are:

1. Direct pressure on the wound

2. Elevation of the affected limb

3. The use of pressure points

4. Splints

5. Pressure splints (air pressure splints or pneumatic anti-shock garments)

6. Tourniquets

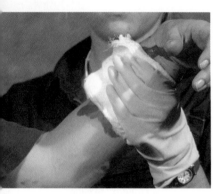

Figure 19.5 *Pack gaping wounds with gauze and apply direct pressure.*

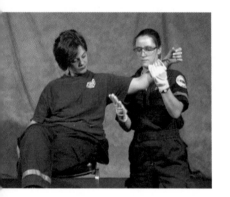

Figure 19.6 *Elevation combined with direct pressure can greatly slow bleeding.*

Pressure Point | *A place where an artery passes near the surface of the body and over a bone; pressure here can stop or reduce bleeding*

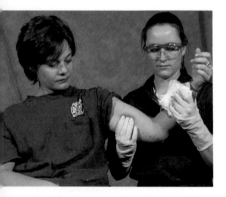

Figure 19.7 *Apply pressure on the brachial artery to control bleeding.*

After bleeding is controlled, apply a sterile dressing. Secure it in place with a snug bandage. Dressings and bandages are discussed further in Chapter 20.

Direct Pressure. Direct pressure is the fastest and most effective means of controlling external bleeding. Using the fingertips of your gloved hand, apply firm pressure to the injury. For a large, gaping wound, pack with sterile gauze (see Fig. 19.5). Then apply direct pressure with your palm. If this is ineffective, remove the dressing, determine the site of bleeding, and apply direct pressure again. If you discover diffuse bleeding, apply additional pressure over the wound.

Sometimes, direct pressure can be applied with a special bandage called a pressure dressing. To create a pressure dressing, firmly place dressings over the wound. Tightly apply a self-adhering bandage to hold the dressings in place. The bandage should extend above and below the dressings. It should be snug enough to control the bleeding, or tight enough so that it takes some effort to lift the bandage.

Elevation. Elevation of an injured limb can be used with direct pressure to slow bleeding. If possible, elevate the extremity above the level of the heart (see Fig. 19.6). Elevation is not recommended if the extremity is swollen, deformed, or very painful. These signs suggest a fracture or dislocation.

Pressure Points. If direct pressure and elevation fail to control bleeding, compressing the appropriate artery against an underlying bone at a **pressure point** may be effective. This reduces the flow of arterial blood to the extremity distal to the injury. For an injury in an upper extremity, feel for the brachial pulse. Compress the artery against the bone with your fingertips (see Figs. 19.7 and 19.8). For injuries in the lower extremities, find the femoral pulse. Use the heel of one hand to compress it, since the size of the artery and surrounding structures require much more force. Direct pressure may still be necessary due to venous bleeding or collateral circulation. This occurs when smaller vessels continue blood circulation after a main vessel becomes obstructed.

Splints. Splints control bleeding associated with painful, swollen, and deformed extremities. These can be due to a fracture, a dislocation, a sprain, or just a severe bruise. The exact injury will be determined later at the receiving facility. In the meantime, you should assume that the extremity is fractured. Splinting helps to control further tissue damage and reduces bleeding by immobilizing broken bone ends. Fractures are discussed in Chapter 21.

Air Pressure Splints. Air pressure splints control bleeding from soft tissue lacerations by applying direct pressure to the wound. They control bleeding from capillaries, veins, and small arteries. To a limited degree, an air splint may help to control bleeding from a fracture site by stabilizing the bone fragments.

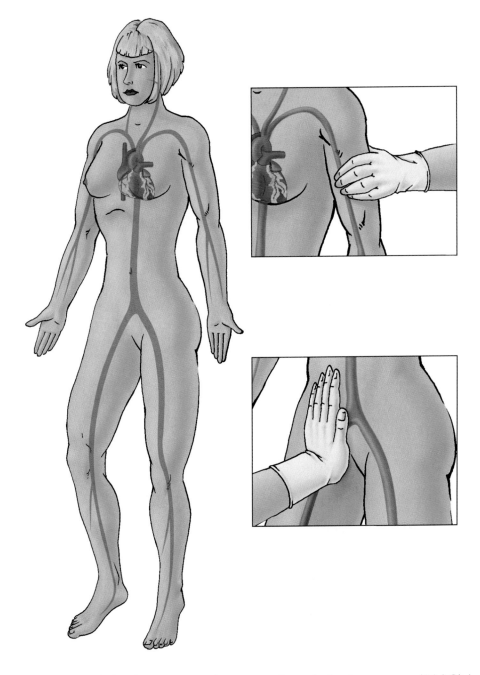

Figure 19.8 *Compression of the brachial artery (upper right) and the femoral artery (lower right) at the pressure points.*

CD-ROM Link

See the series of videos entitled "Bleeding Control" in Chapter 19 and the Video Appendix on the MedEMT CD-ROM for demonstrations of the techniques to control bleeding.

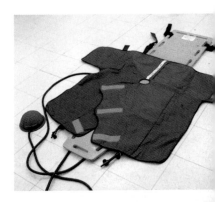

Figure 19.9 *Pneumatic anti-shock garment (PASG).*

Pneumatic Anti-Shock Garments. A pneumatic anti-shock garment (PASG) is also called a military anti–shock trouser (MAST). This is a large garment with three separate, inflatable compartments (see Fig. 19.9). One compartment wraps around the abdomen and pelvis. Separate compartments wrap around each of the lower extremities.

The PASG can be used as a pressure splint. It helps to keep unstable bony structures from moving and causing increased injury. The PASG can also effectively control bleeding from massive soft tissue injuries in the pelvis or lower extremities. As with the air splint, pressure from the PASG can control bleeding from capillaries, veins, and small arteries.

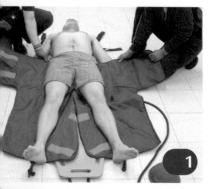

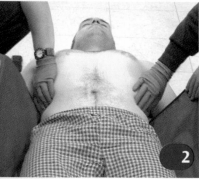

Use of the PASG is controversial. Apply it only if permitted by local protocol. It may also be recommended for patients with hypotension and a history of an abdominal aortic aneurysm. This is a ballooning of a weakened section of the abdominal aorta. Other conditions in which the garment may be useful are:

- Hypotension due to a suspected pelvic fracture
- Anaphylactic shock
- Severe traumatic hypotension

The PASG is contraindicated in cases of:

- Penetrating thoracic injury
- Pulmonary edema
- Rupture of the diaphragm
- Abdominal evisceration
- Acute myocardial infarction
- Cardiogenic shock
- Cardiac tamponade
- Pregnancy

Procedure 19.1 • APPLICATION OF A PASG

Video Appendix   Limit Bleeding   Bloodborne

1. Spread the PASG out flat over a long spine board. Log roll the patient onto the garment and board.

2. Align the upper edge just below the lower ribs. This placement will avoid restricting the lung capacity when the torso straps are applied.

3. Wrap the legs one at a time, securing them with the Velcro straps.

4. Wrap the patient's abdomen and pelvis and secure with the straps.

5. Make sure that the inflating tubes are connected and that the valve for the appropriate compartment is open to allow for inflation. Most stopcock valves have markings that indicate whether they are open or closed.

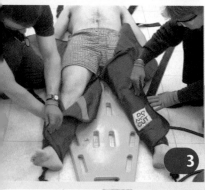

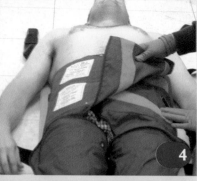

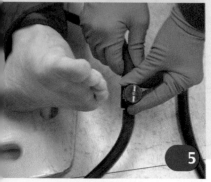

The steps for applying a PASG are shown in Procedure 19.1. Follow local protocols. The preferred method of unfolding is on a long spine board or other rigid lifting device. Smooth out wrinkles that would cause pressure sores if the device was left on for a long time. Undress the patient as much as possible. Bulky clothing or objects in pockets can also cause undue pressure on the skin. Complete your examination of the abdomen, pelvis, and legs, because these areas will not be accessible once the garment is applied.

Do not delay rapid transport of a critically ill patient to apply the PASG. If inflation of the abdominal compartment causes respiratory distress, deflate it immediately and notify medical direction. The distress could be caused by a diaphragmatic rupture. This is a hole in the diaphragm, usually caused by trauma. In this situation, inflation of the abdominal compartment will push the contents of the abdomen into the chest cavity.

Remove the PASG only under the direction and supervision of a physician. Deflate it gradually, beginning with the abdominal compartment. Gradual deflation prevents extreme changes in blood pressure. Monitor the vital signs closely during deflation.

CD-ROM Link

See the video "Pneumatic Anti-Shock Garment" for a demonstration of the application of the PASG.

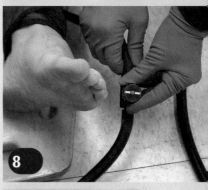

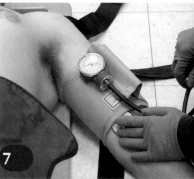

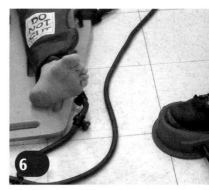

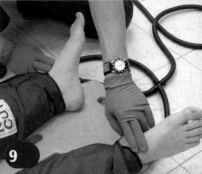

Procedure 19.1 • Application of a PASG (cont.)

6. Inflate the appropriate compartments with the foot pump. Stop when the Velcro straps begin to loosen or the pop-off valve releases. Depending on local protocol, you might only inflate one compartment at a time, checking the blood pressure after each is inflated.

7. If the patient is in severe shock, inflate each compartment in order. Check the blood pressure after each inflation. Attempt to attain a systolic pressure of 100 mmHg. All three compartments should be inflated for suspected pelvic or abdominal hemorrhage. Never inflate just the abdominal compartment.

8. Close the stopcock valves. Record the precise time that the garment was inflated. Recheck the patient's blood pressure every 5 minutes.

9. Check the dorsalis pedis pulses to confirm adequate circulation in the extremities.

Tourniquet | *A device that is wrapped around an extremity to prevent blood flow to or from the distal area*

Tourniquets. A **tourniquet** is a constricting band. It cuts off the distal blood supply in an extremity. It can permanently damage nerves, muscles, blood vessels, and underlying tissue. This may result in loss of the limb. Because of this risk, the tourniquet is used only as a last resort. Use it to control bleeding from an amputated extremity when all other methods have failed.

Application of a tourniquet is shown in Procedure 19.2. Always notify other emergency personnel who will care for the patient that you have applied a tourniquet. After applying one, write a notation indicating the time it was applied on the patient's skin. Use a visible location such as the forehead or abdomen. Also document the presence of the tourniquet and the time it was applied in your prehospital patient care report.

When using a tourniquet, take these precautions:

- Use a wide bandage and secure it tightly. This distributes the pressure over a wide area. A wide band closes the artery, but reduces the risk of cutting into the skin. Avoid using material that will cut into underlying tissue, such as wire, rope, or a belt.

- Leave the tourniquet in open view, so that other medical personnel know that it is in place. Never cover a tourniquet with a bandage or anything that hides it from view.

Procedure 19.2 • APPLICATION OF A TOURNIQUET

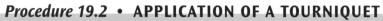

 Limit Bleeding

 Bloodborne

1. Choose a site proximal to the bleeding, but as distal on the extremity as possible. For example, if the wrist is hemorrhaging, applying a tourniquet too high on the arm could cause lack of perfusion and tissue damage to the entire arm.

2. Use a bandage 4 inches wide and 6 to 8 layers deep. Wrap the bandage around the extremity twice.

3. Tie one knot in the bandage. Place a stick or rod on top of the knot. Tie the ends of the bandage over the stick in a square knot.

4. Twist the stick until the bleeding stops. After the bleeding has stopped, secure the stick or rod in position.

5. You can also use an inflated blood pressure cuff as a tourniquet. Monitor it carefully to ensure that it stays inflated.

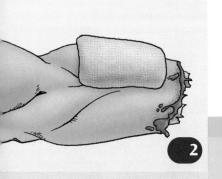

2

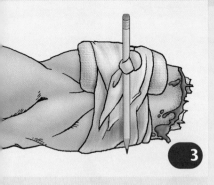

3

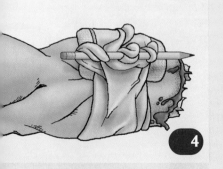

4

- After applying a tourniquet, do not remove or loosen it unless instructed by medical direction.

- Place the tourniquet as close to the injury as possible. However, never place it over a joint.

- Always write the time the tourniquet was applied in a visible place on the patient's body. Include this information in your written report. Follow local protocols.

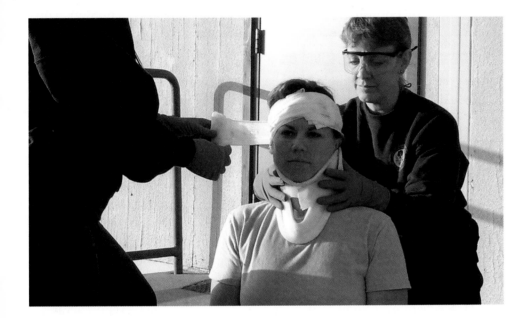

Figure 19.10 *In the case of a skull fracture, carefully wrap the patient's head with a sterile dressing.*

Head Trauma

A skull fracture can cause bleeding and leaking of clear cerebrospinal fluid (CSF) from the ears or nose. If this occurs from head trauma, do not attempt to stop the flow of blood or fluid. Use a loose sterile dressing to collect the fluid (see Fig. 19.10). This also prevents exposure to infection. Recognition and management of head trauma is discussed further in Chapter 22.

Epistaxis

Epistaxis, or nosebleed, may be caused by:

- Direct nasal trauma

- Environmental factors, such as dry air or dry mucous membranes

- Medical conditions, such as hypertension or blood clotting disorders

- Sinusitis or upper respiratory tract infection

- Digital trauma, caused by nose picking

Epistaxis (ep-eh-STAK-ses) | *Hemorrhage from the nose; nosebleed*

A nosebleed is not usually serious, but significant blood loss is possible. This may lead to shock. Patients taking blood thinners may bleed profusely. In this situation, you may have difficulty controlling the bleeding. Be sure to keep the airway open and have suction equipment nearby. Also, keep in mind that as blood pools in the stomach, the patient may become nauseated and vomit.

To care for patients with epistaxis:

1. Have the patient sit up and lean forward.
2. Pinch the fleshy portion of the nostrils together to apply direct pressure. This is effective because most nosebleeds occur near the anterior septum.
3. Keep the patient calm, quiet, and reassured.
4. Instruct the patient to avoid blowing the nose, even if the bleeding has stopped. This could cause a blood clot to break loose, causing further bleeding.

INTERNAL BLEEDING

Internal bleeding can be very serious. Initially, many patients with severe internal bleeding have no external signs or symptoms. Because no blood is visible on the outside of the body, detecting it may be difficult. Internal bleeding can lead to severe blood loss, resulting in shock and death.

Pay close attention to the mechanism of injury for a trauma patient (see Fig. 19.11). Mechanisms of injury were discussed in Chapter 8. Certain fractures, such as those of the pelvis or femur, can cause significant blood loss in the surrounding soft tissues. A bruise the size of a man's fist can contain about 500 mL of blood. Injured or damaged organs can have severe bleeding that is concealed.

Figure 19.11 *Internal bleeding is very common after a motorcycle accident.*

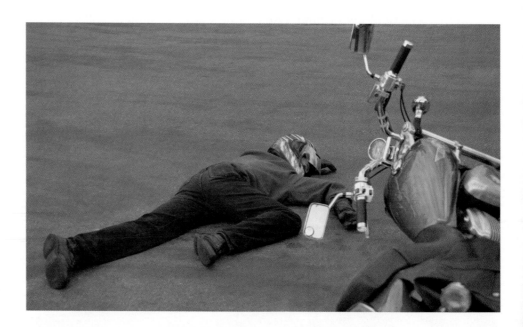

Medical emergencies not related to trauma can also cause internal bleeding. Some conditions, such as gastrointestinal bleeding or a ruptured tubal pregnancy, can sometimes cause external bleeding from an orifice. Assess the clinical signs and symptoms to determine the severity of internal bleeding.

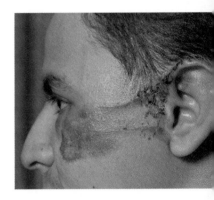

Figure 19.12 *Contusion*.

D.O.T. OBJECTIVE

Establish the relationship between mechanism of injury and internal bleeding.

Mechanism of Injury

Blunt trauma is a common cause of injuries that result in internal bleeding. Typical situations that can cause blunt trauma are:

- Falls
- Motor vehicle accidents
- Cycling accidents
- Pedestrian collisions
- Blast injuries

Signs of blunt trauma are:

- Contusions or bruising (see Fig. 19.12)
- Abrasions
- Deformity
- Edema
- Impact marks (see Fig. 19.13)

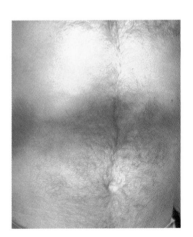

Figure 19.13 *A closed crush injury caused by the tire of a car.*

The location of these signs on the body is important. For example, if you find bruising on the ankle, there is a smaller chance of significant internal bleeding than if you find bruises on the abdomen or the chest wall.

Penetrating injuries from a gunshot wound, stabbing, or impaled object can cause significant internal bleeding. The region of the body penetrated, the proximity of organs and vessels, and the velocity of the projectile all affect the severity of the injury.

D.O.T. OBJECTIVE

List the signs of internal bleeding.

Signs and Symptoms of Internal Bleeding

A patient with internal bleeding will have pain and tenderness upon palpation. A tender, rigid, or distended abdomen is significant. This suggests further internal injuries. Tenderness is especially significant if located over vital organs such as the liver, spleen, or chest. Swelling or bruising may or may not be present at the site of injury.

Internal bleeding may leak outside the body through the vagina or another orifice. Rectal bleeding can indicate gastrointestinal bleeding. The external blood can range in appearance from bright red, to maroon, to a dark, tarry appearance. An emesis containing bright red blood is evidence of upper gastrointestinal bleeding. An emesis that looks like coffee grounds also suggests internal bleeding.

Internal bleeding can be so severe that the patient develops signs and symptoms of shock. This is true for both traumatic and medical causes.

D.O.T. OBJECTIVE

List the steps in the emergency medical care of the patient with signs and symptoms of internal bleeding.

Emergency Care for Internal Bleeding

The following steps outline the emergency medical care of a patient with internal bleeding.

1. Conduct a scene size-up.

2. Complete the initial assessment. Ensure that the airway and breathing are controlled. If the breathing is adequate, provide oxygen at 15 LPM via a nonrebreather mask. If breathing is inadequate, use positive pressure ventilation with supplemental oxygen. Based on the mechanism of injury, take cervical spine precautions if necessary.

3. Complete a focused history and physical exam or a rapid trauma assessment. If permitted in your area, a PASG may be used for uncontrollable hemorrhage or suspected pelvic fractures. The PASG is also recommended for hypotension with a history of an abdominal aortic aneurysm.

4. Rapid transport is indicated if you suspect internal bleeding. Emergency surgery or other lifesaving measures may be necessary.

SHOCK (HYPOPERFUSION)

As mentioned previously, shock is also called hypoperfusion. It is a complex process caused by decreased circulation to the tissues. This results in inadequate perfusion of the cells with oxygen and a build-up of metabolic waste products. Tissue and organ malfunction can occur. At a certain point, shock becomes irreversible and leads to death. The patient's age, underlying medical conditions, and severity of injuries all influence the outcome. Prompt recognition and treatment of shock is essential for patient survival.

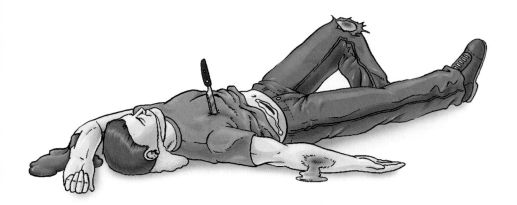

Figure 19.14 *This patient will probably have signs and symptoms of shock.*

Shock is caused by many factors. There are different types of shock that have different causes. **Hemorrhagic shock** is common in trauma patients. Here, hemorrhage causes loss of blood volume (see Fig. 19.14). Blood may be lost externally through a wound, or internally from bleeding due to traumatic internal injuries. This leads to a drop in blood pressure, reducing the body's ability to perfuse vital organs.

Hypovolemic shock is caused by a low volume of fluid circulating in the body. This may be due to blood loss, as in hemorrhagic shock. It may also result from depletion of other body fluids. Significant loss of body fluids can also cause dehydration. The patient will eventually develop hypovolemic shock. Conditions causing fluid depletion are:

• Gastrointestinal diseases with severe vomiting or diarrhea

• Extensive burns with loss of plasma

• Prolonged exertion in hot temperatures causing profuse sweating

• Excessive urination, as seen in diabetics with very high blood sugar and with some other conditions

• Fever

Hemorrhagic (hem-or-AJ-ik) Shock | *Hypoperfusion syndrome caused by excessive blood loss; a type of hypovolemic shock; the most common cause of shock in a trauma patient*

Hypovolemic Shock | *Shock caused by inadequate circulatory volume; may be due to loss of blood or depletion of other body fluids*

You are not expected to diagnose the type of shock your patient is experiencing. Recognize that shock exists and treat it correctly, including rapid transport. Other types of shock are discussed in the Enhanced Study section at the end of this chapter.

D.O.T. OBJECTIVE

List signs and symptoms of shock (hypoperfusion).

Signs and Symptoms of Shock

During shock, the body reduces blood flow to peripheral areas, such as the skin, in order to restore blood volume to vital organs. Blood is shunted to the brain, heart, and kidneys. As this occurs, the skin becomes pale, cool, and clammy.

With hemorrhagic or hypovolemic shock, the body compensates for a loss of blood volume by increasing the heart rate. The respiratory rate becomes rapid and shallow. The kidneys may shut down to reduce water loss and increase blood volume. These mechanisms create a condition called hypoperfusion syndrome. If hypoperfusion syndrome is untreated, decreased perfusion to the brain can lead to agitation, mental confusion, loss of consciousness, and death.

Table 19.1 summarizes the signs and symptoms of shock. Although the stages of shock clearly progress from minor to severe in some patients, many patients quickly move between stages. You may see signs of late and early shock at the same time.

Special Considerations: Infants and Children

Unlike adults, infants and children maintain a normal blood pressure until more than half their blood volume has been lost. By the time a child's blood pressure drops, he or she is near death. A drop in blood pressure is considered a late sign of shock in children. An increased pulse rate is usually an early sign. Depending on blood pressure alone to diagnose shock in children provides a false sense of security. You must rely on other findings. Evaluate capillary refill time, peripheral pulse strength, suspicion of trauma, and mechanism of injury. Remember, even a small amount of blood loss can have very negative effects in an infant or child.

D.O.T. OBJECTIVE

State the steps in the emergency medical care of the patient with signs and symptoms of shock.

Table 19.1 • **SIGNS AND SYMPTOMS OF SHOCK (HYPOPERFUSION)**

Assessment	Signs and Symptoms
Mental Status	Restlessness Anxiety Altered mental status Combativeness
Peripheral Perfusion	Weak, thready, or absent peripheral pulses Pale, cool, clammy skin In infants and children, delayed capillary refill time (more than 2 seconds in normal ambient air temperature)
Vital Signs	Increased pulse rate; pulse weak and thready (an early sign) Increased breathing rate; breathing is shallow, labored, or irregular Dilated pupils Decreased blood pressure (a late sign)
Other	Marked thirst Nausea and vomiting Pallor with cyanosis to the lips Decreased urinary output Weakness, faintness, or dizziness

Emergency Management of Shock

The following steps outline the emergency medical care for managing a patient with signs and symptoms of shock.

1. Conduct a scene size-up.

2. Complete the initial assessment. Ensure that the airway and breathing are intact. Take cervical spine precautions, if necessary. Administer high-flow oxygen to aid perfusion. If the breathing is adequate, use 15 LPM via a nonrebreather mask. If breathing is inadequate, use positive pressure ventilation with supplemental oxygen.

3. Complete a focused history and physical exam or a rapid trauma assessment. Treat life-threatening problems as you discover them. Control external bleeding. If you suspect a pelvic fracture, use the PASG according to local protocol. The PASG may also be used when the patient has a history of an abdominal aortic aneurysm and no chest injury is present.

4. Elevate the lower extremities about 8 to 12 inches, unless the patient has had serious injury to the head, neck, spine, chest, abdomen, pelvis, or lower extremity.

5. Splint any suspected bone or joint injuries (see Chapter 21).

6. Cover the patient with a blanket to prevent loss of body heat.

7. Transport immediately to the nearest appropriate facility. Conduct a detailed assessment while en route to the facility. Conduct ongoing assessments every 5 minutes.

Chapter Nineteen Summary

- Bleeding is a common sign of traumatic injury. Severe bleeding can result in shock. The body normally controls bleeding by constriction of blood vessels and clotting.

- Arterial bleeding, identified by distinct spurting and a bright red color, is difficult to control. This is often a life-threatening condition. Venous bleeding is usually easier to control, but significant blood loss is possible.

- You must consider internal bleeding to be life threatening. Suspect internal bleeding based on the patient's signs and symptoms and the mechanism of injury.

- Control bleeding by direct pressure, elevation, splints, or tourniquet.

- Trauma patients may develop shock (hypoperfusion syndrome) from external and/or internal blood loss. This type of shock is referred to as hypovolemic or hemorrhagic shock.

Key Terms Review

Epistaxis | *page 557*
Hemorrhagic Shock | *page 561*

Hypovolemic Shock | *page 561*
Pressure Point | *page 552*

Tourniquet | *page 556*

Review Questions

1. The term artery refers to:

   a. Any vessel carrying blood
   b. Large systemic vessels that carry oxygenated blood
   c. Any vessel carrying blood toward the heart
   d. Any vessel carrying deoxygenated blood

2. The left side of the heart:

   a. Receives oxygenated blood from the lungs and pumps it through the body
   b. Pumps blood to the pulmonary vein
   c. Is the smallest chamber
   d. Pumps deoxygenated blood to the lungs

3. The average blood volume of an adult male is about:

   a. 5–6 liters
   b. 4 liters
   c. 2–3 liters
   d. 5 gallons

4. Most external bleeding is effectively controlled using:

   a. Pressure points and elevation
   b. Direct pressure and elevation
   c. Direct pressure and pressure points
   d. Pressure splints

5. Bright red blood spurting out of a wound is coming from:

   a. An artery

   b. A vein

   c. The capillary bed

   d. A skull fracture

6. Another name for hypoperfusion syndrome is:

   a. Hemorrhage

   b. Infarction

   c. Aneurysm

   d. Shock

7. Hypovolemic shock results from:

   a. Dilated blood vessels

   b. Loss of blood or body fluids

   c. Failure of the nervous system to control the vascular system

   d. Organ malfunction

8. Which of the following is NOT part of the correct treatment for hypovolemic shock?

   a. Sitting position

   b. Control bleeding

   c. Administer oxygen

   d. Maintain body warmth

9. The right side of the heart pumps blood to the:

   a. Lungs

   b. Body

   c. Brain

   d. Liver

10. Shock is defined as:

   a. Inadequate tissue perfusion

   b. Poor systemic circulation

   c. Myocardial infarction

   d. Altered mental status

11. The term perfusion means:

   a. The adequate flow of blood through an organ structure

   b. An irregular heartbeat

   c. A patient with early signs of Alzheimer's

   d. The movement of a fluid across a membrane

12. You are treating a patient who has had a myocardial infarction and is now in shock. What part of the circulatory system has been compromised in this patient?

   a. Fluid

   b. Tubing

   c. Pump

   d. Hose

13. Your patient has a rigid, distended abdomen after being thrown from a horse. Which injury could be causing internal bleeding?

   a. Liver laceration

   b. Subdural hematoma

   c. Scalp laceration

   d. Pneumothorax

14. A laceration to the carotid artery from a razor blade would probably be categorized as what type of bleeding?

   a. Capillary

   b. Minor

   c. Moderate

   d. Severe

15. The sudden loss of _____ of blood is considered serious in an adult.

   a. 100 mL

   b. 1000 mL

   c. 500 mL

   d. 6 L

CASE STUDIES

Bleeding and Shock

1 You are dispatched to a rural trailer park to treat the victim of an assault. The dispatcher advises you that law enforcement officers have secured the scene and the weapon involved. When you arrive, you find a middle-aged man with multiple stab wounds to the chest, abdomen, and back. After taking BSI and standard precautions, you begin your initial assessment. There is a major bleed on the upper right arm. You find no other potentially life-threatening injuries.

A. What is your initial treatment for the major wound?

B. During your rapid trauma assessment, you note many long, shallow cuts to the torso. These are bleeding mildly. You also notice that your dressing is not adequately controlling bleeding of the right arm. Which wound do you manage next?

C. If direct pressure fails to control the bleeding, what other steps will you take?

2 One morning you respond to an injured child in a home. You find a 6-year-old girl sitting quietly with her mother. A large amount of blood is on the towel the child is holding to her face. The mother informs you that the child has a history of uncontrollable nosebleeds. After taking BSI and SP, you complete the initial assessment. This reveals no life-threatening problems. The focused history and physical exam reveals no active bleeding. The mother wants the child to be taken to the hospital. This upsets the girl. Her nose begins bleeding again.

A. How will you treat the nosebleed?

B. Why is the forward-leaning position important?

3 Your EMS unit is providing coverage for a rodeo event. One of the rodeo clowns accidentally falls and is trampled by a large bull. Your unit arrives to find a 38-year-old man lying on his right side. After taking BSI and SP, you manually stabilize the cervical spine. Your initial assessment reveals no life-threatening injuries. The patient is alert and oriented. Based on the mechanism of injury, you apply high-flow oxygen by non-rebreather mask. Your rapid trauma assessment fails to identify any serious external signs of injury. The patient's initial vital signs are pulse 110, respirations 22, and blood pressure 90/50. His skin is very cool and moist, despite the hot and humid environment. The patient has no previous medical problems. He takes no medications.

A. What condition might you suspect in this patient?

B. Why does internal bleeding warrant rapid transport?

C. While en route to the hospital, the patient's condition worsens. Repeat vital signs show pulse 124, respiration 26, and blood pressure 82/40. The patient is now responsive only to painful stimuli. What other steps can you take to treat this patient's condition?

Stories from the Field
Wrap-Up

A lthough this trauma patient only has one injury, it could be life threatening. Wounds that bleed profusely can result in inadequate perfusion of the body tissues, causing hypoperfusion. This patient has the classic signs and symptoms of shock. He has cool, clammy skin, a fast pulse and respiratory rate, low blood pressure, and mental status changes. When caring for a patient with these symptoms, rapid transport is essential. The patient needs definitive care in the emergency department.

In this case, you and Mark should place the patient in the Trendelenburg position and elevate the injured arm. This reduces blood flow to the injury and keeps more blood circulating to the vital organs. Because the bleeding has only been partially controlled, apply a pressure dressing. If this does not control the bleeding, apply pressure to the pressure point on the brachial artery. Cover the patient with a blanket to prevent heat loss. Transport as soon as possible after completing the rapid trauma assessment.

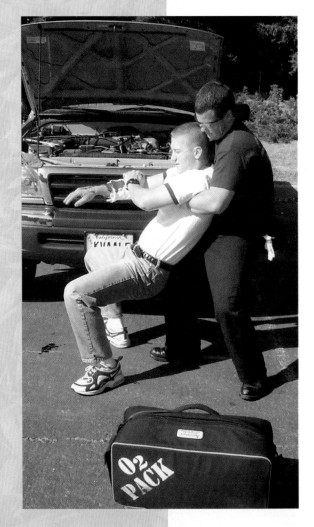

ENHANCED STUDY

Types of Shock

As an EMT-Basic, the most common form of shock you will see is hypovolemic or hemorraghic shock. The following types of shock have other causes. You are not expected to diagnose the type of shock. You must recognize and treat shock when the mechanism of injury or signs and symptoms suggest the possibility of this condition.

Cardiogenic Shock. This condition occurs when the heart cannot pump adequately. Situations that lead to the development of cardiogenic shock are heart muscle damage from a myocardial infarction, dysrhythmias, and other heart diseases. The patient may have signs and symptoms of chest pain and difficulty breathing. On further examination, you may find hypotension and edema of the lower extremities. You may hear fluid in the lungs or crackles. Treatment includes high-flow oxygen and rapid transport. See the section on cardiac emergencies for additional information (Chapter 13).

Distributive Shock. In this general classification of shock, the body has a normal fluid volume. However, fluid is in the wrong place. This is caused by vasodilation, or inappropriate dilation of the blood vessels. Fluid leakage into other tissues also contributes to this condition. Neurogenic shock, septic shock, and anaphylactic shock are examples of this classification.

Neurogenic Shock. If the spinal cord is severely damaged, the sympathetic nervous system will not be able to constrict the blood vessels. Neurogenic shock results from vasodilation. Signs and symptoms are hypotension without tachycardia or vasoconstriction. This condition is often seen in trauma patients with spinal cord injury.

Septic Shock. This condition is caused by release of bacterial toxins into the bloodstream (see Enhancement Fig. 19.1). When this occurs, fluid leaks into the tissues because of vasodilation. Septic shock may not appear until several days after a serious illness or injury.

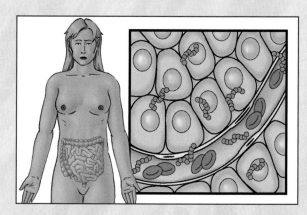

Enhancement Figure 19.1 *In septic shock, bacterial toxins affect the circulation and cause a critical decrease in tissue perfusion.*

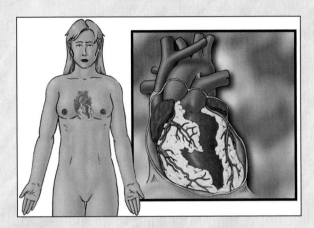

Enhancement Figure 19.2 *Obstructive shock results when blood flow from the heart is blocked.*

Obstructive Shock. In obstructive shock, blood volume is normal. The heart's ability to pump and circulate blood is normal. However, an obstruction to blood flow is present (see Enhancement Fig. 19.2). This may be caused by cardiac tamponade, in which the sac around the heart is filled with fluid. The heart will be unable to fill adequately to pump the blood. Tension pneumothorax is another condition that may cause obstructive shock. This results from an air leak between the lungs and the chest wall. The leak eventually causes the lungs to collapse. The mediastinum shifts, preventing the heart from filling. Management of cardiac tamponade and tension pneumothorax is discussed in the section on chest injuries in Chapter 20.

Anaphylactic Shock. Anaphylactic shock is an extreme allergic reaction to a foreign substance such as a bee sting. The allergen causes blood vessels to dilate and leak fluid into the tissues (see Chapter 15).

Psychogenic Shock. One form of distributive shock is called psychogenic shock. The brain temporarily sends out a signal for the blood vessels to dilate; consequently all the vessels dilate in unison. As the blood pressure drops, the person usually has a syncopal episode (see Chapter 14). Fortunately, the body quickly recognizes the problem, stops sending the signal, and the blood vessels return to their normal state.

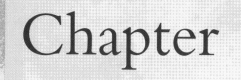

Chapter 20

Soft Tissue Injuries

Stories from the Field

Your volunteer EMS agency participates in many community events throughout the year. Robin and Mark have volunteered to cover the standby ambulance at a local baseball game. They have invited you to go along. Your agency views standbys as an opportunity to educate the public about EMS. These events also provide an opportunity to recruit new members.

While handing out brochures before the game, you hear a loud bang. The noise came from behind the right-field fence. This is the area where the planned post-game fireworks are being set up. A player yells for help and points in the direction of the noise. As you approach, you see an intricate maze of wiring, tubes, and boxes. A man is lying on the ground, tangled in the wires. One of the technicians tells you that the man was working on a launcher tube that detonated prematurely. After ensuring that the scene is safe, Robin and Mark use a two-person carry to move the patient to a safer area. The patient has soot about the face and neck. Most of his exposed skin has been burned. He is conscious and breathing with difficulty.

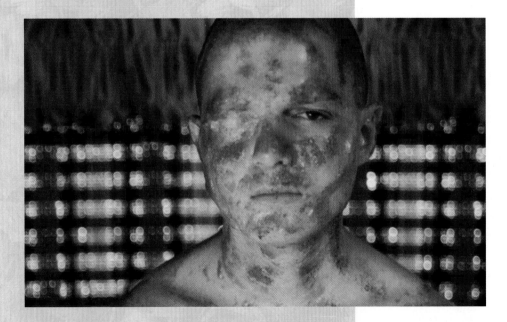

EMT Alert

Treating soft tissue injuries involves a high risk of exposure to blood and body fluids. Always apply the techniques of body substance isolation and standard precautions.

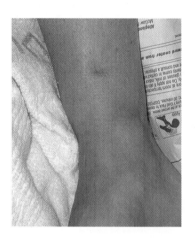

Figure 20.1 *A fractured lower tibia can cause injury to the surrounding soft tissues.*

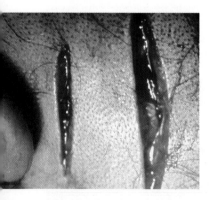

Figure 20.2 *Lacerations of the scalp and the back of the neck.*

Y ou will often treat injuries involving damage to the skin or other soft tissue. In most cases, these injuries are not life threatening. They can involve a tremendous amount of bleeding and pain. In this chapter, we will discuss the types of soft tissue injuries you will encounter and the appropriate prehospital emergency care for each. These include injuries in which the skin remains intact, injuries in which the skin is broken, and burns. The application of dressings and bandages is described in the last section of the chapter.

D.O.T. OBJECTIVES

State the major functions of the skin.

List the layers of the skin.

Establish the relationship between body substance isolation and soft tissue injuries.

SOFT TISSUE INJURIES

The skin, or integument, is a protective barrier. It helps to regulate body temperature, prevents the entry of pathogens, and has receptors that sense heat, cold, pressure, and pain. The skin has three layers:

- Epidermis—the thin, outer layer of skin that offers protection
- Dermis—a thicker, deeper layer of skin, containing sweat and sebaceous glands, hair follicles, blood vessels, and nerve endings
- Subcutaneous layer—consists of fatty cells and connective tissue

Review Chapter 4 for further discussion of the integumentary system.

There are three types of soft tissue injuries: closed injuries, open injuries, and burns. Closed soft tissue injuries usually result from blunt trauma. The skin remains intact, but the underlying structures may be seriously injured (see Fig. 20.1).

In open soft tissue injuries the skin is broken (see Fig. 20.2). These are commonly caused by injury from an external source, such as a knife or broken glass. The skin can also break from the inside outward if the end of a fractured bone tears through it. Broken skin provides an opening for infectious materials to enter the body. It also results in external bleeding.

Burns can cause injury to one or more layers of the skin. Their severity is classified according to the depth of tissue that is affected. Burns can also cause damage to vital body systems.

Soft tissue injuries must be treated promptly. Most of the time, soft tissue injuries should be treated before the patient is moved. However, if rapid transport is indicated, treat only life-threatening injuries before moving the patient. You must learn to recognize and treat major bleeding during your initial assessment.

As with all patient contact, you must take the necessary body substance isolation (BSI) and standard precautions (SP) before and after providing direct care. This includes gloves, eye protection, gowns, and handwashing.

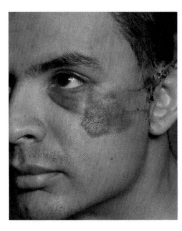

Figure 20.3 *Early phase of a contusion.*

D.O.T. OBJECTIVE

List the types of closed soft tissue injuries.

Closed Soft Tissue Injuries

Closed soft tissue injuries include contusions, hematomas, and crush injuries. All closed soft tissue injuries require similar treatment in the prehospital setting.

Contusions, or bruises, are the most common type of closed wounds. In these injuries, the epidermis remains intact. The cells and blood vessels in the dermis become damaged, resulting in discoloration of the bruised area. A combination of bleeding and tissue damage causes a reddish to purplish discoloration (see Fig. 20.3). This also causes swelling and pain. The blood in the bruise breaks down over time. When this happens, the bruise may become brown to yellow in appearance (see Table 20.1).

Closed Soft Tissue Injury | *Damage to muscle, vessels, or skin; outer skin remains intact*

Contusion | *Bruise; a wound in which the epidermis remains intact, but the cells and blood vessels in the dermis become damaged*

Table 20.1 • PHASES OF BRUISE DISCOLORATION

Age of Bruise	Color
1–2 days	Red
2–5 days	Purple or Blue
5–7 days	Green
7–10 days	Yellow
10–14 days	Brown

Figure 20.4 *Some hematomas progress to gangrene.*

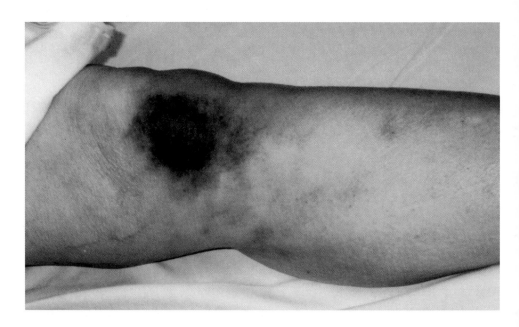

Hematoma (hee-muh-TOE-muh) | *Swelling or mass of blood caused by breaking of a blood vessel*

Hematomas are extravascular collections of blood. They appear under the skin at the site of injury (see Fig. 20.4). The blood leaks out of a damaged blood vessel and clots under the skin. It looks like a raised, bluish discoloration. A hematoma usually involves damage to large vessels. More tissue is involved than with a contusion. A liter or more of blood can be lost.

Crush Injury | *Open or closed soft tissue injury resulting from bilateral blunt trauma forces*

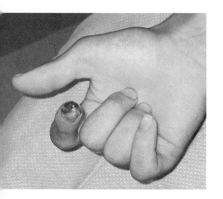

Figure 20.5 *A crushed fingertip.*

Crush injuries are caused by crushing forces from blunt trauma. They may be either open or closed injuries. Closed crush injuries range from very minor, such as a hammer striking a fingertip, to severe, such as a car falling on someone's chest or leg (see Fig. 20.5). Externally, crush injuries may cause swelling, bruising, and deformity. A closed crush injury to the trunk may appear very minor at first. You might only see a small contusion or hematoma. However, solid internal organs such as the liver and spleen could be severely damaged. This will lead to massive internal bleeding and shock. Hollow digestive organs may rupture. If rupture occurs, caustic fluids will leak into the peritoneal cavity.

Always consider crushing injuries to the chest to be life threatening. There is a high potential for injury to the lungs, heart, and major vessels. These injuries are discussed further in the "Special Considerations" section of this chapter.

D.O.T. OBJECTIVE

Describe the emergency medical care of the patient with a closed soft tissue injury.

Emergency Care for Closed Soft Tissue Injuries

These are the steps for the emergency medical care of closed soft tissue injuries:

1. Conduct a scene size-up. BSI precautions should include gloves and hand-washing.

2. Complete the initial assessment. Ensure that the airway is patent and breathing is adequate. Take cervical spine precautions, if necessary. Ventilate or administer oxygen as required. Treat for shock if present, or if you suspect internal bleeding. Use the mechanism of injury and signs and symptoms to guide your treatment decisions.

3. Complete a focused history and physical exam or rapid trauma assessment. Splint painful, swollen, deformed extremities (see Chapter 21). Elevate the extremity, if possible. Apply a cold pack. These measures help to control pain, bleeding, and swelling and to prevent further damage.

4. Complete a detailed assessment. This can be done while en route to the hospital if rapid transport is indicated.

5. Transport as soon as possible. Complete ongoing assessments while en route to the receiving facility.

EMT Tip

Always place a cloth barrier between the patient's skin and a cold pack. Applying a cold pack directly to the skin may cause additional tissue damage. Intense cold could also cause the patient to move suddenly, aggravating the injury.

D.O.T. OBJECTIVE

State the types of open soft tissue injuries.

Open Soft Tissue Injuries

The skin is often torn or damaged during traumatic events. **Open soft tissue injuries** are classified into several types. These include:

- Abrasions—Scratches, scrapes, rug burns, and road rash
- Lacerations—Linear or stellate cuts in the skin
- Avulsions—Flaps of skin that are torn loose or pulled off completely
- Penetration or Puncture Wounds—Breaks in the skin caused by nails, splinters, knives, bullets
- Amputations—Traumatic removal of extremities
- Crush Injuries—Caused by blunt trauma; can be open or closed

The emergency management of all types is similar, with a few specific exceptions.

Open Soft Tissue Injury | Open wound in which muscle, vessels, and/or skin is damaged

Figure 20.6 *An abrasion caused by a motorcycle accident.*

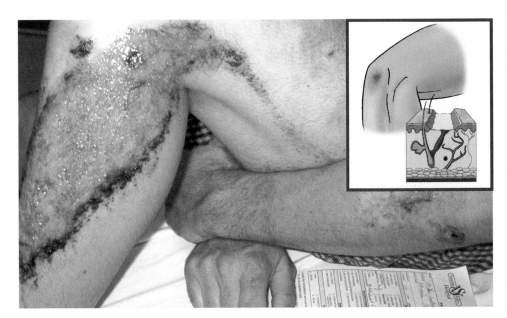

EMT Tip

Remember the term abrasion by thinking of "abrasive," or scraping off the top layers of skin.

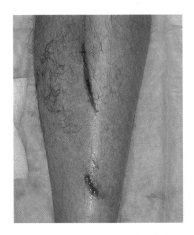

Figure 20.7 *A superficial, linear laceration.*

Figure 20.8 *Severely lacerated lower arm.*

Abrasion | *A superficial scrape injury to the top layer of skin*

Abrasions

An **abrasion** occurs when the outermost layer of skin becomes damaged or is removed by a shearing force. Shearing forces occur when the skin stretches in one direction, while the bone and other underlying structures move in the opposite direction. Scratches, scrapes, and rug burns are abrasions. Road rash is a common term for an abrasion caused by sliding across asphalt or concrete (see Fig. 20.6). These injuries are very painful, because they expose nerve endings in the skin. Abrasions may not bleed, or have only minor oozing from damaged capillary beds. The potential for infection is great in these injuries because dirt and other foreign bodies can become ground into the skin.

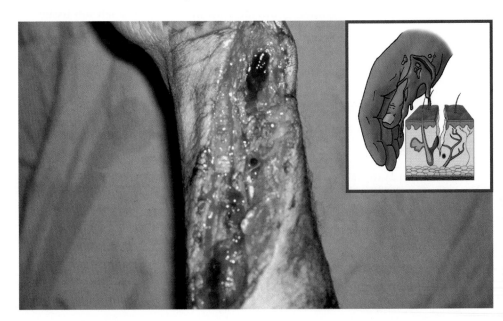

Lacerations

A **laceration** is a cut in the skin of any size, shape, and depth. A linear or regular laceration is usually caused by impact with a sharp object such as a knife or broken glass (see Fig. 20.7). Stellate lacerations are irregularly shaped, and usually caused by forceful impact with a blunt object. Lacerations can be isolated or occur together with other injuries. The bleeding from a laceration can be severe if surrounding blood vessels are cut (see Fig. 20.8).

Laceration | Wound or irregular tear of the skin

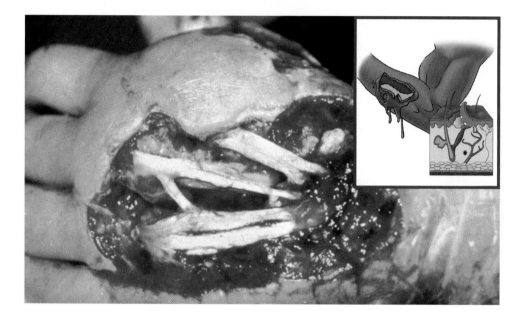

Figure 20.9 *Severe avulsion of the hand.*

Avulsions

An **avulsion** is a flap of skin that has been torn loose or pulled off completely (see Figs. 20.9 and 20.10). The extent and depth of avulsions varies, as does the amount of bleeding. A degloving avulsion is skin that is pulled off an extremity like a glove. The term is also used to describe a part of the body that has been pulled off, such as an avulsed earlobe.

Avulsion | A tearing off or tearing away of a skin flap or body part

Penetration or Puncture Wounds

Penetration or puncture wounds are caused by sharp, pointed objects penetrating the skin and surrounding tissues. Puncture wounds may have little or no external bleeding. However, internal bleeding may be severe. The severity depends on the object involved and the tissues in its path. Common objects that cause puncture wounds are nails, splinters, and knives. Puncture wounds penetrate more deeply than lacerations. There is a potential for internal bleeding or life-threatening injuries to internal organs.

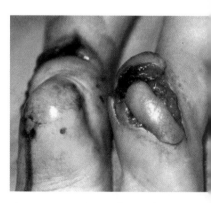

Figure 20.10 *An avulsion of the heels.*

Figure 20.11 *Gunshot wound to the forearm.*

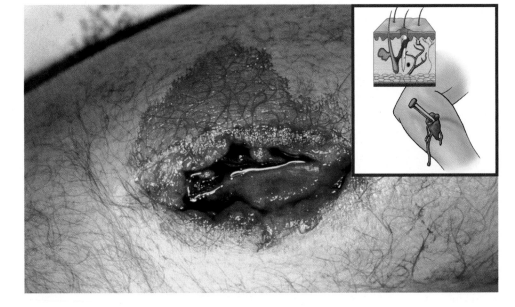

 EMT Tip

As an EMT-B, you will focus on finding and treating all wounds, not on identifying whether the injury is an entrance or exit wound.

A bullet, knife, or other significant force can completely perforate a body part. This creates an entrance and an exit wound. A gunshot may leave powder burns that appear as a black ring on the surrounding skin. A bullet's exit wound is usually larger than the entrance. Remember that guns are high-energy weapons (see Fig. 20.11). Once a bullet enters the body, it can travel in many directions. Always suspect cervical spine injury if the patient has a gunshot wound to the chest, head, neck, or abdomen (see Fig. 20.12).

Figure 20.12 *Gunshot entrance and exit wounds in the face.*

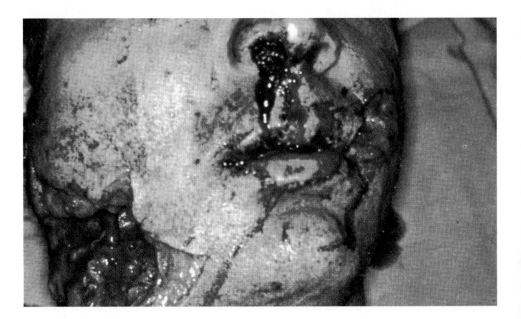

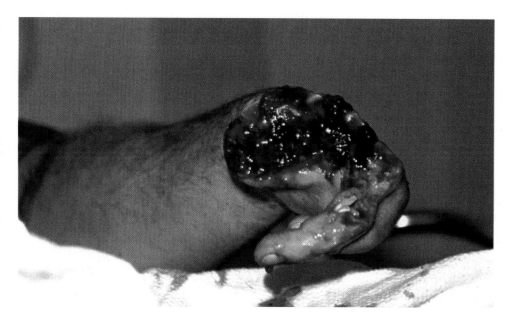

Figure 20.13 *Traumatic amputation of the hand.*

Amputations

Amputations occur when an extremity or other body part has been completely cut through or torn off (see Figs. 20.13 and 20.14). Bleeding can be massive, depending on the size of the extremity. The body tries to control the bleeding by retracting and constricting damaged blood vessels. Edges of the wound may be ragged, with bones or tendons exposed.

Amputation | *Removal of an extremity through trauma or surgery*

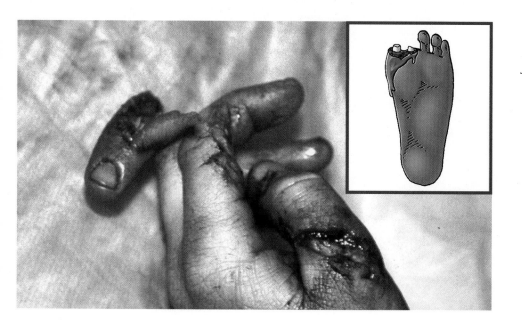

Figure 20.14 *A severely lacerated thumb and amputated finger.*

Figure 20.15 *A severely crushed hand, resulting in a finger amputation.*

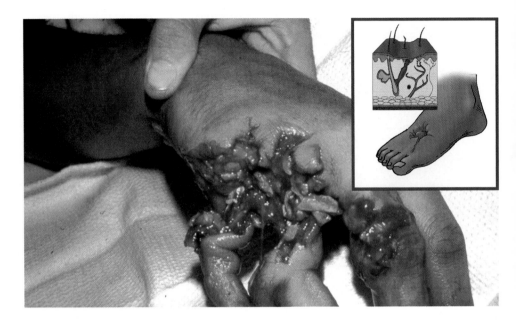

Open Crush Injuries

Crush injuries are caused by extreme pressure from blunt trauma. In open crush injuries, fractured bones may protrude through the skin (see Figs. 20.15 and 20.16). Internal bleeding or severe organ damage may also be present.

Figure 20.16 *Severe crush injury caused by farm equipment.*

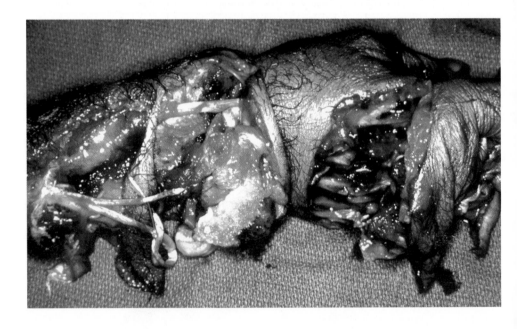

D.O.T. OBJECTIVE

Describe the emergency medical care of the patient with an open soft tissue injury.

Emergency Care for Open Soft Tissue Injuries

These are the steps for managing open soft tissue injuries. The use of direct pressure, elevation, and tourniquets to control bleeding is explained in Chapter 19. There is a section about dressings and bandaging at the end of this chapter.

1. Conduct a scene size-up. Take full BSI and standard precautions.

2. Complete the initial assessment. Ensure that the airway is patent and breathing is adequate. Take cervical spine precautions, if necessary. Ventilate or administer oxygen if needed. Treat for shock if present, or if you suspect internal bleeding. Use the mechanism of injury and the signs and symptoms to guide you.

3. Complete a focused history and physical examination or a rapid trauma assessment. Expose the wound to assess the injury. Remove surrounding debris and cut away clothing. You may have to turn the patient to look for hidden injuries on the back. Check the buttocks and the posterior of the lower extremities, especially if a PASG will be applied. For a patient requiring spinal stabilization, examine the back while log rolling onto a long spine board. Do not turn the patient more than once.

4. Control bleeding with direct pressure and elevation. If this is ineffective, use pressure points. Apply a tourniquet only if all other methods have failed to control bleeding. Prevent further contamination by wiping dirt and other debris away from the wound with a sterile dressing.

5. Once bleeding is controlled, apply a dry, sterile dressing to the wound. Use a bandage to hold the dressing in place. If the injury is to an extremity, make sure that peripheral pulses are not compromised. If diffuse bleeding is discovered, apply additional pressure. The patient may bleed through the original dressing. Remove the dressing, locate the wound, and apply direct pressure. Note that some agencies require leaving the original dressing in place so that the clotting process is not disturbed. Check local protocols.

6. Keep the patient calm, quiet, and reassured. Movement and restlessness aggravate injuries and bleeding. This may also be a sign of impending shock. If shock is present or internal bleeding suspected, treat for shock. Use the mechanism of injury and the patient's signs and symptoms to guide you.

7. Complete a detailed assessment. This can be completed while en route to the receiving facility if rapid transport is indicated.

8. Complete ongoing assessments while en route to the hospital as indicated.

*EMT
Tip*

If you must place the patient on a long backboard, examine his or her back while you perform the log roll.

Injuries with Special Considerations

Some open soft tissue injuries require special consideration. These are penetrating chest injuries, abdominal injuries, genital injuries, impaled objects, amputations, and large open neck injuries.

Open Chest Injuries

Pneumothorax (NU-mo-THOR-aks) | *Air in the chest cavity between the lung and chest wall*

Open chest injuries are caused by penetrating trauma, usually from gunshot wounds, knives, or other sharp objects. A **pneumothorax** can occur from a penetrating wound to the chest. The open wound can cause the lung on the injured side to collapse because the negative pressure inside the chest is lost. This results in a sucking sound on inspiration, so it is also called a sucking chest wound. Ventilation and oxygenation are impaired. Consider any penetrating chest wound to be an open pneumothorax. Signs and symptoms of an open pneumothorax include:

- Presence of an open chest injury
- Sucking sound on inspiration
- Respiratory distress
- Tachycardia
- Tachypnea
- Decreased breath sounds on the injured side
- Subcutaneous emphysema, a crunchy feeling upon palpation due to air under the skin

If air enters the chest cavity from an open wound and then the wound is sealed, the air becomes trapped. This converts an open pneumothorax to a potentially fatal tension pneumothorax. Eventually, tension builds up and collapses the injured lung. This compresses the heart and mediastinum and blocks venous filling of the heart. It also compromises the other lung. The condition results in an obstructive type of shock, which can be fatal. Signs and symptoms of a tension pneumothorax are:

- Respiratory distress

- Decreased breath sounds on the affected side

- Tracheal deviation (away from the injured side)

- Tachycardia

- Hypotension

- Jugular venous distention

- Cyanosis

If an open chest wound is present or pneumothorax is suspected, maintain the ABCs, apply high-flow oxygen, and transport rapidly. Treat for shock, if present. Transport the patient with the injured side down. In this position, gravity pulls down on the mediastinum and the injured lung. This allows maximum inflation and oxygenation of the uninjured lung. Remember the potential for spinal injury with all chest injuries. If suspected, secure the patient to a long spine board. Tilt the board to the injured side while maintaining spinal alignment.

After administering oxygen, apply an occlusive dressing to the open chest wound. Cover the injury with a gloved hand until you can secure the occlusive dressing. Petroleum gauze or a defibrillation pad are excellent for sealing the wound. Tape the occlusive dressing on three sides, providing a flutter-valve effect. This allows air to leave the chest cavity during expiration, but prevents it from entering during inspiration. You reestablish a sealed chest wall and prevent air from entering the chest (see Fig. 20.17). Seal the occlusive dressing as the patient finishes exhaling. This pushes most of the trapped air out of the cavity. Do not tape the fourth side of the dressing. This would cause tension pneumothorax to develop.

Figure 20.17 *Wound dressing for an open pneumothorax.*

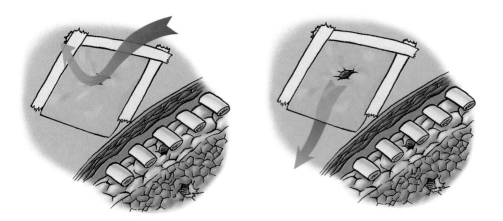

Figure 20.18 *The presence of blood in the chest cavity is a hemothorax.*

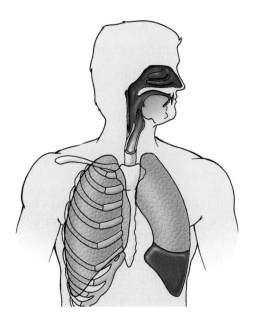

Chest injuries from both blunt and penetrating trauma can cause bleeding from a lung or an injured blood vessel into the chest. As the name implies, hemothorax (hemo = blood, thorax = chest) is a condition in which blood is present in the chest cavity (see Fig. 20.18). If this occurs with a pneumothorax, it is called a hemopneumothorax (blood and air in the chest cavity).

Early recognition of hemothorax is crucial for the patient to survive. Associated rib fractures may be present. Signs and symptoms include:

• Respiratory distress

• Tachycardia

• Tachypnea

• Absent breath sounds on the injured side

If massive bleeding from large vessels occurs, the patient will become hypotensive and quickly go into shock. Treatment involves administering high-flow oxygen and assisting ventilations, if necessary. Treat for shock if present, and take necessary spinal precautions. Transport immediately with the injured side down.

Cardiac tamponade is a condition caused by bleeding within the pericardium, the tough, inelastic tissue surrounding the heart. This can result from injuries to the heart or major blood vessels from chest trauma. As blood fills the space between the heart and pericardium, the atria and ventricles cannot expand fully. Signs and symptoms include respiratory distress, tachycardia, and cyanosis. Neck veins may be distended, heart sounds will be muffled, and blood pressure will drop, causing obstructive shock. Cardiopulmonary arrest eventually occurs because the heart cannot pump blood. Your treatment consists of maintaining the airway, breathing, and circulation. Apply high-flow oxygen and transport rapidly.

Abdominal Injuries

Like chest injuries, abdominal injuries are caused by both blunt and penetrating trauma. Blunt trauma typically causes closed abdominal injuries. These
injuries may cause severe internal bleeding from organ and large vessel damage. Open abdominal injuries are caused by penetrating trauma (see Fig.
20.19). Common mechanisms of injury are gunshot wounds, knives, or other
sharp objects. Besides causing severe bleeding, penetrating injuries that perforate the intestine often cause serious infection in the abdominal cavity.

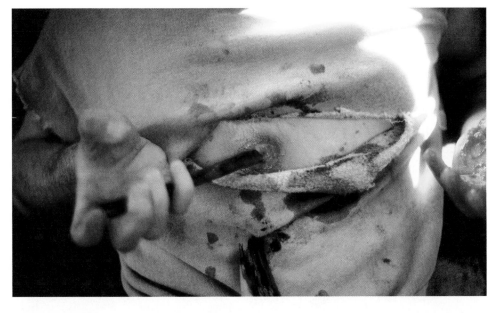

Figure 20.19 *A punctured
sternum.*

Open abdominal injuries may also cause **evisceration**. This is a serious condition in which internal organs protrude through the abdominal wall. Do not
touch or try to replace the exposed organs. Doing so could cause further
damage and contamination. Cover the wound and the exposed organs with a
sterile dressing moistened with sterile saline or sterile water. Never use a
dressing that will adhere to the organs. Secure the moistened dressing with an
occlusive dressing. Petroleum gauze, plastic wrap, or aluminum foil may be
used for this purpose. If no spinal injury is suspected, flex the patient's knees
and hips to relieve tension on the abdominal wall. Provide high-flow oxygen
and maintain the normal body temperature.

*Evisceration (eh-VIS-er-ay-
shun)* | *Abdominal organs
(viscera) protruding through an
open wound*

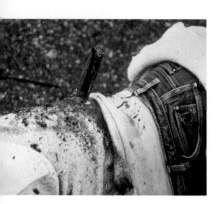

Figure 20.20 *Abdomen impaled by a knife.*

Genital Injuries

Occasionally, you may be called to treat soft tissue injuries to the genital area. These injuries can be very painful. In addition, the patient is often embarrassed. He or she may be reluctant to give you a complete, accurate history of events. If possible, an EMT-B of the same gender should treat the patient.

Lacerations are a common soft tissue injury to the male genitals. Control bleeding with direct pressure. Secure scrotal injuries by using a cravat to make a cradle-type bandage. Men can suffer penile fractures from rupture of engorged blood vessels. Penile amputations should be handled in the same manner as other amputations.

Soft tissue injuries to the female genitalia are discussed in more detail in Chapter 18.

D.O.T. OBJECTIVE

Describe the emergency medical care of a patient with an impaled object.

Impaled Objects

Impaled Object | *An object that pierces the skin*

Some soft tissue injuries involve **impaled objects** that have penetrated the skin and remain embedded in the tissue (see Figs. 20.20 and 20.21). Generally, you should not try to remove an impaled object in the field. Doing so can cause additional bleeding. The impaled object acts as a plug, holding pressure on injured blood vessels. When the object is removed, pressure is released, and bleeding may be profuse. In many instances, patients will have removed impaled objects before EMS arrives.

Figure 20.21 *Leg impaled by a screwdriver.*

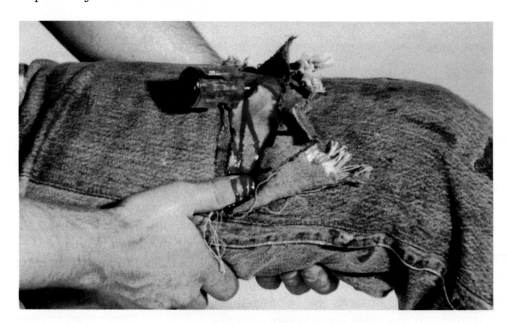

In most cases, expose the wound and manually secure the impaled object in place. Stabilize the object with a bulky dressing. Control bleeding with direct pressure around the wound. Avoid applying pressure to the object. Shortening a long impaled object may be necessary, if it interferes with care. Stabilize the object while someone else carefully cuts it to the necessary length.

You must remove any objects that interfere with airway patency or chest compressions. Rarely, an impaled object interferes with patient transport. Try to reduce its size before attempting to remove it. Consult medical direction. An impaled object in the cheek can dislodge and obstruct the airway. It may also cause bleeding in the oral cavity. This can result in airway compromise, nausea, or vomiting. If other structures are not involved and the airway is endangered, remove an impaled object from the cheek. This is described in Procedure 20.1.

Procedure 20.1 • IMPALED OBJECT IN THE CHEEK

  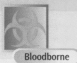
Maintain ABCs   Limit Bleeding   Bloodborne

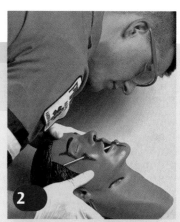

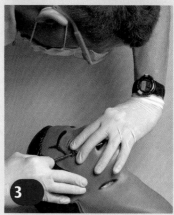

1. Position the patient's head and suction the airway as needed. Spinal precautions may be necessary if trauma is suspected. Continue to monitor the airway.

2. Examine the injured cheek, both inside and out. Look inside the patient's mouth carefully, using a light. Feel inside and out with a gloved finger and pad.

3. If you can see both ends of the object, carefully pull it out. Remove it in the same direction as it entered. If you cannot remove it readily or if it is impaled in deeper structures, stabilize it and leave it in place.

4. After the object is removed, apply pressure to the outside of the wound to control bleeding. Apply a sterile dressing and bandage the cheek. If the patient is alert and cooperative, you may place a gauze pad inside the cheek to control bleeding in the mouth.

Impaled Object in the Eye. An impaled object should not be removed from the eye. After surveying the scene, apply personal protective apparel and complete the initial assessment. Treat as follows:

1. Stabilize the impaled object with bulky dressings or rolled bandages.

2. Place a paper cup or similar item over the object, resting on the bandages (see Figure 20.22). Do not touch the object.

3. Secure the cup by wrapping the base with a rolled gauze or bandage.

4. Because both eyes move together, also place a dressing over the uninjured eye. This will prevent the patient from looking around, thus reducing movement of the injured eye.

Figure 20.22 *Taping a cup around an impaled object in the eye helps to prevent movement of the object. A dressing over the uninjured eye minimizes movement of the eyes.*

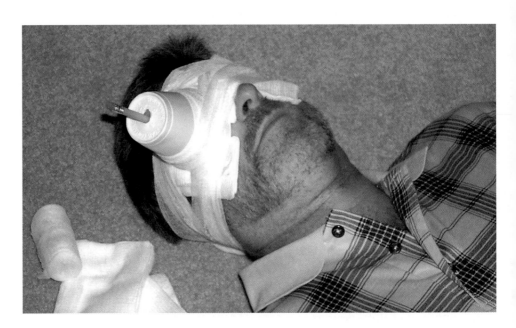

D.O.T. OBJECTIVE

Describe the emergency medical care of a patient with an amputation.

Amputations

Amputation is a serious condition. Blood loss can be great and hypovolemic shock is likely. After surveying the scene, apply personal protective equipment and complete the initial assessment. Manage the airway and breathing. Provide supplemental oxygen immediately. Take spinal precautions as necessary. Control bleeding. Notify medical direction and transport to the closest appropriate medical facility. Transport the patient on the injured side. Carefully monitor the airway.

Procedure 20.2 • **EMERGENCY CARE FOR AMPUTATION**

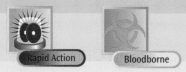
Rapid Action   Bloodborne

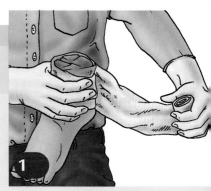

1. Wrap the amputated appendage in a dry, sterile dressing. Avoid immersing the part in liquid. This could cause the tissue to soften to the point of degeneration.

2. Place the part in a plastic bag. Keep it cool. Cooling is necessary to slow the metabolism. A good method of cooling an amputated part is to place the plastic bag in a cooler of water. Place a few ice cubes in the water. However, avoid freezing the part, which will destroy the cellular structure. Never place the amputated part on ice.

3. Do not complete a partial amputation. If the limb is partially amputated, do not cut the tissue holding it to the body. This tissue may aid with reattachment. Immobilize the extremity to prevent further injury, and transport immediately.

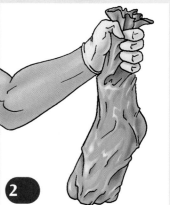

An amputation can result in lifelong disability. Proper emergency care of both the patient and the amputated part increases the potential for successful replantation. Procedure 20.2 describes proper care for the amputated part.

Large Open Neck Injuries

The blood vessels in the neck are very large. Hemorrhage and air embolism are potential problems with neck injuries. In an air embolism, a large air bubble is sucked into an open neck vein. It is transported to the heart where it displaces blood and prevents perfusion of the tissues. The result is often fatal. With large open neck injuries, always suspect spinal cord injury. Follow these steps after completing the scene survey, applying personal protective equipment, and completing the initial assessment:

1. Immediately place a gloved hand over the wound to control bleeding.

2. Cover the wound with an occlusive dressing. Secure the occlusive dressing with another dressing.

3. Apply pressure to the carotid artery only if necessary to control bleeding. Never compress the trachea or both carotid arteries at once.

EMT Tip

Avoid discussing specific replantation possibilities with a patient. If the patient asks you, state that each case is unique and involves many factors. Reassure the patient that your treatment will help with replantation if it is possible.

BURNS

Approximately two million people suffer burn injuries in the United States each year. The source of a burn may be thermal, chemical, radiological, or electrical. The trauma suffered from burns can be much more than skin deep (see Figure 20.23). Burns affect virtually every system in the body. Besides treating the burn itself, you must assess and manage any damage to the:

• Cardiovascular system

• Respiratory system

• Renal system

• Endocrine system

• Gastrointestinal system

• Immune system

• Integumentary system

• Muscular system

In addition to systemic injuries, burn patients may suffer significant scarring. This leaves the patient with a visible reminder of the initial injuries that can have a long-term emotional impact.

Be aware that a medical problem may have occurred before, or be a result of, the burn. For example, a heart attack is a condition that could precede a burn. A burn patient may also suffer traumatic injuries while attempting to escape a fire.

Figure 20.23 *Severely scalded ankle.*

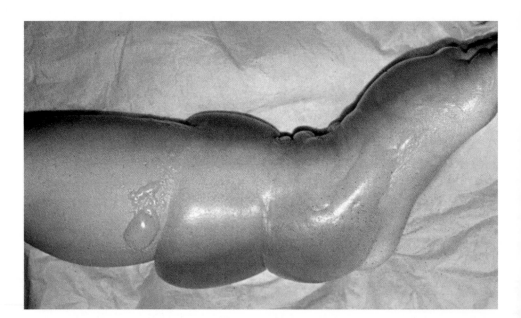

Determining Burn Severity

You must be able to assess the severity of a burn. This is necessary to provide appropriate treatment. Knowing the severity will also help in deciding the best facility to receive the patient. Critically burned patients may benefit from being transported directly to a burn center. Generally, burns are classified as critical, moderate, or minor. Burn severity depends on the following factors:

- Depth and degree of the burn
- Percentage of body area burned
- Location of the burn
- Patient's age and preexisting medical conditions

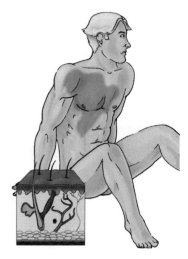

Figure 20.24 *Superficial burn.*

Superficial Burn | *Burn involving only the top layer of the skin (epidermis); first degree burn*

Partial Thickness Burn | *Burn involving both the epidermis and the dermis, but not involving underlying tissue; second degree burn*

Full Thickness Burn | *Burn extending through all dermal layers; may involve the subcutaneous tissues, muscle, bone, or organs; third degree burn*

D.O.T. OBJECTIVES

List the classifications of burns.

Define superficial burn.

List the characteristics of a superficial burn.

Define partial thickness burn.

List the characteristics of a partial thickness burn.

Define full thickness burn.

List the characteristics of a full thickness burn.

Burn Classification by Depth

Burns are classified according to the depth of tissue damage. **Superficial burns** were formerly called first degree burns. **Partial thickness burns** were called second degree burns and **full thickness burns** were described as third degree burns (see Table 20.2 on page 592). Some EMS systems combine depth classification with other characteristics. For example, a burn may be described as a full thickness electrical burn.

A superficial burn involves only the epidermis (see Fig. 20.24). It is characterized by reddened skin and pain at the site. Sunburn is an example of a superficial burn. These burns heal without scarring.

Partial thickness burns damage both the epidermis and the dermis (see Fig. 20.25). They do not injure the underlying structures. Partial thickness burns are characterized by white to red skin. The skin may be moist or mottled,

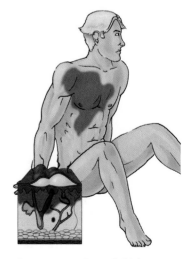

Figure 20.25 *Partial thickness burn.*

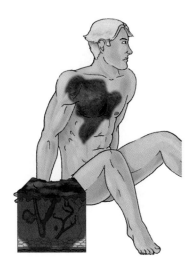

Figure 20.26 *Full thickness burn.*

with patches of red and white. Blisters often develop within the first 2 days. This is caused by fluid leaking from damaged tissue and collecting under the top layer of skin. Partial thickness burns cause intense pain, but usually heal without scarring.

Full thickness burns are severe. These burns extend through all three dermal layers, involving subcutaneous tissue, muscle, bones, and organs (see Fig. 20.26). The skin may appear dry, hard, leathery, or charred. The color can range from white to dark brown. Nerve endings are destroyed, creating a loss of sensation. The patient has little or no pain, except at the periphery. Full thickness burns heal with extensive scar tissue, and often require skin grafting.

Amount of Body Burned (Rule of Nines)

To determine the percentage of body surface area that is burned, the body is divided into regions that contain about 9 percent of the total. The Rule of Nines is the method used for estimating the affected area (see Fig. 20.27).

- The size of a hand is 1 percent of the total body area
- The head and neck comprise 9 percent of an adult's body area and 18 percent of an infant's body
- Each upper extremity (anterior and posterior) is 9 percent of the body
- Each lower extremity (anterior and posterior) is 18 percent of an adult's body and 14 percent of an infant's
- The anterior and posterior trunk each equal 18 percent of the total area
- The genitals are 1 percent of the total

Table 20.2 • CHARACTERISTICS OF BURNS BY DEPTH

Characteristic	Superficial Burn	Partial Thickness Burn	Full Thickness Burn
Skin Layers Injured	Involves only the most superficial layers of the skin	Involves deeper layers including both the epidermis and the dermis	Extends through all the layers of the skin and may involve subcutaneous tissues, muscle, bone, or organs
Skin Color	Reddened skin	White to red skin that may appear moist and mottled	May range from a white to dark brown or charred color
Skin Condition	No blisters	Blister formation is common in the first 2 days	Skin becomes dry, hard, and leathery
Pain	Pain at the site	Intense pain	Nerve endings may be destroyed creating a loss of sensation with little or no pain except at the periphery
Long-Term Damage	Usually heals without scarring	Usually heals without scarring	Extensive scar tissue, often requires skin grafting

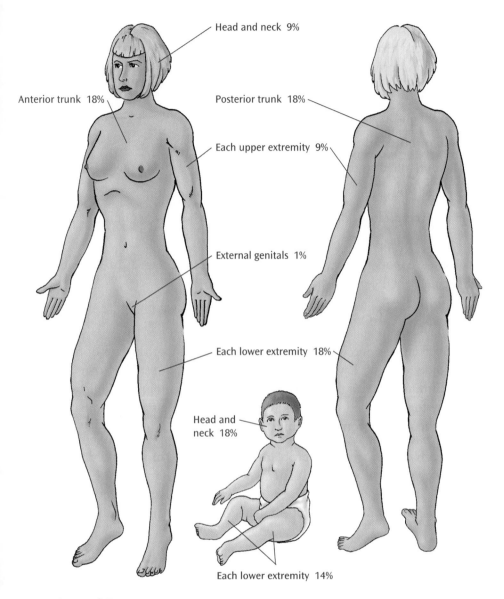

Head and neck 9%

Anterior trunk 18%

Posterior trunk 18%

Each upper extremity 9%

External genitals 1%

Each lower extremity 18%

Head and neck 18%

Each lower extremity 14%

Figure 20.27 *Rule of Nines.*

Location of Burns

The location of a burn affects your care, as well as complications the patient may develop later. Understanding the recovery process and factors that complicate recovery will help the EMT-B to properly gauge the severity of burns.

- Burns to the face may cause airway compromise or eye injuries
- Burns to the hands and feet may cause scarring, limiting function
- Burns to the genitalia and perineum are at high risk for infection
- Circumferential burns (burns that encircle the body or body part) to the chest may compromise respiration
- Circumferential burns to an extremity can compromise circulation

Patients suffering burns to the tissue of the airway, or inhalation injuries, often require aggressive airway management. Their conditions can change quickly. Signs and symptoms of inhalation injuries are:

- Facial burns

- Singed nasal and facial hairs

- Soot and/or burns in the oropharynx

- Dark, carbon-filled sputum

- Shortness of breath, chest tightness, difficulty swallowing

- Evidence of respiratory distress such as stridor, wheezing, coughing, hoarseness, cyanosis

If you observe evidence of airway burns, begin immediate assisted ventilations with supplemental oxygen.

Age and Medical Condition

Age also affects the outcome of the burn. Patients under the age of 5 or patients older than 55 have a higher risk of complications. They may have weaker immune systems, less ability to compensate for rapid fluid loss, or respiratory system overload. These and other factors cause patients to have more difficulty recovering from burn injuries.

Patients with chronic medical problems will also have more difficulty recovering from burns. For example, patients with heart or lung disease, diabetes mellitus, or immune system disorders may have complications related to their underlying condition. The condition may cause the burn to heal more slowly.

Severity of Burns

Once you have determined the depth, location, and percentage of body area burned, you can classify the burn as critical, moderate, or minor.

Critical burns include:

- Burns associated with respiratory injury

- Suspicion of inhalation injuries

- Full thickness burns involving the hands, feet, face, or genitalia (see Fig. 20.28)

- Full thickness burns covering more than 10 percent of the body surface area

- Partial thickness burns covering more than 30 percent of the body

- Burns encompassing an entire body part, such as arm, leg, or chest

- Burns complicated by painful, swollen, deformed extremities or suspected fractures

- Moderate burns in young children or elderly patients

- Burns in patients with severe preexisting illnesses

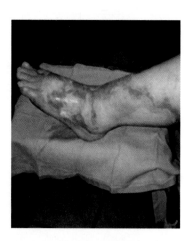

Figure 20.28 *Full thickness burn of the foot and ankle.*

Moderate burns include:

- Full thickness burns of 2 to 10 percent of the body surface area, excluding hands, feet, face, genitalia, or upper airway
- Partial thickness burns of 15 to 30 percent of the body surface area
- Superficial burns of greater than 50 percent of the body surface area

Minor burns include:

- Full thickness burns of less than 2 percent of the body surface area
- Partial thickness burns of less than 15 percent of the body surface area
- Superficial burns of less than 50 percent of the body surface area

Infant and Child Considerations

Children and infants are at a high risk for hypothermia and shock after suffering burns. The destruction of the skin's ability to maintain body temperature leads to rapid loss of heat and fluid after a burn. The risk of airway obstruction after an inhalation injury is also increased because of the smaller size of a child's airway. Consider the possibility of child abuse when evaluating a burned child or infant.

Slightly different criteria are used for determining the severity of burns in infants and children:

- Critical burns are full thickness burns or partial thickness burns involving more than 20 percent of the body surface area, or burns involving the hands, feet, face, airway, or genitalia
- Moderate burns are partial thickness burns involving 10 to 20 percent of the body surface area
- Minor burns are partial thickness burns involving less than 10 percent of the body surface area

---

D.O.T. OBJECTIVES

Describe the emergency medical care of the patient with a superficial burn.

Describe the emergency medical care of the patient with a partial thickness burn.

Describe the emergency medical care of the patient with a full thickness burn.

Emergency Care for Thermal Burns

These are the emergency medical care steps for a patient with a thermal burn.

1. Conduct a scene size-up. Ensure scene safety. Upon approaching a burn victim, the first step is to stop the burning. Water or normal saline can be used. Smothering flames may be necessary.

2. Complete the initial assessment. Ensure that the airway and breathing are controlled. Take cervical spine precautions, if necessary. Provide oxygen. Continually monitor the airway and breathing. Watch for closure of the airway. Be alert for signs and symptoms of inhalation injuries.

3. Complete a focused history and physical exam. During your assessment, remove any smoldering clothing or jewelry that is not adhering to the patient. Classify the severity of the burn.

4. Prevent further contamination by covering the burned area with a dry, sterile burn dressing (see Fig. 20.29). Separate the fingers and toes with sterile gauze, as long as this will not cause further tissue damage. Never break blisters. This will compromise the skin barrier and increase the risk of infection. Do not apply ointments, lotions, or antiseptic. Do not remove grease, tar, or other water insoluble substances.

5. Treat for shock and other injuries as needed.

6. Transport to the closest appropriate facility, based on the patient's condition and local protocols. Complete detailed and ongoing assessments while en route, as dictated by the patient's condition.

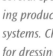

EMT Tip

Several specialized burn dressing products are used in EMS systems. Check local protocols for dressing a burn.

Figure 20.29 *Cover the burned area with a dry, sterile dressing.*

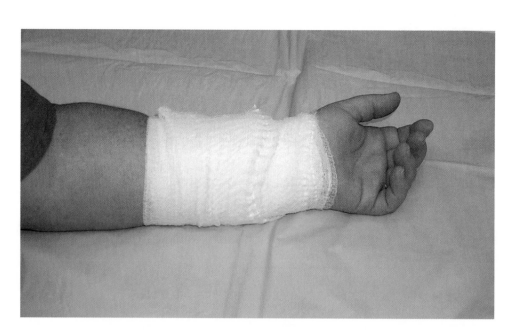

D.O.T. OBJECTIVE

Describe the emergency care for a chemical burn.

Chemical Burns

A chemical burn is caused by contact with acids, alkaline substances, or petroleum products. These agents can damage the skin, eyes, or mucous membranes. The severity of a chemical burn is affected by the particular substance and the amount, concentration, and duration of contact of the agent with the body. Contact with acidic substances, such as hydrochloric or sulfuric acid, coagulates the tissues (see Fig. 20.30). While painful, this limits further damage. Alkaline agents, such as lye or chemicals containing sodium hydroxide, can penetrate deep into tissues. Because of this, they usually cause more serious burns than acids. You may encounter chemical burns during responses to motor vehicle accidents, fires or explosions, and industrial accidents.

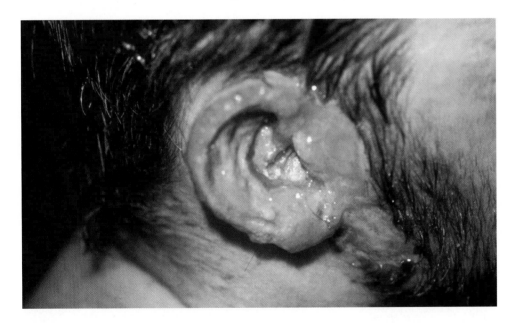

Figure 20.30 *Chemical burn from contact with an acid.*

Treatment of Chemical Burns

The most important aspect of managing chemical burns is personal safety. The Department of Transportation's *Emergency Response Guide* lists information on chemicals and emergency treatments.

For chemical burns to the eyes and the skin, brush off any dry powder remaining on the patient. Lightly brush loose powder away from an eye. Some chemicals, such as dry lime, become more caustic when activated by water. By removing as much of the powder as possible, you reduce the risk of further tissue damage.

Next, use large amounts of water to flush the chemical off the patient. The longer a chemical remains in contact with the skin or eye, the greater the damage. Flushing the contaminated area immediately with a large quantity of water is critical. Water will dilute the chemical and reduce tissue damage. Alkaline burns require longer irrigation than other substances. Continue flushing while en route to the hospital. Make sure you contain the flushed solution with towels or containers. Contact with this solution could contaminate the vehicle or crew.

It may be necessary to remove clothing to reach the affected skin. Maintain patient privacy as much as possible. Avoid contaminating uninjured parts of the body while flushing. If only one eye is affected, turn the patient onto that side. Flush with large amounts of water for at least 15 to 20 minutes. If both eyes are affected, flush with the patient supine.

D.O.T. OBJECTIVE

Describe the emergency care for an electrical burn.

Electrical Burns

Electrical burns can result from lightning or man-made currents. Electricity follows the path of least resistance as it passes through the body to a ground. The extreme heat along this path damages body tissues (see Figs. 20.31 and 20.32). The current may also disrupt the body's own electrical activity. The heart, nerves, and muscles may be affected, causing respiratory and/or cardiac arrest.

Figure 20.31 *Electrical burn from a lightning strike.*

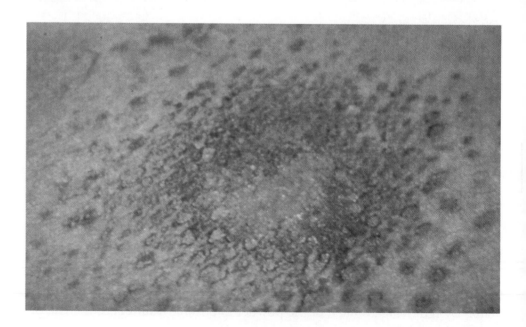

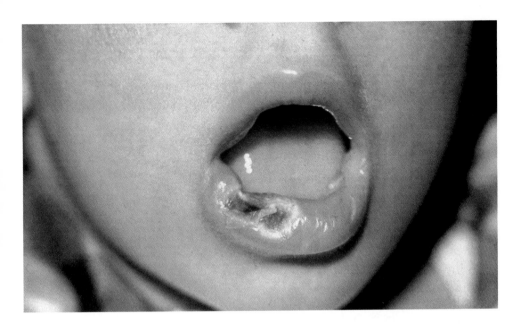

Figure 20.32 *Lip burned by an electrical cord.*

Do not endanger yourself or others at the scene of a potential electrocution. The source of electricity must be turned off by qualified personnel. Do not touch the patient if he or she is still in contact with the electrical source, unless you are trained to do so. The voltage source can use your body as a conduction system. This increases your risk of electrocution. Avoid contacting substances that conduct electricity, such as water or metal. Protect the patient and bystanders from contact, as well.

Once the scene is safe, ensure that the patient's airway, breathing, and circulation are intact. Electrical current can damage the conduction system in the heart. It may paralyze the respiratory muscles, increasing the patient's risk of respiratory or cardiac arrest. If in cardiac arrest, the patient may need automatic external defibrillation. Administer oxygen as needed.

Look for and treat other injuries secondary to the electrocution. The patient's condition may be more serious than externally apparent. Look for entrance and exit burns. Assume that all the tissue in between has been injured. Cool the burn area with water or normal saline. Cover with a sterile dressing, as for thermal burns. Transport the patient as soon as possible.

D.O.T. OBJECTIVE

List the functions of dressing and bandaging.

DRESSING AND BANDAGING

Dressing | Protective covering applied directly to a soft tissue wound

Dressings provide a protective covering for a wound. **Bandages** hold dressings in place. The main reasons for dressing and bandaging an injury are to:

- Control bleeding
- Protect the wound from further damage
- Prevent contamination and infection of the wound

Bandage | Holds a dressing in place (self-adherent, gauze rolls, triangular, air splint)

Sterile Dressings

Sterile | Free of microorganisms (bacteria, viruses, spores) that can cause infection

Sterile dressings are applied directly to an injury. They are used to stop bleeding from an open wound, and will protect the site from further damage and infection.

Common dressings include:

- Universal dressing; also called a multi-trauma or ABD pad. This is a large, bulky dressing, to be used on large areas, such as abdominal wounds.

- Gauze pads; may also be called toppers or sponges. These are made of layered gauze. They come in various sizes, such as 2" x 2", 3" x 3", 4" x 4", and 5" x 9". Gauze pads may be sterile or nonsterile. Sterile gauze pads are packaged in small quantities. Nonsterile gauze is usually wrapped in a large, bulk package.

Occlusive Dressing | A dressing that forms an airtight seal; often applied to open neck, chest or abdominal wounds; items commonly used include defibrillation pads or thick plastic wrap

- **Occlusive dressings**; commonly called petroleum gauze or Vaseline® gauze (see Fig. 20.33). These dressings form an airtight seal when applied to an open neck, chest, or abdominal wound. They are saturated in an ointment or gel that prevents sticking to an open wound. They prevent air movement across the wound.

> **D.O.T. OBJECTIVE**
>
> Describe the purpose of a bandage.

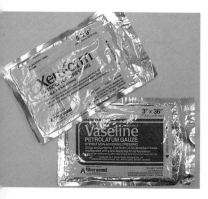

Figure 20.33 *Occlusive dressings.*

Bandages

Bandages are used to hold dressings in place (see Fig. 20.34). Common types of bandages are:

- Self-adherent bandages; commonly called by the brand names Kling® and Kerlix®. These are roller bandages and are available in different sizes. Roller bandages come in various widths, usually from 2 to 6 inches wide. They may be sterile or nonsterile. Since they do not usually come into direct contact with a wound, nonsterile is often used. This type of bandage adheres to itself when applied in layers. The sterile type can also be used as a dressing.

- Gauze rolls are rolls of meshed gauze, available in different sizes.
- Triangular bandages are large pieces of cloth that, when folded, can be used as a bandage or a sling.
- Air splints, when applied to an extremity, can be used to hold a dressing in place.
- Adhesive tape is used to secure dressings or bandages. Note that some people are allergic to the adhesive commonly used in tape. For this reason, most of the tape used in EMS is made of silk, paper, or plastic, and is not true adhesive.

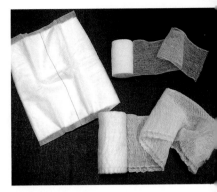

Figure 20.34 *Various types of bandages.*

D.O.T. OBJECTIVE

Describe the effects of improperly applied dressings, splints, and tourniquets.

Dressing and Bandaging Wounds

Various methods and techniques exist for dressing and bandaging soft tissue injuries. A few general guidelines should be closely followed:

- Never treat a soft tissue injury until after you have assessed and treated the patient's airway and breathing.
- A dressing should cover the entire wound. A bandage should cover the entire dressing.
- Do not bandage a dressing in place until bleeding is controlled. Pressure dressings, described in Chapter 19, are an exception. These are designed to help control bleeding.
- Do not cover the tips of the digits, unless burned or amputated. If the tips are exposed, you can assess the sensory, motor, and circulation status of the extremity. Ensure that sensation remains intact. The tip should remain pink, with no evidence of circulatory compromise, such as cyanosis, pallor, or edema.

EMT Tip

Never delay treatment of a life-threatening wound because a proper dressing is not available. You may have to be creative and use immediately available materials to dress a wound. Examples include a clean washcloth, a towel, a T-shirt, a diaper, or a clean sanitary napkin.

Chapter Twenty Summary

- Soft tissue injuries include both closed and open injuries. Hematomas and contusions are examples of closed injuries. Lacerations, abrasions, avulsions, amputations, and punctures are open injuries. Crush injuries may be open or closed.

- Special types of soft tissue injuries include chest wounds, eviscerations, impaled objects, amputations, and open neck injuries.

- Burns can be superficial, partial thickness, or full thickness. The severity of a burn depends on its depth, the amount of the body burned, its location, and the patient's age and medical condition.

- When caring for a burned patient, always stop the burning first. Cover burns with dry, sterile dressings to prevent infection. Because burned skin loses its ability to regulate temperature, treat infants and children for generalized hypothermia.

- Chemical and electrical burns require personal safety precautions and special treatment.

Key Terms Review

Abrasion | page 576

Amputation | page 579

Avulsion | page 577

Bandage | page 600

Closed Soft Tissue
   Injury | page 573

Contusion | page 573

Crush Injury | page 574

Dressing | page 600

Evisceration | page 585

Full Thickness Burn | page 591

Hematoma | page 574

Impaled Object | page 586

Laceration | page 577

Occlusive Dressing | page 600

Open Soft Tissue
   Injury | page 575

Partial Thickness Burn | page 591

Pneumothorax | page 582

Sterile | page 600

Superficial Burn | page 591

Review Questions

1. Which of the following best defines the term hematoma?

   a. Skin discoloration due to bleeding from capillaries

   b. Collection of blood in dermal tissue due to damaged blood vessel

   c. Blood in the chest cavity

   d. Crush injury

2. Your patient was burned on the front of his left arm and his entire back. What percentage of the body was burned?

   a. 22.5 percent

   b. 10 percent

   c. 45 percent

   d. Unable to determine

3. The layer of skin containing the blood vessels, nerves, hair follicles, etc., is called the:

   a. Epidermal ridge
   b. Dermis
   c. Sebaceous layer
   d. Epidermis

4. The term abrasion refers to:

   a. Loss of skin due to rubbing or scraping
   b. A combative, uncooperative patient
   c. Discoloration of the skin due to capillary rupture
   d. Loss of skin from exposure to corrosives

5. Penetrating eye injuries should be treated by:

   a. Covering only the uninjured eye
   b. Covering only the injured eye
   c. Covering both eyes
   d. Not covering the eyes, as this could cause more damage

6. A man has been slashed across his abdomen and his intestines are protruding. The EMT-B should:

   a. Apply a dry sterile dressing and bandage
   b. Replace intestines and apply a moist sterile dressing
   c. Apply a moist sterile dressing without touching the intestines
   d. Apply sterile dressing and heat pack, then bandage

7. A thermal burn is caused by:

   a. Electricity
   b. Heat or flame
   c. Chemicals
   d. Alkaloids

8. Burns caused by chemical agents are generally known as:

   a. Acid burns
   b. Caustic burns
   c. Alkali burns
   d. Chemical burns

9. A partial thickness burn involves:

   a. The epidermis
   b. The epidermis and the dermis
   c. Subcutaneous tissue
   d. Face, hands, feet, or genitalia

10. Which of the following describes a full thickness burn?

    a. Pain and redness
    b. Painless, red-and-white mottled skin
    c. Severe pain and blisters
    d. Leathery skin and little pain

11. Applying a little water to dry lime will:

    a. Turn the lime into a corrosive liquid
    b. Neutralize the lime
    c. Remove the lime before it becomes caustic
    d. Prevent a burn by cooling the skin

12. Once the scene is safe, the first priority in the care of an electrical shock patient is:

    a. Dressing the electrical burns
    b. Tending to airway, breathing, and circulation
    c. Treating associated injuries
    d. Estimating the extent of the burn

13. Sterile dressings:

    a. Hold bandages in place
    b. Are used to protect wounds from further damage
    c. Should be left free at one edge
    d. Should be tightly sealed at the edges

14. The layer of skin where fat is stored for energy is:

    a. Epidermis
    b. Dermis
    c. Terra cotta
    d. Subcutaneous

CASE STUDIES

Soft Tissue Injuries

1 Your crew is dispatched to the elementary school for a student with an eye injury. Upon arrival, you find an 8-year-old girl with a pencil impaled in her right eye. The child is relatively calm. No life-threatening problems are identified during the initial assessment. Your focused history and physical exam reveals no additional problems. The school has been unable to reach the girl's parents. The secretary shows you an emergency treatment form signed by the girl's parents. The parents have authorized emergency treatment in their absence. You request that a copy of the form accompany the patient to the hospital.

A. Should you remove the impaled object? Why?

B. What care is appropriate for the child?

2 Your crew is dispatched to a call for a man down. The call is in a part of the city known for illegal drug activity and gang violence. Law enforcement arrive on the scene and notify you that the scene is safe. There is one patient. He has a large gunshot wound to the abdomen. The young male patient is lying supine on the ground. Your initial assessment reveals that he is not breathing.

A. What are your first steps in treating this patient?

B. Are cervical spine precautions indicated in this case?

C. The gunshot wound has exposed a portion of the patient's intestine. How do you manage the exposed area?

3 You are dispatched to a private residence for a domestic dispute. The time is 2351. When you arrive, the police are present and the scene is secure. A 45-year-old male has been stabbed in the chest by his wife. The patient has a history of alcoholism and spousal abuse. Tonight, the wife feared for her life, stabbed the husband, and then called 9-1-1. The man is lying on the kitchen floor in a pool of blood. An officer is holding a towel to the patient's left chest. A long kitchen knife with blood on it is being sealed in a plastic bag. The patient appears to have labored breathing, although he is cursing loudly. The police officer stands up and removes the towel as you enter. You can hear a sucking, gurgling sound coming from the patient's chest as he breathes.

A. How do you proceed?

B. While performing your initial assessment, you cut away the patient's shirt. You observe a 1-inch stab wound in the left upper chest wall. The wound is making a sucking sound and has blood bubbling from it. You cover it with your gloved hand. What is this chest wound called?

3. What type of dressing should be applied and why?

4. What will you do after applying the dressing?

Stories from the Field
Wrap-Up

You have many issues to consider when caring for patients with soft tissue injuries. When treating soft tissue injuries, always take BSI and standard precautions. This protects both you and the patient. Control external bleeding. Patients with serious burns are very susceptible to infection. Pay special attention to scene safety. Move the patient away from the source of the burn. You may have to delay rescue until a trained and equipped specialist arrives. Additional concerns are preventing hypothermia (especially in infants and children) and assessing for inhalation injuries. Soft tissue injuries can also lead to shock.

Care for the fireworks technician includes a good initial assessment. The presence of soot on the face, nose, and mouth suggests inhalation burns. These can be life threatening. If available, request assistance from advanced life support personnel. Assist ventilations with high-flow oxygen and transport as soon as possible. Remove jewelry or restrictive clothing from injured extremities or around the neck. Cover burns with dry, sterile dressings. Keep the patient warm by covering him with a blanket. Transport the patient to an appropriate facility.

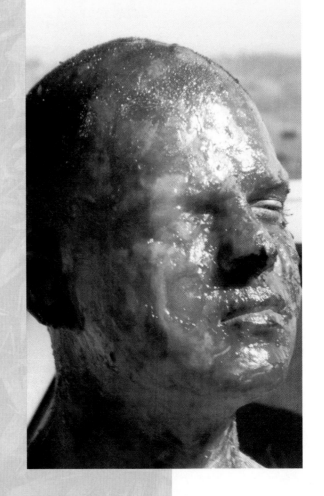

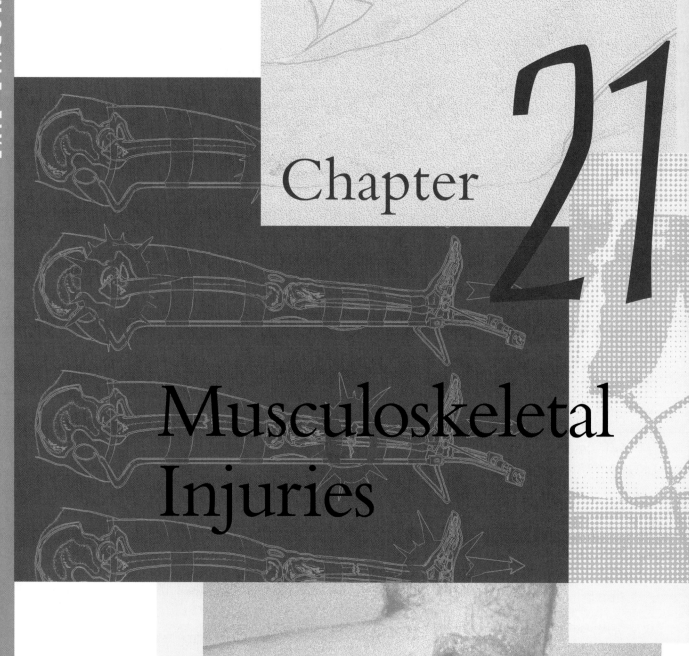

Chapter

21

Musculoskeletal
Injuries

Stories from the Field

One warm afternoon, an elderly woman calls directly to the station. She asks for someone to come evaluate her husband. The couple lives a few blocks away. Mark gets the woman's name, address, and telephone number. He calls the non-emergency dispatch number and advises the dispatcher of the call. After a short drive, you arrive at the house. You find an elderly man sitting on his front porch. The patient explains that as he was walking down the steps, he slipped and injured his knee.

Mark completes an initial assessment and finds no life-threatening conditions. During the focused history and physical exam, Mark discovers that the patient has no pedal pulse in the left foot. The patient also cannot feel a sharp object pressing against his foot. He has a long history of medical problems. He has many allergies and takes multiple medications. The patient states that he became lightheaded and dizzy just before falling. Robin completes the baseline vital signs. The blood pressure is 200/120, with a pulse rate of 94 and a respiratory rate of 22.

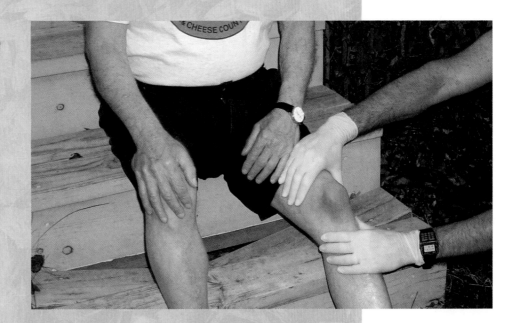

Musculoskeletal injuries are common. They are caused by external forces acting on the body. They include fractures, dislocations, sprains, and strains. Pain and swelling are common to all musculoskeletal injuries. In some cases, obvious deformity is seen. Your treatment will be based on the patient's signs and symptoms, not on a diagnosed problem. You will manage and treat any injury involving a painful and swollen extremity as if it was a fracture, whether or not there is obvious deformity.

Injuries to the spine and skull are skeletal injuries that require special consideration and emergency procedures. Evaluate the mechanism of injury to determine the potential for head and neck injuries. Treat the patient based on your findings. Evaluation and treatment of head and spine injuries are discussed in Chapter 22.

D.O.T. OBJECTIVES

Describe the function of the muscular system.

Describe the function of the skeletal system.

List the major bones or bone groupings of the spinal column; the thorax; the upper extremities; the lower extremities.

MUSCULOSKELETAL SYSTEM REVIEW

The musculoskeletal system consists of the bony framework of the skeleton and the attached skeletal muscles. It provides three key functions. These are:

- Support
- Protection
- Movement

You may wish to refer to Chapter 4 for a more comprehensive discussion of the musculoskeletal system. As a review, the spine supports the head. It contains 33 vertebrae and is the central support for the body. The thorax, or chest, consists of the sternum and ribs. It protects the internal organs of the chest. The shoulders connect the upper extremities to the torso. The humerus connects the shoulder to the elbow. Two distal bones, the radius and ulna, connect to the extensive bony structures of the wrist and hand. The lower extremities are connected to the torso at the pelvis. The femur is the largest bone in the body. It connects to the pelvis at the hip. The femur also connects to the knee. Below the knee are the tibia and fibula, which connect to the ankle. The ankle is connected to the foot, a complicated bone structure.

Muscles, tendons, and ligaments hold the skeletal framework together. Muscles cause movement of the bones. Joints are the points of contact between the bones. They may contain ligaments, tendons, cartilage, or synovial fluid.

INJURIES TO BONES AND JOINTS

You will frequently be called to manage simple injuries to bones or joints. These injuries are often the patient's only complaint. The management of all bone and joint injuries is very similar. Identifying the mechanism of injury helps you to predict the severity and location of musculoskeletal injuries. Information on some specific bone and joint injuries is summarized in the Enhanced Study section at the end of this chapter.

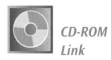

CD-ROM Link

The Authentic Emergency Scenes section in the Video Appendix on the MedEMT CD-ROM contains a video entitled "Broken Femur," which shows a team of EMTs treating an elderly woman who has fallen in her home.

> **D.O.T. OBJECTIVE**
>
> Differentiate between an open and a closed painful, swollen, deformed extremity.

Types of Injuries

There are several types of bone and joint injuries that can occur. For purposes of prehospital care, they are managed based on the signs and symptoms, not on a diagnosed injury. These injuries result in painful, swollen, deformed extremities that must be stabilized to prevent further damage.

Your main consideration with a bone or joint injury is whether it is an open injury or a closed injury. An open injury occurs when a bone end cuts through the skin (see Fig. 21.1). The risk of contamination and infection is great. If the

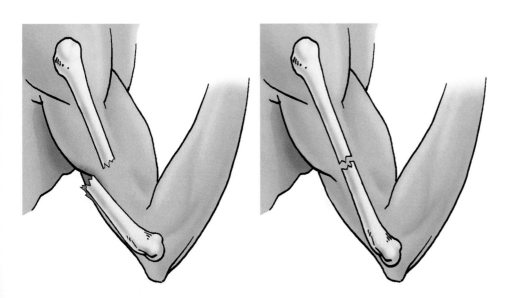

Figure 21.1 *A fractured humerus in an open injury (left) and a closed injury (right).*

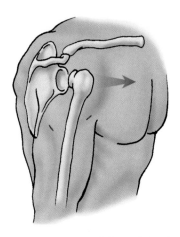

Figure 21.2 *A dislocated shoulder is usually a closed injury.*

skin overlying a fracture is intact, the patient has a closed fracture. The injury will be painful. The skin may be swollen, and the extremity may appear deformed.

The following types of injury can cause a painful, swollen, deformed extremity.

- A fracture is any break in a bone. Bones break in many different ways. The skin over a fracture may be painful, swollen, and deformed. The end of the bone may or may not protrude through the skin. You must determine if the suspected fracture is an open injury or closed injury.

- A dislocation occurs when a bone is dislodged from its normal alignment in a joint (see Fig 21.2). Dislocations of the clavicle are common and can be easily managed. Knee dislocations are seen in falls and motor vehicle collisions. A dislocation can seriously compromise distal circulation, sensation, and motor function of the affected extremity.

- A sprain is a joint injury that involves stretching or tearing of a ligament, the connective tissue that joins bones together (see Fig. 21.3). A strain involves stretching or tearing of a muscle or a tendon, the connective tissue that joins bones to muscles.

Figure 21.3 *Knee sprain (left). Strained biceps tendon (right).*

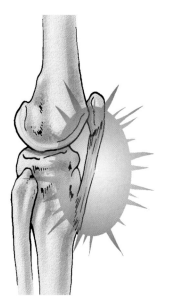
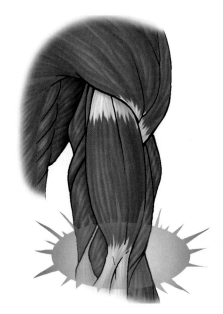

Direct Force | *A force that causes injury to a body part at the site of impact*

Indirect Force | *A transmitted force that causes injury some distance away from the point of impact*

Twisting Force | *Occurs when one part of an extremity remains in place while the rest moves or twists*

Mechanism of Injury

With musculoskeletal injuries, the forces involved in the mechanism of injury play an important role in determining what type of injury occurs. Bone and joint injuries can be caused by direct forces, indirect forces, and twisting forces.

A **direct force** causes injury at the site of impact. **Indirect forces** cause injury some distance away from the point of impact through transmitted force (see Fig. 21.4). For example, a hip or femur can be fractured by transmitted forces when a knee impacts the dashboard during a motor vehicle collision. Injury from a **twisting force** occurs when one part of an extremity remains in place

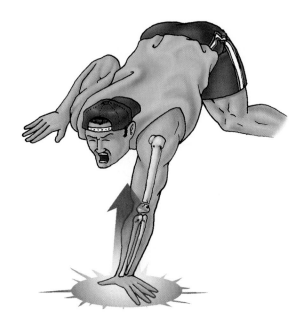

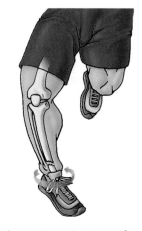

Figure 21.4 *Direct impact on the hand creates an indirect force, which causes injuries further up the arm.*

while the rest moves or twists (see Fig. 21.5). Stepping off a curb the wrong way results in a twisting force that can injure the ankle.

Signs and Symptoms

Signs and symptoms of injuries to the bones and joints are listed below. Not all of these signs and symptoms are present in all bone or joint injuries.

- Deformity
- Angulation (a severe, abnormal bend in an extremity)
- Pain and tenderness
- Crepitation (grating sensation or sound)
- Swelling (see Fig. 21.6)

Figure 21.5 *A twisting force injury is common among athletes.*

Figure 21.6 *Swelling due to an ankle injury.*

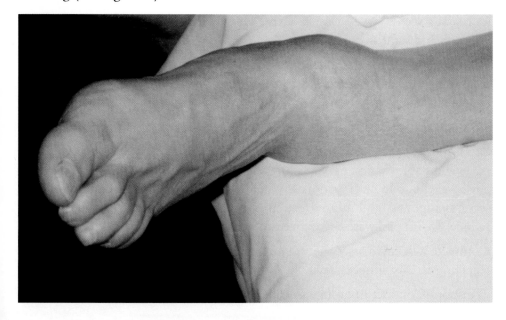

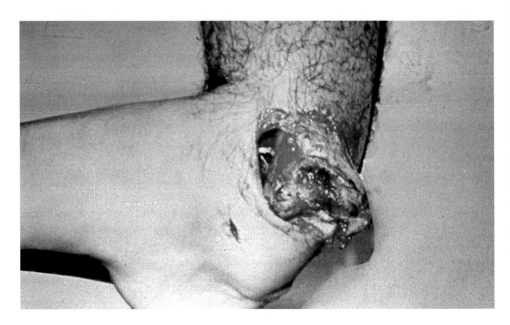

Figure 21.7 *An open ankle fracture with severe angulation.*

- Bruising or discoloration
- Exposed bone ends in an open fracture (see Fig. 21.7)
- A joint that is locked into position

D.O.T. OBJECTIVE

List the emergency medical care for a patient with a painful, swollen, deformed extremity.

Emergency Care for Bone and Joint Injuries

These are the emergency medical care steps for a bone or joint injury:

1. Conduct a scene survey. Ensure scene safety. Use appropriate body substance isolation and standard precautions.

2. Complete the initial assessment. Control the airway and breathing. Take cervical spine precautions, if necessary. Administer oxygen if indicated. Provide life-saving interventions.

3. Complete the focused history and physical exam.

4. Splint musculoskeletal injuries before transport. This keeps the extremity in place and stable, which prevents further injury. Splinting techniques are discussed in the following section. If you are using a long spine board, it can serve as a splint for all injured extremities. Once splinted, apply cold packs to reduce swelling. Elevate the extremity, if possible.

5. Complete a detailed assessment. This can be done while en route to the receiving facility, if necessary.

6. Transport. Conduct ongoing assessments according to patient condition.

SPLINTING

Injuries to bones and joints require splinting before you move the patient, unless life-threatening injuries are present. Patients with life-threatening injuries should have **splints** applied while en route to the hospital. A backboard is often used as a full-body splint when treating severely injured trauma patients. You may use the backboard in place of extremity splints, if necessary.

Splint | *Equipment used to prevent or reduce movement of body joints or injured tissue*

D.O.T. OBJECTIVE

State the reasons for splinting.

Reasons for Splinting

Broken bones result in bone fragments and sharp edges that can damage the surrounding tissue, including muscles, nerves, and blood vessels (see Fig. 21.8). If the injured bones, joints, or bone fragments are moved, further damage occurs. Splinting stabilizes the damaged area by reducing movement. This lowers the risk of injury to surrounding tissue and prevents the bone or joint injury from worsening. Splinting a painful, swollen, deformed extremity helps to:

• Prevent excessive bleeding by reducing damage to nearby blood vessels

• Prevent compression of an artery by a displaced bone which would compromise blood flow distal to the injury

• Reduce the risk that a sharp edge will pierce the skin, thus converting a closed fracture to an open fracture

• Prevent increased pain caused by movement of bone ends

• Reduce the risk of paralysis by immobilizing the cervical spine

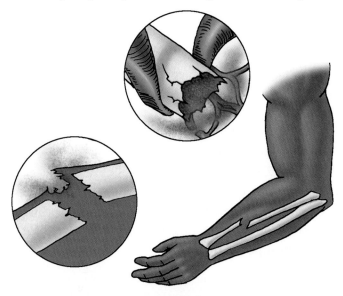

Figure 21.8 *Broken bone fragments can damage the surrounding tissue, including muscles, nerves, and blood vessels.*

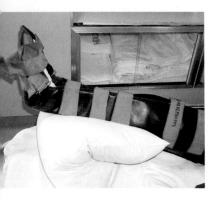

Figure 21.9 *Rigid leg splint secured with Velcro straps.*

Figure 21.10 *Bipolar traction splint with securing straps.*

Types of Splints

Many types of splinting equipment are used in EMS. These include:

- Rigid splints are made of wood, cardboard, plastic, wire, or aluminum (see Fig. 21.9). Some are padded and preformed to fit certain body areas. Others must be molded and padded before application.

- Traction splints are designed to stabilize fractures (see Fig. 21.10). They apply traction (a pulling force) to the muscles surrounding the injury. This reduces pain and prevents further injury. Traction splints are often used to treat femoral fractures.

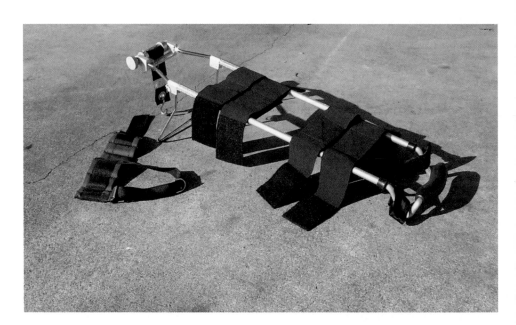

- Air pressure splints (pneumatic splints) are preformed, soft plastic splints (see Fig. 21.11). They become firm when inflated by mouth. The pressure in the splint is low. It can change with temperature and altitude. Air pressure splints are not as rigid as other materials, such as aluminum. They usually cover most of the extremity. Consequently, you cannot assess the pulse distal to the injury after an air splint is applied. For these reasons, rigid splints are the preferred equipment.

- Vacuum splints are another kind of pneumatic splint. They use the extraction of air from a splint to form a kind of mattress around the injury site. In some EMS systems, the vacuum splint is used in place of the long spine board or other rigid splinting device.

- The pneumatic anti-shock garment (PASG) can be used as a pressure splint to stabilize pelvic fractures (see Fig. 21.12). When used for this purpose, all three compartments should be inflated. Review Chapter 19 for application of a PASG. Follow local protocols.

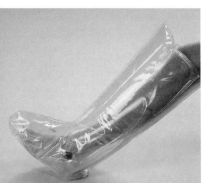

Figure 21.11 *Air pressure splint for the lower leg.*

- A splint can be improvised from any available material that can be used for stabilizing an injured extremity. For example, pillows and magazines can be used for splinting.

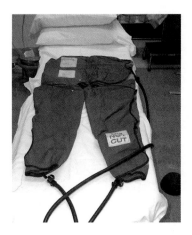

Figure 21.12 *Pneumatic anti-shock garment (PASG).*

D.O.T. OBJECTIVES

List the general rules for splinting.

List the complications of splinting.

General Rules for Splinting

The general procedure for splinting an extremity is described in Procedure 21.1 on page 616. Always assess the pulse, motor function, and sensory status distal to the injury site before and after splinting. A pulse check is accomplished by finding the pulse point below the injury. To check for motor function, ask the patient to move his or her toes or fingers. Check the status of sensory function by lightly pinching or touching the skin distal to the injury. Ask the patient whether he or she feels the touch and the location of the stimulus. For example, lightly pinch the middle finger of an injured arm and ask the patient which finger was pinched. Record your findings.

Splints must be applied correctly and promptly. Failing to do so may cause complications. Excessive movement during splint application can aggravate the injury or damage the surrounding soft tissue, organs, nerves, or muscles. A closed fracture can be converted to an open fracture. Increased bleeding and pain are likely. Permanent damage or disability is possible. A splint that is too loose permits excessive movement, which increases tissue damage. A tight splint may compromise distal circulation or compress nerves and other tissue (see Fig. 21.13).

CD-ROM Link

The video "General Splinting Rules" in Chapter 21 and the Video Appendix on the MedEMT CD-ROM demonstrates the splinting of a tibial fracture.

Figure 21.13 *A loose splint allows bone movement (left). A splint that is too tight can compromise circulation (right).*

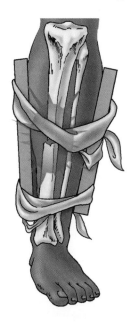
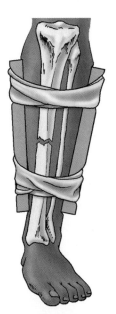

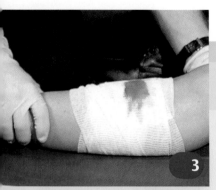

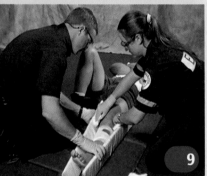

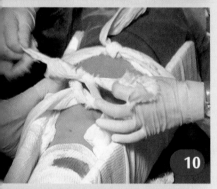

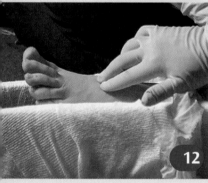

Procedure 21.1 • **GENERAL RULES OF SPLINTING**

Video Appendix

Limit Bleeding

Bloodborne

Stabilize Spine

1. Although bone and joint injuries may be painful and obvious, never treat these injuries until you have managed the patient's airway, breathing, and circulation.

2. Always practice body substance isolation and standard precautions.

3. Manually stabilize the extremity above and below the injury.

4. Assess the pulse, motor function, and sensory status distal to the injury before splinting. Distal pulses may be difficult to find. If a distal pulse is found, mark the location with a pen for future reference. Record your findings.

5. Expose the injury by cutting or removing clothing. Remove rings distal to the injury.

6. If the extremity is severely deformed, or if the distal extremity is cyanotic or pulseless, notify medical direction. You may be instructed to apply gentle traction to align the limb. This may restore circulation. Stop if you observe increased pain, resistance, or crepitation.

7. Cover open wounds with a sterile dressing. This keeps them free of debris and reduces the risk of infection.

8. If bones protrude through the skin, do not try to move them. They may align themselves when you apply the splint.

9. Pad the splint to prevent pressure and discomfort.

10. Immobilize the joints above and below the injury. This prevents excessive movement.

11. If a patient shows signs of shock, treat for shock and transport immediately.

12. Reassess and record the distal pulse, motor function, and sensation every 15 minutes to ensure that the splint has not compromised circulation.

Procedure 21.2 • SPLINTING A LONG BONE

Body Fluids

Stabilize Spine

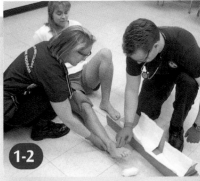
1-2

1. Stabilize the entire bone. Assess the circulatory, motor, and sensory status of the injured extremity.

2. Apply a rigid splint that is sized to immobilize the entire bone.

3. While one EMT stabilizes the extremity and splint, another EMT secures the splint below and above the injury.

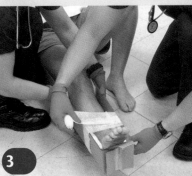

3

4. Once the splint is secured, assess the distal pulse, motor function, and sensation to confirm adequate circulation.

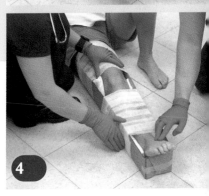
4

Specific Splinting Procedures

Specific splinting procedures depend on the site and type of injury and the type of splint used. Follow the general rules outlined above, with special considerations as described in the following procedures.

- Splinting a long bone is described in Procedure 21.2.

- Splinting an injured joint is described in Procedure 21.3 on page 618.

- The sling and swathe help to immobilize clavicular fractures, shoulder injuries, and arm and forearm fractures (see Procedure 21.4 on page 619). A sling is useful when a rigid splint is applied to an upper extremity. The arm sling further immobilizes the area and reduces weight on the injury. Arm slings may be purchased commercially, fashioned from triangular bandages or cravats, or improvised from other material. A swathe is a folded triangular bandage or other rolled bandage. It is used to bind the injured arm to the chest, providing better immobilization.

EMT Tip

While applying splinting material, ask the patient not to move the injured area.

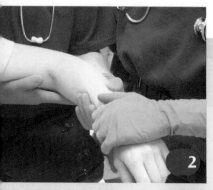

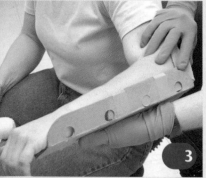

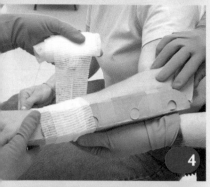

Procedure 21.3 • SPLINTING AN INJURED JOINT

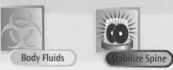

1. Assess the circulatory, motor, and sensory status of the injured extremity.

2. Immobilize the bones above and below the joint.

3. Apply a properly-sized, rigid splint that is configured at an angle that corresponds to the joint position.

4. While one EMT stabilizes the joint, another applies the bandage to secure the splint in place.

5. Once the splint is secured, assess the distal pulse, motor function, and sensation to confirm adequate circulation.

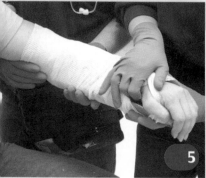

Traction Splinting

Traction splints are used on known or suspected femoral shaft fractures when there are no other suspected joint or leg injuries. A fractured femur is very painful. The patient will usually have swelling and deformity of the mid-thigh. The large thigh muscles may spasm and contract. The strong muscles can pull on the bone ends until they override each other. This shortens the leg, causing severe pain, bleeding, and tissue damage. Significant blood loss may occur at the site of injury. The bleeding may not be readily apparent. For example, a closed femur fracture may result in up to a liter of internal blood loss. Suspect hypovolemic shock in all patients with possible femur injuries. Applying traction will help to control these problems.

Procedure 21.4 • **APPLICATION OF A SLING AND SWATHE**

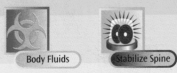

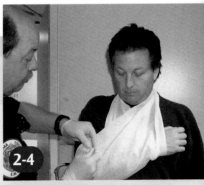

1. Assess the pulse, motor, and sensory status of the injured upper extremity.

2. Bend the elbow, placing the injured extremity comfortably across the chest. Lay the long edge of the triangular bandage along the patient's side opposite the injury. The point of the triangle extends beyond the elbow.

3. Bring the bottom edge of the bandage up over the forearm. Tie the two ends at the side of the neck. Keep the knot away from the center of the neck. Never tie a sling around the neck if you suspect a cervical spine injury. Place thick bandages or padding between the neck and sling for comfort.

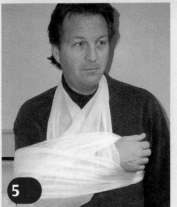

4. Tie or pin the pointed end of the sling to form a cradle. Secure the sling, elevating the hand higher than the elbow. Make sure that the knot is not directly over the cervical vertebrae. This can cause increased discomfort.

5. Wrap one or two wide cravats or other bandages around the chest and over the sling. Tie them firmly in place on the side opposite the injury. Avoid wrapping the uninjured arm.

6. Reassess distal pulse, sensory, and motor status.

Use a traction splint when the patient has a painful, swollen, deformed mid-thigh. Avoid the traction splint if you suspect hip, knee joint, or lower leg injury (see Fig. 21.14). Do not apply a traction splint for:

- An injury that is close to, or involves, the knee
- An injury involving the hip or pelvis as determined by palpation, visualization, or mechanism of injury
- Partial amputation with the distal limb connected by marginal tissue, so that traction would risk separation
- Lower leg or ankle injury

Figure 21.14 *Contraindications to a traction splint (top to bottom): knee injury, hip injury, partial amputation, and ankle injury.*

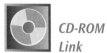

CD-ROM Link

The video "Bipolar Traction Splint" on the MedEMT CD-ROM shows steps in applying this device.

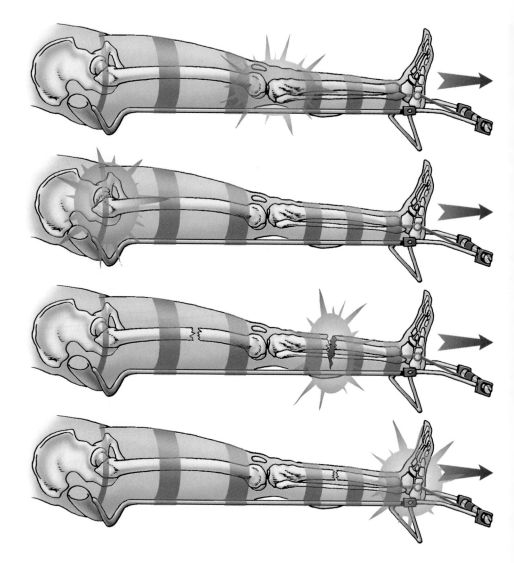

Two basic types of traction splints are used. These are unipolar and bipolar splints. Unipolar splints have one adjustable pole that is secured next to the injured leg (see Procedure 21.5). Bipolar splints have two poles. When using the bipolar traction splint, the leg is secured between the poles (see Procedure 21.6 on page 622). The splint is wedged against the pelvic bone while traction is applied to the ankle strap.

Procedure 21.5 • **UNIPOLAR TRACTION SPLINT**

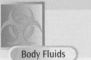
Body Fluids

Stabilize Spine

1. Assess and record the pulse, motor function, and sensory status distal to the injury. Mark the distal pulse point for future reference.

2. Manually stabilize the injured leg by placing one hand directly behind the knee and the other around the ankle.

3. Have your partner apply manual traction. Traction is applied by pulling the leg with both hands along its long axis, toward the toes. Hold the limb in alignment above and below the injury. Maintain manual traction until mechanical traction is in place.

4. Adjust the splint to the proper length.

5. Position the splint along the inside of the injured leg with the ischial pad against the groin.

6. Secure the ischial (proximal) strap. With a male patient, make sure the strap does not entrap the genitals.

7. Secure the ankle (distal) strap, with the foot in an upright position.

8. Attach the hook. Apply mechanical traction until it is equal to the manual traction being applied, and pain and spasms are reduced. If the patient is unresponsive, apply mechanical traction until both legs are of equal length.

9. Secure the support straps. Reevaluate the ischial and ankle straps.

10. Reassess distal pulse, motor, and sensory status.

11. Secure the patient's torso to a backboard to immobilize the hip joint. Secure the splint to the board to prevent movement of the injured leg.

12. If you apply a HARE traction device to an extremely tall patient, you may have to place the patient into the ambulance feet-first to allow for the increased length.

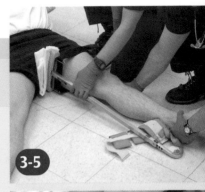
3-5

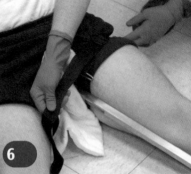
6

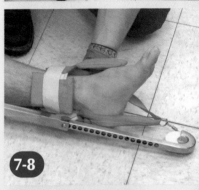
7-8

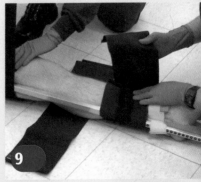
9

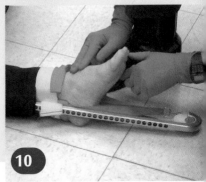
10

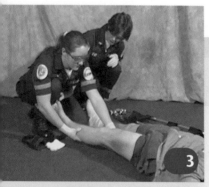

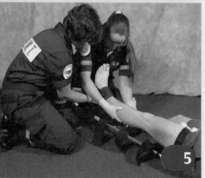

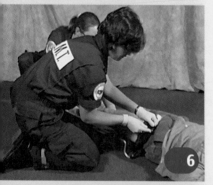

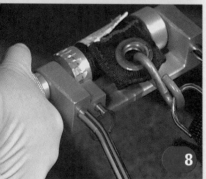

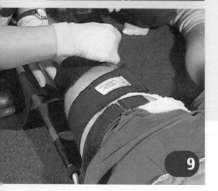

Procedure 21.6 • BIPOLAR TRACTION SPLINT

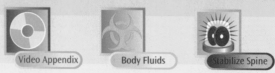

Video Appendix   Body Fluids   Stabilize Spine

1. Assess and record the pulse, motor function, and sensory status distal to the injury. Mark the distal pulse point for future reference.

2. Manually stabilize the injured leg by placing one hand directly behind the knee and the other around the ankle.

3. Have your partner apply manual traction. Traction is applied by pulling the leg with both hands along its long axis, toward the toes. Hold the limb in alignment above and below the injury.

4. Adjust the splint to the proper length.

5. Position the splint under the injured leg with the ischial pad against the bone.

6. Raise the heel stand. Secure the ischial (proximal) strap. With a male patient, make sure the strap does not entrap the genitals.

7. Secure the ankle (distal) strap with the foot in an upright position.

8. Attach the hooks. Apply mechanical traction until it is equal to the manual traction being applied, and pain and spasms are reduced. If the patient is unresponsive, apply mechanical traction until both legs are of equal length.

9. Secure the support straps. Reevaluate the ischial and ankle straps.

10. Reassess pulse, motor, and sensory status.

11. Secure the patient's torso to a backboard to immobilize the hip joint. Secure the splint to the board to prevent movement of the injured leg.

Chapter Twenty-One Summary

- Emergency treatment of suspected musculoskeletal injuries is based on signs and symptoms. Determining whether the injury is a fracture, sprain, or strain is not a priority.

- Splints prevent movement of bone fragments, bone ends, or angulated joints. Preventing motion reduces damage to muscles, nerves, and blood vessels. It prevents a closed injury from becoming an open one. Splints also help to control bleeding and pain.

- Always immobilize the joint above and below the injury. Never secure a tie or strap directly over the injury. Splint an extremity injury only if it can be isolated. If you suspect a severe mechanism of injury and possible spinal injury, splint the extremity to the long backboard during spinal immobilization. Assess the injured extremity for the presence of pulses, movement, and sensation before and after splinting.

- If a deformity is severe, or if the pulse is absent, medical direction may have you attempt to straighten the extremity. Follow local protocols.

Key Terms Review

Direct Force | *page 610*

Indirect Force | *page 610*

Splint | *page 613*

Twisting Force | *page 610*

Review Questions

1. Which of the following is NOT a key function of the skeletal system?

   a. Locomotion
   b. Protection
   c. Temperature control
   d. Support

2. A fracture in which the broken bone ends have penetrated the skin is a(n):

   a. Twisting fracture
   b. Open fracture
   c. Closed fracture
   d. Angulation

3. Splinting can accomplish all of the following EXCEPT:

   a. Prevent a fracture from becoming an open fracture
   b. Accelerate the healing process
   c. Prevent an increase in pain
   d. Reduce tissue damage

4. A sprain is an injury involving:

   a. Muscles
   b. Tendons
   c. Ligaments
   d. Bones

Review Questions (cont.)

5. When caring for a painful, swollen, deformed extremity, immobilize:

   a. The injured bone

   b. The injured bone and the joints above and below it

   c. Only if there is no bleeding

   d. Only with approved splints

6. Which of the following is the best definition of the term closed fracture?

   a. Fracture caused by indirect forces

   b. Fracture where skin is not broken by fractured bone ends

   c. A bone dislodged from its normal alignment in a joint

   d. Incomplete break in a bone

7. A sprain involves:

   a. A joint that has had its ligaments stretched or torn

   b. A bone that is broken

   c. A bone that is out of alignment

   d. A combination of a, b, and c

8. A car's bumper striking a pedestrian's leg is an example of:

   a. Direct force

   b. Indirect force

   c. Twisting force

   d. Psychosomatic force

9. Which of the following is a bone of the upper extremity?

   a. Tibia

   b. Ischium

   c. Mandible

   d. Humerus

10. Which bone helps to protect the heart and lungs?

    a. Sternum

    b. Lumbar spine

    c. Pelvis

    d. Cranium

11. Your patient was struck by a large truck just below the hip. He is unable to bear weight on the leg that was struck. There is no pain to his pelvis on palpation. You note a rapid pulse and the patient's skin is cool and moist. He has no other complaints. You suspect injury to the:

    a. Femur

    b. Ankle

    c. Skull

    d. Rib

12. Your patient was the driver in a motor vehicle collision. She has a painful, swollen, deformed upper left leg. What device should be used to splint her leg?

    a. Traction splint

    b. Cardboard splint

    c. Air splint

    d. Vacuum splint

13. Your patient has an open, painful, swollen, and deformed wrist after falling while ice skating. She is conscious, but obviously in distress. When should you apply an extremity splint to this patient?

    a. While en route to the hospital

    b. After spinal immobilization

    c. Following initial assessment

    d. Immediately upon arrival on scene

CASE STUDIES

Musculoskeletal Injuries

1 You are dispatched to a suburban home in mid-winter. You arrive to find a young woman sitting on a sled in her driveway. She is in good spirits, but complains that her leg hurts. She tells you that her leg got caught on a piece of wood as she was going downhill. You find no life-threatening problems, but the focused history and physical exam reveals an open, deformed right lower extremity and an absent pedal pulse.

A. What is the difference between a deformed extremity with an open fracture and a deformed extremity with a closed fracture?

B. How is the treatment of an open musculoskeletal injury different from one that is closed?

C. If an extremity is pulseless after an injury, what steps should you take and why?

2 Your crew is dispatched to a trucking terminal. Upon your arrival, you are led to a man lying on the terminal floor. According to coworkers, a forklift was moving large barrels into a truck. One fell off, striking the patient on the hip. The patient responds appropriately during your initial assessment. Airway, breathing, and circulation are adequate. Your rapid trauma assessment reveals an unstable pelvis and deformities to both femurs. Initial vital signs are pulse 118, respirations 24, and blood pressure 100/60. The patient's skin is cool and moist.

A. What are the preferred methods for splinting an unstable pelvis?

B. What are possible complications if splinting is done incorrectly?

3 You are helping a neighbor with a backyard party. While you are inside preparing snacks, a child runs in to tell you about an accident on the trampoline. You find a 10-year-old boy crying quietly on the ground. He is holding his right wrist and is in obvious pain. Your initial assessment reveals no life-threatening injuries. You learn from bystanders that the child landed on the rim of the trampoline. His arm was caught in a support. Your neighbor calls the mother, who states that she will come to take her son to the hospital.

A. What type of focused history and physical exam is appropriate for this patient?

B. What should you look for when evaluating this child's arm?

C. You have no splinting materials available other than routine household items. How will you splint the arm using items on hand?

Stories from the Field
Wrap-Up

You will care for many patients with musculoskeletal injuries. Knowing the exact nature of the injury is not critical to your care. Focus on treating the patient's complaints of pain and swelling. When evaluating a trauma patient, check for underlying medical problems that may have triggered the traumatic event. In this case, for example, the patient could have fallen because of his dizziness. Sometimes, a traumatic event will trigger a medical problem. For example, a motor vehicle accident may trigger a heart attack.

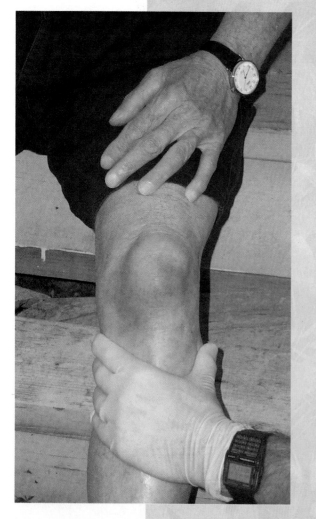

The musculoskeletal system is closely related to the circulatory and nervous systems. Injuries to bones, joints, and muscles can injure the related blood vessels and nerves. Always assess distal neurological function in injured extremities. Your skill in collecting history information is essential. Treatment of this patient includes high-flow oxygen by non-rebreather mask and early transport. Splint and elevate the leg. Apply ice to the injury while en route to the receiving facility.

ENHANCED STUDY

Specific Musculoskeletal Injuries

The following tables describe specific bone and joint injuries to various parts of the body. Typical mechanisms of injury, signs and symptoms, and treatment suggestions are included for each bone or joint.

You will treat all cases of painful, swollen, deformed extremities as if they are fractures. For all injuries, assess the distal pulse, motor function, and sensation before and after applying a splint. Follow local protocols.

Enhancement Table 21.1 • INJURIES TO THE PELVIC REGION

Bone or Joint	Mechanisms of Injury	Signs and Symptoms	Treatment
Hip Dislocation	Major trauma (extended leg and foot on brake pedal before an impact, or knee hitting dashboard) Fall (especially in elderly patients) Crush injury	History of total hip replacement Pain in the hip area Posterior dislocation (common): Hip flexed, adducted, and internally rotated Anterior dislocation (rare): Hip slightly flexed, abducted, and externally rotated Joint feels locked Inability to move leg	Splint in position found or position of comfort Check for other injuries Cold pack
Hip Fracture	Minor trauma (elderly patients) Major trauma (younger patients) Dashboard injury Direct blow to thigh Direct blow to hip	Pain in hip or groin area Severe pain with movement Inability to bear weight External rotation of hip and leg (internal rotation rare) Shortening of the limb	Immobilization Splint with backboard or bind legs together Frequent monitoring of vital signs
Pelvis	Minor trauma (elderly patients) Crush injury Automobile or motorcycle accident Direct trauma Fall from height	Tenderness over pubis or when iliac wings compressed Pain in pelvis when patient squeezes inward with your fist between knees Sacroiliac joint tenderness Pelvic bruising Hematuria Signs of shock	Immobilize spine and legs on long backboard Flex knees to reduce pain and support with pillows Oxygen Frequent monitoring of vital signs Check for other injuries PASG if shock present Rapid transport

ENHANCED STUDY

Specific Musculoskeletal Injuries *(cont.)*

Enhancement Table 21.2 • **INJURIES TO THE LOWER EXTREMITIES**

Bone or Joint	Mechanisms of Injury	Signs and Symptoms	Treatment

Femur	Major trauma
	Direct blow
	Torsion
	Indirect force
	  (knee to dashboard)
	Auto vs. pedestrian collision
	Fall
		Severe pain
		Inability to bear weight on leg
		Swelling
		Deformity
		Angulation
		Crepitus
		Shortening of limb and
		  severe muscle spasms
		Signs of shock
			Maintain airway, breathing,
			  and circulation
			Traction splint only if an
			  isolated femur fracture
			Check for other injuries
			Frequent monitoring
			  of vital signs
			Cold pack

Knee	Dashboard
	Motorcycle accident
	Auto vs. pedestrian collision
	Direct blow
	Fall
	Sports injury
		Pain
		Inability to bend or
		  straighten knee
		Deformity
		Swelling
		Tenderness
			If found straight, rigid splint
			If found angulated, splint
			  in the position found; note
			  compromised circulation
			Check for other injuries
			Frequent monitoring
			  of vital signs
			Cold pack

Tibia and/or
Fibula
	Direct trauma
	  (auto bumper injury)
	Indirect trauma
	Twisting injury
	Fall
		Pain
		Point tenderness
		Swelling
		Deformity
		Crepitus
			Rigid splint as found
			  if pulse is adequate
			Sterile dressing if
			  open fracture
			Cold pack
			Elevation

Ankle or Foot	Automobile accident Athletic injury Crush injury Direct trauma Twisting Fall	Pain Swelling Deformity Hesitancy to bear weight Point tenderness Open fracture	Soft splint Cold pack Elevation

Enhancement Table 21.3 • **INJURIES TO THE UPPER BODY**

Bone or Joint	Mechanisms of Injury	Signs and Symptoms	Treatment

Clavicle	Fall on an outstretched arm
	Blunt force blow
	Direct trauma
	Athletic injury
		Pain in clavicular area
		Point tenderness
		Refusal to raise arm
		Swelling
		Deformity
		Crepitus
		Head tilted toward injury;
		  chin to opposite side
		Dropped shoulder
			Sling and swathe
			Pad the axillary area;
			  avoid damage to the
			  brachial plexus
			  and artery
			Cold pack

Shoulder Fracture or Dislocation	Fall on an
	  outstretched arm
	Direct trauma
	  to the shoulder
		Pain in the shoulder area
		Point tenderness
		Refusal to move arm
		Gross swelling
		Discoloration
		Dropped shoulder
		Holds arm against the chest
		Loss of rounded contour
		  to shoulder
			Sling and swathe
			Cold pack

Upper Arm	Fall on an outstretched arm
	Direct trauma
	Dislocation
		Pain
		Point tenderness
		Swelling
		Inability or resistance
		  to move arm
		Severe deformity or angulation
		Crepitus
			Sling and swathe
			Assess for other injuries,
			  especially the chest
			Cold pack

Elbow	Fall on an extended arm Fall on a flexed elbow Skateboard accident (increasingly common)	Pain Point tenderness Swelling Refusal to move elbow Deformity Decreased circulation to hand	Splint in position found Cold pack
Forearm	Fall on an extended arm Direct trauma	Pain Point tenderness Swelling Deformity or angulation Shortened arm	Rigid splint with sling Cold pack Elevation to avoid accumulation of fluid
Wrist	Fall on outstretched hand	Pain Swelling Deformity	Rigid splint in position found Sling Cold pack Elevation

Chapter

22

Head and Spine Injuries

Stories from the Field

Late one evening you are working in your yard and talking with your neighbor. He is restoring an antique vehicle. While talking to you, he accidentally steps on his son's skateboard, falling to the ground. He lands squarely on his back. His head hits the concrete driveway very hard. You walk over and find him trying to get up. He cannot sit up, and is very confused. You notice a laceration and large hematoma on the back of his head. You call 9-1-1 for an ambulance, although you are not sure whether he will agree to go to the hospital.

While you are waiting for an ambulance, you assume control of your neighbor's cervical spine. You advise him to lie still. He has become very pale and cool. He complains of feeling light-headed, and states he has a bad headache "just behind the eyes." He is becoming very upset because he cannot sit up or move his legs. He says he feels a tingling sensation in his legs, but states repeatedly, "They just don't work." You comfort him and ask him not to move while you maintain cervical spine control.

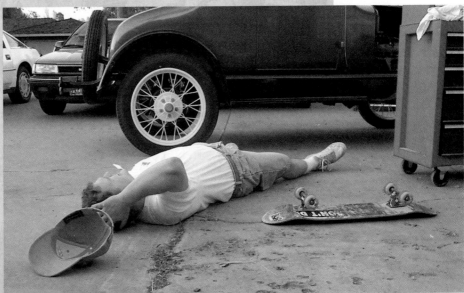

ead and neck injuries are some of the most challenging conditions you will face. Failure to provide appropriate care can have significant, even fatal, consequences for the patient. You must completely immobilize the spine if the mechanism of injury or signs and symptoms suggest possible spinal cord injury. Your initial assessment, including opening the airway, must take into consideration the possibility of spinal injury.

D.O.T. OBJECTIVES

State the components of the nervous system.

List the functions of the central nervous system.

Define the structure of the skeletal system as it relates to the nervous system.

NERVOUS SYSTEM REVIEW

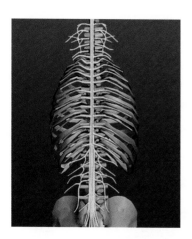

Figure 22.1 *The spinal cord and peripheral nerves.*

The nervous system controls voluntary and involuntary actions. It also senses conditions within and outside of the body. As a review of the description in Chapter 4, the nervous system has two anatomical divisions:

• The central nervous system consists of the brain and spinal cord (see Fig. 4.60 in Chapter 4)

• The peripheral nervous system consists of the sensory and motor nerves that extend from the central nervous system throughout the body (see Fig. 22.1 and Fig. 4.59 in Chapter 4)

The brain is often called the nerve center of the body. It directs the body's response to stimuli. Sensory nerves receive information from the body. They transport the information to the spinal cord and the brain. Motor nerves are triggered by the brain. They transmit instructions to muscle and organ tissues.

The skeletal system cushions and protects the central nervous system. The brain is surrounded by the bones of the skull. The spinal cord is contained within the vertebral column.

D.O.T. OBJECTIVE

Describe the implications of not properly caring for potential spine injuries.

INJURIES TO THE SPINE

Spinal cord injuries are very serious. They can lead to loss of sensation and motor function. Complications may include an inability to breathe adequately and paralysis. Your major concern whenever spinal injury is suspected is to immobilize the patient's spine. This helps to prevent further injury from occurring.

D.O.T. OBJECTIVE

Relate mechanism of injury to potential injuries of the head and spine.

Mechanism of Injury

Mechanism of injury (MOI) was discussed in detail in Chapters 8 and 9. You must maintain a high index of suspicion for spine injuries in instances of:

- Motor vehicle accidents
- Pedestrian vs. vehicle collisions
- Motorcycle accidents
- Falls and jumps
- Diving accidents
- Hangings
- Blunt trauma
- Penetrating trauma to the head, neck, or torso
- Facial trauma
- Unconscious trauma victims

The forces involved in different MOIs produce different types of spinal injuries. Following are the general types of injury you will see.

- Flexion injuries are caused by severe forward movement of the spine. Sudden deceleration in an automobile accident may cause hyperflexion (see Fig. 22.2 on page 634).

- Extension injuries are caused by sudden, severe backward movement of the spine. When a car is hit from behind, the occupant is pushed forward. If the headrest is too low, the head is propelled backward, causing a hyperextension injury of the neck.

CD-ROM Link

The "Fallen Climber" video in the Authentic Emergency Scenes section of the Video Appendix on the MedEMT CD-ROM shows care being given to a victim of a rock climbing accident.

Figure 22.2 *Flexion injuries (left) and extension injuries (right) are common in automobile accidents.*

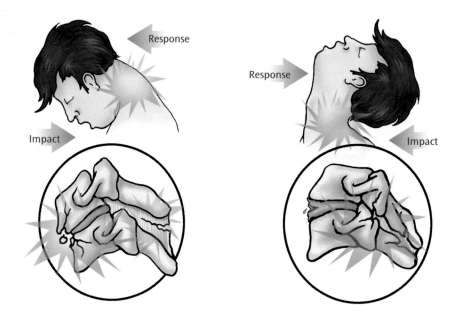

- Extreme movement of the neck sideways can cause lateral bending injuries (see Fig. 22.3).
- Rotation injuries are caused by twisting forces.

Figure 22.3 *Lateral bending injury (left) and rotation injury (right).*

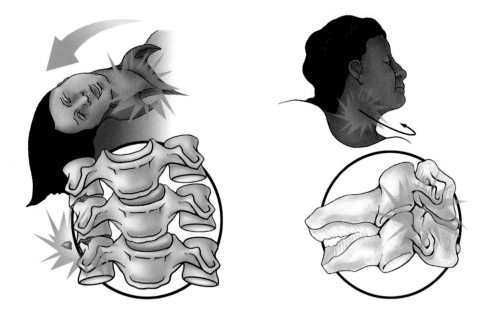

- Distraction injuries are caused by extreme stretching or pulling apart of the spine, spinal cord, and surrounding structures (see Fig. 22.4). These injuries may also cause fractures. For example, the so-called hangman's fracture occurs in hangings. This fracture of the second cervical vertebra is caused by a combination of distraction and extension forces.

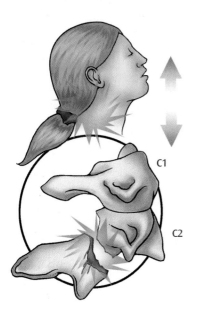

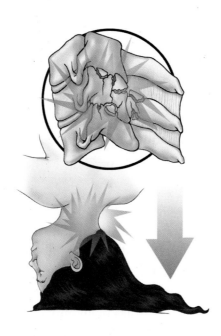

Figure 22.4 *Distraction injury (left) and compression injury (right).*

- **Compression injury** of the spine occurs when a strong force is transmitted up or down the length of the body. Compression injuries are caused by diving accidents, jumps, falls, and motor vehicle accidents.

- Penetration injuries are caused by stabbing and gunshot wounds to the spine (see Fig. 22.5).

Compression Injury | *Spinal injury caused when a strong force is transmitted up or down the length of the body*

D.O.T. OBJECTIVE

State the signs and symptoms of a potential spine injury.

Signs and Symptoms of Spinal Injury

The mechanism of injury may be your only clue to the true nature of an injury. Do not rule out possible spine injury because the patient has no pain or can walk. Patients with some spinal injuries can move the extremities and feel sensations. Suspect cervical spine injury if the patient is injured above the clavicle or if he or she has lost consciousness from a head injury.

Signs and symptoms that a potential spinal injury exists are:

- Tenderness anywhere along the spine.
- Pain associated with movement.
- Pain that is felt anywhere along the spinal column or radiating into the legs. This pain is independent of movement or palpation. It may be intermittent.
- Obvious deformity of the spine on inspection or palpation. This condition is rare.

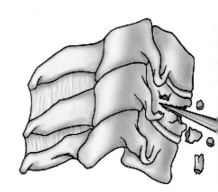

Figure 22.5 *Penetration injury of the cervical spine.*

 EMT Alert

Advise a patient with a potential spine injury not to move while you obtain a history and complete your initial assessment. Do not ask the patient to move or try to move him or her in order to elicit a pain response.

- Soft tissue injuries to the head or neck, the shoulders, the back, the abdomen, or the lower extremities.

- Abnormal sensation or weakness in the extremities. This can indicate possible neurological problems. Sensations such as numbness or tingling in the extremities are called **paresthesia**.

- Loss of sensation or paralysis inferior to the level of suspected injury.

- Loss of sensation or paralysis in the upper or lower extremities.

- Incontinence.

- Inadequate breathing effort, indicating respiratory muscle paralysis. The diaphragm may remain functional even though chest wall muscles are paralyzed. This results in shallow breathing with little or no abdominal movement.

- Neurogenic shock, caused by an inability of the blood vessels to constrict and raise the heart rate to compensate for loss of fluid. Signs of neurogenic shock are hypotension and bradycardia with no obvious blood loss.

- Priapism in males, a constant, abnormal erection of the penis that is caused by injury to nerves supplying the genitals.

Paresthesia (pair-as-THEEZ-e-uh) | *Abnormal sensations of tingling, numbness, burning, coldness, pain, or tightness in the extremities*

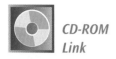

CD-ROM Link

The "Spine Immobilization–Initial Patient Assessment" video in Chapter 22 and the Video Appendix on the MedEMT CD-ROM demonstrates the steps for determining whether a patient has a spine injury.

Patient Assessment in Potential Spine Injuries

Besides stabilizing life-threatening conditions, you must ensure that no further spinal injury occurs. Upon arrival, assess the patient for potential spine injuries. Observe the mechanism of injury and the signs and symptoms. Always err on the side of caution. Treat and immobilize any patient with a suspected head or spine injury. Failure to assess the need for spinal immobilization can result in death or permanent disability.

Whenever a potential spinal injury is suspected, regardless of the location of injury, you must secure the entire spinal column to prevent additional movement and injury. You cannot provide adequate and safe spinal precautions if you secure only the cervical spine or only the lumbar spine. Each area that is not secured can move freely and might bend at the point where immobilization ends. This would increase the risk of significant spinal injury.

Unresponsive Patient

When caring for an unresponsive patient, obtain as much information as possible from bystanders. Determine the mechanism of injury and the patient's mental status prior to your arrival. Assume head or spine injury is present in all unresponsive trauma patients. Perform your initial assessment and physical exam after manually stabilizing the spine.

Describe the method of determining if a responsive patient
may have a spine injury.

Responsive Patient

When assessing a responsive patient with a potential spine or head injury, do
not cause the patient to move the head or neck in order to see you. Approach
the patient from the front. Advise the patient not to move his or her head
while answering your questions.

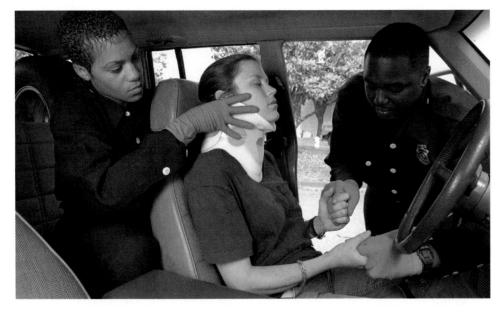

Figure 22.6 *Assessing for
equal grip strength.*

- Ask the patient, "What happened?" "Does your neck or back hurt?" "Where
  does it hurt?" "Can you move your hands and feet?"

- Complete a sensory exam. As you touch each extremity, ask if the patient can
  feel your touch. Ask whether he or she can localize the sensation.

- Complete a motor exam. Check for equal grip strength in the upper extremities. Have the patient grip two fingers from each of your hands simultaneously, using both of his or her hands (see Fig. 22.6). For the lower extremities,
  check for push/pull strength of the feet against your hands. If you detect differences in strength between the two sides, the patient may have a spinal cord
  injury. However, be sure to establish whether he or she has a past history of
  motor weakness on one or both sides.

- Complete a DCAP–BTLS evaluation (see Fig. 22.7).

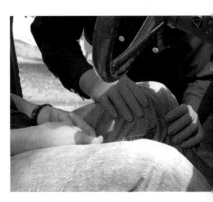

Figure 22.7 *Assessing the
lower extremities for deformities.*

D.O.T. OBJECTIVE

Relate the airway emergency medical care techniques to the patient with a suspected spine injury.

Emergency Medical Care: Potential Spine Injury

These are the emergency medical care steps for a patient with a potential spinal injury:

EMT Tip

Remember to always practice body substance isolation and standard precautions when caring for patients with suspected spinal injury.

1. Complete the scene survey.

2. Immediately establish and maintain manual in-line stabilization. Place the head in a neutral position, in a straight line with the spinal column. If the patient complains of pain with movement, or the head is not easily moved, secure the patient in the position in which he or she was found. Maintain manual stabilization until the head and body are completely secured to a backboard.

3. Complete the initial assessment. If necessary, control the airway and assist ventilations while cervical spine precautions are in place. Use the jaw-thrust maneuver to open the airway.

4. Complete the appropriate focused history and physical exam.

5. Assess pulses, motor function, and sensory status in all extremities. Use the AVPU scale to assess the level of responsiveness. Record your initial findings and reassess after any movement. Documenting changes in the patient's neurological status is especially important.

EMT Alert

For any patient with suspected head or spine injuries, open the airway using the jaw-thrust maneuver.

6. Assess the cervical region. Gently palpate the neck and cervical spine. Check for tender areas. Also check for trauma to the spine using DCAP-BTLS.

7. Properly size and apply a rigid cervical collar. The procedure is outlined in the "Immobilization" section of this chapter. You must apply the correct size. The wrong size will do more harm than good. If the collar does not fit, place a rolled towel around the neck, tape it to the board, and maintain manual in-line stabilization.

8. Immobilize the patient to a long or short spine board as described in the "Immobilization" section of this chapter. The type of device and the procedure for moving the patient are determined by the injury, the scene, and the resources available. The primary goal is prevention of further injury. Keeping the patient's movements to a minimum will help you to meet this goal.

9. Conduct detailed and ongoing assessments. Transport to the closest appropriate facility.

INJURIES TO THE SKULL AND BRAIN

Patients can sustain many types of injuries to the head, including lacerations, contusions, and fractures. Less obvious injuries to the brain may cause permanent neurologic impairment or death. Recognizing these potential injuries is important to providing definitive care.

Injuries to the Scalp and Skull

Scalp wounds are like other soft tissue injuries. However, the scalp is very vascular, and may bleed profusely when cut (see Fig. 22.8). Bleeding can usually be controlled with direct pressure. Bleeding beneath the scalp can form a hematoma, distorting the appearance of the head.

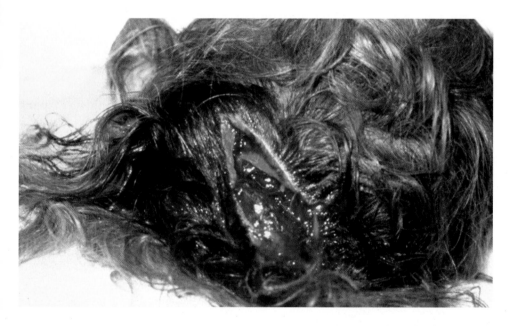

Figure 22.8 *Severely lacerated scalp.*

Skull injuries can be open or closed. In an **open head injury**, the skull is fractured, exposing the brain to the outside. This is a severe injury with a high risk of contamination and infection. In a **closed head injury**, the skull remains intact. The scalp may or may not be lacerated.

Knowing the mechanism of injury will help you to identify the nature of the patient's injuries. Signs and symptoms of scalp or skull injury are:

- Contusions, lacerations, or hematomas to the scalp
- Deformity of the skull
- Blood or **cerebrospinal fluid (CSF)** leaking from the ears or nose
- Bruising or discoloration around the eyes (raccoon eyes)
- Bruising or discoloration behind the ears (**Battle's sign**)

Open Head Injury | *A severe traumatic head injury in which the skull is fractured*

Closed Head Injury | *Trauma to the head in which the skull remains intact; scalp may or may not be lacerated*

Cerebrospinal Fluid (CSF) | *Fluid that fills the ventricles and cavities of the brain and surrounds the spinal cord*

Battle's Sign | *Bruising behind the ears or mastoid process due to basilar skull fracture*

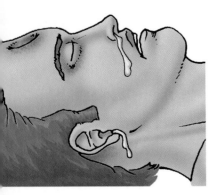

Figure 22.9 *Battle's sign, raccoon eyes, and CSF leakage from the nose and ears are signs of a skull fracture.*

Raccoon eyes, Battle's sign, and blood or CSF leaking from the ears or nose suggest a fracture at the base of the skull (see Fig. 22.9). The discoloration is caused by internal bleeding behind the ears or around the eyes. Bruises may take several hours to appear. An alert, seated patient may complain of a salty taste at the back of the throat. This is caused by leaking CSF.

Underlying brain damage may be present with scalp or skull injuries. Bleeding into the skull or injury of the brain tissue causes an increase in pressure within the skull.

Injuries to the Face and Jaw

Facial injuries are caused by blunt or penetrating trauma to the face. These injuries are commonly seen in MVCs, falls, or assaults (see Figs. 22.10, 22.11, 22.12, and 22.13). The injuries are rarely life threatening. However, airway obstruction or hemorrhage can occur. The patient may also have associated head, neck, or brain injuries.

Figure 22.10 *Knife laceration.*

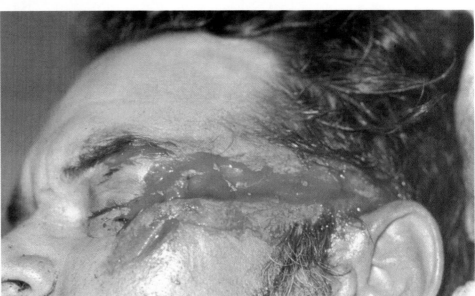

Signs and symptoms of facial injury include swelling, deformity, discoloration, bleeding, and tenderness upon palpation. The mandible may be fractured or dislocated. In this case, the patient will have difficulty moving the jaw or speaking. He or she will not be able to clench the teeth. The upper and lower teeth may not align properly.

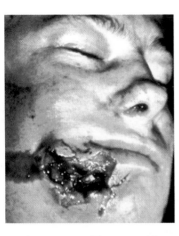

Figure 22.11 *Face grazed by a bullet.*

Blood, secretions, bone fragments, and teeth may cause airway obstruction. Establishing an open and patent airway is your first priority. Be prepared to suction blood or secretions, control bleeding, and remove debris. Use the jaw-thrust maneuver to open the airway. Secure the spine with a cervical collar and backboard. Position the patient to allow drainage from the mouth. Treat for a suspected head injury.

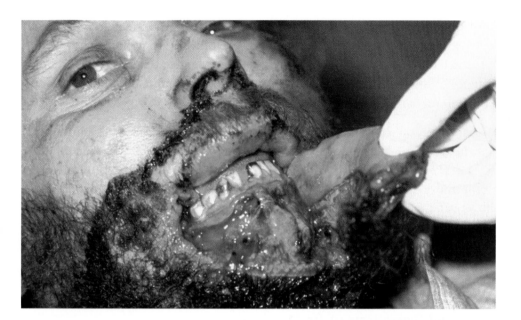

Figure 22.12 *Severely avulsed chin.*

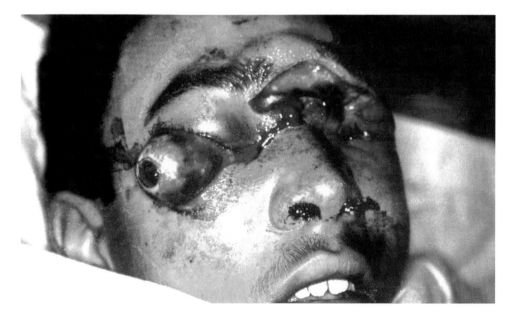

Figure 22.13 *Avulsed eye protruding from the bony orbit.*

Injuries to the Brain

Brain injuries range from mild **concussions** to more serious conditions requiring emergency surgery. The major problem with brain injuries is the potential for bleeding within the rigid skull. Bleeding creates pressure which causes changes in the patient's level of responsiveness. It can lead to permanent brain tissue damage. Although you will not identify the type of brain injury your patient might have, the Enhanced Study section at the end of this chapter describes different types of brain injuries.

Concussion | *Temporary disruption of normal brain function, usually caused by blunt trauma to the head*

Most brain injuries result from trauma. However, nontraumatic brain injury can also occur. This can be caused by blood clots or hemorrhage within the brain. Medical conditions such as a cerebrovascular accident are usually the cause. This condition is also called a stroke, CVA, or brain attack (discussed in Chapter 14).

You must recognize when a patient has signs and symptoms of a brain injury and treat him or her appropriately. Signs and symptoms include altered mental status and loss of sensory or motor functions. Patients with nontraumatic brain injury display similar signs and symptoms to a head trauma patient. However, there will be no evidence of trauma or obvious mechanism of injury. Treatment for brain injuries includes controlling the airway and cervical spine, administering oxygen, and rapid transport. Transport the patient in the recovery position, in case vomiting occurs. In the case of nontraumatic brain injury, spinal immobilization may not be necessary.

Signs and Symptoms of Brain Injury

Whenever the mechanism of injury suggests head trauma, suspect associated brain injury. If signs and symptoms of a brain injury exist but the skull appears intact, suspect a possible closed head injury.

Dementia | *A loss of cognitive and intellectual functions caused by a variety of disorders*

Altered or deteriorating mental status is an excellent indicator of brain injury. The patient may be confused or disoriented, asking repetitive questions. Or he or she may be completely unresponsive. Note that some patients may have a history of **dementia**, a chronic condition with a baseline mental state that is not normal. Confirm this with the family, if possible. Other signs and symptoms of brain or head injury are:

- Physical signs of trauma about the head, such as contusions, lacerations, or hematomas of the scalp, or deformity of the skull
- Pain or tenderness of the scalp
- A soft area or depression felt upon palpation of the skull
- Exposed brain tissue or bleeding from an open skull injury
- Raccoon eyes
- Battle's sign
- Nausea and/or vomiting (caused by increased pressure on the brain)
- Irregular breathing pattern
- Clear cerebrospinal fluid or blood leaking from the ears or nose
- Unequal pupil size with altered mental status
- Paralysis or disability on one side of the body
- Seizures
- Very high blood pressure with slow pulse

Assessment of the Head-Injured Patient

When assessing a patient with a suspected head injury, include the following:

- Note the mechanism of injury during the scene survey. Look for helmet or windshield deformities or evidence of a fall (see Fig. 22.14).

- If a patient is or has been unconscious, obtain as much information as possible from bystanders. Try to confirm the history of the event and the length of time he or she was unconscious. Remember that unresponsive patients cannot adequately control their airways and require close monitoring.

- Complete a rapid assessment of mental status using the AVPU scale. Deteriorating mental status is one of the best indicators of brain injury.

- Complete a physical exam of the head, palpating the entire scalp if possible. Maintain cervical spine control. Look for broken facial bones or penetrating trauma. Note tenderness, contusions, lacerations, or other signs of trauma. Do not press on open head injuries or skull deformities. Do not attempt to remove an object impaled in the skull.

- Examine the eyes for responsiveness and equal pupil size. Look for raccoon eyes.

- Examine the ears and nose for blood or cerebrospinal fluid. Look for Battle's sign behind the ears.

- Assess motor and sensory function as you would for a spine-injured patient.

- If time allows, use the **Glasgow Coma Scale (GCS)** to evaluate the patient's mental status. The GCS is an objective evaluation of the patient's level of responsiveness on a numeric scale. It is more descriptive than using subjective terms such as "groggy" or "altered mental state." The Enhanced Study section at the end of this chapter describes evaluation using the GCS.

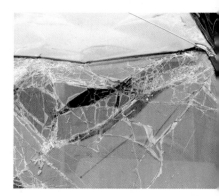

Figure 22.14 *Evidence of a vehicle rollover crash.*

Glasgow Coma Scale (GCS) | *A tool for assessing a patient's level of responsiveness*

Emergency Medical Care: Traumatic Head Injury

These are the steps for treating a patient with trauma to the head.

1. Complete the scene survey.

2. Open the airway using the jaw-thrust maneuver. Maintain an open airway.

3. Assume a patient with a severe head injury or who is unconscious also has a neck injury. Provide and maintain manual in-line stabilization in a neutral position.

4. Insert an oral airway adjunct if the patient is unconscious. Have suction available to prevent aspiration in case of secretions or vomitus.

5. If the patient is breathing adequately, provide oxygen at 15 LPM by non-rebreather mask. If the patient is not breathing or respirations are inadequate, use positive pressure ventilation with oxygen. Check your local protocols.

6. Quickly complete a circulatory check. Look for major bleeding. Ensure the patient has a pulse.

7. Always suspect spinal injury in head injury patients. Immobilize the neck and spine using a rigid collar and backboard (described in the following section).

8. Complete the appropriate focused history and physical exam. If you suspect closed head injury, transport the patient to a trauma center immediately.

9. Complete a detailed physical exam and ongoing assessments while en route to the hospital. Closely monitor the airway, breathing, pulse, and mental status.

Consider the following points during your care of a head-injured patient:

- Do not apply pressure to external bleeding from the skull if there is evidence of skull injury. Signs of skull injury are depressed segments, bone fragments, or protruding brain tissue. Apply a loose gauze dressing.

- Do not try to stop bleeding or CSF leakage from ears or nose. Apply a loose gauze dressing.

- Do not remove an object impaled in the head. Stabilize it with bulky dressings.

- Monitor the patient's condition closely for changes, including seizures, vomiting, or decreasing mental status. Be prepared to treat changes in condition if they appear.

EMT Alert

Whenever manual stabilization is provided, the EMT holding the patient's head is in charge of making the calls for any move (unless that responsibility has been shifted to someone in a better position to manage and see all movements).

IMMOBILIZATION

The key to managing suspected spinal injuries is preventing further damage. Sometimes cervical fractures are not complete and have not injured the spinal cord. Proper immobilization is essential for avoiding future injury. Standard ambulance stretchers are not designed to protect the damaged spine from further injury. Specific spinal immobilization devices are required to properly secure and protect the spine. You cannot always determine whether the spine has been injured. Spinal immobilization is only a precaution in the majority of patients you will care for. However, for those who have been injured, it is one of the most important treatments you will provide.

When moving a spine-injured patient, the crew must work in unison with one individual as the leader to avoid any additional injury. The EMT-B at the patient's head is generally the one given the duty of counting out the cadence for any log roll or patient repositioning. Be sure that everyone understands that the patient must be moved as a unit on the call of the person at the head.

Cervical Spine Immobilization Devices

Apply a cervical collar any time you suspect a spine injury. Consider the patient's history, mechanism of injury, and signs and symptoms. Maintain a high index of suspicion in patients with:

- Head injury and loss of consciousness
- Injuries above the clavicle

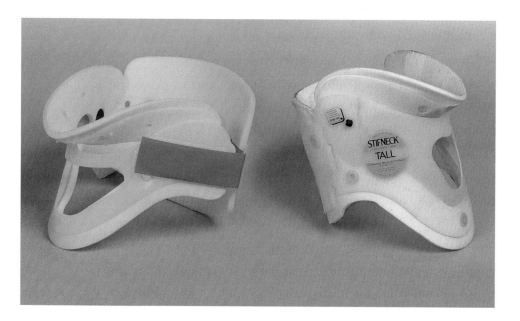

Figure 22.15 *Examples of rigid cervical collars. Note that some cervical collars are color-coded for size.*

A rigid cervical collar should always be used (see Fig. 22.15). Soft collars permit too much neck movement and are not used in EMS. The steps for applying a cervical collar to a supine patient are shown in Procedure 22.1 on page 646. Procedure 22.2 on page 647 shows how to apply a cervical collar to a seated patient.

A cervical collar alone does not provide adequate spinal immobilization. Cervical collars are used together with short and long backboards. The best rigid cervical collars only reduce motion by 50 percent. You must always immobilize the entire spine, even if the neck is the only injured area. Have one EMT-B complete manual in-line stabilization while a second applies the collar. Maintain manual stabilization until the patient is completely secured to a backboard (see Fig. 22.16).

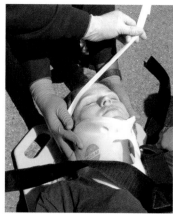

Figure 22.16 *Maintain manual stabilization until the patient is completely secured to a backboard.*

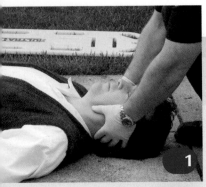

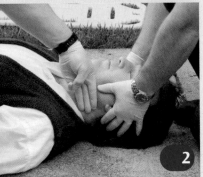

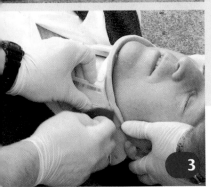

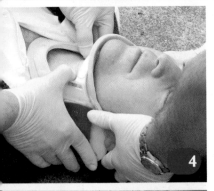

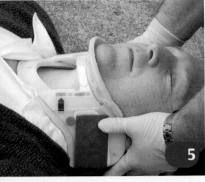

Procedure 22.1 • CERVICAL COLLAR: SUPINE PATIENT

Video Appendix

Stabilize Spine

Body Fluids

1. Manually maintain the neck in a neutral, in-line position before applying a rigid cervical collar. Position yourself at the patient's head. Place your index fingers at the base of the neck, just below C7.

2. Support the mandible with your thumbs. Avoid compressing the blood vessels under the mandible. Cradle the occiput and posterior neck with the remaining fingers. Keep your elbows pointed outward. This prevents inadvertent flexion of the neck when lifting.

3. Have a second EMT-B slide the back portion of the collar behind the patient's neck. Place the front piece under the chin. Double-check the collar size.

4. Adjust the collar, using the trachea hole as an anchor point. Pull laterally to tighten and secure the Velcro strap.

5. Continue manual stabilization while transferring the patient to a long board.

D.O.T. OBJECTIVES

Discuss indications for sizing and using a cervical spine immobilization device.

Describe a method for sizing a cervical spine immobilization device.

Cervical Collar Size

A cervical collar that is too small will not adequately stabilize the neck. A collar that is too large permits too much movement. The length of a patient's neck and the design of the collar determine the correct size. To be effective, a rigid cervical collar must rest on the shoulder girdle. This firmly supports both sides of the jaw, without obstructing the airway or interfering with ventilation.

To determine the proper size for a cervical collar, measure the distance between an imaginary line drawn across the top of the shoulders where the collar will sit and the bottom plane of the patient's chin. To measure the collar, place

Procedure 22.2 • **CERVICAL COLLAR: SEATED PATIENT**

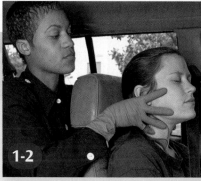

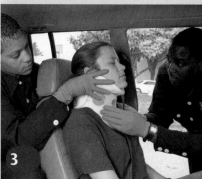

1. Move behind a seated patient, if possible. Tell the patient not to move the head or neck for any reason.

2. Establish neutral in-line stabilization. Position your hands over the patient's ears. Place your thumbs against the posterior aspect of the skull. Position your little fingers just under the angle of the mandible. Avoid the soft tissue under the chin. Bring your arms in toward your body. Rest them against the back of the seat, headrest, or your ribs. This position reduces movement and provides support. Some extrications will be lengthy, causing rescuer fatigue.

3. A second EMT slides the chin piece up the chest wall. Make sure that the chin extends far enough onto the chin piece. With the chin piece in place, slide the flat portion of the collar behind the neck. When positioned correctly, the sides will rest on the shoulders. Using the trachea hole as an anchor point, pull the Velcro strap laterally until the collar is secured.

your outstretched fingers next to the patient's neck. The finger width should equal the distance on the collar between the imaginary lines, corresponding to the curve that rests on the shoulder and chin support.

D.O.T. OBJECTIVES

List instances when a short spine board should be used.

Describe how to immobilize a patient using a short spine board.

 CD-ROM Link

For a demonstration of sizing and applying a cervical collar, see the video, "Initial Assessment of a Spine Injury" in Chapter 22 and the Video Appendix on the MedEMT CD-ROM.

Short Backboard Immobilization Devices

Short backboard immobilization devices are used to stabilize noncritical patients with suspected spinal injuries who are found in a sitting position. You will need materials such as tape, backboard straps, and padding to secure the patient. Short boards are interim devices that stabilize the head, neck, and torso. A short device does not fully immobilize the patient. Secure him or her to a long spine board as soon as possible.

CD-ROM
Link

The video, "Spine Immobilization–Sitting Patient" in Chapter 22 and the Video Appendix on the MedEMT CD-ROM shows the steps for applying a KED.

The two main types of short boards are the rigid board and the flexible vest-style device. The short spine board was the first device designed for patients found in a seated position (see Fig. 6.19 in Chapter 6). However, modern automobiles have contoured seats which do not easily accommodate the rigid board. Today, most agencies use a vest-type device such as the Kendrick Extrication Device or KED (see Figs. 6.20 and 6.21 in Chapter 6). Because this is a flexible piece of equipment, it can be used with contoured car seats or in other confined spaces where a rigid spine board will not fit.

Whether you use a short spine board or a flexible vest, you will follow the same steps to immobilize a sitting patient. You will secure the torso first and the head last. Application of a KED to a seated patient is shown in Procedure 22.3.

EMT
Tip

After securing the middle and lower straps on the KED, you can keep the device from slipping down on the patient's torso by adding two straps or cravats. Thread them through the loops in the back, then over the shoulders. Fasten to the top chest strap.

You will not apply a short spine device if a patient requires an urgent move because of injuries, limited access to other patients, or an unsafe scene. Instead, manually stabilize the head and lower the patient directly onto a long board. Continue manual stabilization until the patient is secured to the board. Refer to the section "Moving Patients" in Chapter 6.

Long Backboard Immobilization Devices

Long board immobilization devices are full body spinal immobilization devices (see Fig. 22.17 and Fig. 6.18 in Chapter 6). They stabilize and immobilize the head, neck, torso, pelvis, and extremities. Use the long backboard for patients found in lying, standing, or sitting positions. Long boards are used to stabilize the entire spinal column during transport. Sometimes they are used together with short backboards. Several different types of long boards are available. The boards must be padded and secured with tape, Velcro, or backboard straps.

Figure 22.17 *Securing a patient to a long spine board.*

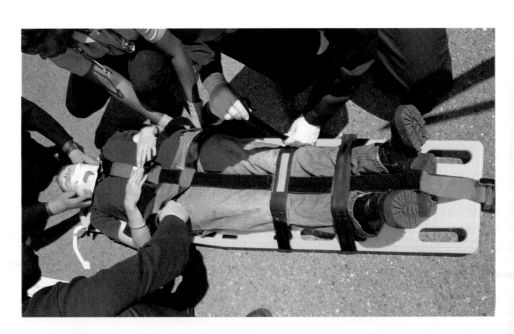

Procedure 22.3 • KENDRICK EXTRICATION DEVICE

  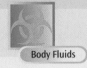

Video Appendix Stabilize Spine Body Fluids

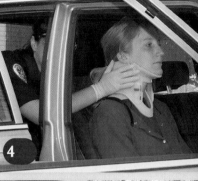
4

1. Provide manual in-line stabilization.

2. Complete an initial assessment including pulses, motor, and sensory functions in all extremities.

3. Assess the cervical area, back, scapula, clavicles, and arms. Check for penetrating objects, lacerations, and bleeding.

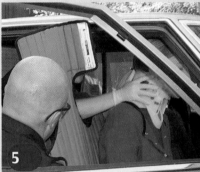
5

4. Apply a rigid cervical collar.

5. Slip the KED in place behind the patient.

6. Fasten the top strap across the chest. Avoid tightening straps too much, which may exacerbate chest or abdominal injuries.

7. Secure the middle and lower straps. Leave enough room to slip two or three fingers under the straps.

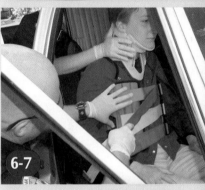
6-7

8. Position the groin straps across the pelvis. Fasten them to the buckle on the same side from which they originated, forming a loop. Avoid entrapping the genitalia in males. These straps keep the device from sliding up or moving from side to side.

9. Pad between the head and headpiece, if necessary. Then, bring the flaps to the sides of the head. Secure the head with Velcro straps or wide tape.

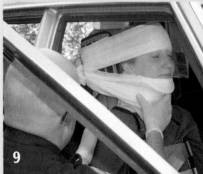
9

10. Place a long spine board under or near the patient's buttocks. Lift or rotate the patient, then lower him or her onto the long board. If lifting is required, hold the legs close to the knees. The patient and KED are lifted as a unit. Lifting on the device alone will cause it to move up the torso and can flex the patient's body unnecessarily.

11. Secure the patient to the long board.

12. Reassess pulses, motor, and sensory status.

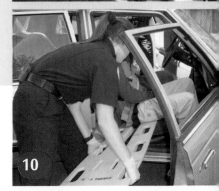
10

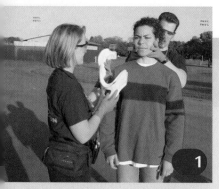

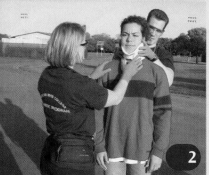

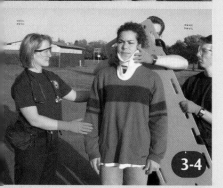

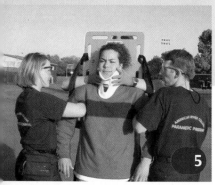

Procedure 22.4 • LONG SPINE BOARD: STANDING PATIENT

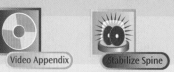

Video Appendix   Stabilize Spine   Back Safety   Body Fluids

1. Maintain manual stabilization of the spine until the patient is fully secured to the board.

2. Complete the initial assessment and focused physical exam. Apply a rigid cervical collar.

3. One EMT-B stands on each side of the patient. Additional rescuers stand in front of and behind the patient. Place the long spine board behind the standing patient.

4. The EMT-B behind the patient reaches around the board, holding the patient's head between his or her palms. While this rescuer manually stabilizes the neck from behind, two others support the sides of the long board. Center the board behind the patient.

5. The EMT-Bs on the patient's sides reach under the patient's arms, grasping the board at the level of the patient's armpit or higher. With their free hands, the rescuers secure the head to the board.

6. After positioning the board and patient, slowly lower the patient and board backward as one unit. The EMT-Bs on the patient's sides each place one leg behind the board. They slowly tip the board backward. The EMT-B in front secures the patient's ankles to the board to prevent the patient from slipping down as the board is lowered. Move the board into a level horizontal position. The EMT-Bs on the sides take a step and shift their weight behind the patient for support.

D.O.T. OBJECTIVES

Describe how to secure a patient to a long spine board.

Describe how to log roll a patient with a suspected spine injury.

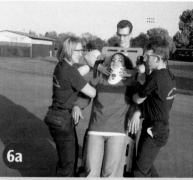

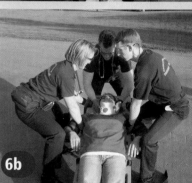

Procedure 22.4 • Long Spine Board: Standing Patient *(cont.)*

7. Pad void spaces between the patient and the board.

8. Fasten the patient's torso to the board. The straps should be snug, but must not restrict breathing. Fasten straps at the armpit level across the chest. Strapping techniques vary widely. Follow the manufacturer's suggestions and local protocols.

9. Secure the pelvis to the board. Padding between the legs will provide more comfort for the patient.

0. Position a head immobilization device on each side of the head. Secure the head with a strap over the forehead and a second strap over the cervical collar. Never obstruct access to the airway.

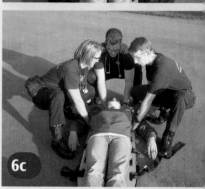

1. Tie the patient's wrists together loosely with a wide bandage. This helps to immobilize the arms and discourages the patient from reaching for anything. Avoid using material that will cut into the patient's wrists.

2. Secure the legs proximal and distal to the knees.

3. Head trauma victims frequently vomit. If the patient is secured to the board correctly, he or she can be turned on one side to clear the airway. Check for proper securing and padding. Carefully tilt the board without changing the patient's position.

4. Transport as soon as possible. Reassess the pulses and motor and sensory functions.

Immobilizing a Patient on the Long Spine Board

The long board is used to immobilize patients from a standing or lying position. The steps for securing a standing patient are described in Procedure 22.4.

CD-ROM Link

The video, "Spine Immobilization–Standing Patient," in Chapter 22 and the Video Appendix on the MedEMT CD-ROM shows the steps for securing a standing patient to a long spine board.

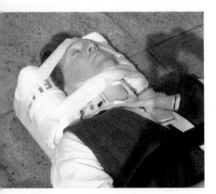

Figure 22.18 *Additional padding can eliminate excess movement of the head. Secure the head to the spine board for maximum stability.*

CD-ROM Link

The video, "Spine Immobilization–Reclining Patient" in Chapter 22 and the Video Appendix on the MedEMT CD-ROM demonstrates a four-person log roll onto a long spine board.

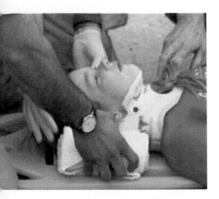

Figure 22.19 *A rolled towel on the sides of the head and neck helps to eliminate space, further reducing the chance of movement.*

These are the steps for immobilizing a patient from the supine position:

1. Maintain manual in-line stabilization.
2. Complete an initial assessment. Assess pulses and motor and sensory functions in all extremities.
3. Complete a focused physical exam or an assessment of the cervical area, back, scapula, clavicles, and arms. Check for penetrating objects, lacerations, and bleeding.
4. Apply a rigid cervical collar.
5. Position the long board on the ground, parallel to the patient.
6. Transfer the patient onto the board by log rolling, lifting, or sliding. Determine which method to use based on the situation, scene, and available resources. Choose the method that keeps spinal movement to a minimum. One EMT-B must stabilize the neck during all movement. He or she gives the commands to move the patient. Log rolling a patient is described in Procedure 22.5.
7. Pad void spaces, if necessary. Avoid padding behind the cervical collar, which may hyperextend the neck when the head is secured to the board.
8. Secure the torso and pelvis to the board.
9. Immobilize the head to the board. Avoid airway obstruction (see Fig. 22.18).
10. Secure the wrists and legs.
11. Transport the patient as soon as possible. Reassess the pulses and motor and sensory functions in all extremities while en route. Document your findings.

Padding

When a patient is immobilized on a backboard, the contours of the body create spaces. This can occur at the head, neck, lumbar region, and knees. Space between the patient and a backboard is uncomfortable and may permit movement. Eliminate space with layers of firm, folded padding such as towels, blankets, or foam. An air splint may also be considered to fill voids and act as padding. Avoid moving the patient while applying padding.

Use a thin pad beneath an adult's head, if necessary. This can provide comfort against the hard board. Be sure that the head remains in a neutral position. Never place a pillow under the head, because this may cause too much flexion. Avoid padding behind the cervical collar in adults and children. This could cause hyperextension of the neck when the head is secured to the board. Padding behind the torso may be necessary to support the vertebral curvature. Place padding under an infant's or child's body from the shoulders to the toes. This establishes a neutral position.

Position a head immobilization device on each side of the head to maintain position and prevent side-to-side movement (see Fig. 22.19). You can improvise with foam blocks, rolled towels, or other lightweight padding.

Procedure 22.5 • LOG ROLLING A PATIENT

 Video Appendix Stabilize Spine Back Safety Body Fluids

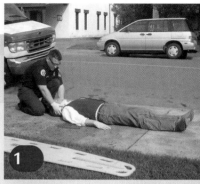

1. EMT-B #1 kneels at the patient's head and places his or her palms on both sides of the patient's face. This limits patient movement while maintaining the head in a straight line with the spine. This EMT-B controls the cervical spine until the patient is fully immobilized on the long spine board.

2. Ideally, four people will be involved in the log roll. Two EMT-Bs prepare for the roll by kneeling along one side of the patient. If possible, they should kneel along an uninjured side. Leave enough room to complete the roll. They position their hands on the far side of the patient. Control the upper arm, waist (belt line), thighs, knees, and feet. EMT-B #2 places one hand on the patient's thigh and one on the upper arm. EMT-B #3 places one hand on the knee and one near the mid-torso.

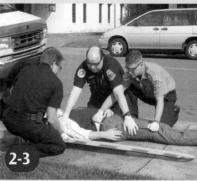

3. EMT-B #1 directs the roll, giving a signal such as "On a count of three...". He or she maintains continuous manual stabilization of the head. On the signal, the other EMT-Bs roll the patient towards them as one stable unit. If the patient complains of pain while attempting to move the neck, or if the head is not easily moved, do not attempt the log roll. Secure the patient in the position found, with as little movement as possible.

4. While the patient is on one side, assess the back if this was not done previously. Look for DCAP-BTLS and other injuries.

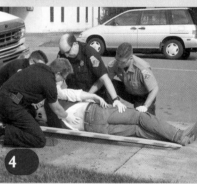

5. EMT-B #4, who is on the opposite side of the patient, positions the long board beneath the patient. As a unit, under the direction of EMT-B #1, all EMT-Bs gently roll the patient onto the board.

6. Pad the voids and the board as needed. Secure the patient to the board. EMT-B #1 maintains manual in-line stabilization until the patient is fully secured for transport.

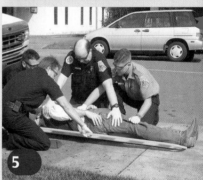

7. An alternate procedure is for EMT-B #4 to assist with the roll. He or she kneels next to EMT-B #3 and places one hand on the ankles and the other on the upper thigh or pelvis. While the patient is on one side, EMT-B #3 reaches over the patient to position the board.

8. If only two or three rescuers are available, one EMT-B manually stabilizes the head and neck. The others control and roll the patient's body as described.

EMT Tip

It can be difficult to center a side-lying patient on the long board. Position the head of the board 12 to 18 inches above the patient's head. After completing the log roll, the patient will be about two-thirds of the way onto the board. From here, you can slide the patient into position, using a diagonal motion to center him or her on the board. This prevents strictly vertical or horizontal movement, which may aggravate injuries.

SPECIAL CONSIDERATIONS

There are some special circumstances to be aware of with head and spine injuries. Some situations require you to perform a rapid extrication without first providing full spinal stabilization. Immobilizing an infant or child requires special care. If a trauma patient is wearing a helmet, you must decide whether or not to remove it and use the proper procedure.

D.O.T. OBJECTIVES

Describe the indications for the use of rapid extrication.

List steps in performing rapid extrication.

Rapid Extrication

An urgent move or rapid extrication may be necessary in cases where:

- The patient is critically injured or his or her condition is unstable
- The patient is blocking access to another, more seriously injured patient
- The scene is not safe or secure (see Fig. 22.20)

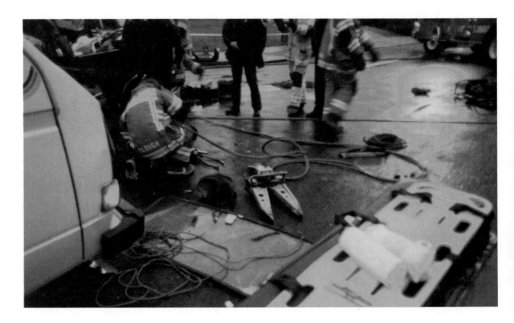

Figure 22.20 *A rapid extrication is required when a patient's or a crew member's life is in immediate danger.*

Review Chapter 6 for the guidelines for performing an emergency or urgent move. Procedure 6.2 describes the steps for rapidly extricating a seated patient from a car. Since time is critical, you must transfer the patient directly to a long spine board. After cervical stabilization, align the patient's body, then lower him or her directly onto the long board. Maintain manual stabilization while moving the patient. Transport immediately, completing assessments while en route.

Immobilizing Infants and Children

An infant or child with a potential spine injury must be immobilized on an appropriately sized board. Use a short board, long board, or padded splint. Follow the same immobilization procedure as for an adult. An infant or child has a large head in relation to body length. The neck has a natural tendency to flex when the infant is supine. Padding elevates the body and reduces the flexion. Pad beneath the body from the shoulders to the heels. This will immobilize the neck and spine in a neutral position. The cervical collar must also fit an infant or child correctly. An improperly fitting device will do more harm than good. If you do not have a collar that fits, roll a towel, then tape it to the board. Manually support the head.

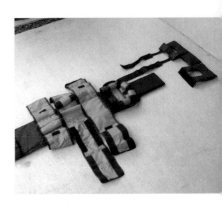

Figure 22.21 *The Pediatric Extrication Device is used for children with suspected head or spine injuries.*

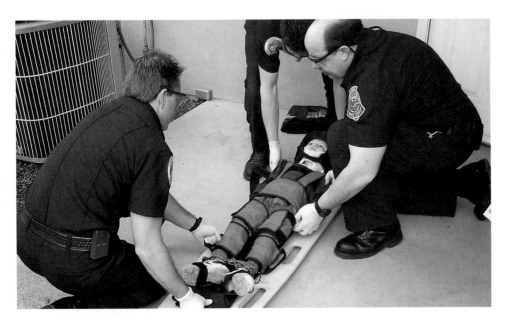

Figure 22.22 *A cervical collar is applied before the PED. Fully immobilize the child and the PED on a long board.*

The preferred device for extricating children is the flexible Pediatric Extrication Device or PED (see Figs. 22.21 and 22.22). The PED is designed and sized for full-body immobilization of a child. You will encounter motor vehicle collisions that require caring for an infant or child who is in a child safety seat. Methods for immobilizing a child to the seat and extricating a child from the seat are described in the Enhanced Study section at the end of this chapter.

D.O.T. OBJECTIVES

Identify different types of helmets.

Describe the unique characteristics of sports helmets.

Discuss the circumstances when a helmet should be removed.

State the circumstances when a helmet should be left on the patient.

Explain the preferred methods to remove a helmet.

Discuss alternative methods for removal of a helmet.

Describe how a patient's head is stabilized to remove the helmet.

Differentiate how the head is stabilized with a helmet compared to without a helmet.

Helmet Removal

A patient who sustains a head or spine injury while wearing a helmet requires special assessment and treatment. Leaving certain styles of helmet in place can cause a problem with stabilization. This is particularly true in children. The helmet may interfere with your ability to maintain the head in a neutral position.

CD-ROM
Link

The video "Helmet Removal" in Chapter 22 and the Video Appendix on the MedEMT CD-ROM demonstrates the steps for helmet removal.

The two basic types of helmets are sports helmets and vehicular helmets. Football helmets and bicycle helmets are examples of sports helmets. Injury prevention programs have stressed the need for both children and adults to wear helmets when riding bicycles. Most sports helmets are open in the front or have face masks that can be cut away or unsnapped. The design permits easy access to the airway. A motorcycle helmet is a vehicular helmet. Vehicular helmets often have full-face shields. The shield reduces the risk of facial injuries, but prevents immediate access to the airway.

When assessing an injured patient, you must decide whether or not to remove the helmet. If a helmet interferes with proper stabilization of the spine or prevents clear access to the airway, it must be removed immediately. Ask yourself these questions:

• Is the airway open? Is breathing adequate? Is the airway accessible? Can I suction or provide ventilations without interference from the helmet?

• Can I effectively immobilize the head and neck with the helmet in place?

Procedure 22.6 • HELMET REMOVAL

Video Appendix

Stabilize Spine

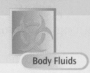
Body Fluids

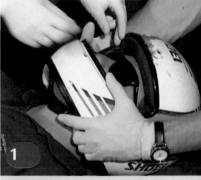
1

1. If the patient is wearing eyeglasses or large earrings, remove them to prevent further injury.

2. EMT-B #1 kneels at the patient's head, holding the sides of the helmet in both hands. He or she manually stabilizes the helmet, keeping the neck in a neutral position. Extend the fingers to support the mandible on both sides. This stabilizes the head and neck

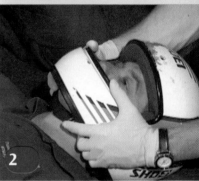
2

3. EMT-B #2 approaches from the foot. He or she loosens the chin strap or face shield. Cutting the straps may be necessary.

4. With one hand, EMT-B #2 stabilizes the mandible at the angle of the jaw just in front of the ears. He or she supports the back of the head at the base of the skull with the other hand.

5. While EMT-B #2 supports the head, EMT-B # 1 pulls laterally on the sides of the helmet. This stretches the helmet slightly so it will clear the ears. Gently slip the helmet halfway over the head.

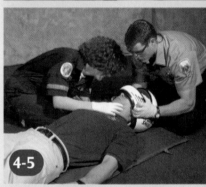
4-5

6. EMT-B #2 continues to stabilize the neck, preventing the head from extending backward. He or she readjusts the hand position to ensure that the back of the head is secure as the helmet comes off.

7. EMT-B #1 pulls the helmet straight off, avoiding flexion or extension of the neck. Slightly rotating a helmet with an attached face mask may be necessary to clear the nose. You can also push the nose down momentarily to allow the helmet to pass. Never turn or move the neck laterally during this procedure.

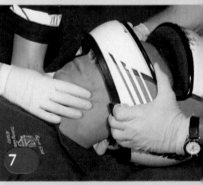
7

8. Proceed with spinal immobilization. EMT-B#2 manually stabilizes the head until a cervical collar is in place and the patient is secured to a backboard.

• Will taking the helmet off aggravate the injury?

• How tight is the helmet? How much movement is possible inside the helmet? The head must be immobilized to prevent neck injury. If a neck injury is present, movement within a loose helmet can lead to further spinal damage.

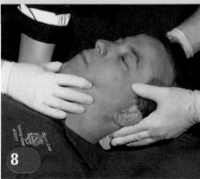
8

Leave the helmet in place if:

- The patient has no airway or breathing problems and airway access is not restricted
- The helmet does not interfere with assessment or reassessment of the airway and breathing
- The helmet fits well, limiting movement of the head inside the helmet
- Proper spinal immobilization can be completed
- Removal of the helmet will significantly aggravate or worsen the patient's injuries

Remove the helmet if:

- It interferes with your ability to assess or manage the airway and breathing
- The helmet does not fit tightly, allowing excessive head movement
- You cannot immobilize the spine correctly with the helmet in place
- The patient is in cardiac arrest
- The helmet is unstable

General rules for helmet removal are described in Procedure 22.6. When you remove a helmet, manual stabilization of the head and neck must be maintained. A two-rescuer procedure is recommended for helmet removal. The specific technique used depends on the type of helmet involved. If a helmet is left on a patient, padding may be needed to prevent neck extension, depending on the helmet size. Sports shoulder pads may also interfere with maintaining a neutral position of the neck.

Chapter Twenty-Two Summary

- Management of the airway and breathing are essential to the patient's survival and recovery from head or spine injuries.

- A patient may have a spinal injury even if he or she can walk, move extremities, or feel sensation. Absence of pain in the back or spinal column does not rule out the possibility of injury.

- Loss of movement or sensation in extremities is a key indication of spinal cord injury. Spinal cord injuries may cause paralysis and inadequate breathing.

- Indicators of possible head injuries are alteration in mental status (especially combativeness), skull deformity, blood or CSF draining from the ears or nose, raccoon eyes, Battle's sign, contusions, lacerations, or hematomas.

- If the mechanism of injury suggests spinal injury, immediately control the cervical spine. Adequate stabilization is essential. This prevents worsening or aggravation of hidden spinal injuries during transport.

- Apply a rigid cervical collar any time you suspect a spinal injury. To be effective, a rigid cervical collar must fit properly. The rigid cervical collar alone does not adequately immobilize the spinal column. It must be used in conjunction with a long board, short board, or vest-type immobilization device.

- The rigid short board and the flexible vest-style device are interim devices used to stabilize the head, neck, and torso. Because the KED is a flexible piece of equipment, it can be used in confined spaces where a short spine board will not fit. With both devices, secure the torso first and head last.

- Long board immobilization devices are full-body spinal immobilization devices.

- Remove a helmet if it interferes with your ability to assess or manage the patient's airway or breathing, or if the helmet is loose.

Key Terms Review

Battle's Sign | *page 639*
Cerebrospinal Fluid (CSF) | *page 639*
Closed Head Injury | *page 639*

Compression Injury | *page 635*
Concussion | *page 641*
Dementia | *page 642*

Glasgow Coma Scale
(GCS) | *page 643*
Open Head Injury | *page 639*
Paresthesia | *page 636*

Review Questions

1. The term Battle's sign means:

   a. Bruising behind the ears

   b. Bruising under the eyes

   c. CSF leaking from the nose

   d. Depression on the skull

2. Which skeletal structure protects the brain?

   a. Rib cage

   b. Thoracic vertebrae

   c. Skull

   d. Sternum

Review Questions *(cont.)*

3. A nerve that carries a message from the brain to an organ or muscle is called a:

   a. Sensory nerve

   b. Motor nerve

   c. Peripheral nerve

   d. Sympathetic nerve

4. Which of the following is NOT a proper way to assess for spinal injury?

   a. Sensory exam

   b. Hand grip strength

   c. Move legs to assess for pain

   d. Observe cervical deformity

5. Which of the following injuries could be involved when a patient dives into a shallow pool of water?

   a. Compression

   b. Distraction

   c. Penetration

   d. Extension

6. You arrive to find a victim of an assault lying in an alley, crumpled up in the fetal position. To prevent further spinal damage, you should first:

   a. Apply a cervical collar

   b. Log roll onto a long board

   c. Reposition head in-line with spine, as long as no pain is reported and the head is moved easily

   d. Rapidly move patient onto a stretcher for transport

7. When should you release manual spinal stabilization while securing a patient to a long spine board?

   a. After cervical collar is measured and applied

   b. When extra hands are needed for patient care

   c. After head and body are secured to board

   d. After patient is placed on ambulance stretcher

8. Which of the following is NOT an indication for cervical spine immobilization?

   a. Fall with a depressed section of skull

   b. Unresponsive patient trapped in an MVA

   c. Suicide by hanging

   d. Kidney pain

9. What is a Kendrick Extrication Device?

   a. A vest used to stabilize the head and neck

   b. A tool used to pull steering wheels off patients

   c. A small lock pick device to open cars

   d. A wire basket used to move patients

10. To size a cervical collar for a patient, you:

    a. Make an educated guess

    b. Use your fingers to measure the patient's neck

    c. Fit the collar to your own neck first

    d. Try different sizes until one fits

11. When a patient has external bleeding from the skull, you should NOT:

    a. Apply a loose dressing

    b. Apply pressure

    c. Immobilize the patient

    d. Transport as soon as possible

12. Priapism is:

    a. A constant, abnormal erection of the penis

    b. A constant, annoying sound only the patient hears

    c. The inability to move the lower extremities

    d. Loss of auditory function

13. A stable patient in a car complains of neck pain after a minor collision. Which method is best to use?

    a. Short spine board or KED

    b. Long spine board

    c. Rapid extrication

    d. Self-extrication

14. What should you do first before extricating a patient using a short spine board?

    a. Assess distal extremity function

    b. Hold manual stabilization

    c. Apply cervical collar

    d. Secure the head to a long board

15. Which condition does not require rapid extrication?

    a. Patient has open femur fracture

    b. Patient blocks access to critical patient

    c. The vehicle is in danger of exploding

    d. The patient is unconscious

CASE STUDIES

Head and Spine Injuries

1 You are dispatched to a baseball field for a report of a child down. When you arrive, a 12-year-old girl is on the ground, unconscious. Team members identify her as Linda. She was pitching when she was hit in the head by a line drive. The girl is lying on her back. She does not respond when you call her name. Your partner maintains in-line cervical spine stabilization. The airway is open and the patient is breathing well. Linda responds to a painful stimulus. You provide oxygen and apply a rigid cervical collar. The rapid trauma assessment shows a large hematoma on the right temple. The pupils are equal and reactive to light. No other signs of trauma are noted. Initial vital signs are BP 145/86, pulse 70, and respirations 20. With the help of the coach, you log roll the girl and secure her to a long spine board. You transport her immediately to the nearest receiving hospital. While en route, Linda has snoring respirations and makes gagging sounds. Her breathing pattern is irregular. Suddenly, she begins to vomit.

A. What do you do next?

B. Linda now has snoring respirations at a rate of 10, a pulse of 45, and blood pressure of 180/110. She no longer responds to pain. What is your next step?

C. When you arrived, what indications suggested that you should stabilize Linda's cervical spine?

2 You respond to a report of an injured athlete at a high school football practice. A coach meets you at the gate. A player is lying on the ground, still wearing a helmet. The team trainer is stabilizing his cervical spine. While making a tackle, the player hit a fence post head first. He was very confused for several minutes after the impact. Now, he is awake and oriented. He states, "I just want to get up." The coach provides a parental permission form authorizing consent for treatment. The patient has no life-threatening conditions. He is moving his head inside the helmet.

A. Is cervical spine immobilization indicated?

B. How will you determine whether or not to remove the helmet?

C. Is removal of the helmet indicated? Why?

D. What other treatments are indicated for this patient?

3 You are dispatched to a motor vehicle accident with one person injured. You arrive to find two vehicles in a parking lot. The patient was sitting in his parked car. A van backed into the rear of the car. The patient is awake, alert, oriented, and very talkative. He is sitting in the driver's seat, complaining of neck and upper back pain.

A. Is rapid extrication indicated in this case? Why or why not?

B. What devices will you use to remove the patient without compromising the cervical spine?

C. In addition to DCAP-BTLS, how will you assess the patient's neurological status?

Stories from the Field
Wrap-Up

For injuries to the head, neck, or back, your care in the field can mean the difference between full recovery and a life of disability. Immobilizing the spine is the best way to minimize the damage from a neck or spinal injury. It also ensures that the patient's injuries will not be aggravated during transport. The mechanism of injury may be your only clue to the presence of a head, neck, or spine injury. Carefully evaluate the mechanism of injury and treat for the worst injuries possible.

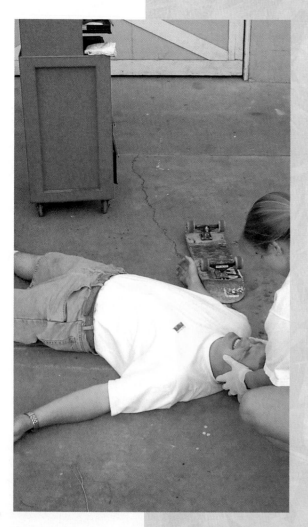

Quickly controlling your neighbor's spine is a key step in treatment. Based on the mechanism of injury, he may have head, neck, or spinal injuries. He may also have a combination of the three. The patient's altered mental status, skin color, and condition indicate the need for rapid transport after EMS arrival. The crew will administer high-flow oxygen by nonrebreather mask if breathing remains adequate. Manual stabilization, application of a cervical collar, and securely immobilizing the patient to a long spine board are essential for preventing further damage.

ENHANCED STUDY

Brain Injuries

This section describes different types of brain injuries that can occur.

Increased Intracranial Pressure. The skull is a fixed, rigid container that protects the brain. The brain and surrounding structures occupy most of the skull, leaving little room for expansion. Because space is limited, bleeding or swelling in or around the brain can be very serious. Both conditions increase pressure on the brain and brainstem. This is called increased intracranial pressure. The signs and symptoms are a decreasing level of consciousness, elevated blood pressure, and slow pulse. Respiratory depression and death may follow. Increased intracranial pressure is serious and requires immediate treatment. Ventilate the patient with high-flow oxygen at a rate of 16 to 24 ventilations per minute. Be sure to allow enough time for exhalation to occur. This will help to reduce the amount of carbon dioxide being retained in the bloodstream. This helps to decrease the brain swelling. Transport to the most appropriate trauma center. Follow local protocols.

Concussion. A concussion is usually caused by blunt head trauma. The injury causes a brief loss of brain function. The signs and symptoms vary from being momentarily stunned to complete unresponsiveness. Loss of consciousness lasting a few minutes or less is common. The condition does not recur. Another common symptom is headache. The patient may have some memory loss. He or she may not remember the details of the accident. Other signs and symptoms are:

- Confusion
- Combativeness
- Repetitive questioning
- Dizziness
- Nausea and vomiting

The patient usually improves in a short time. He or she may recover before arrival at the emergency department. Deterioration in the patient's mental status suggests a more serious brain injury.

Brain Contusion. A contusion is bruising of the brain tissue. It may be caused by blunt or penetrating trauma to the head. The force of the blow is sufficient to cause bleeding and swelling. An acceleration/deceleration injury can also cause a brain contusion. This type of injury is common in motor vehicle accidents. The force of the injury causes the brain to bounce off the inside of the skull. Bruising can occur at the point of impact or on the opposite side of the brain.

Contusions are usually associated with serious concussions with prolonged symptoms. The patient may also have:

- Weakness or paralysis of the extremities
- Unequal pupils
- Vomiting
- Mental status changes

If the contusion is large or associated with edema, the injury may cause increased intracranial pressure.

ENHANCED STUDY

Brain Injuries (cont.)

Brain Laceration. A laceration of the brain may be caused by blunt or, more commonly, penetrating trauma. Injured brain tissue and vessels usually bleed. Patients with lacerations of the brain usually have severe brain injuries.

Stabilize the patient immediately and transport. Never remove an impaled object (see Enhancement Fig. 22.1). Stabilize it with a bulky dressing.

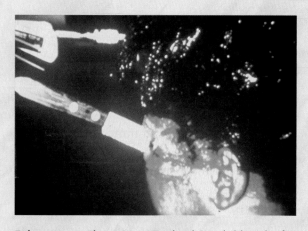

Enhancement Figure 22.1 *Forehead impaled by a knife.*

Epidural Hematoma. A hematoma may occur anywhere within the cranium. The exact location and size is determined in the hospital by a CT scan. An epidural hematoma is a collection of blood between the dura (the protective covering of the brain) and the skull (see Enhancement Fig. 22.2). This injury is usually caused by a head injury with an associated skull fracture and arterial bleeding. It is relatively rare, but can be rapidly fatal. Immediate surgical intervention is necessary.

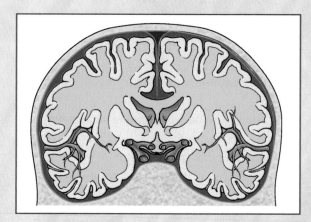

Enhancement Figure 22.2 *Epidural hematoma (thin red line beneath the skull on the upper right).*

Typical signs and symptoms of an epidural hematoma are:

- Loss of consciousness followed by a period of responsiveness

- A secondary decrease in the level of consciousness

- Hemiparesis on the side opposite the injury

If the patient is responsive, he or she may be groggy and complain of a headache. A classic sign is a fixed and dilated pupil on the side of the injury, with a groggy or unresponsive patient.

Subdural Hematoma. A subdural hematoma is a collection of blood between the brain and the dura (see Enhancement Fig. 22.3). A blow to the head or an acceleration/deceleration accident usually causes this injury. Bleeding occurs as the result of a ruptured vein on the brain's surface. A skull fracture may or may not be present. Subdural hematomas are much more common than epidural hematomas. The underlying brain injury is often significant, resulting in high mortality. Surgery is usually required, unless the hematoma is very small.

Intracerebral Hematoma. An intracerebral hematoma is a collection of blood within the brain tissue (see Enhancement Fig. 22.4). This type of hemorrhage may be caused by trauma or by spontaneous bleeding, such as a stroke. The signs and symptoms depend on the size and location of the hematoma.

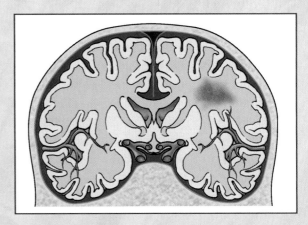

Enhancement Figure 22.4 *Intracerebral hematoma.*

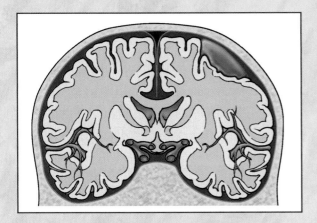

Enhancement Figure 22.3 *Subdural hematoma.*

The extent of the damage depends on the size and location of the hematoma. Signs and symptoms of a subdural hematoma are:

• Altered level of consciousness

• Headache

• Nausea/vomiting

• Hemiparesis

• Dilated pupil

ENHANCED STUDY

Glasgow Coma Scale

The Glasgow Coma Scale is a numeric evaluation of a patient's level of responsiveness. The GCS score is the sum of three general functions. These are eye opening (E), verbal response (V), and motor response (M). The values to assign for different responses are shown in Enhancement Table 22.1 for adults and Enhancement Table 22.2 for pediatric patients. A patient with a GCS score less than or equal to 8 probably has a serious head injury. A person with a GCS score of 9 to 12 has a moderate head injury, while a GCS score of 13 to 15 suggests minor head injury.

For example, an adult patient whose eyes open only to voice commands (E = 3), whose verbal response is the use of inappropriate words (V = 3), and whose best motor response is withdrawing from pain (M = 4), has a total GCS score of E + V + M = 10.

Exercise. You arrive on scene where a three-month old female fell from a couch onto the floor. Her father believes she stopped breathing for a few seconds. She turned blue from head to toe. The infant appears to be in moderate respiratory distress. She opens her eyes and cries when you pinch her hand. She pulls away when you try to assess her capillary refill. What is the GCS score for this infant?

Answer. Eye opening: responds to painful stimuli = 2. Verbal: cries to painful stimuli = 3. Motor: withdraws to touch = 5. GCS = 10 (moderate head injury).

Enhancement Table 22.1 • ADULT GLASGOW COMA SCALE

Eye Opening	Verbal Response	Motor Response
Spontaneous = 4	Oriented and talking = 5	Obeys commands = 6
To speech = 3	Disoriented and talking = 4	Localizes pain = 5
To pain = 2	Inappropriate words = 3	Withdraws to pain = 4
No response = 1	Incomprehensible sounds = 2	Flexion to pain = 3
	No response = 1	Extension to pain = 2
		No response = 1

Enhancement Table 22.2 • PEDIATRIC GLASGOW COMA SCALE

Eye Opening	Verbal Response	Motor Response
Spontaneous = 4	Coos and babbles = 5	Spontaneous = 6
To speech = 3	Irritable or cries = 4	Withdraws to touch = 5
To pain = 2	Cries to pain = 3	Withdraws to pain = 4
No response = 1	Moans to pain = 2	Flexion to pain = 3
	No response = 1	Extension to pain = 2
		No response = 1

ENHANCED STUDY

Child Safety Seats

When the condition of an infant or child does not require that they be placed in a supine position, a car safety seat can be used as an immobilization device (see Enhancement Procedure 22.1). Some infants or children must be rapidly extricated from a safety seat, then immobilized in a supine position (see Enhancement Procedure 22.2). Manual stabilization of the head and neck must be maintained throughout this two-rescuer procedure.

Enhancement Procedure 22.1

SAFETY SEAT IMMOBILIZATION

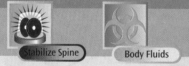

Stabilize Spine   Body Fluids

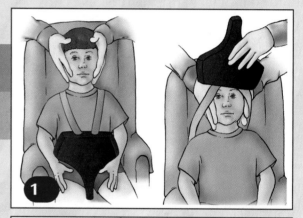

1. One EMT applies manual stabilization of the head and neck. A second EMT detaches the seat restraint and measures for the proper cervical collar.

2. The second EMT applies the cervical collar. Once the collar is applied, the first EMT continues to hold manual stabilization. If there is no properly sized collar for a newborn, an infant, or a small child, small rolled towels can be taped in place.

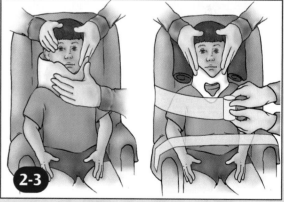

3. After placing a blanket or other padding on the child's lap, the second EMT secures the pelvis and torso to the seat with tape.

4. The forehead is padded and taped by the second EMT. To fill the spaces, towels or pads can be placed on the sides of the child's head. Finally, the second EMT tapes across the cervical collar and under the chin, to avoid putting pressure on the neck.

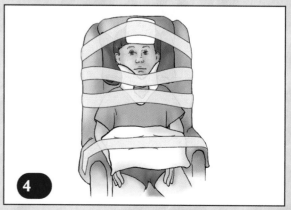

ENHANCED STUDY

Child Safety Seats (cont.)

Enhancement Procedure 22.2
SAFETY SEAT RAPID EXTRICATION

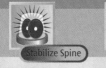 Stabilize Spine Body Fluids

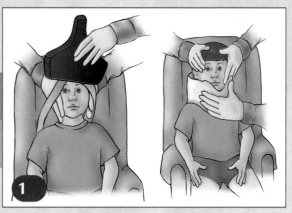

1. One EMT holds manual stabilization while the other removes the seat restraints. The second EMT applies the proper cervical collar.

2. While the first EMT holds manual stabilization, the second EMT places the safety seat on the center of a backboard and slowly tips it back to a supine position, making sure that the child does not slip out of the seat. A rolled towel can be placed in the shoulder position to fill any potential gap between the neck and board.

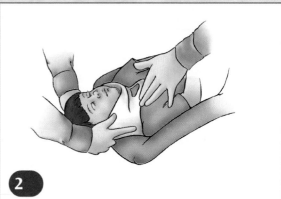

3. The EMT holding manual stabilization coordinates a smooth, long-axis transfer from the seat to a spine board or PED. The shoulders are positioned over the rolled towel.

4. Once the move is completed, the first EMT maintains stabilization while the other EMT straps the child's upper chest, pelvis, and legs onto the board. Do not strap across the abdomen. Rolled towels are placed to fill gaps around the head. The forehead and collar are then strapped. The chin is not secured, because this would put pressure on the neck.

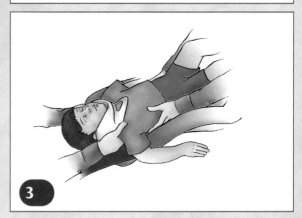

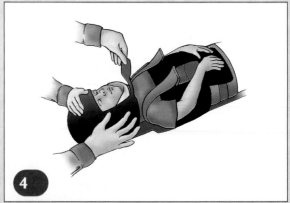

D.O.T. Module
Infants and Children

6

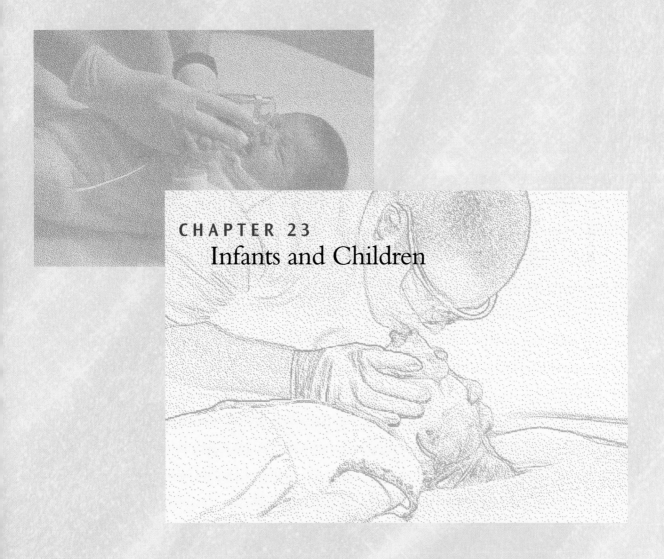

CHAPTER 23
Infants and Children

Chapter

23

Infants and Children

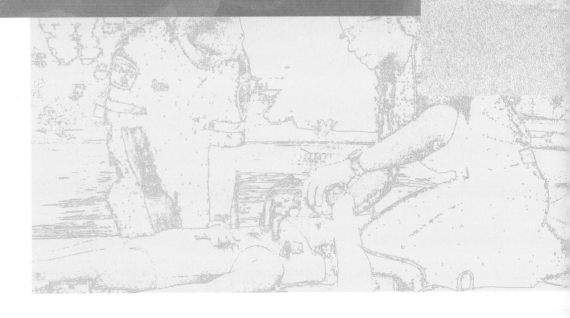

Stories from the Field

You and your partner Mark respond to a call involving a child with burns. You arrive to find a 3-year-old child in his mother's arms, crying violently. The mother states that he accidentally pulled a pot of boiling water off the stove. The child's airway is open. His breathing is fast but adequate. His pulse is rapid. There is significant red splotching on his back and chest. His left forearm is bright red.

At Mark's direction, you place the child on high-flow oxygen by non-rebreather mask. When you apply the mask, the child becomes more agitated. He frantically pulls it away. He has no burns on the face, but the injuries on his body appear very serious. After only 15 minutes, small blisters are forming over most of the burned skin. Mark reminds you that the burns are critical because of the percentage of skin burned, and because the arm burn is circumferential. As you prepare the child for transport, you notice the father sitting on the living room floor. He is muttering, "I didn't mean to do it." When you ask Mark if you should question the father, he tells you to document it later, after providing care for the child.

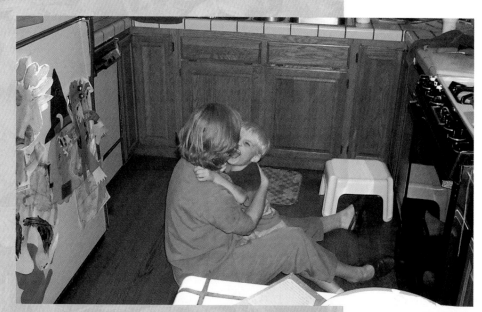

ediatric cases involving infants and children account for 10 percent of pre-hospital calls. Fortunately, most are minor emergencies that do not require lifesaving measures. Many prehospital caregivers have little opportunity to care for pediatric emergencies. This may lead to a lack of confidence and anxiety about pediatric calls. Understanding the unique characteristics of the pediatric patient will help you to feel more prepared.

Until recently, most EMS systems treated children as small adults. Attention to the adult cardiac or trauma patient was foremost, with little consideration to the special needs of children. Now, field personnel are provided with the appropriate training and equipment to care for children. This chapter will emphasize the special assessment and treatment methods required when working with infants and children.

EMT
Tip

Even if an infant or child has no previous medical history and no obvious signs of infectious disease, BSI and standard precautions are always necessary. Appearances can be deceiving and deadly.

THE PEDIATRIC PATIENT

Children are physiologically, anatomically, and psychologically different from adults. Becoming familiar with these differences will improve your effectiveness in communicating, assessing, and treating children.

It can be difficult to assess and treat a child. A child's condition may change quickly. Procedures that are simple on adults may be difficult in children because of their small size. When you are called to a pediatric emergency, you usually have to rely on parents or caregivers for information about what happened. The child probably cannot tell you what is wrong. You will need to rely on this history and your own observations and assessment. Children also tend to resist interventions by strangers. If possible, involve the parents in your assessment and management. A parent can help to maintain a position of comfort for the child. Caregivers can hold a mask to administer oxygen. And they are the best resources for keeping their children calm.

> ### D.O.T. OBJECTIVES
>
> Identify the developmental considerations for the following age groups: infants, toddlers, preschool, school age, and adolescent.
>
> Differentiate the response of the ill or injured infant or child (age specific) from that of an adult.

Developmental Differences

Pediatric patients grow through different stages called newborn, infant, toddler, preschool, school age, and adolescent (see Table 23.1). Each stage of a child's growth and development is unique. Being familiar with age-related differences is important. This will help you to understand the emotional and physical needs for each age group. It will also improve your ability to speak and respond to a child.

Table 23.1 • **PEDIATRIC PATIENT AGE GROUPS**

Age	Development Stage
Birth to 1 month old	Newborn
Up to 1 year old	Infant
1 to 3 years old	Toddler
3 to 6 years old	Preschooler
6 to 12 years old	School-aged
12 to 18 years old	Adolescent

Four golden rules when dealing with children are:

- Never lie to a child, especially if he or she asks, "Will it hurt?"
- Assume that any child can hear and understand everything that is said.
- Tell the child everything you are going to do before doing it.
- Involve the parents in the child's care as much as possible. This relieves the child's fear and anxiety. It also increases the parent's confidence in you and gives them some control over the situation.

Newborns and Infants

Within 6 months of birth, infants recognize a primary caregiver's face and voice. By the end of the first year, children have clearly bonded with the primary caregiver. They are usually very distressed by separation. Children this age may be afraid of strangers. Initially observing the child from a distance may be beneficial. However, remember that an infant's condition can deteriorate very quickly.

As you approach the child, observe the chest rise and fall and count the breathing rate. Monitor the infant's color, and note the level of activity. If it is safe, have a familiar caregiver hold the infant while you perform your assessment. This may help to calm the infant. Speak with a soothing voice and relaxed facial expression.

Figure 23.1 It is difficult to assess the vital signs of a crying infant.

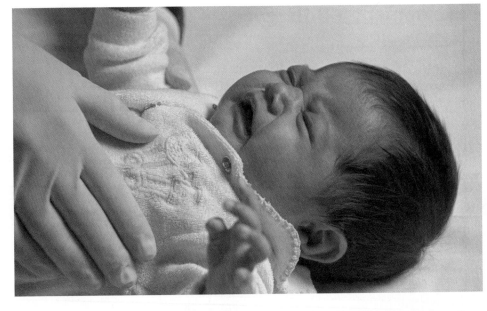

Figure 23.1 It is difficult to assess the vital signs of a crying infant.

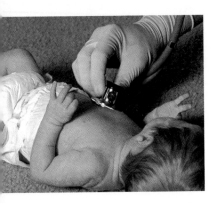

Figure 23.2 A warmed stethoscope relieves some of the discomfort felt by the infant.

Toddler | *Child who is 1 to 3 years old*

If the infant remains quiet when you approach, assess the heart and lungs first. When the infant realizes you are a stranger, he or she may become agitated and cry (see Fig. 23.1). This makes taking vital signs much more difficult. Most infants will resist being held for a brachial pulse check. Listen to the heart to count the pulse. This is easier than trying to hold the arm still.

Use the trunk-to-head approach for assessment. Gently examine the chest, abdomen, and extremities first. Warm your hands and stethoscope to avoid startling the child (see Fig. 23.2). Let the child play with the end of your stethoscope while you begin the assessment. Infants are highly sensitive to stimulation around the face, so examine the head last. They will also resist being confined by an oxygen mask.

Toddlers

Toddlers have a sense of body awareness and know what they like and dislike. They can be more challenging to assess because they are feisty. Most toddlers are uncooperative when healthy. They may become even more so when sick or injured. Toddlers fear pain, needles, and being shamed or at fault. You probably cannot comfort a toddler with a verbal explanation.

In general, toddlers do not like:

- To be touched
- To be separated from their parents
- To have clothing removed
- To feel suffocated by an oxygen mask

A toddler may believe that his or her injury or illness is a punishment. Reassure the child that he or she is not bad, and that the incident was not his or her

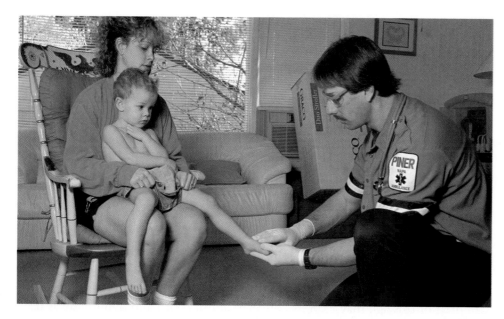

EMT Tip

Preschoolers and young school-aged children take everything literally. They think in relative terms. Be very careful when conversing with children. Common words may be misinterpreted. "A little bit" to you may seem like a lot to a 3-foot-tall child.

fault. Speak in a calm, soothing voice. Distract the child with a favorite toy or object, if possible. Toddlers are very inquisitive. Arousing the child's curiosity during care may be helpful. Allow the child to play with harmless equipment while you complete the exam. Children may also cooperate better if you allow them to participate in care. For example, let them plug in the oxygen tubing while you set the flow rate.

When examining a toddler:

- Complete a focused assessment quickly, before the child becomes agitated
- Examine the child using the trunk-to-head approach (see Fig. 23.3)
- Speak with a soothing voice and maintain a relaxed facial expression
- Remove the clothing, examine the child, then replace the clothes
- Allow the child to hold a security object

Preschool Children

Preschoolers can think concretely, understand, and follow instructions. Slowly explain what you are going to do. Use simple terms. Avoid anatomical or medical terminology.

Preschooler | *Child who is 3 to 6 years old*

Preschoolers may be modest and resist being undressed. They also have a sense of body integrity. They are afraid of pain, permanent injury, and being shamed or at fault. In general, preschoolers do not like:

- To be touched
- To be separated from their parents
- To have clothing removed
- To feel suffocated by an oxygen mask

When examining a preschooler:

- Use the trunk-to-head approach for assessment.
- Remove clothing, examine the child, and then replace the clothes.
- Cover bleeding injuries after assessment and stabilization. For preschoolers, out of sight is out of mind.
- Allow the child to hold a security object.
- Reassure the child that you are going to the hospital, "where they can help to fix you."

School-Aged Children

School-Aged | *Child who is 6 to 12 years old*

School-aged children can reason. They have a simple understanding of anatomy. They usually understand that you are there to help them, and often try to cooperate. Use simple words when speaking with school-aged children. Children of this age may express concerns about death and dying. This is usually due to a death within the family. Children of this age fear:

- Pain
- Blood
- Disfigurement
- Permanent injury

When examining school-aged children:

- Be honest and informative while keeping the information simple
- Direct questions to the child rather than the parent, if possible
- Cover bleeding injuries after assessment and stabilization
- Respect the child's modesty

Adolescents

Adolescent | *Child who is 12 to 18 years old*

Adolescents can think concretely and abstractly. However, they often do not consider the consequences of their actions. Adolescents may feel immortal. They believe that nothing bad can happen to them. Consequently, they take risks leading to injury. At the same time, they fear disfigurement and permanent injury.

Getting an adolescent to reveal information about events, sexual history, personal habits, drug use, or possible illegal activities may be challenging. Peer approval, issues of identity, autonomy, and rebellion may block communication. Be conversational, if possible. Treat an adolescent as an adult. Make sure he or she knows that everything discussed is confidential and will only be released as allowed by law. Remember that history taking is not a criminal investigation.

Adolescents want to appear tough. They may have difficulty admitting pain or fear when injured. They may want to be assessed privately, away from parents and guardians. Allow them the option of being assessed in a private or semi-private area with a parent close by. Be careful not to anger the parents by suggesting privacy for the adolescent. Adolescents respond well to same-gender providers. Always have a second EMT-B present when interviewing a teenager of the opposite gender.

When examining an adolescent:

• Be honest and informative

• Respect modesty and privacy

• Speak to the patient as an adult

D.O.T. OBJECTIVE

Describe differences in anatomy and physiology of the infant, child, and adult patient.

Anatomy and Physiology Concerns

Most of the underlying principles of emergency care are the same for children as for adults. In many cases, the assessment and treatment techniques are the same as you have learned so far. However, infants and children have some important anatomical and physiological differences (see Table 23.2). You must be aware of these differences so you can modify your care.

Table 23.2 • **PEDIATRIC ANATOMICAL DIFFERENCES**

Structure	Characteristics in Infants and Children
Head	Proportionally larger than adults Infants have soft spots, or fontanelles
Tongue	Proportionally larger; easily blocks airway
Airway	Small airway; easily blocked by secretions or swelling Infants are usually nose breathers
Circulation	Smaller volume increases risk of shock
Skin	Large surface area increases risk of hypothermia

The most significant differences have to do with the airway. See the sections "Special Considerations for Infants and Children" in Chapter 4 and "Anatomical Differences in Children" in Chapter 7 for a review. The airway differences to keep in mind are:

- Infants and children have smaller airways. They are easily blocked by secretions and airway swelling. A small amount of swelling or obstruction will readily block the airway. Infants may need frequent nasal suctioning.

- The tongue in an infant or child is large compared with the mandible size. It can easily block the airway in an unconscious infant or child.

- The positioning for opening the airway is different from adults. Excessive hyperextension or flexion of the neck may block the airway.

- Infants are usually nose breathers. Suctioning a secretion-filled nasopharynx usually improves breathing problems.

PEDIATRIC AIRWAY MANAGEMENT

The most important aspect of prehospital care for infants and children is proper airway and breathing management and adequate oxygenation. Following is a brief review of specific techniques for airway management that were discussed in Chapter 7 and Appendix B. Review this material, especially the sections on treatment of pediatric patients.

Opening and Maintaining the Airway

If a child is not breathing, open the airway immediately. When a child becomes unconscious, oral muscles relax. The tongue may slip back in the throat, obstructing the airway. Perform the head-tilt/chin-lift maneuver or the jaw-thrust maneuver. Remember that for infants and small children, the head-tilt/chin-lift maneuver is slightly modified (see Fig. 23.4). Avoid hyperextending the neck, which could collapse the airway. If you suspect a cervical spine injury, you must perform the jaw-thrust maneuver (see Fig. 23.5).

Figure 23.4 *Avoid overextending the neck when performing the head-tilt/chin-lift maneuver on a child.*

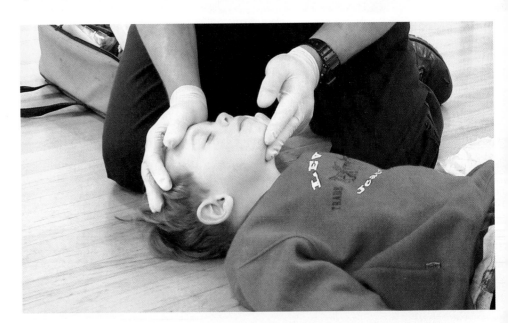

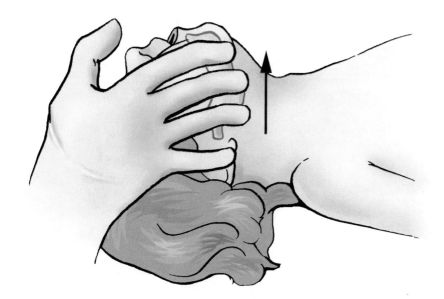

Figure 23.5 *The jaw-thrust maneuver opens the airway without tilting the head or extending the neck.*

Suction any secretions, vomitus, or blood from the airway. Flexible plastic suction catheters are useful for removing thin secretions. A wide-bore suction catheter is more effective for removing thick secretions, such as vomitus. A wide-bore suction catheter may also be called a Yankauer tip, a tonsil tip, or a tonsil sucker. Always use sterile technique when suctioning. Avoid suctioning for more than 5 seconds at a time. Administer 100 percent oxygen before and after suctioning to prevent hypoxia.

Airway adjuncts are used to maintain an open airway when a patient is unable to do so. Use the oropharyngeal airway adjunct (OPA) for an unresponsive patient who has no gag reflex. If the patient is responsive, the OPA may trigger gagging or vomiting. Recall that for an infant or child, you should insert the OPA right side up. Do not rotate it, as for an adult patient. A tongue depressor may be used to assist insertion. Insert the tongue blade as far as the base of the tongue. Push down against the tongue while inserting the adjunct.

A nasopharyngeal airway (NPA) provides a channel for airflow between the nasal passages and the back of the oropharynx. It may be used with responsive patients. Airway adjuncts must be properly sized for the patient. Avoid using either the NPA or OPA in patients with head trauma.

Assisted Artificial Ventilation

In the following situations, provide assisted artificial ventilation as soon as practical:

- Severe respiratory distress
- Altered mental status
- Cyanosis, despite supplemental oxygen by a non-rebreather mask
- Decompensated respiratory failure or arrest

Figure 23.6 *Ventilating with a pocket face mask.*

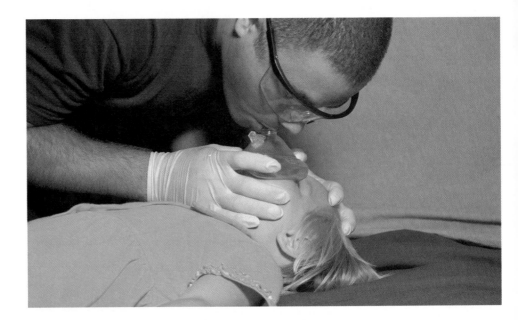

When a bag-valve mask is not immediately available, a pocket face mask may be used to provide ventilations (see Fig. 23.6). Ventilate infants and children once every 3 seconds. While inhaled room air contains 21 percent oxygen, our exhaled breath contains approximately 16 percent oxygen.

When supplemental oxygen is available and the child is receptive, supplemental oxygen should be attached to a ventilation device. Use a bag-valve mask to assist ventilations (see Fig. 23.7). Squeeze the bag slowly and evenly to make the chest rise adequately. Avoid hyperinflation. Deliver 100 percent oxygen using an oxygen reservoir at a rate of 20 breaths per minute.

Figure 23.7 *Ventilating a child with a bag-valve mask.*

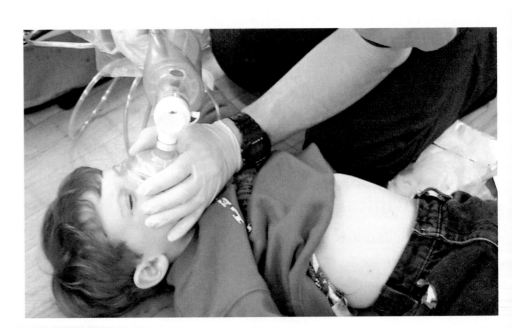

Two techniques can be used for sealing the mask. The two-hand technique is the preferred method, because it seals more tightly (see Fig. 23.8). This technique requires a second person to ventilate the child. A single rescuer can ventilate using the one-hand technique. Hold the mask in place with one hand, using the other hand to squeeze the bag. Avoid pressing on the neck with your fingers.

Pediatric Oxygen Therapy

Several devices and methods may be used to provide supplemental oxygen therapy to infants and children. These are:

- Non-rebreather mask
- Blow-by techniques
- Nasal cannula

Non-Rebreather Mask

A non-rebreather mask delivers 90 percent oxygen upon inspiration (see Fig. 23.9). Administer oxygen at 15 liters per minute. Indications for use of the non-rebreather mask are:

- Signs of early respiratory distress
- Pediatric patient who is receptive to placement of the non-rebreather mask

Ventilation face masks can be used for both oxygen administration and assisted artificial ventilation. The rim of the mask has a soft seal to prevent air leakage. Proper sizing and placement are critical to ensure an airtight seal. The mask should fit over the bridge of the nose and under the chin (see Fig. 23.10). Avoid applying pressure to the eyes.

When placing a mask on a patient with suspected trauma, use the jaw-thrust maneuver to maintain the airway. Provide manual in-line stabilization of the cervical spine.

Blow-By Techniques

Another method for oxygen delivery is the blow-by technique (see Fig. 23.11 on page 682). Indications for using a blow-by technique are:

- Spontaneous and adequate breathing
- Signs of early respiratory distress
- Child resists placement of non-rebreather mask

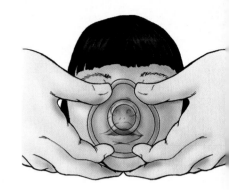

Figure 23.8 *Two-hand placement of the mask seals it more tightly.*

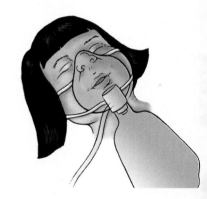

Figure 23.9 *Child's non-rebreather mask.*

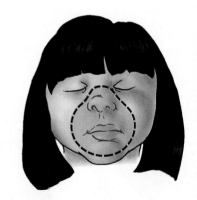

Figure 23.10 *An airtight seal is critical when sizing a mask.*

Figure 23.11 *The blow-by technique is one way of delivering oxygen without having to strap a mask to the infant's face.*

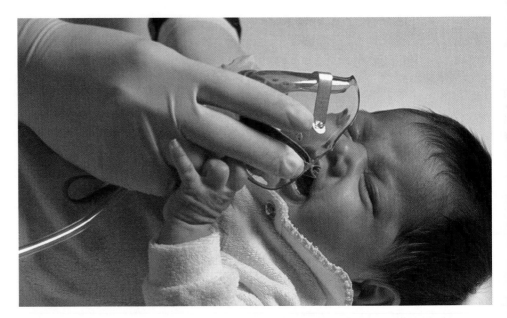

To use the blow-by technique, hold the end of the oxygen tubing approximately 2 inches from the child's nose and mouth (see Fig. 23.12). You can also insert the oxygen tubing into a paper cup and hold it near the face.

Figure 23.12 *Two blow-by methods.*

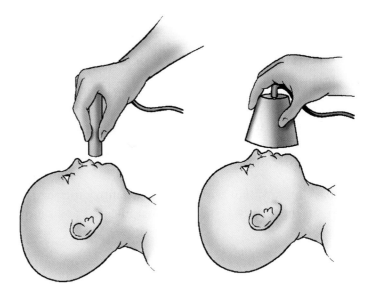

If a child has a favorite toy, be creative. A stuffed animal can hold oxygen tubing under a paw or arm. Delivering some oxygen using this method is better than not delivering any. Use the $KidO_2$ device if available in your agency (see Fig. 12.11 in Chapter 12).

Nasal Cannula

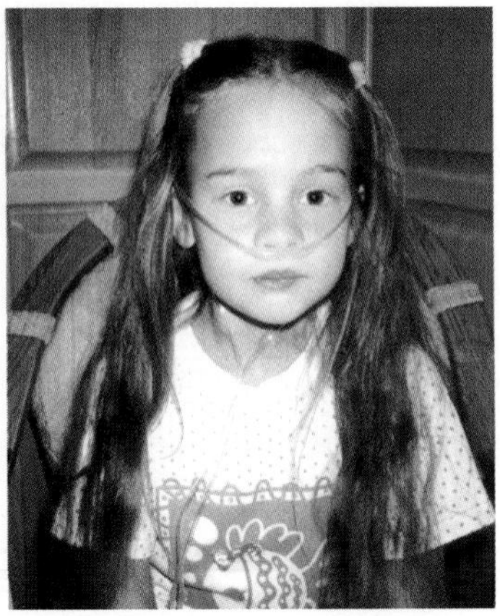

Another method for oxygen delivery is the use of a nasal cannula (see Fig. 23.13). Use the cannula only when a child resists your efforts to place the mask. When used, administer oxygen at 4 liters per minute.

Figure 23.13 *Nasal cannula on a child.*

GENERAL PEDIATRIC ASSESSMENT

Complete a scene size-up, initial assessment, and appropriate focused history and physical exam on every call, whether the patient is an infant, a child, or an adult. To assess the condition of an infant or child, you must look at the big picture. Evaluate the entire child. Begin your assessment from across the room, before approaching the child. Note the surroundings. Look for a mechanism of injury or signs of trauma.

Your general impression of whether an infant or child seems well or sick can be obtained from the overall appearance (see Table 23.3). Observe the following:

- Note the interactions with the parent and with you. Is the level of responsiveness and behavior normal for a child of this age?

- Is breathing normal or labored? What is the quality of cying or speech?

- What is the skin color and body position?

- What is the emotional state?

Table 23.3 • GENERAL IMPRESSION: INFANTS AND CHILDREN

Characteristic	Well Child	Sick Child
Emotional State	Calm, or cries but can be comforted by parent	Cannot be consoled
Quality of Crying	Strong	Whimpering, weak, or high-pitched
Activity	Playful, active	Lethargic, refuses to play, exhausted
Responsiveness	Attentive, responds to parents and EMTs, makes eye contact	Inappropriate or absent
Skin Color	Pink	Pale or cyanotic
Skin Tone and Body Position	Normal for age	Resistant, limp, flaccid

---

D.O.T. OBJECTIVE

Describe the methods of determining end organ perfusion in the infant and child patient.

Airway, Breathing, and Circulation

Your first priority is to manage the ABCs. Look for airway or breathing problems by observing the child's respirations (see Table 23.4). Listen to the breath sounds with a stethoscope. Auscultate along the chest, below both armpits.

Table 23.4 • OBSERVATION OF BREATHING

Characteristic	Adequate Breathing	Inadequate Breathing
Rate	Normal	Rapid, slow, or absent
Chest Expansion	Full; equal and symmetric	Shallow; unequal
Effort of Breathing	Normal	Labored
Flaring of Nostrils	Absent	Present
Breath Sounds	Quiet	Stridor, crowing, or noisy
Retractions	Absent	Present
Grunting	Absent	Present on expiration
Position	Relaxed	Tripod position

Abnormal breath sounds may offer clues to the nature and severity of a problem. Some examples of abnormal sounds are:

- Coughing, gagging, or gasping
- Stridor, wheezing
- Noisy breath sounds
- Diminished or unequal breath sounds

Chapter 5 describes how to measure and evaluate the pulses and blood pressure. For infants and children, assess circulation and perfusion by observing the:

- Pulses
- Capillary refill (in children under 6 years)
- Blood pressure (in children older than 3 years)
- Skin color, temperature, and moisture

Capillary Refill Time | *Time required for the capillary beds to refill with blood after blanching; used for assessing perfusion in infants and children*

Capillary refill time is useful for assessing circulation in children. It is an excellent indication of perfusion. When circulation is decreased, the time it takes for blood to refill is diminished. To conduct this test, grasp the child's fingertip. Squeeze the nail bed enough to make it turn white. Quickly release the pressure. Observe how long it takes for the nail bed to return to its original color. Normal capillary refill occurs in less than 2 seconds. In some infants and very small children, you may have to use the palms, soles of the feet, or toes instead of a nail bed (see Fig. 23.14). Delayed capillary refill is an early sign of shock in children.

Focused History and Physical Exam

After assessing and managing the ABCs, you may have adequate information to determine a child's needs for emergency care and transport. If not, obtain a focused history, including information provided by witnesses and caregivers. Complete the appropriate physical exam and measure vital signs. Follow the

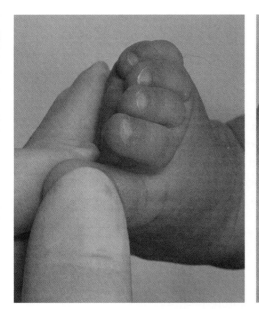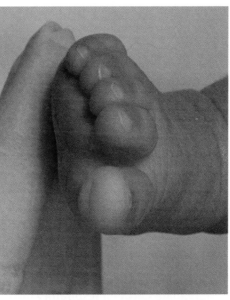

Figure 23.14 *The large toe is a good location for assessing an infant's capillary refill.*

general patient assessment strategy discussed in Chapters 8 and 9. Modify the procedures as required for the situation and the child's age. Use the toe-trunk-head approach to reduce the child's anxiety. Check the:

- SAMPLE history
- OPQRST history
- DCAP-BTLS indicators of body injury
- Well versus sick appearance
- Vital signs

Recall from Chapter 5 that normal vital signs vary by age. For example, infants have faster breathing and heart rates. Table 5.1 in Chapter 5 lists average ranges of vital signs for different age groups. Remember that children can compensate for poor circulation and respiration. However, they may become exhausted and deteriorate suddenly.

COMMON PEDIATRIC PROBLEMS

You will see certain problems when providing emergency medical care to infants and children. These are:

- Airway obstruction
- Respiratory diseases
- Seizures
- Altered mental status
- Poisoning

- Fever

- Shock

- Near drowning

- Sudden infant death syndrome (SIDS)

Children do not usually have the same disease processes as adults. For example, a child does not have the buildup of fatty plaque that contributes to heart attacks in adults. The patient assessment and emergency medical care for each condition presented in the following sections are meant to highlight the differences and special considerations you will encounter on calls involving infants and children.

D.O.T. OBJECTIVES

Differentiate between respiratory distress and respiratory failure.

State the usual cause of cardiac arrest in infants and children versus adults.

EMT
Tip

Any child who does not resist ventilation with a bag-valve mask probably needs continued ventilatory support.

Early Respiratory Distress | Respiratory problem in which patient can compensate for decreased oxygenation or circulation by increasing breathing rate and effort

Pediatric Respiratory Problems

You will care for infants and children in various stages of respiratory distress. Initially, they compensate well by increasing their breathing rate and effort. As the child becomes fatigued, he or she may decompensate quickly. With respiratory decompensation, the body is unable to manage the respiratory malfunction. Other body systems begin to fail, resulting in respiratory failure or arrest. Learn to identify the various types of respiratory problems. This will enable you to anticipate and recognize respiratory problems before they worsen. See Chapters 7 and 12 for more information on respiratory distress, failure, and arrest.

You must be able to identify signs of **early respiratory distress**, also known as compensated respiratory failure. When you observe increased breathing rate and effort, suspect early respiratory distress. Any of the following signs indicates an increased breathing effort:

- Nasal flaring

- Retractions of the muscles between the ribs

- Neck or abdominal muscle retractions

- Stridor

- Audible wheezing

- Grunting

Anticipate that respiratory distress can worsen and take early corrective measures. A child in early respiratory distress may become exhausted and suddenly progress to the advanced stage called decompensated respiratory failure. A child is in respiratory failure when the signs and symptoms of early respiratory distress are present together with any of the following signs:

- Respiratory rate over 60
- Cyanosis
- Decreased muscle tone
- Severe use of accessory muscles
- Poor peripheral perfusion
- Altered mental status
- Grunting

The most common cause of cardiac arrest in the infant or child is respiratory arrest. Respiratory arrest occurs when the respiratory rate drops below 10 per minute, muscle tone is lost, the child loses consciousness, or the pulse or heart rate is absent or decreasing.

Provide supplemental oxygen to all children with respiratory emergencies. In addition, assist ventilations for children who are in severe respiratory distress or with any signs of respiratory failure. Provide oxygen and ventilate with a bag-valve mask if a child is in respiratory arrest.

D.O.T. OBJECTIVES

Indicate various causes of respiratory emergencies.

Summarize emergency medical care strategies for respiratory distress and respiratory failure.

List the steps in the management of foreign body airway obstruction.

Airway Obstruction

In children, respiratory problems are usually caused by airway obstruction. This means that a blockage is preventing air movement. It is often due to swallowing foreign objects. Asthma and some respiratory infections may also cause airway obstruction.

You have learned that an airway obstruction may be partial or complete. When the airway is partially obstructed, some air moves past the obstruction. Signs of a partial airway obstruction, or early respiratory distress, are:

- Child is alert
- Sitting in tripod position
- Concentrating on breathing
- Stridor, crowing, or noisy breathing
- Pink skin color
- Good peripheral perfusion
- Retractions are present

A child with a partial obstruction may be able to clear the obstruction without intervention. Encourage the child to continue attempts to relieve the obstruction naturally. Assist the child to assume a comfortable position (not supine). Ask the parent to help while you offer oxygen. Perform a limited exam. Do not assess blood pressure. Avoid agitating the child. Transport immediately.

A complete airway obstruction is a critical condition, requiring immediate interventions and possible resuscitation. Signs of complete airway obstruction are:

- No audible crying or speech
- Ineffective or absent cough
- Increased respiratory distress
- Stridor
- Altered mental status
- Loss of consciousness
- Cyanosis

For complete airway obstruction, follow the foreign body removal procedures for an infant of child. These skills were learned as part of your BLS course and are reviewed in Chapter 7 and Appendix B. Clear any visible foreign body. Deliver abdominal thrusts for a child older than 1 year. Use back blows and chest thrusts for an infant. After dislodging the foreign body, deliver oxygen at 15 liters per minute by non-rebreather mask. If the child is not breathing adequately, assist ventilations while you provide supplemental oxygen.

Respiratory Diseases

Infants and children are subject to chronic and acute respiratory diseases. These can cause airway obstruction or respiratory distress. Respiratory diseases are discussed in more detail in Chapter 12. You must be able to recognize the difference between upper airway obstruction and lower airway disease. With upper airway obstruction, stridor is present on inspiration. With lower airway diseases such as asthma or epiglottitis, the child will wheeze. Exhalation will be very difficult. You may also observe rapid breathing without stridor. A child with a chronic disease generally has medications or equipment in the home. He or she may be less anxious about the episode. A child with an airway obstruction will probably appear nervous or scared.

D.O.T. OBJECTIVES

List the common causes of seizures in the infant and child patient.

Describe the management of seizures in the infant and child patient.

Seizures in Children

Seizures are most commonly caused by fever in infants and children, especially those under the age of 2. Other causes are epilepsy, infections, head injury, decreased levels of oxygen, poisoning (including drug overdose), or low blood sugar. Seizures are frightening to caregivers, but are usually harmless. In children who have frequent seizures, they are rarely life threatening. However, all seizures should be considered life threatening by the EMT.

A seizure may be brief or prolonged. Most seizures last only a few minutes, resolving spontaneously. You will usually arrive after the seizure. Assess for the presence of injuries sustained during the seizure. During the SAMPLE history, ask the caregiver:

- Has the child had seizures before?
- If so, is this the child's normal seizure pattern?
- Has the child taken any anti-seizure medication?

Inadequate breathing and/or altered mental status may occur following a seizure. Keep in mind that seizures can be caused by a more dangerous underlying condition, such as a head injury. See Chapter 14 for more information on seizures.

The emergency care steps for pediatric seizures are basically the same as for adults. Recall that you should never place anything in the patient's mouth during a seizure. Never attempt to restrain a patient who is actively seizing.

- Assure airway patency
- Have suction ready
- Administer high-flow oxygen by non-rebreather mask
- If necessary, assist ventilations with a bag-valve mask
- Consider immediate transport

Altered Mental Status

A child's mental status may be altered due to low blood sugar, poisoning, a post-seizure state, infection, head injury, decreased oxygen levels, or shock. Emergency medical care must be directed toward caring for life-threatening conditions in patients with altered mental status. Remember that respiratory compromise is a common cause of an altered mental state.

The emergency care steps for an infant or child with altered mental status are similar to those for an adult (see Chapter 14):

- Monitor airway patency closely
- Have suction ready
- Administer high-flow oxygen by non-rebreather mask
- Assist ventilations, if necessary
- Consider immediate transport

Poisoning

Accidental poisonings are common in children because of their inquisitive nature. As with adult poisonings, identify the route of entry when assessing for possible poisoning. You learned in Chapter 16 that poison may enter the body by ingestion, inhalation, absorption, or injection. Attempt to find and bring the container to the hospital, if possible.

Always contact medical direction for a responsive patient who has been poisoned. They will determine whether or not to administer activated charcoal. In addition:

- Monitor the airway and breathing carefully. Administer high-flow oxygen by non-rebreather mask or assist ventilations, if necessary.
- Transport the patient. Complete a detailed examination while en route to the hospital. Continue to monitor the level of responsiveness.

If the child is found unresponsive, or becomes unresponsive during transport, be prepared to provide positive-pressure ventilations with supplemental oxygen if the breathing becomes inadequate.

Fever

Fever in infants and children is a common reason for an ambulance call. Fevers are usually caused by infection, dehydration, or heat exposure. Occasionally, a **febrile** seizure may occur when the fever rises quickly. Fever with a rash is a potentially serious condition. An example of a severe cause is meningitis.

Febrile (FEE-bril) | *Having a fever*

Besides the usual SAMPLE history and physical assessment, look for signs of dehydration:

- Weak, rapid pulse
- Sunken eyes
- Dry mucous membranes
- Dry skin that remains "tented" when pinched
- Rash
- Crying without tears
- Sunken fontanelles

Follow local protocols for lowering the temperature of pediatric patients. Monitor the airway and breathing carefully. Anticipate febrile seizures. Transport the patient.

D.O.T. OBJECTIVE

Identify the signs and symptoms of shock (hypoperfusion) in the infant and child patient.

Pediatric Shock

Hypovolemic shock is the most common form of shock in infants and children. This is caused by inadequate circulatory volume. Hypovolemic shock in children is usually caused by severe blood loss. It may also be caused by dehydration after a period of vomiting or diarrhea. Other causes of shock are trauma, infection, and abdominal injuries. Less common causes in pediatric patients are allergic reactions, poisoning, and cardiac events.

The signs and symptoms of shock in infants and children are:

- Rapid respiratory rate
- Pale, clammy, cool skin
- Weak or absent peripheral pulses
- Delayed capillary refill
- Sunken fontanelles in infants less than 18 months old
- Decreased urine output (reported by caregivers); dry diaper
- Altered mental status
- Absence of tears, even when crying

The emergency medical care for shock is discussed in detail in Chapter 22. Review the following general emergency care steps. Keep in mind that an infant or child may deteriorate faster and more severely than an adult who is suffering from shock.

1. Administer oxygen and maintain the airway. Assist ventilations with a bag-valve mask, if necessary.
2. Manage the patient's bleeding, if present.
3. Elevate the legs.
4. Keep the patient warm.
5. Transport immediately. Compete the detailed exam while en route, if time permits.

Near Drowning

In a near drowning, the patient survives for at least 24 hours following the episode. This can occur in any amount of water (see Fig. 23.15). Death by drowning usually results from hypoxia, not fluid in the lungs. When water contacts the glottic opening, it induces a reflex action that closes the airway. Assisted artificial ventilation is the first priority when managing a near drowning. Treat the patient even if he or she is unresponsive and pulseless. Begin resuscitation (see Figs. 23.16 and 23.17). Be persistent, especially in cold water submersion. Always consider the possibility of trauma, hypothermia, and/or alcohol ingestion (especially in adolescents). See Chapter 17 for a complete discussion of drowning and near drowning.

All near-drowning patients should be transported to the hospital. The child may develop secondary drowning syndrome, even if breathing normally. Secondary drowning syndrome is general deterioration after normal breathing resumes. This is due to complications associated with systemic failures minutes to hours after the event. This can cause cardiac arrest.

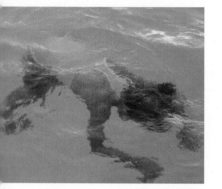

Figure 23.15 *A near drowning can occur in any amount of water.*

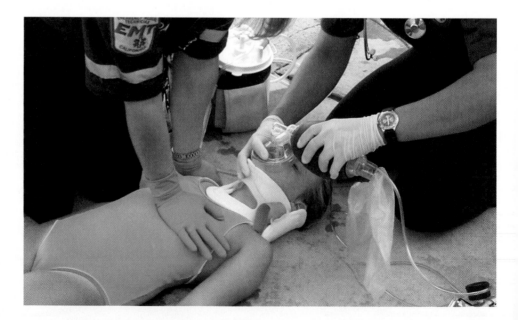

Figure 23.16 *Immediately begin CPR when near drowning is suspected.*

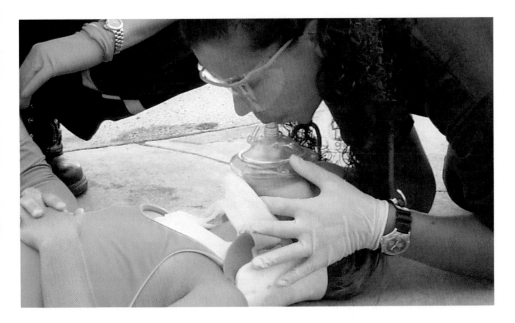

Figure 23.17 *An unresponsive and pulseless drowning victim still requires resuscitation.*

Sudden Infant Death Syndrome (SIDS)

A frequent cause of death in infants between 1 month and 1 year of age is **sudden infant death syndrome**, or **SIDS**. Another term for this condition is crib death (see Fig. 23.18). Every year in the U.S., nearly three thousand infants die from SIDS. Most who die are between 1 and 4 months old. The cause of SIDS is currently unknown, although some predisposing factors have been identified, such as respiratory illness, premature birth, gender, and race. The parents most commonly discover the baby early in the morning.

When you arrive on a SIDS scene, you will find an infant in cardiac arrest. Do not delay resuscitation, but try to obtain a brief history, including:

- Physical appearance of the infant
- Position of the baby in the crib
- Physical appearance and objects in the crib
- Presence of dangerous or suffocating objects in the room
- Circumstances surrounding the discovery of the infant
- General health and any recent illnesses

Attempt to resuscitate the suspected SIDS-arrested infant. This helps the grieving parents feel that everything possible was done. The exception is if rigor mortis is present. With rigor mortis, the joints become rigid. If present, leave the infant in the position found (follow local protocols). Contact authorities according to local protocols and standing orders.

With SIDS, the primary concerns are supporting the parents and assisting with the grieving process. If possible, at least one crew member should remain with family members after the infant is transported. Some agencies

Sudden Infant Death Syndrome (SIDS) | *Crib death; cause unknown*

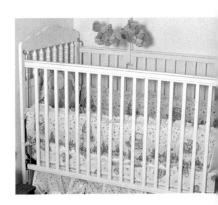

Figure 23.18 *SIDS patients are usually discovered in the morning.*

EMT Tip

When questioning family members about possible SIDS deaths, avoid using the word "you." Simple, open-ended questions such as "What happened?" work well.

CD-ROM Link

The "Pedestrian Accident" animation in Chapter 23 and the Video Appendix on the MedEMT CD-ROM illustrates the mechanism of injury when a child is struck by a car.

will dispatch a clergy member or a supervisor to the scene to work with family members and caregivers. One of the first steps in the grief process involves talking about events, so you should allow them to speak freely. Parents may display great emotional distress, grief, or imagined guilt. Avoid any comments that may make the parents feel blamed. Avoid false reassurances. Do not dismiss the parents' or your own emotional turmoil.

D.O.T. OBJECTIVE

Differentiate between the injury patterns in adults, infants, and children.

PEDIATRIC TRAUMA

Trauma is the number one cause of death in infants and children. Blunt trauma injuries are the most common. The number one killer in pediatric trauma is the automobile. Many children who survive collisions are permanently disabled.

Pediatric trauma requires special consideration because of anatomical differences from adults. The pattern of injury will be different. For an introductory discussion about blunt trauma and mechanism of injury (MOI), see Chapter 8. Table 23.5 lists common MOIs and typical injuries that will be seen in an infant or child.

Table 23.5 • PEDIATRIC TRAUMA

Mechanism of Injury	Typical Injuries
Motor Vehicle Passenger	If unrestrained, head and neck injuries from striking the dashboard If an airbag has been deployed, head and neck injuries from being struck by the airbag If restrained, abdominal and lower spine injuries from the restraints
Struck while Riding Bicycle	Head, spinal, and abdominal injuries
Pedestrian Struck by Vehicle	Head, chest, and lower extremity injuries; abdominal injuries with possible internal bleeding
Fall from Height	Head and neck injuries
Diving into Shallow Water	Head and neck injuries
Burns	Skin and inhalation injuries
Sports	Head and neck injuries
Child Abuse	Head, extremity, and internal organ injuries

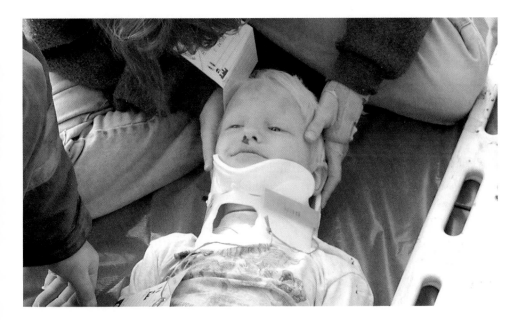

Figure 23.19 *When children are passengers in vehicle collisions, head, neck, spine, and abdomen injuries are common.*

Many children involved in motor vehicle collisions (MVCs) are injured because they are not restrained. This is often because parents failed to secure the child's safety seat. Other reasons are improper application of the restraint or improper seating in relation to an airbag. Such accidents may cause head, neck, spine, and abdominal injuries (see Fig. 23.19).

Children who are not riding in vehicles are also frequently injured in MVCs. Thousands of children are hit annually while walking on roadways (see Fig. 23.20). Many are injured when riding bicycles, skateboards, or roller blades. These accidents cause head, neck, spine, abdominal, or lower extremity injuries.

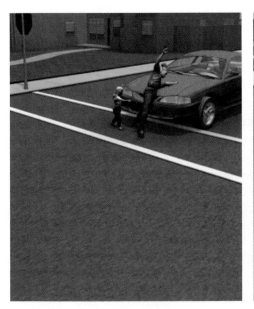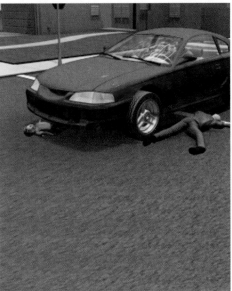

Figure 23.20 *In a pedestrian accident, children are usually bumped and thrown forward because of their low centers of mass.*

Specific Body Systems

The following sections highlight specific differences for assessing and treating an infant or child when trauma is sustained.

Head Assessment

When caring for an infant or child with a head injury, closely monitor and maintain the airway. Use the modified jaw-thrust maneuver if a head or spine injury is suspected. Keep the head and neck in an in-line position. In infants and small children, this may be difficult because the oversized skull forces the child into a chin-down position. Be particularly careful to avoid spinal injury when immobilizing children. Never use sandbags to stabilize the head. The weights may further injure the child if the board needs to be turned for vomitus.

When assessing the head of an infant or child, consider:

- Respiratory arrest is common secondary to head injuries
- Nausea and vomiting are common signs and symptoms of head injury
- Shock in a head injury patient can indicate other internal injuries
- Hypoxia in children is usually caused by the tongue obstructing the airway due to loss of consciousness

Chest Assessment

A child's ribs are soft and pliable, making them more resistant to fracture. They are more likely to transmit the force of an injury to underlying internal organs. Children with internal injuries may not show signs of external rib injury or fracture. Suspect heart, lung, or spleen injury whenever the mechanism of injury suggests blunt trauma to the chest.

Abdomen Assessment

The abdomen in children is thinner and provides less protection against blunt trauma than in adults. Blunt trauma commonly causes hidden internal injuries. The only sign may be rapid deterioration in condition. Be suspicious if the child is deteriorating quickly without signs of external injury.

Younger children are diaphragmatic breathers. When excessive pressure causes stomach distention to push the diaphragm up, the lungs cannot expand fully. When assisting ventilations, avoid high pressures that may force air into the stomach.

Extremity Assessment

Injuries to the extremities of infants or children are assessed and managed in the same way as for adults. See Chapter 21 for more information about emergency care for extremity injuries.

Emergency Care for Pediatric Trauma

These are the general emergency care steps to follow when you respond to a trauma call involving an infant or child:

1. Establish and maintain an airway. Use the jaw-thrust maneuver if a head or neck injury is suspected.
2. Suction as needed with a large bore catheter. Deliver oxygen at 15 liters per minute by non-rebreather mask. Assist ventilations if the infant or child is in respiratory distress. Ventilate with a bag-valve mask for respiratory arrest. Consider early transport if the mechanism of injury is severe, or if the patient shows signs or symptoms of respiratory distress.
3. Provide spinal immobilization and transport the child immediately. Complete a detailed examination while en route to the hospital.

Pneumatic Anti-Shock Garment (PASG)

When shock is suspected in an infant or child, consider using a pneumatic anti-shock garment only if it fits the child. Avoid placing the infant or child in one leg of an adult garment. Indications for use of an anti-shock garment are:

• Trauma with signs of severe hypoperfusion
• Pelvic instability

Do not inflate the abdominal compartment of an anti-shock garment on an infant or child, because this may cause further injury.

Burns

Burns are a common pediatric injury that can require major treatment. Infants and children are at high risk for hypothermia and shock after suffering burns. When treating burns on infants and children, cover the burned area with a non-adherent sterile dressing. Sterile sheets may also be used.

Identify the patient as a candidate for transport to a burn center according to local protocols or standing orders. Review the section on burns in Chapter 20.

CD-ROM Link

The video "Child Trauma" in the Authentic Emergency Scenes section of Chapter 23 and the Video Appendix on the MedEMT CD-ROM shows the importance of gentle treatment during immobilization and transport of an injured child.

CHILD ABUSE AND NEGLECT

Disturbingly, child abuse and neglect are growing causes of death and injury to children in the United States. Child abuse is improper or excessive action leading to injury or harm. Central nervous system injuries are the most lethal. These usually occur when the infant or child is violently shaken. This condition is called shaken baby syndrome. You must be aware of the possibility of physical child abuse in order to recognize it. Signs and symptoms of physical abuse include:

- Multiple bruises in various stages of healing
- Injury inconsistent with mechanism described
- Repeated calls to the same address
- Fresh burns; small burns to the hands, feet, face, or abdomen from cigarettes or cigars
- Caregivers inappropriately unconcerned
- Conflicting stories
- Child is fearful of describing how the injury occurred
- Caregivers complain about irrelevant problems unrelated to the injury
- Human bite marks
- Bruises or lacerations with a pattern (such as a belt buckle or loop marks)
- Rope, electrical, or immersion burns

Another situation you may encounter is suspected sexual abuse of a child. Some signs and symptoms are:

- Discharge from the vagina or penis, perhaps associated with a sexually transmitted disease
- Lacerations indicating vaginal and/or anal penetration
- Semen on the clothes or body
- Bruising on the genitalia

Child neglect is defined as giving insufficient attention or respect to someone who has a claim to that attention. Neglect usually involves ignoring the child's basic needs for food, shelter, and clothing. Some signs and symptoms of child neglect are:

- Lack of adult supervision
- Malnourished appearing child
- Unsafe living environment
- Untreated chronic illness (e.g., no medication for an asthmatic)
- Delay in reporting injuries

- Poor skin hygiene
- Severe insect infestation
- Lack of medical attention for serious injuries
- Repeated calls to the same residence for pediatric injuries

Physical abuse and neglect are the two forms of abuse that the EMT-B is most likely to suspect. Emotional abuse, while prevalent, is less visible and more difficult to determine in an emergency situation.

D.O.T. OBJECTIVE

Describe the medical and legal responsibilities in suspected child abuse.

Medical and Legal Considerations

If you suspect a child is a victim of abuse, avoid taking the child's history in front of the parents. Do not leave the child alone with a suspected abuser. In dealing with caregivers, do not suggest abuse. Avoid making accusations. Doing so will delay treatment of the child and create a potentially unsafe scene. Take a history from the caregivers separately from the child. Objectively report details of the situation to the hospital personnel. In your documentation, quote statements from the involved parties, if necessary. Provide an assessment of what you saw and heard, not your opinion. Document the:

- Condition of the home
- Behavior of caregivers
- Patterns and location of injuries

In some states, EMS providers are required to report suspicions of child abuse to social service agencies or law enforcement. Follow the child abuse and neglect reporting requirements of your state. See the section on "Confidentiality" in Chapter 3 for more information on cases that are reportable under law in most states.

SPECIAL PEDIATRIC NEEDS

Many infants and children with special medical needs are living at home. They are cared for by family members and home care providers. They have complicated medical conditions and require mechanical support equipment. Occasionally, these children will have an acute emergency or malfunction of their mechanical support equipment. You will be called to provide emergency medical care. Examples of conditions in which infants and children with special needs are cared for in the home are:

- Premature babies with lung disease
- Infants and children with heart disease
- Infants and children with neurologic disease
- Children with a chronic disease or altered function from birth
- Children who become brain-damaged as a result of trauma or near drowning

Medical Support Equipment

Calls related to complications of medical support equipment are common in homebound infants and children. The child's family will usually be familiar with the support device and can be a good resource. Equipment commonly used in the home is:

- Tracheostomy tubes
- Home artificial ventilators
- Central intravenous lines
- Gastrostomy tubes and other gastric feeders
- Shunts

Figure 23.21 *A tracheostomy tube provides unobstructed access to the trachea.*

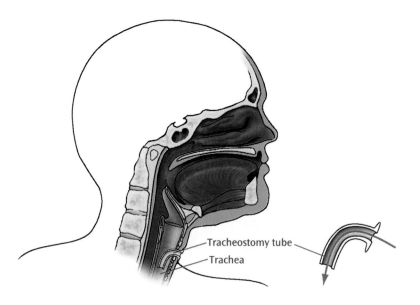

Tracheostomy tube
Trachea

Tracheostomy Tubes

A tracheostomy tube is a short, rigid plastic tube. It is surgically inserted through an opening in the neck (see Fig. 23.21). The tube provides unobstructed access to the trachea. Tracheostomies are performed on children who need ventilator assistance. They are also common in children with neurologic disease who have difficulty managing secretions. Common complications of tracheostomy tubes are:

- Obstruction
- Bleeding
- Air leak or dislodged tube
- Infection around the tube

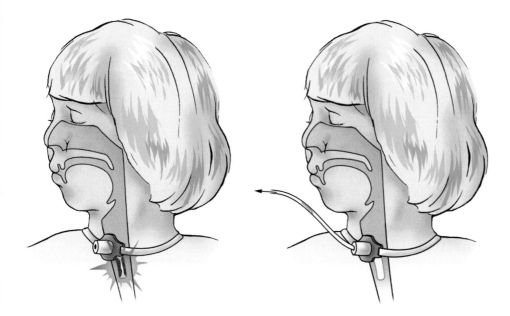

Figure 23.22 *Mucus can be cleared from a blocked tracheostomy tube by suctioning.*

The most common cause of obstruction in tracheostomy tubes is accumulation of mucus. Suctioning with a suction catheter that is half the diameter of the tracheostomy tube can clear mucus (see Fig. 23.22). Avoid suctioning for more than 5 seconds. If frequent passes are necessary, hyperventilate the child before, between, and after suctioning with 100 percent oxygen to prevent hypoxia. Repeat until clear. Assist the child in maintaining a position of comfort and consider transport.

An air leak or dislodged tracheostomy tube may cause a compromised airway. If this occurs, you may have to assist ventilations with a bag-valve mask. For a review of bag-valve mask ventilation of a tracheostomy tube, see Chapter 7. Most pediatric tracheostomy tubes have a standard 15/22 adapter that will connect to a standard bag-valve device. There are two methods for ventilating a stoma. If you are unable to artificially ventilate through the stoma, suction the tube. Then seal the bag-valve mask around the infant's mouth and nose and ventilate. To be effective, you must completely obstruct the stoma with your hand. The second option is to use the bag-valve mask directly over the stoma opening or tube. Cover the infant's mouth and nose with your hand so that the ventilations do not escape through the mouth or nose. Transport the child promptly.

Sometimes an infection may develop at a stoma site. Signs of infection are:

- Redness

- Increased warmth

- Swelling

- Purulent or malodorous drainage

Occasionally, a patient may have bleeding around the stoma. This is usually caused by excessive coughing. The irritation from coughing may cause bleeding into the adjacent soft tissue. Suction the airway frequently to prevent aspirating blood.

The general care for problems with a tracheostomy tube is:

1. Maintain an open airway.

2. Suction mucus and any foreign material.

3. Place the infant or child in a position of comfort.

4. Provide high-flow oxygen with a bag-valve mask. Ventilate once every 3 seconds.

5. Transport. The transport decision should be based on the level of respiratory distress and any other signs of respiratory or cardiac compromise.

Home Artificial Ventilators

A home ventilator automatically assists a patient to breathe. You may be called if a home artificial ventilator malfunctions. Usually, the caregivers know quite a bit about the equipment and can help you troubleshoot. The most common reasons that home ventilators malfunction are:

- Mechanical failure

- Power outage

- Low oxygen supply

Backup batteries may briefly sustain functioning during a power outage. However, in a prolonged outage, the child may need to be transported to a facility with an available power supply. If you are unable to get the ventilator up and running, the patient care steps to follow are to:

- Maintain an open airway

- Provide artificial ventilation with supplemental oxygen

- Transport the child

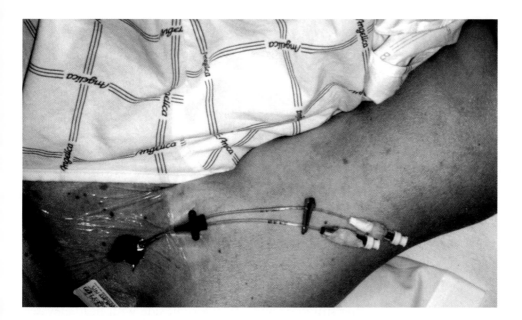

Figure 23.23 *An intravenous line allows immediate access to the bloodstream.*

Central Intravenous Lines

Central intravenous (IV) lines provide permanent intravenous access. A central line is a way to get medications into the bloodstream by tapping into a vein (see Fig. 23.23). Common brand names for venous access devices are Hickman®, Broviac®, Port-a-Cath®, Groshong®, Mediport™, and Infus-A-Port™. Intravenous access is outside the scope of practice for EMT-Bs. However, you may be called to assist in some situations. Common complications of central lines are:

• Cracked line

• Infection

• Clotting off

• Bleeding

• Dislodged line

When providing emergency care for a central line, control bleeding by applying direct pressure to the device. If a line is broken, or if blood is coming through a port on the catheter, apply a clamp to stop the flow of blood. Apply the clamp between the body and the break or port. Transport the patient as soon as possible.

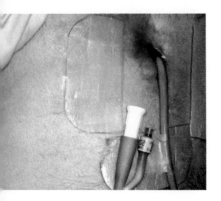

Figure 23.24 *Gastrostomy tube.*

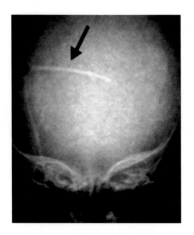

Figure 23.25 *X-ray of a pediatric shunt.*

Gastrostomy Tubes

Many special needs children cannot be fed by mouth. Instead, they are fed directly into the stomach through a gastrostomy tube (see Fig. 23.24). A gastrostomy tube is a flexible, plastic tube. It is surgically placed through an incision in the abdominal wall into the stomach. The child is fed a liquid formula directly through the tube. Infection and a dislodged tube are common complications. Provide the following emergency care for problems resulting from the malfunction of a gastrostomy tube:

1. Establish and maintain an airway.
2. Have suction available.
3. Be alert for altered mental status in a diabetic child. The child will become hypoglycemic quickly if he or she cannot be fed.
4. Provide supplemental oxygen.
5. Transport the child either sitting or lying on the right side with head elevated to reduce the risk of aspiration.

Shunts

Some children have a condition that causes accumulation of excess cerebrospinal fluid in the brain. This condition is called hydrocephalus. Hydrocephalus is treated with a shunt, a device that runs from the brain to the abdomen to drain excess cerebrospinal fluid (see Fig. 23.25). You will usually find a reservoir on one side of the skull. Complications of shunt malfunction are mental status changes and respiratory arrest. When caring for patients with shunt malfunction, establish and maintain an airway. Be prepared to artificially ventilate, suction, and transport.

> **D.O.T. OBJECTIVE**
>
> Recognize the need for EMT-Basic debriefing following a difficult infant or child transport.

EMOTIONAL CONSIDERATIONS

Emergency calls for infants and children can be very emotional situations. Besides the primary patient, you are involved with family members. They may be afraid, harbor feelings of guilt, or feel helpless. Some are injured themselves. Parents may respond to EMT-Bs with agitation, anger, or hysteria.

When your patient is an infant or child, you should strive for a calm, supportive interaction with the family. Calm parents are better able to keep their child calm. Remember that the parents' anxiety arises from concern over the child's pain and well-being. Involve the parents in your care unless medical conditions require separation. Let them hold the child in a position of comfort and try to reduce the child's anxiety. Even though parents may not have medical training, they are the experts on what is normal or abnormal for their children.

Pediatric emergencies can also be difficult for the EMT-Bs who respond. You must recognize your own emotional reactions. You may feel inadequate to provide care because you haven't treated many infants or children. Remember that most of what you know about treating adults applies to children, with the differences you have learned in this course.

Emergency calls involving severely ill or injured children are events that may automatically trigger a CISD session in your system. The CISD process is discussed in Chapter 2. Many EMT-Bs find these calls particularly troubling. Factors that contribute to the high stress levels associated with these calls are:

- Anxiety from a lack of experience treating pediatric patients
- Stress from identifying the patient with your own children or family members
- Emotional distress from assisting others with the grieving process

Chapter Twenty-Three Summary

- Children are very different from adults. Be open and honest when caring for them. Approach them at their level. Be aware of the concerns of children in each age group. Fear is the motivating factor in a child's behavior. Newborns through school-aged children may have difficulty communicating.

- A child's airway is smaller and anatomically different from an adult's. Airway passages are smaller and more easily obstructed.

- Children compensate very well for a lack of oxygen for a short time, then decompensate very quickly.

- Your general impression of a child is very important. A child that looks sick usually is. When forming your general impression, look at how the child interacts with the parents and environment. Listen to the quality of the child's cry or speech. Note how the child responds to your presence.

- Cardiac arrest in children is usually caused by respiratory arrest.

- Respiratory emergencies, seizures, alterations in mental status, and poisonings are frequent causes of EMS calls in children. Evaluate and manage the child's airway and breathing carefully.

- SIDS is the sudden death of an infant during the first year of life. The causes are not clearly understood. Try to resuscitate suspected SIDS patients unless rigor mortis is present. Follow local protocol. Provide emotional support for the parents.

- Trauma is the number one cause of death in infants and children. Blunt injury is most common. Children can sustain serious internal injuries but show few external signs because the protective bone structure is very pliable. Care of a pediatric trauma patient should focus on managing the airway and breathing and rapid transport.

- Child abuse and neglect are serious problems in today's society. Be aware of the signs and symptoms of abuse and neglect. Learn the specific reporting requirements of your state. When caring for children when abuse is suspected, focus on providing emergency care. Do not question or accuse the parents. Document carefully, and provide objective information to the hospital.

- Because of advances in technology, many children with special needs are being cared for at home. Children may have feeding tubes, tracheostomy tubes, home ventilators, central IV lines, or shunts. Use the parents as resources for managing these patients. They often know more about the equipment than you do.

- The best way to interact with parents of an injured or ill child is to involve them in the child's care as much as possible. This gives them a measure of control over the situation.

Key Terms Review

Adolescent | page 676

Capillary Refill Time | page 684

Early Respiratory
  Distress | page 686

Febrile | page 690

Preschooler | page 675

School-Aged | page 676

Sudden Infant Death
  Syndrome (SIDS) | page 693

Toddler | page 674

Review Questions

1. What is the age range of an infant?

   a. Birth to 6 months

   b. Birth to 12 months

   c. Birth to 18 months

   d. Birth to 24 months

2. When examining an adolescent:

   a. Assume that he/she is mature enough to give full and accurate information

   b. Answer questions honestly

   c. Be sure a parent observes all procedures

   d. Tell the patient that he/she should have known better

3. To remove a foreign body from the airway of a conscious 18-month-old patient, use:

   a. Back blows

   b. Chest thrusts

   c. Abdominal thrusts from behind the patient

   d. Abdominal thrusts from beside or in front of the patient

4. Keep the following in mind when performing bag-valve mask ventilation on a child:

   a. A one-hand technique gives the best seal

   b. Avoid thoracic hyperinflation

   c. Do not ventilate if cyanosis is seen

   d. Exhaled air has a high oxygen concentration

5. In young children, fever is a common cause of:

   a. Seizures

   b. Respiratory distress

   c. Death

   d. Shock

6. The cause of SIDS is:

   a. Unknown

   b. Related to child abuse

   c. Related to child neglect

   d. Related to specific preexisting diseases

7. Which of the following is NOT part of the treatment for a pediatric shock patient?

   a. Administer oxygen

   b. Give fluids by mouth

   c. Control bleeding

   d. Keep warm

8. The age group most concerned with disfigurement and permanent injury is:

   a. Toddler

   b. Preschool

   c. Adolescent

   d. Adult

9. Most cardiac arrests in children and infants occur as a result of:

   a. Plaque buildup

   b. Respiratory arrest

   c. Drug overdose

   d. Trauma

10. Provide blow-by oxygen to an infant or child with:

    a. Altered mental status

    b. Decompensated respiratory failure

    c. Cardiac arrest

    d. Signs of early respiratory distress

11. Febrile seizures in children under age 2 are almost always:

    a. Fatal

    b. Harmless

    c. Diabetes-related

    d. Harmful

12. One of the most critical anatomical differences between infants and adults is:

    a. Children and infants have smaller airways

    b. Children and infants have larger airways

    c. Children and infants have less mass in their heads

    d. Children and infants have proportionally smaller tongues

Review Questions *(cont.)*

13. A 13-year-old victim of a car accident will probably be most concerned about:

    a. Disfigurement
    b. Guilt
    c. Embarrassment
    d. Pain

14. Which age group does not like to be touched, have clothing removed, or be separated from their parents?

    a. Infant
    b. Toddler
    c. Preschooler
    d. Adolescent

15. The primary cause of death in children over 1 year of age is:

    a. Complete airway obstruction
    b. Trauma
    c. Poisoning
    d. SIDS

16. If you suspect child abuse, you should:

    a. Report your suspicion to the receiving facility doctor
    b. Ask the child if his parents ever hurt him
    c. Tell the parents of your suspicions, encourage them to seek help
    d. Discuss the case with people you respect to get their opinions

CASE STUDIES

Infants and Children

1 You are dispatched to a retail store in an urban part of town. The dispatcher advises you that the patient is a child with respiratory distress. You find a 4-year-old male sitting with his mother. The mother states that the child ate a large leaf from a plastic display plant. The child has noisy, high-pitched breathing and retractions. He appears to be in acute distress.

A. What is your general impression of the child?

B. What interventions are appropriate for the signs and symptoms?

C. You are able to remove some plastic from the patient's upper airway. He is now crying softly and able to talk, but cannot cough. He is irritable and clings to his mother. Should you transport the child to the hospital? How?

D. If the patient doesn't tolerate a mask, how will you provide supplemental oxygen?

2 Your crew is dispatched to a residence for difficulty breathing. You recognize the address of a young girl with asthma. The mother meets you in the driveway with a limp child in her arms. Your initial assessment reveals a 7-year-old female who appears very sick. The girl is lethargic and will not talk to the EMS crew. Her airway is clear and easily opened. Respirations are very shallow, with a rate of 50. The patient makes a grunting noise with each breath and appears blue about the lips.

A. What is the patient's chief complaint?

B. If her condition is not stabilized, what might occur?

C. What treatment is immediately indicated?

3 You are off duty and shopping at a local grocery store. You hear an announcement requesting any doctor in the store to come to the office. You identify yourself as an EMT-B and offer assistance. The manager directs you to a preschool child lying in his mother's lap, apparently sleeping. The mother left the child for a few minutes and returned to find he had opened a bottle of cough syrup. He told her he took some medicine to feel better. Then he fell asleep in the shopping cart.

A. What should your first action be?

B. You determine that the child is not breathing and has a slow, bounding pulse. His airway is patent. What should you do to prevent cardiac arrest?

C. A first responder unit arrives and continues ventilations with supplemental oxygen. How can you be of further assistance?

Stories from the Field
Wrap-Up

Respiratory compromise is often the cause of cardiac arrest in children. With this child, providing supplemental oxygen despite his resistance to the mask is important. Try placing the oxygen tubing under the arm of a favorite stuffed animal. Have the mother help. The child's injuries require rapid, early transport to a burn center. Treat the burns as you would for an adult patient. Cover the child, keeping him as warm as possible. Burned children can become hypothermic very quickly.

Continually monitor the airway, breathing, and responsiveness. Respiratory burns can cause life-threatening airway problems.

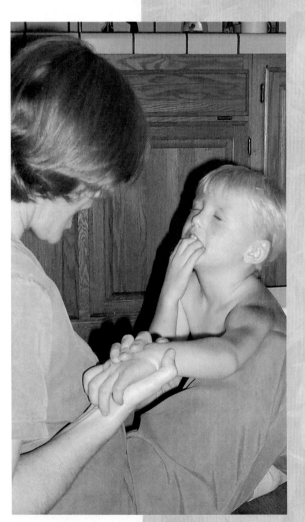

Later, objectively document the father's location and statement and the mother's account of events. Burn injuries may be associated with child abuse. Your first priority is caring for the child, not investigating the incident. Follow the reporting requirements in your area. Do not make accusations. Inform the hospital staff upon arrival. Do not mention causes of the accident in the radio report, which anyone with a scanner can hear.

D.O.T. Module
Operations

7

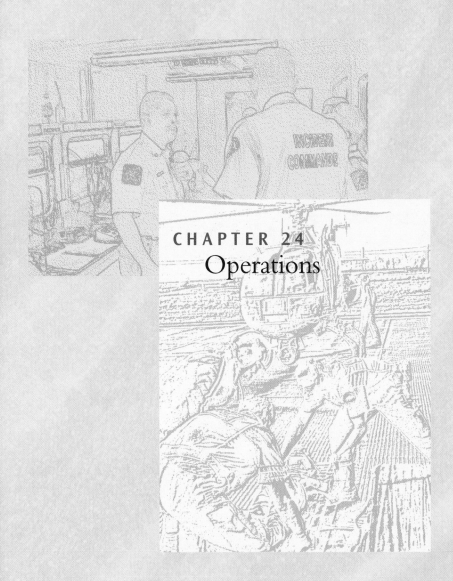

CHAPTER 24
Operations

Chapter

24

Operations

Stories from the Field

Today is one of your last shifts as a student. You are dispatched to a train vs. motor vehicle collision. Because the accident is close to the station, your unit will be one of the first to arrive. No other information is available. As you approach, you see that a train has collided with a tanker truck. The truck was hit just behind the tractor section. Dark, thick smoke is billowing from the tanker.

As you assess the scene from inside your vehicle, a police officer arrives. He begins walking toward the truck. Moments later, the officer falls to the ground and suffers a seizure. Immediately, Robin and John radio for assistance. They move the ambulance out of the area. From your new position, you see several patients on the other side of the train lying on the ground.

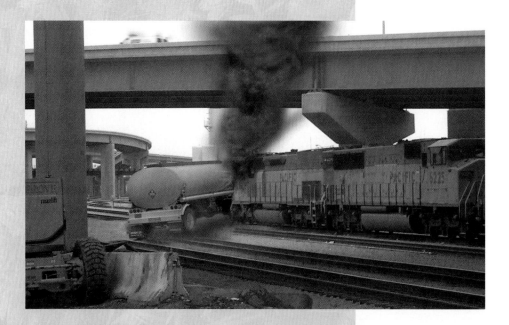

As an EMT-B, you function primarily in the prehospital or out-of-hospital environment. You will respond to many different types of emergencies. Every call involves specific stages. This chapter reviews your responsibilities at each stage. In order to respond at a moment's notice, the medical and nonmedical equipment for patient care and ambulance operations must be systematically maintained. Ambulance operations and driving safety are discussed in this chapter.

In addition to basic patient care, you must also be familiar with special situations including rescues, hazardous materials, and multiple casualty incidents. When multiple casualties are involved, incident management systems are used by EMS to help control and coordinate emergency resources. Patients are triaged based on priority for treatment and transportation. This chapter provides an overview of these specialized EMS responses.

D.O.T. OBJECTIVE

List the phases of an ambulance call.

PHASES OF AN AMBULANCE CALL

The phases of an EMS response can vary. In general, the phases of each call are:

- Vehicle maintenance, preparation, and equipment checkout
- Dispatch to a call
- En route to the scene
- Arrival at the scene
- Transferring the patient to the ambulance
- En route to the receiving facility
- Arrival at the receiving facility
- En route to the station
- Post run

For a successful response, you must manage each phase of the call safely and consistently. Never disregard a phase or leave a stage incomplete. This could reduce the quality of care and increase your risk of legal action. An omission may also cause injury to you, your crew, the patient, or the public.

As you study the following sections, review what you have learned throughout this course. Chapter 1 discusses the roles of an EMT-Basic during all phases of a call. For information on appropriate communications and documentation during a response, review Chapter 10.

Preparation for a Call

The preparation phase involves your duties before receiving a request for services. A properly maintained, well-stocked emergency vehicle is fundamental to response readiness. Illness and injury are unplanned events. You must be prepared to respond to any type of call on a moment's notice. Your vehicle must be ready to roll at all times. You must be able to respond in many conditions. This will help you to reach, care for, and transport the patient in a safe, timely, and professional manner.

Personnel

The qualifications of personnel determine how scene, patient, and transport decisions are managed. In some systems, you will provide initial care until a more qualified EMS provider arrives and assumes control. Learn your local requirements for personnel qualifications and specialized training. All personnel must be prepared to respond to a call and must follow all safety procedures.

The staffing requirements for ambulances vary. The minimum staffing is one EMT-Basic in the patient compartment and one EMT-B or other qualified driver in the front (see Fig. 24.1). Some areas require two EMT-Bs in the patient compartment. This is the preferred minimum level of staffing for an ambulance.

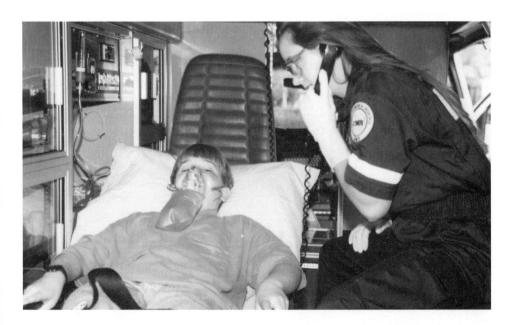

Figure 24.1 *Minimum staffing of an ambulance requires one EMT-Basic in the patient compartment.*

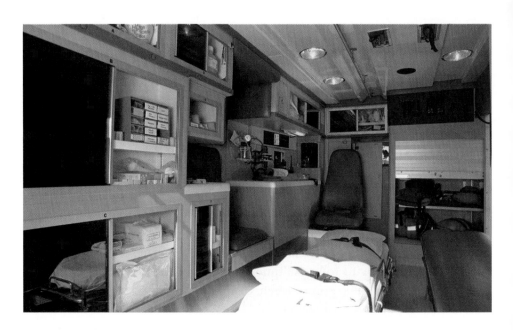

Figure 24.2 *All ambulances are required to carry certain equipment and supplies.*

Equipment

A variety of equipment is needed to manage emergencies. Ambulances carry both medical and nonmedical supplies (see Fig. 24.2). Equipment requirements for ambulances vary by state and municipality. The equipment required will depend on the specific needs of your system, agency, and geographical area. At a minimum, an ambulance must carry:

- Basic supplies
- Patient transfer equipment
- Airway adjuncts
- Suction equipment
- Artificial ventilation devices
- Oxygen delivery equipment
- Cardiac compression equipment
- Basic wound care supplies
- Splinting supplies
- Childbirth supplies
- Medications
- Automated external defibrillator (AED)

  Nonmedical supplies may include:

- Comprehensive maps of the service area showing preplanned routes
- Protocols and standing orders
- Basic mechanical tools

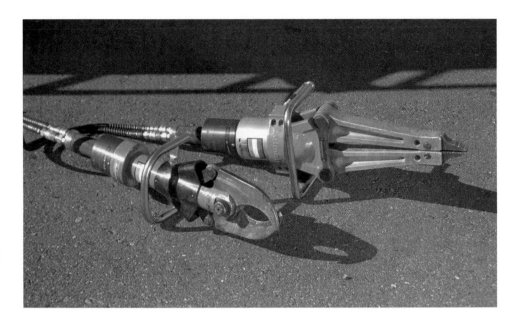

Figure 24.3 *Some emergency vehicles carry specialized rescue equipment such as this power hydraulic spreader.*

- Personal safety equipment
- Equipment for gaining access or extricating victims that is used by personnel with specialized training (see Fig. 24.3)

Never respond to an emergency without the required equipment. A patient's life could hang in the balance. Check all supplies daily. They should be ready to use before each call and they must be restocked, cleaned, or maintained after each run.

Daily Inspection of Equipment

One of your daily duties is to prepare the ambulance and its medical equipment (see Fig. 24.4). A good method is to use an inspection checklist when you come on duty. The list confirms that you have the necessary supplies and equipment. It also helps you to confirm that the ambulance is in safe operating condition.

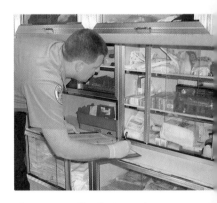

Figure 24.4 *Daily inspection of the vehicle's supplies and equipment is an important EMT-B responsibility.*

Always check, maintain, repair, and restock the ambulance equipment and supplies at the beginning of the shift. Never assume that the previous crew has restocked the vehicle or checked its condition. Check the batteries that power the AED, suction, oxygen, and other critical equipment. Batteries are a leading cause of equipment failure. Become familiar with all equipment and where it is stored.

A systematic and standardized inspection also helps to identify potential problems with the vehicle. Many EMS providers use aggressive preventative maintenance programs to reduce the number of mechanical failures in the field. Some agencies require you to inspect the vehicle for potential problems (see Figs. 24.5 and 24.6). Mechanical maintenance and inspection helps to identify problems before they become serious. A serious problem can endanger

Figure 24.5 *Regularly scheduled inspection of vehicles helps to minimize mechanical breakdowns.*

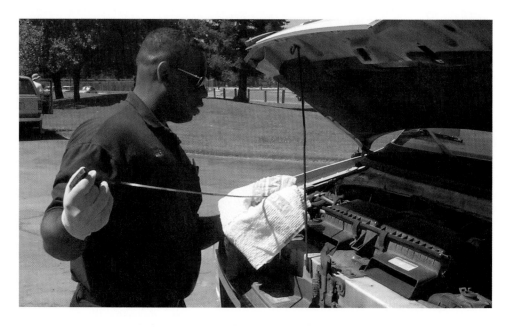

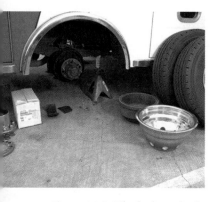

Figure 24.6 *The brakes, wheels, and tires must be in excellent condition. Qualified personnel perform this maintenance.*

passengers. Preventing mechanical failure is an important part of the preparatory phase. At a minimum, a mechanical checklist should include:

- Fuel, oil, and brake fluid levels
- Engine cooling system
- Battery and power systems
- Radiator hoses and fan belts
- Brakes, wheels, and tires
- Headlights, stoplights, turn signals, and emergency warning lights
- Horn and siren
- Wipers
- Door closing and latching devices
- Seat belts
- Dash lights
- Air conditioning, heating, and ventilation systems
- Communication system and radio
- External electrical connectors or shorelines
- Extra oil, brake fluid, and other supplies carried on the unit
- Interior and exterior cleanliness

Your agency will have procedures for reporting problems found during inspections. Always err on the side of safety. If you think a problem will affect safety or patient care, report it immediately. Follow local procedures for submitting problems in writing. You can be held legally accountable for not reporting your concerns.

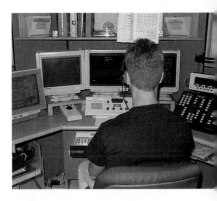

Figure 24.7 *Emergency dispatch center.*

Dispatch

The next phase of a call begins with a request for services. The request is relayed through an emergency dispatch center (see Fig. 24.7). Emergency dispatch centers are also called public safety answering points. They are a central link between members of the public and EMS responders. Dispatch centers provide 24-hour access to EMS through public access telephone numbers. Many communities use 9-1-1. Others have a local seven-digit number to call. Note that cellular telephones do not allow direct access to the local emergency dispatch center. In most regions of the country, 9-1-1 calls from cellular phones are first routed to a commercial phone company or a statewide public safety organization such as the highway patrol. Information is then passed on to local jurisdictions.

In many areas, the dispatch center is staffed by specially trained personnel called Emergency Medical Dispatchers (EMDs). These individuals can advise a caller on how to begin emergency care. They provide step-by-step instructions to callers who have little or no medical knowledge. The information provided by EMDs is directly responsible for saving countless lives. The role of EMDs is discussed in Chapter 1.

When you are contacted by the dispatch center to respond to an emergency, you will usually be told the:

- Nature of the call
- Location of the patient
- Number of patients and potential severity of conditions
- Other special problems

Dispatch may also inform you about additional equipment that will respond to the scene. Some systems notify each unit of the location and route of other vehicles responding. Knowing the location of others enables the driver to choose an alternate route or be aware of converging resources. This information increases your awareness of potential problems that you may encounter.

Ask the dispatcher to repeat or restate information, if necessary. If something is unclear, ask for clarification. Most dispatch information is accurate, but errors may occur. Be open-minded enough to change your plans after you arrive on the scene.

EMT Tip

Repeating information received from the dispatch center to verify accuracy is useful. This technique is called echoing. Writing the information down as you receive it is also helpful.

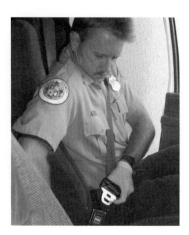

Figure 24.8 *Always wear your seat belt when riding in an emergency vehicle.*

En Route to the Scene

The next phase of the call is the response to the scene. Before leaving the station, you should:

• Quickly check the vehicle

• Make sure the outside compartment doors are closed and secure

• Disconnect external electrical cords

• Retrieve and properly store jump kits

• Fasten your seat belts (see Fig. 24.8)

• Adjust all mirrors and seats

• Scan the instruments for normal operation

Always follow safe driving guidelines as discussed later in this chapter. As you are rolling, prepare for events at the scene. While en route, the crew should:

• Notify dispatch that you are responding to the call.

• Confirm and clarify essential dispatch information. This should include the nature and location of the call, the number of patients (if known), and the severity of injuries (if known).

• Obtain additional information about special conditions or problems, updates on the situation, and other units en route to the same scene.

• Predetermine team member responsibilities and duties.

• Assess equipment needs.

• Call for advanced life support units, if necessary.

• If needed, request additional resources such as law enforcement, special rescue teams, or aeromedical response units.

In many EMS systems, the EMD updates the call information while you are en route.

Arrival on Scene

Arrival at the scene should be orderly and safe. Maintaining scene control is one of the most difficult skills to master. Your actions should be timely, organized, and efficient. Your primary goals are to:

• Assess the patient

• Provide immediate interventions

• Prepare for safe transport to the appropriate facility

When you arrive, notify the dispatcher. Take BSI and standard precautions before patient contact. Use gloves, gowns, and eyewear as appropriate. Assess the scene for hazards. Do not become part of the problem. Review the information on personal and scene safety in Chapter 2. Evaluate the situation on a risk versus benefit basis. Ask yourself:

- Is the emergency vehicle parked in a safe location?
- Is it safe to approach the patient?
- Should the victim be moved immediately because of hazards?
- Can the patient self-evacuate? If not, then call for appropriate assistance and wait.

To save valuable time, consider possible injuries and a potential course of action before leaving your vehicle. The mechanism of injury or nature of illness provides clues to the actions you should take. Immediately integrate any new information into your plan. For example, you might arrive on a scene where an unconscious elderly man is lying outside his garage. At this point, you might suspect syncope, stroke, or a medication problem. As you approach, you notice a small pool of blood coming from his nose. A stepladder is leaning against the garage. With this new information, you would consider that the man may have fallen from the ladder.

Chapters 5, 8, and 9 detail further steps for assessing a patient's condition. Review Chapter 7 for management of the airway. Treatment methods for patients with medical conditions are covered in Chapters 12–15. Procedures for stabilizing traumatic injuries are found in Chapters 19–22.

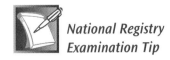

National Registry Examination Tip

Recognize the importance of scene safety awareness. Remember the steps for scene safety. Be able to recognize and use dispatch information. This will give you valuable clues about scene safety and patient condition.

D.O.T. OBJECTIVE

Differentiate between the various methods of moving a patient to the unit based upon injury or illness.

Transferring the Patient to the Ambulance

As you care for a patient, you will prepare to transfer him or her to the ambulance. Patient packaging is usually done during the focused history and physical exam or the rapid assessment. Select a moving technique based on the patient's illness or injury and location. Consider each situation carefully. Make sure you do not compromise the quality of patient care. Review Chapters 6, 21, and 22 for considerations while immobilizing, lifting, and moving a patient.

Choose the most suitable device for moving the patient. Secure him or her correctly. Determine the best position for transport. Often, the patient can be transported in a sitting position. However, the patient's condition may require special positioning. Consider the need to maintain a clear airway, apply direct pressure, or perform chest compressions. Some patients must be transported in a supine position to maintain cervical spine immobilization (see Fig. 24.9).

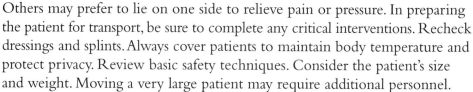

Figure 24.9 *Choose an appropriate method and position to move your patient.*

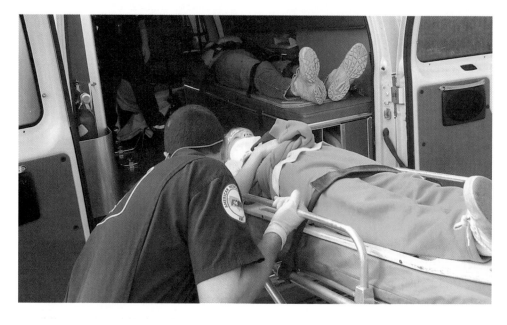

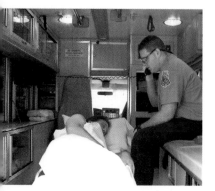

Figure 24.10 *Communicate the patient's condition to the receiving facility.*

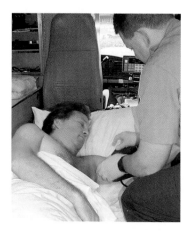

Figure 24.11 *Continue to assess and manage your patient while en route to the receiving facility.*

Others may prefer to lie on one side to relieve pain or pressure. In preparing the patient for transport, be sure to complete any critical interventions. Recheck dressings and splints. Always cover patients to maintain body temperature and protect privacy. Review basic safety techniques. Consider the patient's size and weight. Moving a very large patient may require additional personnel.

En Route to the Receiving Facility

Quickly check the unit before leaving the scene. Make sure that outside compartment doors are closed. Check for obvious mechanical problems. While en route to the hospital, your crew must:

- Follow all safe driving guidelines and show due regard for other motorists.
- Notify dispatch of your destination and the level of response.
- Notify the receiving facility of your estimated time of arrival. Provide them with clear, accurate information about the patient's condition (see Fig. 24.10).
- Continue ongoing assessments and repeat vital sign measurements. Perform a detailed assessment as necessary (see Fig. 24.11).
- Reassure the patient.
- Notify the receiving facility if the patient's condition deteriorates or improves. Keep your partner informed of the patient's condition. Work as a team.
- Complete prehospital care reports if the situation allows.

Family Members

Family members may ask to ride in the ambulance with the patient. This is particularly true when the patient is an infant or child. Your local policies and agency procedures will help you to decide how to handle the request. If family members accompany the patient, give them clear directions before moving the vehicle. Advise them about where to sit and what is expected of them during the transport. Insist that passengers wear their safety belts.

The patient's family or friends may want to follow the ambulance to the hospital. In this situation, tell them the following:

- Give directions to the receiving facility.
- Instruct the driver not to follow too closely behind the ambulance or to try and keep up with you. This presents a risk to the patient, your ambulance crew, and the driver of the vehicle.
- Advise the driver that he or she must obey all traffic laws. He or she must not follow you through intersections.
- Reassure the family that you will provide the best care possible during transport.

CD-ROM Link

The video "Paramedic in the Ambulance" in the Authentic Emergency Scenes section of the Video Appendix on the MedEMT CD-ROM shows the sense of urgency and professionalism despite the cramped quarters in the rear of an ambulance.

D.O.T. OBJECTIVE

Apply the components of the essential patient information in a written report.

Arrival at the Receiving Facility

When you arrive at the hospital, notify the dispatch center. To complete the call and transfer care, additional steps are required. Continue care until you transfer the patient to hospital personnel. In some situations, this may be an EMS professional of equal or higher certification. A written prehospital care report (PCR) must be completed and left at the receiving facility before you return to service (see Fig. 24.12). Review the material in

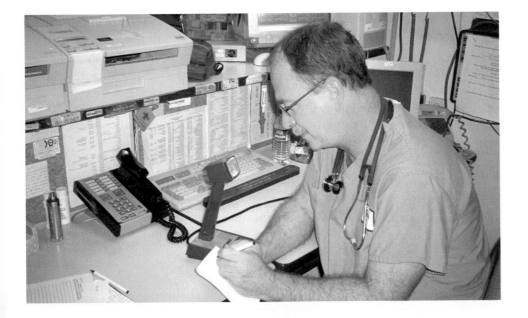

Figure 24.12 *Provide a report on your patient to the health care professional assuming care at the receiving facility.*

Chapter 10 for components of your written and verbal reports to hospital personnel. Remember that failure to transfer care properly may be considered patient abandonment (see Chapter 3).

Tiered Emergency Response

Some EMS systems have a tiered emergency response protocol. This is true for many areas in which few providers have advanced EMT training. In a tiered response, an EMT-Basic crew initially cares for and transports the patient. In the meantime, an advanced crew is dispatched to the scene or to a designated meeting place. In some systems, one or more advanced providers move to the basic ambulance. They will assume responsibility for patient care and continue to the hospital in this vehicle. In other tiered systems, the patient is transferred from the basic ambulance to an advanced-care ambulance.

If you are transferring care to another EMS provider, supply him or her with all the information that you would normally give to the staff at the receiving facility. Also furnish written documentation from the scene. Make sure the transporting crew knows how to contact you in case additional information is required. Transfer the patient's valuables or personal effects. Write the disposition of belongings on your report. You cannot complete the final steps in the response until hospital personnel or another EMS provider assumes care.

> **D.O.T. OBJECTIVE**
>
> Identify what is essential for completion of a call.

En Route to the Station and Post Run

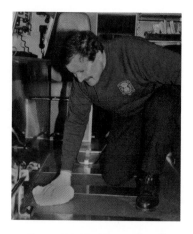

Figure 24.13 *Preparation for the next call includes cleaning the ambulance.*

Preparing the ambulance after a call is a critical step in call completion. Remember that requests for service have no pattern. In many systems, an ambulance may not return to the station immediately. You may not return at all during a busy shift. You may be dispatched to another call directly from the hospital. The unit must be ready to respond immediately after every call.

Before returning to your station, prepare for the next call. Clean and disinfect the ambulance and equipment (see Fig. 24.13). Restock disposable supplies. Preparing your unit before returning to the station makes you available immediately. This benefits the next patient and the other units in the system. If you are not able to adequately restock any required medical or nonmedical supplies, you must notify the dispatch center immediately. They must know that your unit is out of the system until the issue is resolved. Waiting for several minutes before you notify the EMD makes system management more difficult.

During the post-run phase, you may find yourself in a parking lot, station house, or hospital ambulance bay. Many systems have time limits on preparing the unit for the next call. After the run, you should:

- Collect equipment left at the hospital by your unit or others in your agency
- Exchange linens, spine boards, and other equipment that must be left at the hospital (if this is local policy)
- Inspect the ambulance and equipment
- Clean and disinfect the ambulance
- Clean and disinfect equipment
- Replenish used supplies and restock disposable supplies
- Return and secure equipment to the proper storage areas
- Refuel the unit
- Complete run reports
- Notify dispatch that the unit is ready for another call

Notify dispatch before leaving the hospital. Advise them if you cannot adequately clean and restock your ambulance. Follow local protocols for cleaning the vehicle. Never respond to an emergency call until the ambulance is 100 percent ready.

EMT Tip

Most seasoned EMS providers will tell you that any missing equipment or supplies are commonly needed when you least expect it. Even if you have not used a piece of equipment for months, if you do not have it, you can bet it will be urgently needed on the next call.

D.O.T. OBJECTIVES

Summarize the importance of preparing the unit for the next response.

Distinguish among the terms cleaning, disinfection, high-level disinfection, and sterilization.

Describe how to clean or disinfect items following patient care.

Decontamination

Decontamination is an important part of preparing the ambulance for the next call. Cleaning the vehicle, equipment, and supplies is essential to infection control. You do not want to be exposed to an infectious disease. Likewise, you do not want subsequent patients to be exposed. The CDC have identified four levels of decontamination:

1. Sterilization
2. High-level disinfection
3. Disinfection
4. Cleaning

Sterilization is a process that destroys all microbes. It involves using pressurized steam, gas, or immersion in an approved chemical solution. High-level disinfection, like sterilization, eliminates all microorganisms. However, it cannot eradicate large numbers of bacterial spores. It is used for instruments that have come in contact with mucous membranes. High-level disinfection involves hot-water pasteurization with a water temperature of 176° F to 212° F. Soaking times are determined by manufacturer's recommendations.

Disinfection | *Removal of germs, bacteria or other potentially infectious materials*

Disinfection destroys most pathogens, including the tuberculosis bacterium. It does not destroy bacterial spores. Disinfection is done by wiping the area with an approved chemical germicide. A common solution used in ambulances is 1:100 chlorine bleach in water.

Cleaning is similar to disinfection. It destroys most bacteria and some viruses and fungi. It cannot destroy the tuberculosis bacterium or bacterial spores. Cleaning is done by wiping the surface with a common disinfectant (see Fig. 24.14).

Figure 24.14 *Cleaning is an important part of preventing the spread of illness from one patient to another.*

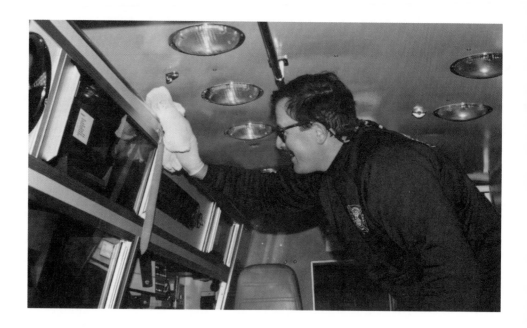

EMT Alert

Wash your hands immediately after cleaning the ambulance patient compartment.

DRIVING SAFETY AND LAWS

Safe driving is essential for a successful response and good patient care. You must be physically and mentally fit to operate an emergency vehicle safely. The ability to work under stress, a positive attitude, and knowing your abilities and limitations are important. You must be tolerant of other drivers. However, you must also anticipate unpredictable or dangerous actions.

Most localities or states recommend or require emergency vehicle drivers to attend an approved emergency vehicle operator's course. While operating an emergency vehicle, you are subject to special driving laws, ordinances, and regulations. You also have a special responsibility to ensure the safety of your crew and the public. You must always operate an emergency vehicle with a due regard for the safety of other motorists.

D.O.T. OBJECTIVE

Describe the general provisions of state laws relating to the operation of the ambulance and privileges in any or all of the following categories: speed, warning lights, sirens, right-of-way, parking, and turning.

Laws and Regulations

Most states have similar laws, regulations, and ordinances governing the operation of an emergency vehicle. Usually, special rules address:

- Specific emergency or disaster routes
- Speed limit regulations
- Direction of traffic flow or specified turns
- Procedures at red lights, stop signs, and intersections
- Procedures near school buses
- Use of audible warning devices or sirens
- Use of visual warning devices or lights
- Vehicle parking and standing

Some state and local governments have additional rules and regulations. You must learn and understand the laws, regulations, and ordinances in your area before operating an emergency response vehicle.

Emergency vehicle operation regulations provide exemptions from the normal traffic laws in very specific circumstances. Strict conditions must be met before using these exemptions. You must follow the regulations in your area. If these conditions are met, then you may usually:

- Exceed posted speed limits
- Drive through red lights, flashing red lights, stop signs, and stop signals
- Drive against the right-of-way at uncontrolled intersections
- Drive through "Yield" or "Merge" signs
- Disregard "No Turn" signs for right or left turns

- Disregard proper traffic lanes
- Drive the wrong way on a divided highway or one-way street
- Drive left of the center line
- Cross double or single solid lines
- Pass on the right side of other moving vehicles
- Change directions
- Continue past a school bus that is loading; however, you may not pass a bus that is unloading, unless directed by a crossing guard
- Disregard emergency or disaster routes or blockades
- Disregard parking and standing regulations

Before using these exemptions, most states mandate that the situation must be a true emergency. Continually evaluate whether the time you save will affect the patient's outcome. If so, then using red lights and the siren during exemptions may be justified. If the time saved will not affect the patient's well-being, routine transport without red lights and siren is appropriate. When operating an ambulance under normal conditions, you must obey all applicable laws, rules, and regulations. Normal conditions exist when you are driving, but not responding in an emergency mode.

D.O.T. OBJECTIVE

Discuss "Due Regard for Safety of All Others" while operating an emergency vehicle.

Due Regard for the Safety of Others

Despite the permitted exemptions, you must always drive with due regard for the safety of others. If you disregard this standard, you are endangering lives and you may be held legally and financially accountable for the consequences of your actions. It is important to remember that your actions may be evaluated and criticized years after an accident, by individuals unfamiliar with the stresses and realities of EMS. They will apply the standard of "Due Regard for the Safety of Others" when examining your behavior behind the wheel.

D.O.T. OBJECTIVE

List contributing factors to unsafe driving conditions.

Safe Driving Practices

Safe driving directly affects your ability to provide skilled care. To ensure the safety of everyone involved:

- Be sure the driver and all passengers wear safety belts.
- Know the characteristics of your vehicle, such as acceleration, braking, and cornering. Many ambulances, particularly vans and sport utility vehicles, are top-heavy and will tip or overturn easily.
- Select an appropriate route.
- Drive with due regard for safety of other drivers and pedestrians at all times.
- Maintain a 3- to 4-second following distance between the ambulance and the vehicle in front of you.
- Be alert to changes in weather and road conditions.
- Exercise caution when using red lights and siren. Know when to use them. Know when not to use them.
- Keep the headlights on at all times; they are the most visible warning devices on an emergency vehicle.
- Use a spotter to guide you when you are backing up.

Many things contribute to unsafe emergency vehicle operation. However, certain elements are most commonly cited after the fact. They are:

- Failure to show due regard for other motorists
- Excessive speed
- Reckless driving
- Failure to obey traffic signals or posted warnings
- Failure to consider weather and road conditions
- Failure to heed dispatch warnings
- Inadequate dispatch information
- Multiple emergency vehicle response
- Miscommunication with escorts

D.O.T. OBJECTIVE

Describe the considerations that should be given to: intersections, request for escorts, and following an escort vehicle.

Intersections

Be especially cautious at intersections. They are the most common sites of emergency vehicle collisions. A motorist may run a red light, or other vehicles may obstruct your vision as you enter the intersection. In a response involving multiple emergency vehicles, waiting motorists may mistakenly assume that the first emergency vehicle is the only one. They resume movement into the intersection as the second vehicle approaches, increasing the risk of a crash.

Vehicle Escorts

Sometimes you will need an escort while traveling to or away from the scene. Use escorts only if you are unfamiliar with the location of the patient or receiving facility. Avoid escorting one emergency vehicle with another. You may think that this will clear a path and speed up transport. However, it does not save time. Multiple vehicles traveling at high speeds with lights and sirens can be a factor in serious accidents.

When a multiple-vehicle response is necessary, the D.O.T. recommends that none of the vehicles use lights or sirens. When traveling with an escort, maintain a safe following distance. Follow at least 500 feet behind the escort car. Agree on a communications channel with other drivers. Clearly communicate with each other during the escort.

D.O.T. OBJECTIVE

Discuss various situations that may affect response to a call.

Other Potential Hazards

A number of factors can negatively affect your emergency response. Some depend on your geographic location. Be aware of potential problems in the following situations.

Ignorant, aggressive, or abusive drivers. Unfortunately, not everyone respects the needs of emergency vehicles. Some individuals blatantly disregard traffic rules. This creates major safety problems for you and other drivers. During many EMS responses, these drivers endanger themselves and the ambulance. They may pull to your right, chase the ambulance, or stop suddenly. This increases the risk of serious accidents. If another driver's actions are placing you at risk, immediately contact dispatch. Request law enforcement assistance.

Detours. You should be familiar with major road construction and repairs in your area. If you see major detours that affect response routes, notify dispatch immediately. They can relay this information and recommend alternate routes to other responders.

Time of day. Traffic patterns change with the time and day of the week. Traffic jams may be a problem. A good method for avoiding traffic jams is to listen to the local traffic reports during your shift.

Holiday seasons. In urban and suburban areas, holiday seasons can disrupt traffic patterns. Shopping malls are a particular problem. Be aware of these changes and plan alternate routes.

Railroads. In some areas, railroad tracks crisscross the landscape. If you don't know the train schedules, you could be caught at a crossing waiting for a long, slow train. If railroad tracks lie along your normal response routes, plan alternate routes.

Schools and school buses. Avoiding areas where young children and school buses are common is always best, if possible. Children are notorious for dodging into traffic. Know when the schools in your immediate area are in and out of session. Slow down when passing schools, or any areas in which children congregate.

Weather. Adverse weather conditions may affect a safe response. If snow or ice is a factor in your area, be familiar with routes that are cleared frequently. Most areas designate snow routes. Make sure your vehicle is equipped for rapidly changing weather conditions. Avoid surprises. Change to snow tires or four-wheel drive units early in the season. Monitor the condition of wiper blades. Check the antifreeze, heaters, and other supplies needed in difficult weather.

Positioning the Unit at the Scene

Upon arrival at the scene, position the ambulance for safe and timely patient access. Park in a driveway or on the shoulder of the road, if possible. Take up the entire road on narrow or no-parking roads. Avoid parking in a location that might impede your safe exit.

As you approach the scene in your vehicle, look for clues suggesting potential hazards. For example, after a motor vehicle accident, leaking fuel can burn or explode. To be safe, always park at least 100 feet in front of or beyond the scene of a MVC (see Fig. 24.15). Hazardous materials can leak and spilled fluids travel downhill. In this situation, park at least 2,000 feet upwind and uphill from the accident.

Figure 24.15 *Park emergency vehicles at a distance that protects your working area.*

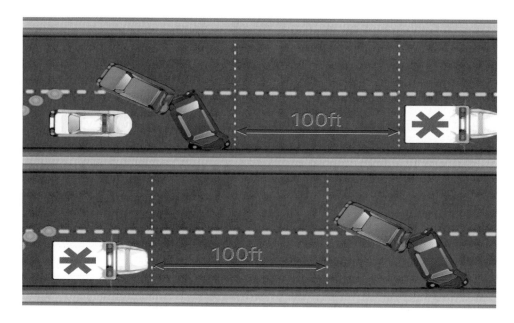

Always set the parking brake to prevent the ambulance from rolling. Also, shut off the headlights unless you must illuminate the scene. Follow local laws for using warning lights and signals. Learn the ordinances regarding emergency vehicle parking and standing. In many areas, ambulance security is also a concern. The ambulance and equipment can be stolen or vandalized while unattended. To reduce the risk, park in well-lighted areas, remove the keys, and lock the doors.

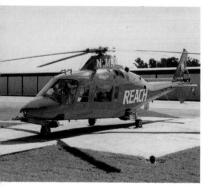

Figure 24.16 *Aeromedical helicopter.*

AEROMEDICAL SERVICES

In many areas, helicopter transport is a standard of care (see Figs. 24.16 and 24.17). They are used routinely for certain medical problems and traumatic injuries. The helicopter is an extension of the emergency department. Statistics show that many lives are saved as a direct result of rapid transport and emergency care given in the helicopter.

Consider using aeromedical services for patients with significant mechanisms of injury, such as:

• A vehicle rollover in which the passengers are unrestrained

• A collision causing the death of an occupant in the same vehicle

• Ejection of a patient from the vehicle

• A rider thrown from a motorcycle at a speed greater than 10 m.p.h.

• A pedestrian struck by a car at a speed of greater than 10 m.p.h.

• A fall of greater than 20 feet for an adult or 10 feet for a child

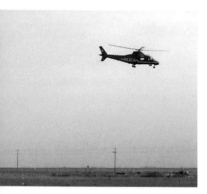

Figure 24.17 *Rapid transport is a major benefit of helicopter transportation.*

Helicopters are invaluable as a rapid transport option. Consider time and distance in situations in which:

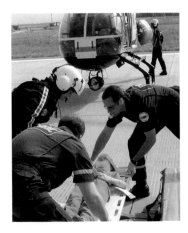

Figure 24.18 *Preparing the patient for aeromedical evacuation.*

- The time for ground transport to an appropriate facility is more than 15 minutes. This is true even if ground transport to a hospital without a trauma center would require less time than air transport to a trauma center. Follow local protocols.
- The patient is entrapped and extrication will take longer than 15 minutes.
- The resources of local ground units are limited, and ground transport will deprive the area of EMS personnel.
- The patient will benefit from rapid delivery to more advanced in-hospital care.

Aeromedical response reduces the time between an injury and definitive hospital care (see Figs. 24.18 and 24.19). This is a major benefit to patients. However, avoid delaying ground transport to use aeromedical services. If you must wait for air transport, consider using ground transport. If the difference in arrival time between the two methods is small, consider immediate ground transport. Know and follow your local policies.

Figure 24.19 *Arriving at the receiving facility.*

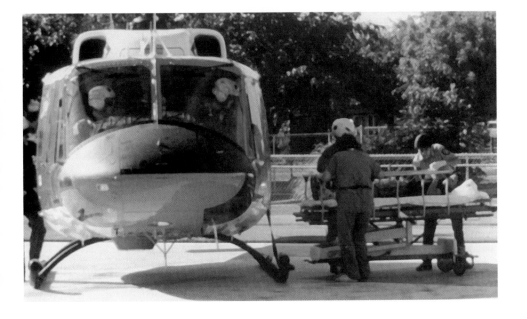

Helicopter Scene Safety

You must know basic safety procedures even if you have little contact with helicopters. Safety around an aircraft is everyone's responsibility. General considerations are:

- Stay at least 100 feet away from the landing zone. Keep spectators at least 200 feet away (see Fig. 24.20).

Figure 24.20 *Helicopters create special hazards for rescuers.*

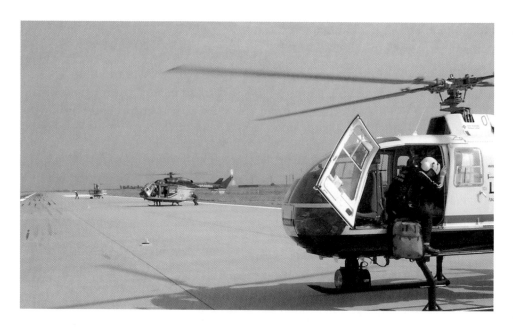

- Never point spotlights at an aircraft. Turn off white or clear lights in the landing area. Lights may blind the pilot or affect his or her vision on final approach.

- Never approach a helicopter until the pilot signals that it is safe. Always follow the helicopter crew's directions.

- Crouch down when approaching the rotor blades.

- When a helicopter gets close to the ground, the rotor blades pull air upwards. This causes dust, rocks, grass, and other loose items to blow around, creating potentially hazardous rotor wash. Keep the patient and crew clear of the rotor wash area. Secure loose items that might blow away.

- Do not permit smoking within 100 feet of the aircraft. This reduces the risk of fire.

- Always stay clear of the tail rotors. This is true even when patients are loaded from the rear. Remember that the rotors may be invisible when turning.

Contact your local aeromedical team to learn about special courses on helicopter safety in your area.

Landing Zone

After requesting a helicopter, immediately prepare for its arrival. Establishing a safe landing zone is essential. More than one person will be needed. You cannot be in charge of patient care and establish the landing zone. Doing this endangers everyone. Use the following steps to prepare a landing zone:

1. Identify a communications person. He or she should have a good sense of direction and be familiar with the immediate area. This person should not be directly involved in patient care.

2. The communications officer contacts the air dispatch center to provide information. Inform the dispatcher of the unit calling and their call sign, the radio frequency to use, and the number of aircraft needed. Tell them the location of the incident and any prominent landmarks in the area.

3. Set up a landing zone. The area must be free of obstructions. The ideal size is 100 feet by 100 feet. The minimum acceptable size is 60 feet by 60 feet. The landing zone must be on level ground at least 50 feet from parked vehicles. Mark each corner of the landing zone with an independent lighting system. Put a fifth lighted warning device on the upwind side to specify wind direction (see Fig. 24.21).

4. If the landing zone is on a roadway, stop traffic in both directions.

5. If conditions are dusty or dry, try to wet down the landing area. Blowing dust may be a problem for the pilot and others on the ground. Wetting the area also reduces the risk of fire.

6. The communications officer radios information to the helicopter about power lines, poles, antennas, or trees. Lights may be used to illuminate these hazards.

7. Assign one person to guide the pilot in. Wearing eye and ear protection, this person stands near the wind direction marker. He or she faces the touchdown area, back to the wind. The guide raises his or her arms overhead to signify the landing direction. Follow the exact instructions of the pilot or crew.

8. If possible, have fire personnel and equipment standing safely nearby the landing zone.

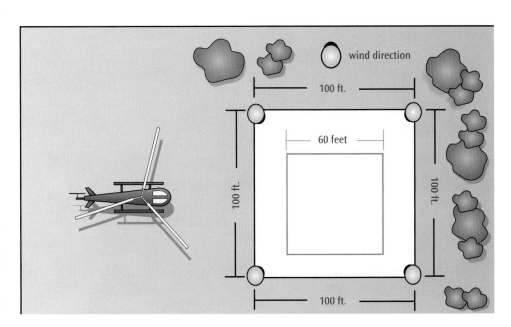

Figure 24.21 *Place lights at the corners of the landing zone.*

PATIENT EXTRICATION

Extrication is the process of removing a patient from entanglement. Safe and efficient procedures must be used. Extrication services are needed in many situations. Examples of extrication scenes are:

• Vehicle crashes

• Industrial accidents

• Structure collapses

• Trench collapses

• High-angle falls

Most of the time, items that surround and entrap a patient must be removed or disentangled. This is done using cutting, spreading, or prying equipment (see Fig. 24.22). Disentanglement provides a passage for patient access and removal.

Figure 24.22 *Disentanglement allows access to and removal of the patient.*

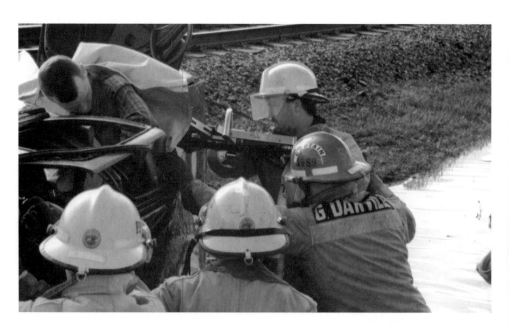

Safe, effective extrication requires proper knowledge, skills, and equipment. Three fundamental components of extrication are:

- Safety
- Equipment
- Patient management

Specially trained EMTs, firefighters, or law enforcement personnel may be responsible for extrication. In some systems, EMT-Basics are responsible for extrication, rescue, and medical care. Special classes on extrication techniques are available. You may not be responsible for rescue and extrication. However, you must understand the actions, safety, and medical aspects of the process. Become familiar with your local protocols. Solid communication and excellent teamwork are essential.

D.O.T. OBJECTIVE

Discuss the role of the EMT-Basic in extrication.

Role of the EMT-Basic

As an EMT-B, your role will vary with local protocols and the circumstances of the call. Patient care is always your first priority, unless delays would endanger the life of a patient or rescuer. Personnel involved in an extrication must establish a chain of command or incident command system. Following the chain of command ensures good patient care. The incident command system for situations involving multiple casualties is discussed later in this chapter.

When other personnel handle a rescue, you will be responsible for patient care before and during extrication. You must ensure that he or she is removed without further injury. Work together with the other rescuers. Coordinate your interventions with their activities. Extrication must not interfere with patient care.

In some situations, you may be responsible for extrication operations (see Fig. 24.23). In this case, your role changes. Rescue EMT-Bs focus on careful and efficient patient removal. Other responders will manage the patient's medical needs. If you must function in both roles simultaneously, make patient care your first priority.

Figure 24.23 *You may be involved in the extrication or rescue process.*

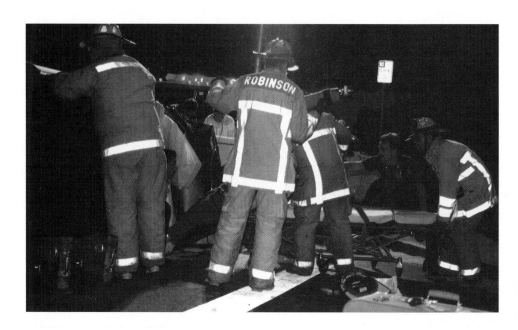

D.O.T. OBJECTIVES

Identify what equipment for personal safety is required for the EMT-Basic.

State the steps that should be taken to protect the patient during extrication.

Rescue Scene Safety

Personal and patient safety is important during extrication. Be aware of hazards on the scene:

- Sometimes, hazardous materials prevent you from gaining access. Become familiar with your local hazardous materials response plan.

- Because of the nature of extrication, the risk of fire is increased. Someone must focus on reducing the chance of fire. This may be as simple as turning off a car's ignition. It may be as complicated as shutting down power lines or gas meters.

- Unstable vehicles pose a risk for the patient and rescuers. Assess the stability of each vehicle before moving too close to it. Stabilize vehicles if necessary before beginning patient care or extrication (see Fig. 24.24).

You are responsible for your own safety and the safety of patients and bystanders (review Chapters 2 and 8). Your personal safety takes priority. Wear personal protective equipment suitable for the level of potential hazards (see Fig. 24.25). For extrication, appropriate PPE may include:

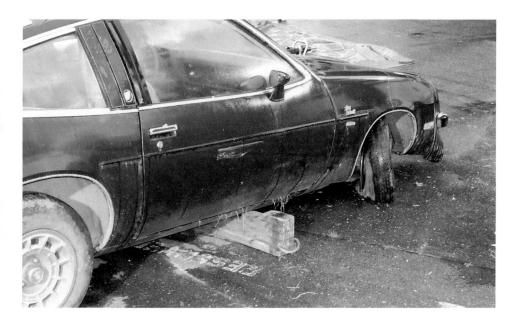

Figure 24.24 *Place wood blocks under a vehicle to prevent it from shifting during a rescue.*

- Impact-resistant helmet with ear protection and chin strap
- Protective eye wear, ideally with an elastic strap and vents to prevent fogging
- Lightweight, puncture-resistant turnout coat
- Leather gloves or other OSHA-approved hand protection
- Calf-high boots with steel insoles and steel toes
- Body substance isolation and standard precautions equipment such as latex gloves, face shields, eye protection, and HEPA filters

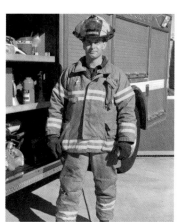

Figure 24.25 *Appropriate PPE for extrication procedures.*

In many extrication situations, an inner circle or boundary is established around the patient. The circle concept helps to maintain a safe scene and reduces the risk of injury to the responders. Within the circle, all personnel must wear the necessary PPE. Outside the circle, EMS crew members are not required to wear the same PPE as those inside the inner circle.

After personal safety precautions, patient safety is your next priority. As you provide initial care and the extrication efforts begin, follow these guidelines to maintain a safe and efficient scene:

- Communicate with the patient. Explain what is happening, including sounds, smells, and possible movements. The patient is probably frightened and unfamiliar with all the sounds usually found on the scene of an extrication effort.
- Protect the patient throughout the extrication. Cover him or her with a blanket to protect against broken glass, sharp metal, the environment, and other hazards (see Fig. 24.26). If possible, get under the blanket with the patient. Continue your assessment using a small light.

Figure 24.26 *A blanket or tarp helps to protect the patient during extrication operations.*

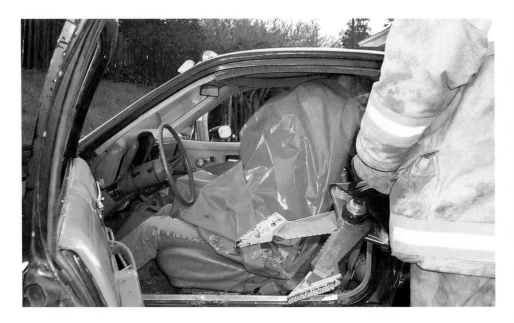

- Limit the number of people who interact with the patient. He or she is already frightened. Additional people asking questions or talking loudly adds unnecessary confusion and stress.

- Limit bystanders' access to the scene. Bystanders increase the risk for additional injuries and communication problems (see Fig. 24.27).

Figure 24.27 *Bystanders' motives may include concern for the patient, a desire to help, or plain curiosity. Keep them away from the scene.*

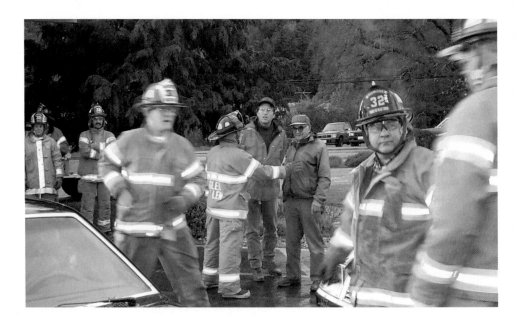

Extrication Equipment

Specialized equipment is fundamental to extrication. The most important equipment is an EMS vehicle equipped for rescue. There are three types of rescue vehicles. Light duty units are basic rescue units. They carry simple hand tools and basic

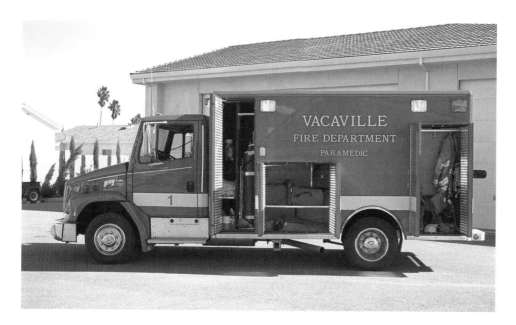

Figure 24.28 *Light-duty rescue units are equipped with basic rescue tools.*

hydraulic tools (see Figs. 24.28 and 24.29). The tools are used to help remove patients from simple entanglement. They are useful when patients need immediate removal and care. Many ambulance services stock their units with basic hand tools.

Medium-duty units carry all the equipment carried by light-duty units. In addition, they have specialized equipment such as:

* Port-a-powers, or manually operated hydraulic spreaders
* Powered hydraulic spreaders and cutters (see Fig. 24.30)
* Hydraulic rams

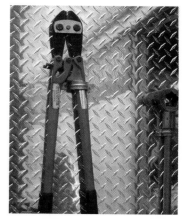

Figure 24.29 *A typical hand tool mounted in the equipment compartment.*

Figure 24.30 *Medium-duty units carry more specialized equipment.*

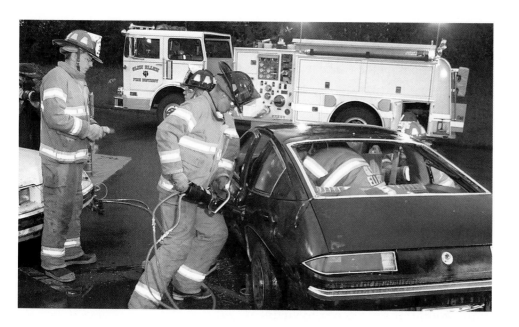

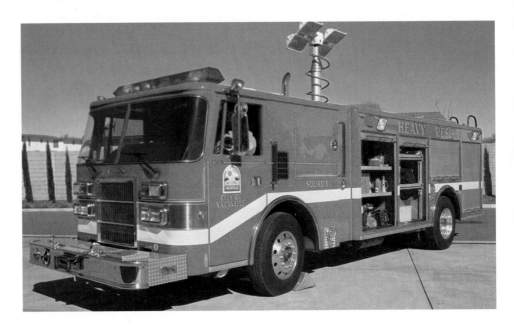

Figure 24.31 *Heavy-duty units are used in more complex rescues.*

Heavy-duty units are the most advanced rescue vehicles (see Fig. 24.31). They are equipped for complex rescues. Rescues requiring specialized tools require a heavy-duty vehicle. They carry the same equipment as light- and medium-duty units, as well as:

• High- and low-pressure air bags

• Cutting torches

• Dive equipment

• Rigging

• High-angle rescue equipment

D.O.T. OBJECTIVES

Evaluate various methods of gaining access to the patient.

Distinguish between simple and complex access.

Gaining Access to the Patient

Proven techniques are used for gaining access to patients during extrication. Patient access is categorized as simple or complex. This helps to identify the level of equipment and staff needed. Use common sense to decide which methods will work best. Always consider the patient's condition and level of entrapment.

• Slightly trapped patients are able to be removed by lifting or moving debris from around or on top of the victim.

- Moderately entangled patients require more advanced extrication procedures. Specialized tools will be needed. Patients in this situation can usually be disentangled in a short time.

- Severely entangled patients are pinned by heavy or complex debris. Extrication requires highly sophisticated equipment. Removing the patient may take hours or days.

Simple access does not require sophisticated equipment and can be done by all EMT-Bs. In these situations, attempt simple solutions. Avoid unnecessary property damage and wasted time. Try to open each door, window, gate, or other device. For example, in an auto accident, the patient may be able to safely unlock a door or roll down a window. If glass might break, use a spring-loaded center punch to gain access (see Figs. 24.32 and 24.33). This removes the glass safely, providing immediate access.

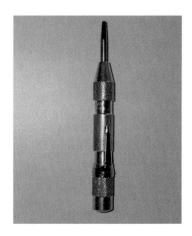

Figure 24.32 *Spring-loaded center punch.*

Figure 24.33 *The impact from a center punch causes the window to crumble.*

Simple Access | *A rescue that does not require sophisticated equipment*

Complex Access | *A rescue requiring specialized skills and equipment*

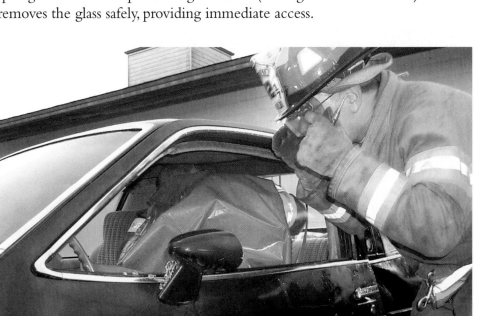

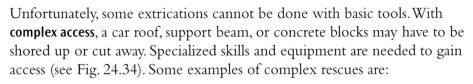

Unfortunately, some extrications cannot be done with basic tools. With **complex access**, a car roof, support beam, or concrete blocks may have to be shored up or cut away. Specialized skills and equipment are needed to gain access (see Fig. 24.34). Some examples of complex rescues are:

- Water rescues
- Motor vehicle crashes involving significant entrapment
- High-angle rescues
- Trench, cave, or structure collapses

In these situations, highly trained staff must assist in the rescue. These specialized skills are taught in separate programs (trench, high-angle, and basic vehicle rescue). Without additional training, you are responsible for emergency care.

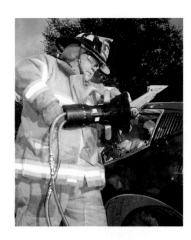

Figure 24.34 *Cutting into a car to reach the patient is a complex rescue.*

Figure 24.35 *Stabilize the patient's spine as soon as you can reach him.*

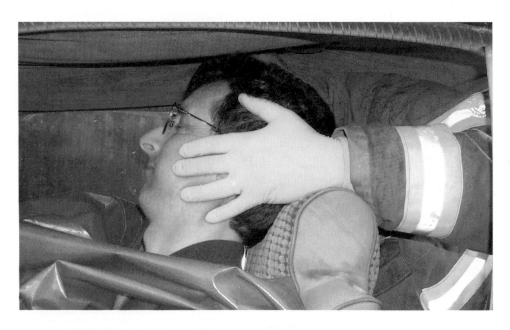

Removing the Patient

Once physical contact with the patient is safe, stabilize the spine immediately (see Fig. 24.35). Pay particular attention to the cervical spine. Complete an initial assessment and provide critical interventions. If the ABCs are compromised, consider rapid extrication procedures (see Chapter 6).

After the patient is secured and critical care has been given, extrication can begin (see Fig. 24.36). Select the exit path of least resistance that reduces the risk of further injury. Be sure enough personnel are available for the job. During patient removal, continue protecting yourself, the crew, and the patient from hazards.

Figure 24.36 *Removal of the patient after disentanglement.*

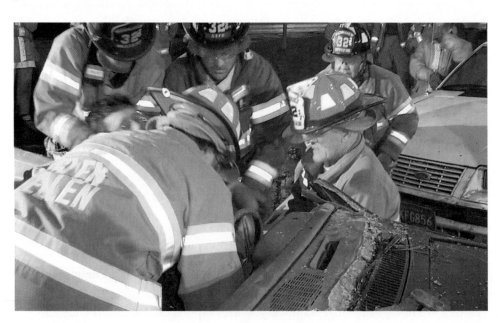

HAZARDOUS MATERIALS

Hazardous materials, abbreviated **HAZ-MAT**, include chemicals and substances that are potentially harmful. They increase the risk of injury, health problems, or significant property damage if not controlled properly. Recognizing hazardous materials is an important part of scene size-up and patient care. Billions of tons of hazardous materials are produced each year. The exact extent of uncontrolled exposures is unknown. Hazardous material exposures are a common problem. Always consider hazardous materials when responding and during scene size-up.

Becoming an expert in hazardous materials is not necessary to perform the duties of an EMT-Basic. Dealing with a hazardous material emergency requires specialized training and equipment. You must quickly recognize that a hazardous substance is present and prevent further illness or injury. You must also learn how, when, and who to contact when arriving on the scene of a possible hazardous materials call.

Most hazardous materials events involve man-made substances. However, you may also respond to a scene involving natural hazardous materials. For example, if underground mining is common in your area, natural gases are a constant threat. In other areas, flash floods could be hazardous. Floods can quickly kill people and destroy property. Preplanning is the key to preparing for natural hazards.

For any HAZ-MAT response, focus your attention on scene safety. First ensure personal and crew safety. Patient safety is your next concern, followed by the well-being of the general public. Begin forming an impression of the scene as you approach. If you are not sure that you will be safe, do not enter. Bystanders should be asked to leave the area. Once appropriate personnel declare that the scene is safe, continue with the response.

Hazardous Material (HAZ-MAT) | *Substance that is potentially harmful or that presents an unreasonable risk for injury, health problems, or significant property damage if not properly controlled*

D.O.T. OBJECTIVES

Describe what the EMT-Basic should do if there is reason to believe that there is a hazard at the scene.

Break down the steps to approaching a hazardous situation.

Approaching the Scene

As you know, each scene is unique. Learn to trust your senses when you suspect hazardous materials. Your sense of smell works well in many emergencies. However, you cannot rely on this alone to detect the presence of hazardous materials. Many hazardous materials are odorless, colorless, or both, and can be rapidly fatal. Some visual clues suggesting a problem are:

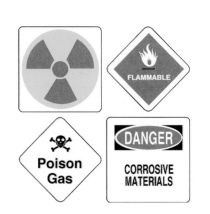

Figure 24.37 *Signs or placards like these indicate the presence of hazardous materials.*

- Smoldering or self-igniting materials
- Boiling or active chemicals
- Color waves or vapors over the scene
- Frost near a container
- Unusual or rapid deterioration of a container or items in contact with the material
- Dead animals or obviously injured patients
- Presence of warning signs on vehicles or labels on containers (see Fig. 24.37)
- Multiple unconscious people in the same location

Adapt your approach to a hazardous material scene to ensure safe arrival. Never assume anything when hazardous materials are present. Always treat the scene as potentially dangerous until a HAZ-MAT expert advises you it is safe. The steps for approaching a potentially hazardous situation are:

- Park a safe distance away from the scene, upwind and uphill
- Avoid contact with the materials
- Notify law enforcement early
- Keep all unnecessary people away from the area
- Isolate the area

When approaching a hazardous materials scene, quickly attempt to identify the material causing the problem. Then look for patients who may be affected by the substance. If they are safe, ask them about the materials involved and what happened. Secure the scene and limit the exposure of rescuers and bystanders. Do not enter the scene unless you are specifically trained in HAZ-MAT operations. Wear the appropriate personal protective equipment.

This may include a full-body suit or a **self-contained breathing apparatus or SCBA** (see Fig. 24.38). Only after the substance has been identified and the scene is secured should you remove patients to an established safe zone.

Identifying the Material

The size and shape of a container may offer clues to the material inside. Look for labels listing the name of the material or the type of hazard. Shipping papers provide specific information for vehicles that are transporting hazardous materials. These describe the material, list the hazard classification, and show a four-digit identification number for the substance. Shipping papers must be in the driver's possession at all times. Look for them in the cab on a clipboard or inside an envelope.

The U.S. D.O.T. requires vehicles transporting a large amount of hazardous materials to display highly visible labels or placards. These labels are color-coded to describe specific hazards (see Fig. 24.39). The colors indicate the following hazards:

- Red signifies flammable material
- Yellow indicates reactive material or oxidizers
- Green symbolizes nonflammable gases
- White denotes poisons
- Orange signifies explosives
- Blue means water-reactive material
- White/red striped symbolizes flammable solids
- Yellow/white indicates radioactive material
- White/black represents corrosive material

Self-Contained Breathing Apparatus (SCBA) | *Equipment that provides clean air to a rescuer and protects him or her from hazardous vapors*

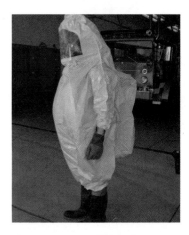

Figure 24.38 *A full-body HAZ-MAT suit may be necessary for hazardous materials incidents. This suit includes SCBA equipment.*

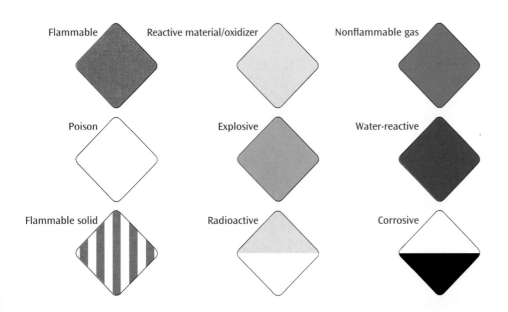

Figure 24.39 *Color-coded hazard placards.*

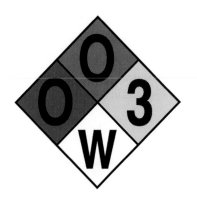

Figure 24.40 *NFPA 704 placards use numbers and symbols to indicate dangers. This material has no health or fire hazard, but there is a significant reactivity hazard (3) with water (W).*

In addition to color codes, the placards may display a four-digit identification number. A legend may state whether the material is flammable, radioactive, explosive, or poisonous. Not all vehicles carrying hazardous materials have placards. If the quantity of material is small, labels may not be required.

The National Fire Protection Association (NFPA) has also adopted a labeling system for hazards called NFPA 704. Materials are divided into four hazard categories (see Figs. 24.40). Substances are rated according to the degree of danger. Nonhazardous substances are rated 0. The most hazardous substances are rated 4. These labels are also color-coded:

- Blue for health hazard
- Red for fire hazard
- Yellow for reactivity hazard

A white area contains information regarding radioactivity, oxidation hazards, or special protective equipment requirements. Refer to Figure 2.10 in Chapter 2 for the complete NFPA 704 key.

> **D.O.T. OBJECTIVE**
>
> Explain the methods for preventing contamination of self, equipment, and facilities.

Containing Contamination

EMS responders have a major responsibility to contain and control the spread of the dangerous materials. You must ensure that patients, equipment, and personnel are decontaminated before leaving the scene. Decontamination is the process of physically removing contaminants and/or converting them to harmless substances.

If medically required, a patient may be transported before decontamination is complete. In this situation, the transport must not endanger the EMS crew or the general public. Confirm that the receiving hospital is prepared to receive a contaminated patient. They must be able to decontaminate the EMS staff, patient, equipment, ambulance, and other materials used on scene. Be overly cautious when transporting contaminated patients, staff, or equipment.

Your local EMS system will have a designated decontamination plan. Follow the plan exactly. Each HAZ-MAT event has specific steps for decontamination. A typical plan usually includes the following basic steps, which may be set up at separate stations.

1. Segregated equipment drop. Place external equipment in decontamination pools with plastic liners.

2. Wash and rinse outer garments. Showers are used to wash external clothing, such as boots and gloves.

3. Outer boot and glove removal. External boots and gloves are deposited in lined containers.

4. Tank change. This step occurs here only if the responder has left a hot zone for a tank change. Subsequent stations are designed to remove additional equipment. Otherwise, this will be the last station.

5. Self-contained breathing apparatus removal. SCBA removed and stored in plastic containers.

6. HAZ-MAT suit and boot removal. Removal of external environmental suits and boots.

7. Field wash. Shower to wash completely.

After following the required steps, complete a written report of the event. Describe your steps and exposure levels in detail.

HAZ-MAT Resources

As hazardous material emergencies become more common, **HAZ-MAT teams** are being trained to manage these emergencies. HAZ-MAT teams consist of personnel specially trained to manage emergencies involving hazardous materials. Your first resource is your local hazardous materials response team.

HAZ-MAT Team | Personnel specially trained to manage emergencies involving hazardous materials

Many EMS providers are required to participate in specialized training for hazardous materials. Two federal agencies, the Occupational Safety and Health Administration (OSHA) and the Environmental Protection Agency (EPA) have developed regulations to protect responders. These agencies make recommendations for controlling hazardous substances. OSHA CFR 1910.120 identifies four levels of hazardous materials training:

• First Responder Awareness—Personnel are trained to identify problems and notify the proper authorities.

• First Responder Operations—Designed for personnel responsible for protecting life, property, and the environment.

• Hazardous Materials Technician—Training for personnel who will contain and manage the hazardous materials.

• Hazardous Materials Specialist— A level of training designed for responders with advanced knowledge and skills. This person provides command and support activities on the scene of actual hazardous material events.

The U.S. D.O.T. provides a valuable publication entitled *Hazardous Materials: The Emergency Response Handbook* (DOT P5800.6). This guide illustrates the standard shapes and colors used for coding hazardous materials signs. Every emergency vehicle should be equipped with this book.

EMT Tip

Always think of personal, crew, patient, and bystander safety first. If something at a scene does not seem right, be suspicious and do not enter the area. Always use proper personal protective equipment.

Another resource is the Chemical Transportation Emergency Center (CHEMTREC). This center is a public service division of the Chemical Manufacturers' Association. They maintain a 24-hour, 7-day-a-week hotline at (800) 424-9300. The center provides current information on managing and controlling hazardous substances. CHEM-TEL Inc. is a similar information resource center. They can be reached at (800) 255-3924. When accessing these resources, be prepared to provide the:

- Identification number of the material
- Nature of the problem
- Location of the emergency
- Call-back number and your name
- Guide number
- Shipper or manufacturer of the product
- Type and condition of the shipping container
- Rail, car, or truck number

D.O.T. OBJECTIVES

Describe the basic concepts of incident management.

Define the role of the EMT-Basic in a disaster operation.

INCIDENT MANAGEMENT SYSTEMS

Incident Management System (IMS) | A system designed to control, direct, and coordinate emergency responders and resources in case of a disaster

At a large-scale or dangerous emergency scene, a simple, efficient, task-based management structure is critical. In many areas, disaster operations require the implementation of an **incident management system (IMS)**. These systems are designed to control, direct, and coordinate the allocation of emergency responders and resources (see Fig. 24.41). An IMS:

- Provides an orderly way to communicate information vital to decision making
- Facilitates interactions among allied agencies using a single command structure

Once a major incident is reported, an incident manager is assigned. This person assigns all personnel to specific sectors as they arrive. The incident manager might also be called a branch director or incident commander. He or she is usually the senior EMT on the scene. The incident manager establishes specific EMS divisions or sectors for the incident (see Fig. 24.42). These include:

- Extrication
- Treatment

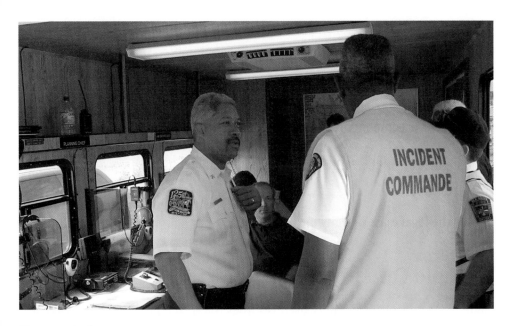

Figure 24.41 *The command post is a key part of an Incident Management System.*

- Transportation
- Staging
- Supply (personnel and equipment)
- Triage
- Mobile command center
- CISD
- HAZ–MAT

After you are assigned to a specific sector, immediately report to the sector officer for your duties (see Fig. 24.43). Report back to the sector officer after completing each assigned task. Stay within your assigned area. Avoid moving from one sector to another without specific instructions.

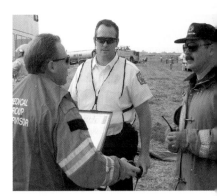

Figure 24.42 *Individual sectors are established to oversee key aspects of the incident.*

Figure 24.43 *Communicate with your sector commander when finished with each assignment.*

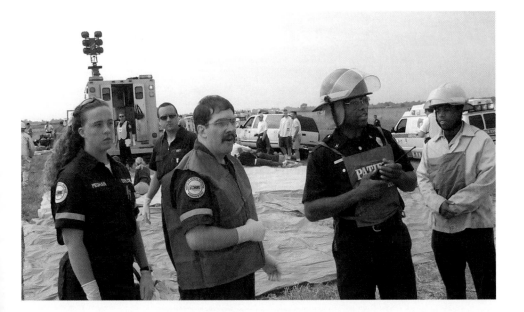

Multiple Casualty Incidents

Multiple casualty incidents (MCIs) are responses that place great demands on the equipment and personnel within a local EMS system. An MCI is also referred to as a multiple casualty situation (MCS). An MCI can involve a few serious injuries or several hundred patients (see Fig. 24.44).

Figure 24.44 *Staging area for a mass casualty incident.*

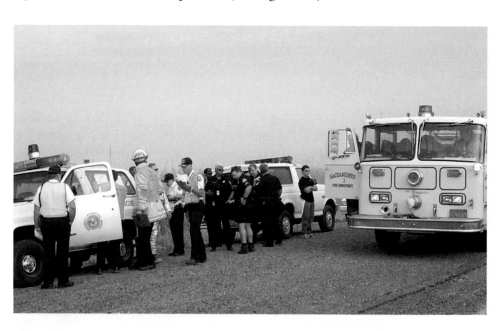

Multiple Casualty Incident (MCI) | *Response that can involve a few serious injuries or several hundred patients; can place great demands on a local EMS system*

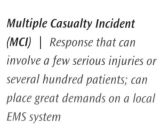

When arriving on the scene of an MCI, quickly estimate the number of patients. Identify the need for, and type of, additional help to request. The first arriving and most knowledgeable EMS provider begins triage. Follow the local MCI policy. Basic triage involves sorting multiple casualties into priority levels for emergency care and transportation (see Fig. 24.45). Triage helps you to determine the:

• Number of injuries
• Severity of injuries

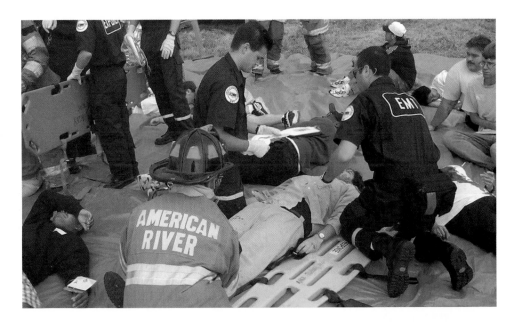

Figure 24.45 *During triage, patients are quickly assessed and prioritized for treatment.*

- Resources needed to care for the patients
- Priority of each patient for care or transport

Sorting and triaging multiple patients is a difficult and emotional process. START is an acronym for "simple triage and rapid treatment or transport." In this triage model, EMT-Basics are trained to quickly determine the status of each patient. Every patient is given a very quick assessment in a very short amount of time. There are four levels of priority used for patient triage. Based on their priority, each patient receives a color-coded tag. Patients are sometimes placed on color-coded tarps corresponding to their priorities (see Fig. 24.46).

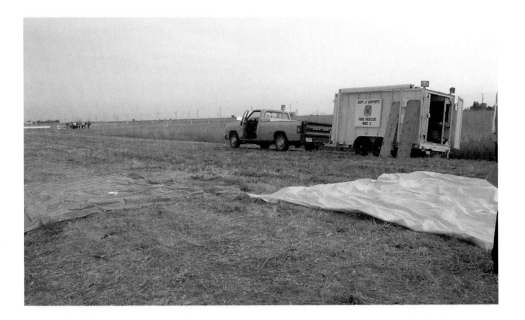

Figure 24.46 *Tarps are used to identify various MCI sectors or patient priorities.*

Each patient's priority level is recorded on a color-coded triage tag that is attached to him or her (see Fig. 24.47).

Figure 24.47 *Triage tags are used to record patient information during an MCI. They are usually two-sided.*

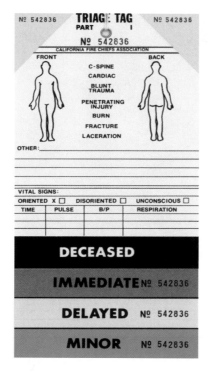

Highest priority patients require immediate care. This level is color-coded red (see Fig. 24.48). Most personnel and equipment will be concentrated on treating or transporting patients in the highest priority category. These patients have:

- Airway and breathing difficulties
- Uncontrolled or severe bleeding
- Decreased mental status
- Severe medical problems
- Shock
- Severe burns

Figure 24.48 *Rapid identification of priority patients is an important part of MCI management.*

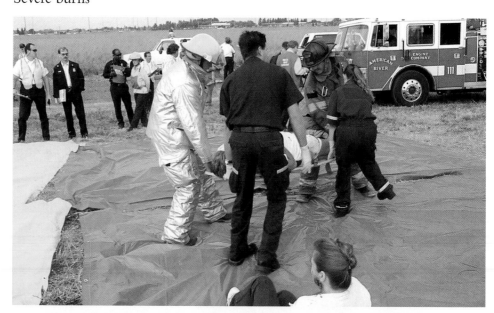

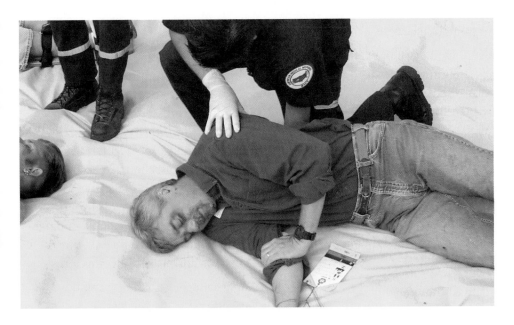

Figure 24.49 *A rapid assessment helps to determine the patient priority.*

Second priority patients can have care delayed. They are color-coded yellow (see Fig. 24.49). These include patients with:

- Burns but no airway problems
- Major or multiple bone or joint injuries
- Back injuries, with or without spinal cord damage

Lowest priority patients require minor care. These injuries are color-coded green (see Fig. 24.50). The conditions include:

- Minor painful, swollen, deformed extremities or fractures
- Minor soft tissue injuries

Deceased patients are color-coded black. This assessment is based on:

- Obvious or imminent death due to vital organ failure, total body incineration, and so forth
- Absence of vital signs
- Massive blood loss
- Very severe head injuries
- Major chest trauma

The triage officer completes the initial assessment. He or she will continue to assign and coordinate personnel, supplies, and patient transport (see Fig. 24.51). Transportation decisions are based on a variety of factors, including:

- Patient prioritization
- Destination facilities and capabilities
- Transportation resources

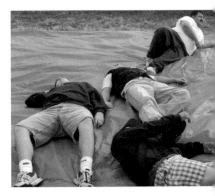

Figure 24.50 *Some patients with minor injuries can be grouped for mass transport.*

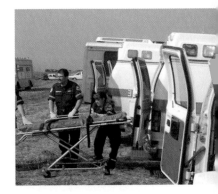

Figure 24.51 *Proper utilization of ambulances and hospital resources is important in making a transport decision.*

Chapter Twenty-Four Summary

- Every EMS call has specific stages, from preparation to post run. Learn your responsibilities during each stage. Carefully plan for the next stage as you handle each call.

- Air medical services are an excellent resource for managing critically ill or injured patients. They provide advanced care and rapid transport to receiving facilities. Safety is your first priority when dealing with air medical services.

- Your role may include rescuing a patient. Patient care takes priority over rescue unless delayed movement will endanger the life of the patient or rescuers. You are responsible for your own safety and the safety of your crew, the patient, and bystanders.

- When trying to gain access to a patient, try simple things first, such as unlocking doors, rolling down windows, or opening doors. Choose the path of least resistance. Be sure to have sufficient personnel to rescue the patient safely. Protect the patient from hazards created during the rescue. Use available resources for special rescue situations.

- Hazardous materials are transported by air, land, rail, and water. Safety is your primary concern. Never enter a hazardous materials scene without proper training and protective equipment. Always park upwind and uphill of a hazardous material scene. Secure the scene to keep bystanders away. As you approach the scene, look for evidence of hazardous materials. Shipping containers, placards, container labels, and shipping papers provide information. Use resources such as CHEMTREC for additional information.

- Incident management systems help to control and coordinate emergency resources during disasters. Sectors or divisions are established to support EMS operations. The incident commander assigns responsibilities to individuals based on a preestablished plan.

- Mass casualty incidents place a great demand on resources. The goal is to provide the greatest good for the most people possible. Patients are triaged based on their priority for treatment. This is determined by the initial assessment or an abbreviated assessment. After triage, patients are treated and transported based on priority, available resources, and destination hospitals.

Key Terms Review

Review Questions

1. Emergency equipment and medical supplies should be checked:

   a. Hourly
   b. Daily
   c. After each run
   d. Weekly

2. Decontamination that uses hot water treatment is called:

   a. Sterilization
   b. High-level disinfection
   c. Disinfection
   d. Cleaning

3. CHEMTREC provides:

   a. 24-hour information on hazardous materials
   b. Spill clean-up equipment and personnel
   c. Media coverage of HAZ-MAT incidents
   d. Compensation for losses due to HAZ-MAT incidents

4. If you encounter a HAZ-MAT incident, the first thing you should do is:

   a. Attempt to rescue the patient
   b. Isolate the area and keep people away
   c. Determine if there has actually been a spill
   d. Retrieve the shipping papers

5. The major purpose of an incident management system is to provide:

   a. Independent functioning of EMTs on the scene
   b. A separate command post for each agency involved
   c. Single, integrated control and communication
   d. Physicians as incident commanders

6. The first emergency unit to arrive on the scene of a multiple casualty incident should immediately:

   a. Assess patients for treatment priority
   b. Complete a size-up scene, report conditions, and request needed resources
   c. Begin treatment of the most critical patients
   d. Move patients to appropriate treatment areas

7. You arrive on the scene of a cardiac arrest to discover that the batteries in your defibrillator are dead. Who is responsible for ensuring that properly working equipment is present on your ambulance?

   a. You
   b. The crew you relieved
   c. Your supervisor
   d. Equipment officer

8. What information should you provide to hospital staff during transfer of patient care?

   a. Next of kin
   b. Chief complaint
   c. Occupation
   d. ETA

9. Which of the following is NOT part of the minimum medical equipment to be carried on an ambulance?

   a. Airways
   b. Ammonia inhalants
   c. Suction equipment
   d. Splinting supplies

10. What should you do if you believe a problem with the ambulance might adversely affect safety or patient care?

    a. Explain your concerns to the patient
    b. Report concerns in writing to the proper staff
    c. Abandon the ambulance immediately
    d. Advise the nearest law enforcement officer

11. When transferring care to hospital staff, report all of the following EXCEPT:

    a. The patient's name
    b. Additional treatment provided
    c. Additional radio frequencies used
    d. Repeat the chief complaint

Review Questions *(cont.)*

12. A(n) _____ can assist in identifying the material or type of hazard that a vehicle is carrying.

    a. Emblem
    b. Billboard
    c. Placard
    d. PCR

13. Which of the following conditions would be considered high priority in a multiple casualty situation?

    a. Cardiac arrest
    b. Severe bleeding
    c. Multiple fractures
    d. Nausea and vomiting

14. Triage of patients involves sorting patients into _____ levels.

    a. 2
    b. 3
    c. 4
    d. 6

15. EMT personnel should stay at least _____ feet away from an incoming helicopter.

    a. 10
    b. 25
    c. 30
    d. 50

CASE STUDIES

Operations

1 Crew change is always a hectic time. Several ambulances arrive and depart within minutes of each other. Today is no different. As you begin the unit inspection checklist, dispatch informs your partner that all ambulances are busy. Your unit is the only one available in the entire county. During your hurried inspection, you discover the ambulance is low on fuel. The tubing for the in-house oxygen system is cracked. It is leaking continuously. Your partner advises you that this is an ongoing problem with this rig.

A. How will you handle this situation?

2 You are responding to a man down near the chemical facility just outside city limits. Until today, the production plant has operated without any major incidents. As you arrive, you notice a large tractor in a field. A man is waving at you wildly. There appears to be a layer of fog lying close to the freshly-tilled ground. You smell a strong odor of ammonia. The man tells you that his friend is in the tractor. The operator is unresponsive and breathing very heavily. You realize that this is an unsafe scene and that your personal safety is endangered.

A. List the visual clues suggesting a hazardous materials event.

B. What are your immediate actions?

C. State the cardinal rule for approaching the scene of a potential hazardous materials event.

3 You are dispatched to a serious MVC at one of the worst intersections in the county. While en route, you learn that one of your company's ambulances is involved. A good friend of your partner is injured. Several emergency vehicles are converging on the same intersection from different directions. Your partner is driving too fast for road conditions.

A. What actions should you take immediately?

B. Describe conditions that adversely affect an emergency response.

4 Early in the morning, you are dispatched to a multiple vehicle crash. This is very unusual in your rural area. Several tractor trailers and twenty passenger vehicles are involved. En route, dispatch advises you that several of the big rigs are on fire. Bystanders report multiple fatalities. Your unit is the first to arrive on the scene. As you approach, you can see the fires. Your partner grabs some triage tags and heads toward the accident scene. As you get out trauma gear, you hear sirens approaching in the distance.

A. As the first unit to arrive, what initial actions will you take?

B. Describe the basic purpose of an incident management system.

C. Define multiple casualty situation.

D. Describe the concept of triage.

E. What factors must be considered when making transport decisions at a scene with multiple casualties?

Stories from the Field
Wrap-Up

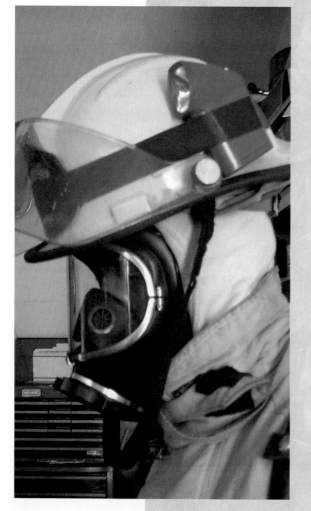

You must consider many safety issues when approaching this scene. Personal safety is your first priority. Because there is evidence of hazardous materials, you immediately move your vehicle and crew uphill and upwind. You can often identify a hazardous material from placards on the carrier vehicle. Never enter a hazardous material scene unless properly trained and equipped. Call for assistance from specialized services or teams. Secure a perimeter around the danger area. With the assistance of the HAZ-MAT team, establish a decontamination area. Also set up areas for initial treatment and transport for multiple patients.

After the victims have been removed by trained personnel, be prepared to assess and treat them. Use a triage system to assign each patient a priority. Good communication among providers, incident commanders, and receiving hospitals is essential. Ensure that receiving facilities are aware of the suspected chemical exposure. Your patient care is based on signs and symptoms. Also obtain information from material safety data sheets or the chemical manufacturer.

Appendices

Advanced Airway Management

T he most efficient method for maintaining the airways of unresponsive patients who require continuous positive pressure ventilations is endotracheal intubation, also known as orotracheal intubation. Endotracheal intubation is an advanced technique for intervening and maintaining a patient's airway and breathing. Review the basic information on airway anatomy and physiology before studying advanced airway management (see Fig. A.1). The anatomy and physiology of breathing and management of the airway are discussed in Chapter 4, Chapter 7, and Chapter 12. Special considerations for infants and children are found in Chapter 23.

Figure A.1 *The anatomical structures of the respiratory system.*

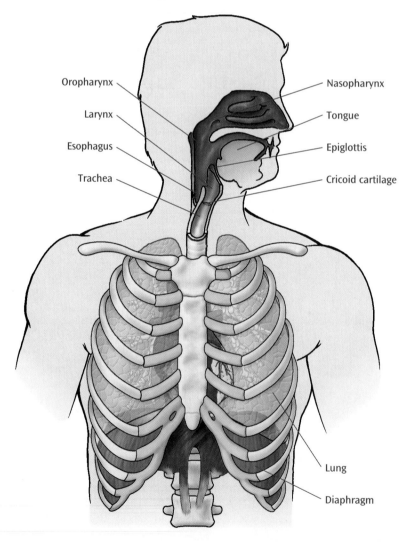

Oropharynx

Larynx

Esophagus

Trachea

Nasopharynx

Tongue

Epiglottis

Cricoid cartilage

Lung

Diaphragm

Explain the pathophysiology of airway compromise.

AIRWAY OBSTRUCTION

Airway obstruction often occurs because the pharynx is blocked. The tongue can cause airway obstruction if it falls to the back of the throat in an unconscious patient. Other causes of pharynx obstruction are vomitus or secretions, tissue swelling from trauma or an allergic reaction, and occlusion by a foreign object.

The epiglottis blocks the lower airway during swallowing to prevent food and liquid from entering. An unresponsive patient can lose this protective mechanism, increasing the risk for aspiration. The epiglottis can swell rapidly in a condition called epiglottitis. This occurs most commonly in young children, and can cause complete airway obstruction.

Identify and describe the airway anatomy in the infant, child and the adult.

Differentiate between the airway anatomy in the infant, child, and the adult.

Infant and Child Anatomy Considerations

Overall, the airway structures in the child's mouth and nose are small in comparison to an adult's. Consequently, they are more easily obstructed. The tongue takes up proportionally more space in the pharynx of the child. This increases the potential risk of airway obstruction. It also makes visualization of the cords more difficult during endotracheal intubation. The trachea and bronchi in children are narrow. Airway obstruction from foreign bodies or tissue swelling, such as in croup, is more likely to occur. The narrowest part of the airway is the cricoid cartilage.

Cartilage has not yet developed its full rigidity in infants and children. The trachea and cricoid cartilage are soft and flexible. Excessive hyperextension or flexion of the neck can cause airway blockage. A soft chest wall causes infants and children to rely more heavily on the diaphragm for breathing. In addition, the stomach can be easily overinflated during artificial ventilation. The gastric distention that results inhibits full inflation of the lungs, decreasing oxygenation.

Opening and Maintaining the Airway

The goal of airway management is to establish and maintain a patent airway so the patient can be adequately oxygenated. Use the head-tilt/chin-lift maneuver or the jaw-thrust maneuver if spinal injury is suspected. Basic airway adjuncts (the OPA and the NPA) and the use of oxygen therapy in airway management are covered in Chapter 7.

You must suction before placing an advanced airway such as an endotracheal tube. Indications for suctioning are obvious secretions and difficulty ventilating the patient with a bag-valve mask. Gurgling sounds suggest that the patient needs immediate suctioning of liquid secretions. The lack of a gag reflex in any patient should be the first clue that aggressive suctioning may be necessary. Chapter 7 describes suctioning units and the procedure for suctioning the oropharynx. Later in this appendix, you will learn about deep suctioning of the trachea.

Nasogastric Tubes

Nasogastric (NG) Tube | *Tube inserted into the nasal passage for decompression of the stomach or proximal bowel or for gastric lavage*

Nasogastric (NG) tubes are occasionally used to decompress the stomach or proximal bowel. The NG tube is technically not an airway tube because it is used for the gastrointestinal system. Decompression using an NG tube is necessary when abdominal distention makes it difficult to ventilate a patient. In the prehospital setting, gastric distention is usually caused by internal injuries, overly aggressive artificial ventilations, or both. Gastric distention can be a problem with a patient of any age. However, it is most often seen in infants and children due to their smaller airway structures.

The NG tube can be used for gastric lavage. This procedure washes out the stomach in upper GI bleeding and ingestion of toxins. The tube is also used as a route for administration of medications and nutrition. Use of an NG tube is contraindicated for patients with major facial, head, or spinal trauma. In this situation, orogastric tube insertion is preferred for relieving gastric distention.

The NG tube is a safe device. However, placement of NG tubes is associated with some complications. These are:

- Inadvertent tracheal intubation
- Nasal tissue damage
- Emesis
- Passage of the tube into the cranium in cases of basilar skull fractures

Table A.1 • PEDIATRIC NASOGASTRIC TUBE SIZES

Age Range	Tube Size
Newborn/Infant	8.0 French
Toddler/Preschool	10.0 French
School-Age	12.0 French
Adolescent	14.0–16.0 French

Before inserting an NG tube, prepare, assemble, and check all your equipment. You should have a variety of tube sizes available. Typical sizes are listed in Table A.1. Other equipment you must have includes:

- 20 mL syringe
- Water-soluble lubricant
- Suction unit and connecting tube
- Stethoscope
- Emesis basin
- Tape

Before you begin insertion of the NG tube, always make sure that the patient is adequately oxygenated. The steps for inserting a nasogastric tube are described in Procedure A.1.

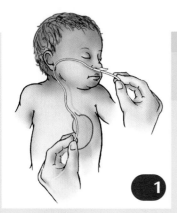

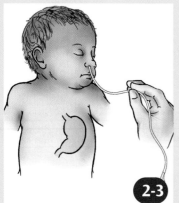

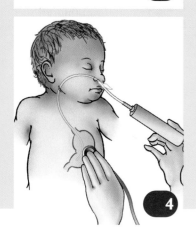

Procedure A.1 • PEDIATRIC NASOGASTRIC TUBE

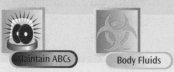

Maintain ABCs   Body Fluids

1. Measure the tube length from the tip of the patient's nose, to the tip of the earlobe, to the tip of the xiphoid process. Begin the measurement at the lips if an orogastric tube is used. Mark the correct tube length with a piece of tape. This will ensure the tube is not inserted too far. Lubricate the distal end of the tube.

2. If trauma is not suspected, position the patient supine with the head turned to the left side.

3. Gently pass the tube along the nasal floor until the tape mark is reached.

4. Check tube placement. This is important because the tube may have entered the lungs accidentally. Inject 10–20 mL of air into the tube while auscultating over the epigastrium with a stethoscope. You will hear a gurgling sound if the tube is placed correctly.

5. Aspirate the stomach contents by attaching the syringe to the tube and pulling back on the plunger. This also ensures correct placement.

6. Secure the tube in place with tape.

D.O.T. OBJECTIVES

Describe the indications for advanced airway management.

List complications associated with advanced airway management.

OROTRACHEAL INTUBATION

Orotracheal intubation is an advanced airway procedure. During orotracheal intubation, a tube is inserted into the trachea through the mouth (oro = mouth and tracheal = trachea) (see Fig. A.2). The tube is called an endotracheal tube because the distal end is placed into the trachea (endo = into). Often the terms orotracheal intubation and **endotracheal intubation** are used interchangeably. The endotracheal tube provides a direct route for artificial ventilation and medication administration. It protects the lower airway against aspiration of foreign materials.

Orotracheal Intubation | Technique involving insertion of a tube through the mouth and into the trachea; also endotracheal intubation

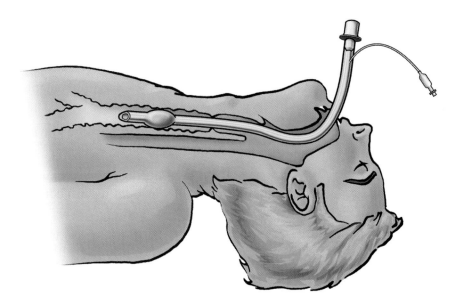

Figure A.2 *The orotracheal tube provides a route for artificial ventilation and medicine administration, while preventing aspiration with a barrier cuff.*

Endotracheal Intubation | Orotracheal intubation

Orotracheal intubation is the most effective means of controlling the airway in an apneic patient because it:

• Completely controls the airway

• Reduces the risk of aspiration

• Reduces the risk of gastric distention

• Allows for better oxygen delivery and ventilation

• Delivers air directly to the trachea and lungs

• Provides a quick, easy route for deep suctioning of the trachea and bronchi

Indications for orotracheal intubation are:

• Inability to ventilate the apneic patient

• Patients who are unable to protect their own airways

• No gag reflex or coughing

• Unresponsive to painful stimuli

- Respiratory or cardiac arrest
- Hypoxia
- Poor air movement
- Poor chest wall excursion
- Toxic inhalation emergencies or airway burns

  Intubation is a life saving procedure. However, several complications can have severe or fatal consequences. Some complications associated with advanced airway management are:

- Soft tissue trauma to the airway, broken teeth, or lacerated lips
- Hypoxia from prolonged attempts at intubation
- Hypoxia from inadvertent and uncorrected esophageal intubation
- Vomiting or dry regurgitation from stimulation of a partially active gag reflex
- Right mainstem bronchus intubation from excessive distal placement of the endotracheal tube

Vagus Nerve | Tenth cranial nerve; controls smooth muscles of the lungs, heart, and abdominal viscera

- Slowing of the patient's heart rate from **vagus nerve** stimulation; during the procedure, monitor the heart rate continuously
- Accidental extubation (removal or dislodging) during movement and transport; particularly in infants, children, or when a patient regains consciousness and self-extubates
- Collapse of a lung

> **D.O.T. OBJECTIVE**
>
> List the equipment required for orotracheal intubation.

**EMT
Alert**

Always apply the principles of BSI and standard precautions during orotracheal intubation. You will look directly into the patient's mouth and airway. This exposes you to blood, emesis, and other secretions. You will need gloves, a mask, and protective eyewear.

Intubation Equipment

Orotracheal intubation requires proper equipment. This includes:

- BSI equipment
- Laryngoscope
- Endotracheal tubes in various sizes
- Stylet
- Water-soluble lubricant
- 10 mL syringe
- Securing device or tape
- Suction unit
- Towels or padding to position the patient

Laryngoscope

The **laryngoscope** is used for lifting and holding the tongue. This enables you to visualize the vocal cords, allowing tube placement. The instrument has two main components (see Fig. A.3). The handle houses the batteries. The laryngoscope blade contains a small light. Lifting the blade upward enables you to see the vocal cords. The laryngoscope is designed for use in the left hand.

Laryngoscope | *An instrument with a light and interchangeable blades, used for holding the tongue out of the way for intubation*

Figure A.3 *Laryngoscope blades and handle.*

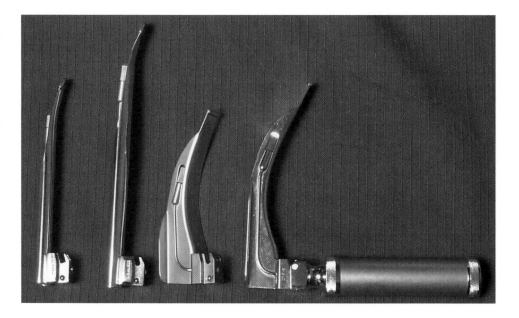

Two types of blades are used for the laryngoscope—curved and straight. The main difference between the blades is where the distal end is placed within the airway. The straight blade lifts the epiglottis directly, allowing visualization of the glottic opening and the vocal cords (see Fig. A.4 on page 770). The curved blade fits into the vallecula, the space between the base of the tongue and epiglottis. The blade selected depends on your training and preference. Both are available in assorted sizes. The smallest is size 0, which is used for an infant. A size 4 is used for a large adult. Because of anatomical differences, the straight blade is preferred for infants and small children. It enables you to see the cords better by providing greater tongue displacement.

Figure A.4 *The laryngoscope allows visualization of the vocal cords. The straight blade (left) lifts the epiglottis. The curved blade (right) fits into the vallecula.*

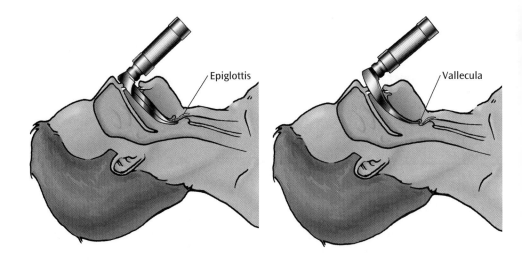

Most laryngoscopes require the user to assemble the handle and blade. A locking bar at the end of the handle fits into a notch on the blade. The two parts slip together. When the blade is lifted up, it locks into place at a 90-degree angle to the handle. This turns on the light. Check the laryngoscope daily to ensure that it works properly. The light should be bright, white, and fit tightly inside the blade. Spare batteries and bulbs must be available. Store them with the laryngoscope.

D.O.T. OBJECTIVE

Describe the methods of choosing the appropriate size endotracheal tube in an adult patient.

Endotracheal Tubes

The endotracheal tube is a clear, flexible, hollow tube. Oxygen is delivered through the tube after it has been passed through the vocal cords. The tubes come in an assortment of sizes (see Table A.2). A general rule in an emergency is that a 7.5 mm endotracheal tube fits an adult. Having extra tubes available during intubation is helpful. Select extra tubes one size larger and one size smaller than estimated. Have these tubes available in case the first tube does not fit.

The endotracheal tube has several components (see Fig. A.5). The proximal end remains outside the patient. It has a standard 15 mm adapter on the end which attaches to a bag-valve mask or other ventilation device. The distal end passes into the trachea. The tip of the endotracheal tube is beveled. This permits easier passage through the vocal cords. The Murphy eye is a small hole opposite the bevel. This hole is a safeguard to allow ventilation if the tip becomes obstructed.

Table A.2 • ADULT ENDOTRACHEAL TUBE SIZES

Patient Size	Tube Diameter
Average Adult Female	7.0–8.0 mm
Average Adult Male	8.0–8.5 mm
Largest Adults	10.0 mm

A cuff at the distal end of the tube holds about 10 mL of air. When inflated, the cuff provides an airtight seal around the tube. It prevents air from leaking out around the edges of the tube while ventilating the patient. The cuff is inflated using a 10 mL syringe through a one-way inflation valve. The syringe is connected to the cuff by an inflation tube. The cuff helps to prevent the tube from dislodging from the airway. It seals the airway to prevent aspiration in case of vomiting. To verify that the cuff is inflated, a pilot balloon is positioned just past the valve. The pilot balloon inflates when the cuff is inflated. If the cuff leaks, the pilot balloon will deflate.

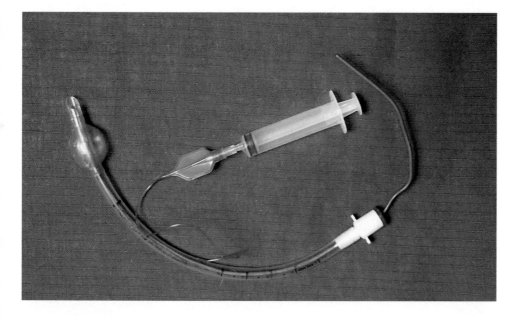

Figure A.5 *Endotracheal tube.*

Cuffed tubes are sized at 6.0 mm and up. They are used for larger children (age 8 and older) and adults. Use uncuffed tubes in sizes 2.5 to 5.5 mm for infants and smaller children. The cricoid ring is the narrowest part of the airway in younger children and infants. It provides a seal, making cuffed tubes unnecessary. The tube without a cuff is more easily dislodged and must be carefully monitored.

The standard length of an adult endotracheal tube is 33 cm. The tube has centimeter markings indicating distance from the tip. When properly placed, the tip of the tube should end about midway between the vocal cords and the carina. If it is placed too high, it may become dislodged when the patient moves. Placement that is too deep generally results in **right mainstem intubation**. This is a common occurrence. The tube preferentially travels into the right

Right Mainstem Intubation |

Placement of an endotracheal tube beyond the carina and into the right mainstem bronchus; results in ventilation of the right lung only

EMT Tip

Remember: "Teeth and tube at 22." Have someone monitor the endotracheal tube before, during, and after tube placement. Practice holding the tube at the maximum length you will use. Use an effective tie-down method to keep the tube at the proper depth. As with all technical EMS skills, practice your intubation skills frequently.

mainstem bronchus, which branches from the trachea at a straighter angle than the left. If right mainstem intubation occurs, you will ventilate only the right lung. The breath sounds will be diminished on the left.

Knowing a few key measurements is one way to help prevent right mainstem intubation. A general rule is that the endotracheal tube should be placed 22 cm beyond where the teeth and tube meet. Use this as a general rule only. The exact distance depends on the patient's size. Other helpful measurements for an average adult are:

- 15 cm from the teeth to the vocal cords
- 20 cm from the teeth to the sternal notch
- 25 cm from the teeth to the carina

D.O.T. OBJECTIVE

State the reasons for and proper use of the stylet in orotracheal intubation.

Stylet

The stylet is made of malleable metal (see Fig. A.6). It is inserted into the endotracheal tube to provide stiffness and shape, making intubation easier. Lubricate the stylet with a water-soluble lubricant for easy removal. The stylet must never extend past the end of the tube, because it could traumatize the airway. Keep the stylet just above the proximal end of the Murphy eye. Once inserted, shape the stylet so it looks like a hockey stick. This shape makes it easier to pass the tube through the vocal cords. After placing the tube, hold it firmly with the left hand so it will not dislodge. Remove the stylet with your right hand.

Figure A.6 *The stylet provides stiffness and shape to the endotracheal tube.*

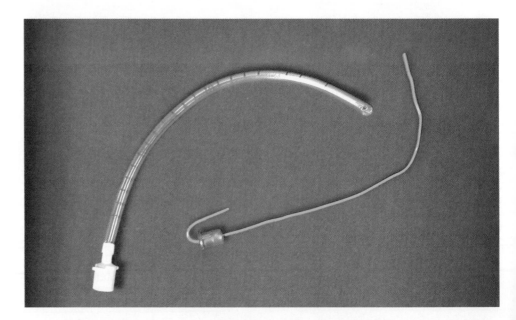

Syringe

A 10 mL syringe is needed to inflate the cuff after the tube is placed. Use the syringe to test the cuff for leakage before insertion. Inject 10 mL of air into the cuff. Verify the integrity of the cuff and the pilot balloon. Then deflate the cuff by pulling back on the plunger while pushing down on the one-way inflation valve and pilot balloon. Leave the syringe attached to the valve while intubating so you can readily inflate the cuff. Once the cuff is inflated, remove the syringe and keep it close by in case you must add more air.

Other Equipment

After intubation, positioning the tube, and inflating the cuff, you must secure the tube in place. This is necessary because the tube can easily become dislodged with patient movement. The tube can be secured by many methods. Commercial devices are available or cloth tape may be used. The particular method used is determined by local medical direction. After taping, insert an oral airway adjunct or bite block to prevent the patient from biting down on the tube.

During orotracheal intubation, secretions or other debris may obstruct your view of the vocal cords. A suction unit must always be available. Use a large bore catheter to clear the airway. Later, a soft French catheter can be used to suction through the endotracheal tube.

Towels may be used to elevate the shoulders or head. This will help to align the airway during intubation. If cervical spine injury is suspected, you must maintain in-line immobilization during intubation. In this situation, avoid elevating the shoulders, neck, or head.

D.O.T. OBJECTIVE

Describe how to perform the Sellick maneuver (cricoid pressure).

Sellick's Maneuver

Gastric distention resulting in regurgitation and aspiration of vomitus can be a serious complication during intubation and artificial ventilation. An effective method of preventing this is to apply pressure directly over the cricoid cartilage. Apply pressure posteriorly during intubation. This is called **Sellick's maneuver** or cricoid pressure. The maneuver was developed for use during intubation of patients in the operating room. It prevents passive regurgitation caused by medication-induced paralysis. Use Sellick's maneuver during intubation in unresponsive patients without a cough or gag reflex.

Sellick's Maneuver | *Pressure applied directly over the cricoid cartilage; also cricoid pressure*

To find the cricoid cartilage, first palpate the thyroid cartilage or Adam's apple in the anterior neck. Then move your finger inferior to feel the depression of the cricothyroid membrane. The firm ring forming the inferior border of the cricothyroid membrane is the cricoid cartilage. The esophagus is soft and pliable, and located directly posterior to the trachea. Applying cricoid pressure closes the esophageal opening. Another benefit is that it pushes the vocal cords down. This makes them easier to visualize during intubation.

Figure A.7 *Sellick's maneuver is also known as applying cricoid pressure.*

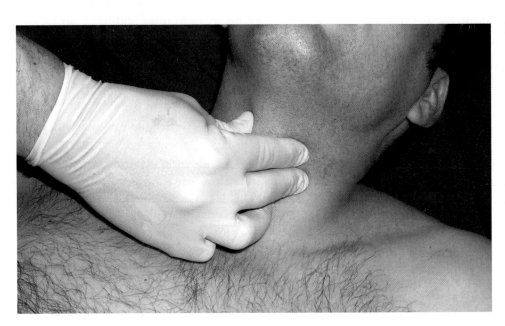

EMT Tip

Judging how much pressure to apply during Sellick's maneuver may be difficult. This exercise will help you to understand how much pressure is needed. Pinch your thumb and index finger together. Push on the bridge of your nose, or your partner's nose, until it hurts. Pressure applied during Sellick's maneuver is about equal to the pressure it takes to cause pain.

Having a third EMT available during Sellick's maneuver is best. Intubation, ventilation, and spinal immobilization require two people. The third rescuer finds the cricoid cartilage with the thumb and index finger (see Fig. A.7). Spread the fingers lateral to the midline. Apply firm pressure backward, or posteriorly, to occlude the esophagus. Maintain pressure until intubation is complete and the cuff is inflated. The EMT applying cricoid pressure may feel the tube passing through the trachea. This helps to confirm tube placement.

Sellick's maneuver can be very beneficial during intubation. However, you must consider some drawbacks. You must be able to identify the correct anatomy to avoid damaging other structures. Identifying the cricoid cartilage in children, small adults, and patients with thick necks may be difficult. Applying excessive pressure to the cricoid cartilage may cause tracheal obstruction in infants and children. Another drawback is the need for an extra rescuer who is trained and available to do the maneuver. Because some patients will require immediate airway management, you may not have time to apply cricoid pressure.

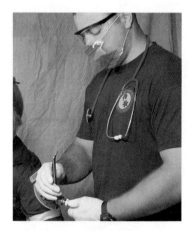

Figure A.8 *Prepare and check your equipment before starting intubation.*

Procedure for Adult Orotracheal Intubation

Several techniques and routes are used to place the endotracheal tube. The visualized orotracheal route is presented in Procedure A.2 on page 776. Follow local protocols when inserting an endotracheal tube by different routes or using a different technique. Although truly sterile procedures are almost impossible in the out-of-hospital setting, keep the procedure as sterile as possible. Keep the tube in its wrapping until absolutely necessary and do not place it on the floor before or after an intubation attempt.

The following items are used in an endotracheal intubation. The equipment must be checked and prepared prior to starting the procedure (see Fig. A.8).

- Suction must be working. Attach a large bore rigid tip. Keep the unit within easy reach of your right hand.

- Lubricate and insert the stylet to the proper position. Mold it to a hockey stick shape.

- Select the correct size endotracheal tube. Have tubes one size larger and one size smaller immediately available. Test the integrity of the cuff by injecting 5 to 10 mL of air. Deflate the cuff, keeping the syringe attached to the inflation valve.

- Apply a water-soluble lubricant around the distal end of the tube. Keep the tube free of any debris (carpet, dirt, vomitus, etc.).

- Select the correct shape and size blade for the laryngoscope. Connect it to the handle. Test the bulb. Make sure it is tight and shines brightly (see Fig. A.9).

- Have a securing device ready for use after inserting the tube.

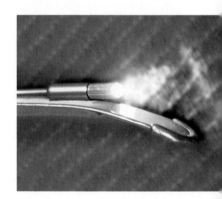

Figure A.9 *The laryngoscope light should be bright and tight.*

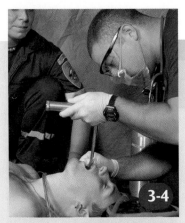

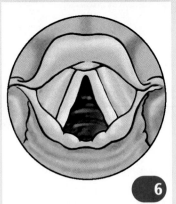

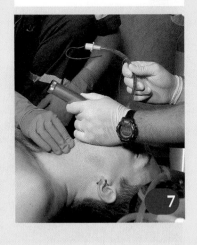

Procedure A.2 • **OROTRACHEAL INTUBATION**

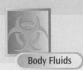

Maintain ABCs   Body Fluids

1. Position yourself directly behind the supine patient's head. Place the suction unit and endotracheal tube on your right and the laryngoscope on your left.

2. Stop ventilations, remove the OPA, and attempt to see the vocal cords.

3. Holding the laryngoscope in your left hand, lift the patient's jaw anteriorly with your right hand. Insert the blade into the right corner of the mouth. Do not interchange the hands. Insert a straight blade directly past the epiglottis. Insert a curved blade into the space between the base of the tongue and the epiglottis.

4. Lift the scope up and away from the patient. Direct the force along the axis of the handle. Avoid pulling the handle back toward you. This creates a fulcrum and may injure the teeth.

5. If a third EMT is available, ask him or her to apply Sellick's maneuver. This will improve visualization of the vocal cords and reduce the risk of gastric distention or aspiration. The maneuver is especially helpful during spinal immobilization. Maintain cricoid pressure until intubation is complete.

6. Visualize the white, V-shaped vocal cords. Suction any time your view of the cords is obstructed by secretions or emesis. Once the cords are in view, do not lose sight of them during your intubation attempt.

7. With the endotracheal tube in your right hand, gently advance it between the two cords until the cuff is just past them. Do not let go of the tube until it is secured. If you cannot see the cords, cannot pass the tube between the cords, and/or it takes longer than 30 seconds to intubate, withdraw. Immediately hyperventilate the patient before trying again.

8. Remove the laryngoscope blade. Turn the light off by pushing the blade down with your left hand.

9. Holding the tube in place, carefully remove the stylet. Be careful; it may be difficult to dislodge the stylet from inside the tube. Inflate the cuff with 5 to 10 mL of air. Remove the syringe.

10. Have your partner attach the bag-valve mask, then provide a few artificial ventilations. Note the markings on the tube at the teeth or gum line. Record this later.

The patient must be adequately oxygenated and ventilated prior to starting the intubation procedure. This helps to compensate for the lack of oxygen during the procedure. First secure the airway manually using basic adjuncts. Ventilate with a bag-valve mask, using high-flow oxygen (see Fig. A.10). Assess the baseline lung sounds and chest rise. Hyperventilate the patient at a rate of 24 breaths per minute for 1 to 2 minutes before attempting to intubate.

You must have a clear view of the vocal cords in order to place the tube correctly. If you do not suspect spinal trauma, hyperextend the patient's neck by tilting the head and lifting the chin. If you cannot visualize the cords, raise the patient's shoulders an inch with a small folded towel or sheet. Vary the position according to the age and size of the patient. Attempt to see the cords again. If spinal trauma is suspected, intubate with the head and neck in a neutral position. This will make alignment and visualization of the cords more difficult. Ask another EMT to perform the jaw-thrust maneuver while maintaining spinal stabilization. This may make seeing the cords easier.

The patient will become hypoxic and deteriorate rapidly if the tube is placed incorrectly. There will be an increase in the heart rate, poor skin color, and a decrease in the level of responsiveness. Visualization of the tube passing through the vocal cords is the only accurate way of confirming correct placement. Other ways to verify the placement are:

- Assess for chest rise and fall during each ventilation.

- Auscultate for breath sounds. Listen first over the epigastrium, which is located above the umbilical region. You should not hear sounds here during ventilation. Next, listen over the left axilla, or apex (see Fig. A.11). Compare with the breath sounds over the right axilla. Breath sounds should be equal bilaterally. Listen over the left base. Compare with the breath sounds over the right base. Breath sounds should be equal bilaterally.

- Observe the patient for signs of hypoxia. The patient may be combative or cyanotic. He or she will deteriorate if the esophagus is intubated. To assess general deterioration, evaluate the heart rate, skin color, and level of responsiveness.

- Other methods for detecting complications can be used, if available and allowed by local protocols. Pulse oximetry, end tidal carbon dioxide detectors, and esophageal intubation detectors are excellent indicators.

- If you hear a gurgling sound over the epigastrium during ventilation, the tube was inserted into the esophagus. Stop ventilation immediately. Deflate the cuff and remove the tube. Have suction available. Vomiting may occur from gastric distention. Immediately begin to hyperventilate the patient for 2 to 5 minutes, before your second and final attempt. An unrecognized esophageal intubation is fatal.

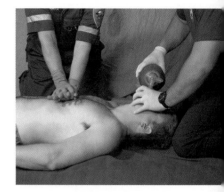

Figure A.10 *Perform bag-valve mask ventilation prior to intubation.*

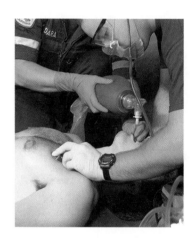

Figure A.11 *Equal breath sounds help to confirm placement of the endotracheal tube.*

EMT Alert

Intubation should take 30 seconds or less. Avoid taking longer than 30 seconds without ventilating the patient. To judge the time, hold your breath while intubating. If you need to breathe before the patient has been successfully intubated, stop and ventilate the patient before another attempt.

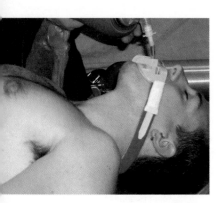

Figure A.12 *Secure the tube after confirming its placement.*

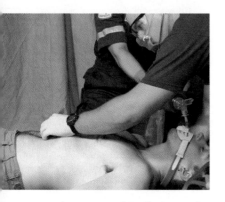

Figure A.13 *Ventilation and assessment of breath sounds can be done simultaneously.*

• If breath sounds are diminished or absent on the left, the right mainstem bronchus was probably intubated. Deflate the cuff. Slowly and gently withdraw the tube, about 1 cm at a time. Take care not to completely remove the tube. Continue artificial ventilations and auscultation over the left chest. Continue this procedure until equal breath sounds are heard. Be careful not to accidentally extubate the patient. Reinflate the cuff, if present.

If no air sounds are heard over the epigastrium and breath sounds are equal bilaterally, placement is correct. Secure the tube using tape or a commercial device that is approved by local medical direction (see Fig. A.12). After securing the tube, artificially ventilate the patient at a rate appropriate to his or her age (see Fig. A.13). Note the distance that the tube has been inserted. If appropriate, insert an oral airway to act as a bite block.

Reassess breath sounds frequently, especially after every major move or if the patient deteriorates suddenly. Major moves take place from the scene to the ambulance and from the ambulance to the receiving facility.

Orotracheal Suctioning

Orotracheal suctioning is also called deep suctioning. In this procedure, suctioning is done through an endotracheal tube. Suctioning is done in the trachea, usually to the level of the carina. A long, soft, flexible catheter is used. The catheter must be sterile. Select a French catheter or a whistle tip catheter. The diameter of the catheter must be small enough to fit through the endotracheal tube. Suction is applied as the catheter is withdrawn. This procedure differs from basic airway management. Basic suctioning does not go beyond the level of the posterior pharynx.

You will need to provide orotracheal suction when there are obvious secretions in the endotracheal tube. You will hear gurgling sounds with respirations, or you may see secretions in the tube. In extreme cases, secretions can bubble over the top of the tube when the bag-valve mask is not attached.

In some situations, secretions will not be obvious, yet you will have difficulty ventilating the intubated patient. This may be caused by secretions or mucus deep in the trachea, the bronchi, or the endotracheal tube. Orotracheal suctioning will help to clear the airway if secretions are obstructing it. However, complications may occur. Potential complications are:

• Cardiac arrhythmias

• Hypoxia

• Damage to the mucosa, the tissue lining of the airway

• Coughing and bronchospasm (wheezing)

Most of these complications are caused by a lack of oxygen during suctioning. Direct trauma and stimulation of the respiratory tract from the catheter can also cause problems. Limit complications by adhering to the guidelines and time limits for suctioning.

Follow these steps for orotracheal suctioning:

1. Set up the equipment. Turn on the unit to ensure that suction is working. Use sterile technique. Keep the catheter in the package until ready for use.

2. Preoxygenate the patient with high-flow oxygen. Hyperventilate by giving 5 breaths with the bag-valve mask before and after suctioning (see Fig. A.14). This helps to compensate for the lack of oxygen during suctioning.

3. Measure the length of the catheter from the corner of the ear to the lips, then down to the nipple line. This length approximates the level of the carina.

4. Insert the catheter into the endotracheal tube the desired distance (see Fig. A.15). Do not apply suction.

5. Cover the hole in the whistle-tip catheter to apply suction. Suction for no more than 15 seconds in adults. In infants and children, suction for 5 seconds. Withdraw the catheter using a twisting motion.

6. Hyperventilate the patient at least 5 times after suctioning. If further suctioning is needed, repeat the procedure.

7. Carefully observe the patient for signs of deterioration or complications during suctioning. This is particularly important in children. A slow, rapid, or irregular heart rate suggests a dangerous decline in oxygen. Stimulation from the catheter may also cause this. Remove the catheter immediately. Ventilate with oxygen for at least 30 seconds.

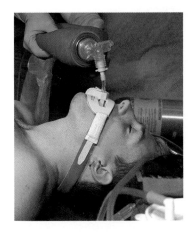

Figure A.14 *Hyperventilating prior to suctioning helps to compensate for lack of oxygen during suctioning.*

Figure A.15 *The suction catheter should never be inserted beyond the carina.*

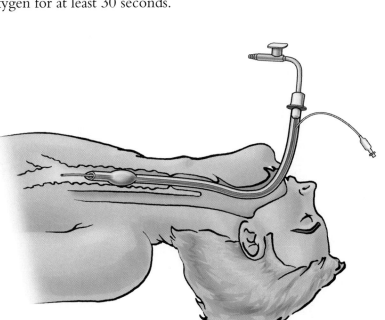

Pediatric Orotracheal Intubation

The purpose of orotracheal intubation in children is the same as for adults. The technique is similar. You have learned the anatomical differences in the pediatric airway. These differences require special consideration, and are important to know when intubating a child.

Creating a single, clear visual plane from the mouth through the pharynx to the glottis is difficult in children. This is because of the larger tongue. The glottis is also more anterior in children. Infants and children are more likely to develop bradycardia from airway stimulation during intubation. They are also more sensitive to hypoxia, creating further challenges.

The equipment for intubation in infants and children is the same as for adults. The only differences relate to sizing the equipment to fit the pediatric airway (see Fig. A.16). The size of the endotracheal tube is based on the size of the cricoid ring, rather than the glottic opening. The cricoid ring creates a cuff for the endotracheal tube. Uncuffed tubes are used in children under 8 years old.

The advantages and complications of orotracheal intubation are the same in infants or children as they are in adults. Orotracheal intubation in children is indicated:

- When prolonged artificial ventilation is required
- When adequate artificial ventilation cannot be achieved by other methods
- In unresponsive patients without a cough or gag reflex
- If the patient is apneic

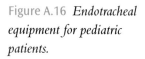

Figure A.16 *Endotracheal equipment for pediatric patients.*

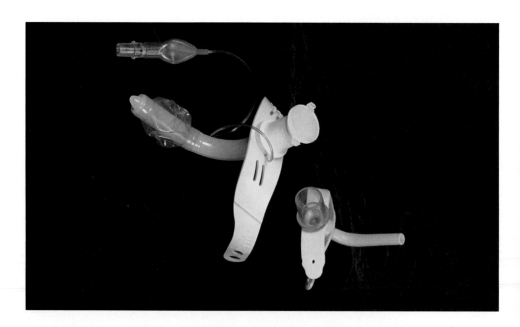

State the formula for sizing an infant or child endotracheal tube.

Define the various alternative methods for sizing the infant and child endotracheal tube.

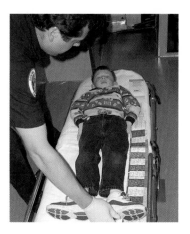

Figure A.17 *The size of the endotracheal tube can be estimated based on the height of the child.*

Equipment

Chose equipment sizes appropriate to the child's size. Remembering to use the correct size bag-valve mask is important. This ensures a tight seal while ventilating before intubation.

Select the laryngoscope blade you are most comfortable with. Because of anatomical differences, the straight blade is preferred for infants and small children. It provides greater tongue displacement, giving you a better view of the vocal cords. In older children, the curved blade is preferred. This has a broader base and flange. It permits greater displacement of the tongue in older children.

Have a selection of endotracheal tubes available in different sizes when intubating an infant or child. The average sizes for infants and children are listed in Table A.3. Several other methods can be used to determine the appropriate size tube. Having a chart or tape device available to help you size the endotracheal tube is best. A commercial device is the Broselow tape (see Fig. A.17). This tape uses the patient's height to calculate the correct size endotracheal tube. It also lists other equipment and medication dosages.

Other methods used to estimate tube size are:

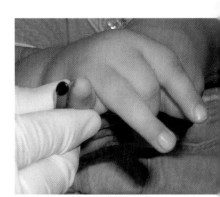

Figure A.18 *Estimate tube size from the size of the patient's little finger.*

- Size of the little finger—the outside diameter of the tube equals the diameter of the patient's little finger (see Fig. A.18). Use this method as a starting point for determining endotracheal tube size.
- Nasal sizing—the internal diameter of the nares equals the outside diameter of the tube.

Whatever method is used, having tubes that are one size larger and one size smaller than estimated is helpful.

Table A.3 • ENDOTRACHEAL TUBE SIZES IN CHILDREN

Age Range	Tube Diameter
Neonate	2.5–3.5 mm
Infant	3.5–4.0 mm
Child	4.0–6.0 mm

Figure A.19 *Cuffed endotracheal tube.*

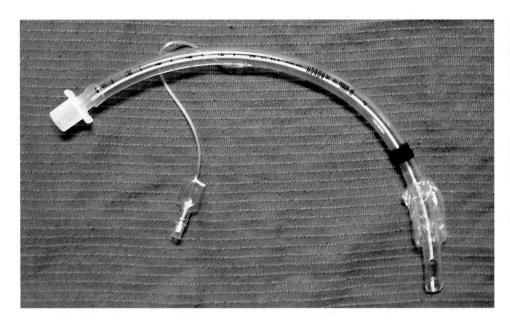

EMT Tip

A helpful formula to determine tube size in children older than 1 year is to add 16 to the child's age in years and divide by 4. Thus the tube size for a 4-year-old child is 5.0.

Use cuffed tubes for patients 8 years of age or older (see Fig. A.19). The tube is inserted until the cuff is just past the vocal cords. Use the uncuffed endotracheal tube and small stylet in patients less than 8 years old (see Fig. A.20). In this age group, a cuffed tube is not needed because the cricoid cartilage holds the tube in place.

Figure A.20 *Uncuffed endotracheal tube.*

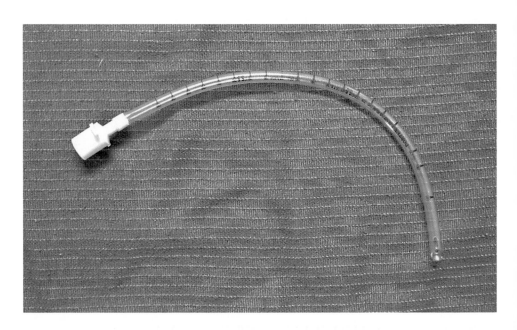

Right mainstem intubation can easily occur in infants and children. In neonates and infants, the distance between midtracheal and right mainstem intubation is only a few centimeters. Average distances between the teeth and the midtrachea are shown by age group in Table A.4. The uncuffed endotracheal tube should have a vocal cord marker. This ensures that the tip of the tube is placed in the

Table A.4 • ENDOTRACHEAL TUBE LENGTHS FOR CHILDREN

Age Range	Distance from Teeth to Midtrachea
6 months to 1 year	12 cm
2 years	14 cm
4 to 6 years	16 cm
6 to 10 years	18 cm
10 to 12 years	20 cm

midtracheal position. In very small patients, the best indicator of correct tube placement is symmetrical respirations. Breath sounds may be misleading. They are easily transmitted through the small chest, and can be heard in both lungs and the epigastrium.

D.O.T. OBJECTIVE

Describe the skill of orotracheal intubation in the infant and child patient.

Procedure for Pediatric Orotracheal Intubation

The procedure for orotracheal intubation in infants and children is the same as intubating adults except for special considerations that are due to anatomical differences. Follow the general methods detailed in Procedure A.2, with the following variations:

- Hyperventilate the patient at an age-appropriate rate for 1 to 2 minutes before beginning. The rate should be greater than 30 breaths per minute for infants and greater than 24 breaths per minute for children.

- Continuously monitor the heart rate when attempting to insert the tube. Mechanical stimulation of the airway may cause bradycardia in infants and children. If the heart rate drops to less than 80 in infants or less than 60 in children, stop immediately. Ventilate before proceeding.

- Be gentle when intubating infants or children. Little force is needed to visualize the cords or place the endotracheal tube.

- Insert straight blades directly past the epiglottis. Insert curved blades into the vallecula. Remember that the cartilage of the epiglottis is less developed in infants and children. This makes it more flexible and more likely to obscure the airway. Consequently, more attention is necessary to visualize the cords in this age group.

- As with adults, visualization of the tube passing through the cords is the only accurate way of confirming correct placement. In addition, you can assess for symmetrical rise and fall of the chest. This is the best indicator in infants and children because breath sounds may be misleading. Also assess for improvement in heart rate and skin color. The color will quickly improve in infants and children, increasing the heart rate to normal levels. Auscultate for breath sounds. Listen first over the epigastrium. Compare breath sounds over the left axilla with the breath sounds over the right axilla. Listen over the left base. Compare with the breath sounds over the right base. Breath sounds should be equal bilaterally. Listen at the sternal notch. If the tube is too small, a large air leak will be heard.

- After the tube is secured, position and secure the child to an appropriate device to reduce head movement. With infants and children, even small head movements may dislodge the tube.

If the tube is properly placed but inadequate lung expansion occurs, check for the following causes:

- The tube is too small, causing a large air leak at the glottic opening. This can be detected by auscultating over the neck, above the sternal notch. Replace the tube with a larger one. If the patient is older than 8, use a cuffed tube. If a cuffed tube was used, add more air to the cuff. Check the integrity of the pilot balloon.

- The pop-off valve on the bag-valve mask has not been deactivated as it should be, and air escapes with each ventilation. This suggests a leak in the bag-valve device.

- The endotracheal tube is blocked with secretions. This is treated with orotracheal suctioning. If suctioning fails, replace the tube.

- The EMT-B ventilating the patient is delivering inadequate breaths.

Barotrauma | *Ruptured lung resulting from over-aggressive ventilations*

All the complications described for adult patients may also be seen in children. If ventilated too aggressively, lung tissue ruptures more easily. This condition, called **barotrauma**, creates an air leak. It leads to a collapsed lung or pneumothorax. Slow, easy ventilations are key when using the endotracheal tube in pediatric patients. If you are uncertain of tube placement, remove the tube and ventilate the patient with basic airway adjuncts. Remember that an unrecognized esophageal intubation is fatal.

Key Terms Review

Basic Life Support

The heart may stop beating for many reasons. In infants and children, it usually follows respiratory arrest. In adults, heart disease is the main cause. Other causes of cardiac arrest include:

- Sudden death
- Respiratory arrest (especially in children)
- Medical emergencies, such as stroke, epilepsy, diabetes, and allergic reactions
- Electrical shock
- Poisoning
- Drowning and suffocation
- Congenital abnormalities
- Trauma and bleeding

Whatever the cause, the emergency care for cardiac arrest is CPR. CPR is effective because it circulates oxygen-rich blood. The time between clinical death and the beginning of irreversible brain cell changes can be prolonged by applying CPR. Without CPR, the patient quickly progresses from clinical death to biological death.

The Chain of Survival

The American Heart Association (AHA) has identified a series of critical interventions for cardiac arrest. This chain of survival includes links that must fit together during a successful resuscitation event (see Fig. B.1 on page 786). The four links in the chain of survival increase the likelihood of survival for a cardiac arrest patient:

1. Early access to the EMS system
2. Early CPR
3. Early defibrillation
4. Early ACLS

If a link in the chain is missing or is not done correctly, the chain is broken. This significantly reduces the patient's chance of survival.

Early access means that the public is educated to recognize a cardiac emergency early and activate the EMS system before starting CPR. Emergency medical dispatchers can provide pre-arrival instructions and direct the performance of CPR.

Figure B.1 *Chain of survival.*

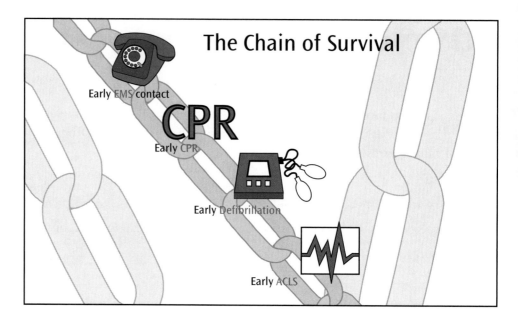

Early CPR is a key step in the success of further interventions. Family members, bystanders, first responders, and EMT-Basics can provide CPR before advanced EMS teams arrive. The longer CPR is performed, the less effective it becomes. It cannot sustain life indefinitely. Frequently, a patient needs defibrillation to survive. CPR increases the amount of time in which defibrillation will be effective. It can help prevent brain damage until advanced cardiac life support arrives. CPR must be started as early as possible.

Early defibrillation represents the third link in the chain of survival and is definitive treatment for life-threatening cardiac arrhythmias. Defibrillation must be done within a few minutes of cardiac arrest to be effective. Many EMT-Bs, first responders, and law enforcement personnel are trained to use automated external defibrillators (AEDs) with great success. In many communities, on airplanes, and in places of mass gathering, AEDs are used by laypersons. Chapter 13 describes use of the AED in detail.

EMT-Intermediates and EMT-Paramedics provide early advanced cardiac life support (ACLS). They continue CPR, defibrillate, give medications, and use specialized airways to increase the patient's chance of survival. ACLS providers represent the fourth and final link in the chain of survival.

Although not officially included as a link in the chain, rapid transport to an emergency department is important. Here, the patient will receive early definitive care. This is an essential factor to increasing the incidence of survival.

Initial Patient Assessment

Upon arrival, check for scene safety and apply the personal protective principles of BSI and standard precautions. These include wearing latex gloves and using a barrier device during CPR. Also consider using a gown, mask, and/or eye shield to avoid contact with blood or body fluids, thus reducing the risk of infection. Follow these steps to perform an initial assessment of the patient and to provide basic life support interventions:

1. Establish unresponsiveness. Pinch the patient gently or shout, "Are you OK?"

2. Activate the EMS system immediately if the patient is an adult. If the patient is an infant or a child, give CPR for 1 minute before calling EMS.

3. Position the patient. The patient should be supine on a firm, flat surface for resuscitation to be effective. If the patient is prone, carefully roll him or her so that the head, shoulders, and torso move as a unit, without twisting. If possible, have others help you with the roll. Keep the patient's neck and back in a straight line.

4. Assess the patency of the airway. If necessary, open the airway as described in the following section.

5. Establish breathlessness. Look, listen, and feel for breathing for 3 to 5 seconds. If breathing is absent, provide rescue breathing (see the following section).

6. If the patient is breathing, with no evidence of spinal injury, position him or her in the recovery position (see Fig. B.2). Roll the patient onto one side. Be sure the head, shoulders, and torso move simultaneously, without twisting. Position the patient's top hand directly under the chin. Bend the top leg slightly at the knee. The bottom arm can also be placed upward, as if raising the hand. This offers more stability while lying on the side. Ultimately, this position should allow the patient to maintain an open airway and allow fluids to drain from the airway.

7. If the patient is not breathing, establish pulselessness. If the pulse is absent, begin chest compressions.

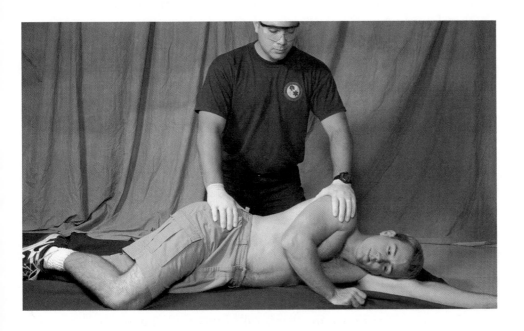

Figure B.2 *Patient in the recovery position.*

Figure B.3 *Head-tilt/chin-lift maneuver.*

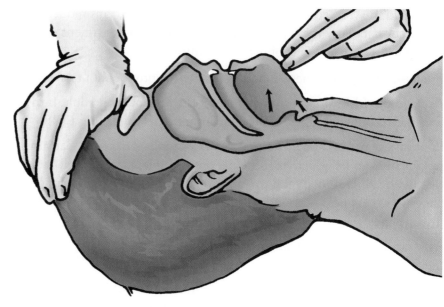

Figure B.4 *Jaw-thrust maneuver for possible spinal injury.*

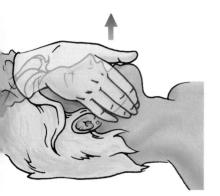

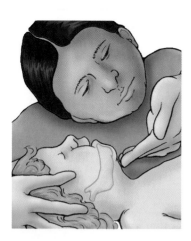

Figure B.5 *The head-tilt/chin-lift maneuver is slightly modified for a child to avoid overextending the neck.*

Airway and Breathing

You must provide interventions for a patient who does not have a patent airway or is not breathing.

Open the Airway

If there is no evidence of head or neck trauma, open the airway using the head-tilt/chin-lift maneuver (see Fig. B.3). Use the jaw-thrust maneuver if spinal injury is suspected (see Fig. B.4). For adults, these procedures are described in Chapter 7. The maneuvers are slightly modified for pediatric patients.

For infants and small children, follow these steps to perform the head-tilt/chin-lift maneuver:

1. Place one hand on the child's forehead.
2. Gently tilt the head back to a neutral position.
3. Avoid overextending the neck, because this could kink the airway closed.
4. Place the fingers of your other hand under the bony part of the chin; lift the mandible upward and outward (see Fig. B.5). Do not use your thumb.

If you suspect a cervical spine injury, open the airway without tilting the head or extending the neck. To do this, perform the jaw-thrust maneuver:

1. Place two or three fingers under each side of the child's lower jaw at the mandibular angle.
2. Lift the jaw upward and outward.
3. If the child is supine, the airway is best maintained by placing a thin roll behind the upper back and shoulders. This position allows the neck to remain aligned and the airway open in what is called the sniffing position.

Rescue Breathing

If a patient (adult, child, or infant) is not breathing, rescue breathing helps to provide oxygen to the body.

EMS personnel must use a barrier device when doing rescue breathing by mouth. This technique is called mouth-to-barrier device breathing or mouth-to-mask breathing. Barrier devices are face masks or face shields with one-way anti-reflux valves (see Fig. B.6). The one-way valves prevent air or body fluids from entering the rescuer's mouth. Mouth-to-mask breathing is usually done when you are alone. Most of the time you will have a partner to help with CPR. The bag-valve mask (BVM) is usually used in this case (see Fig. B.7). Use of the BVM is described in Chapter 7. You may need to use a barrier device in other cases, such as when equipment is not available or is malfunctioning.

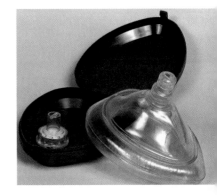

Figure B.6 *The pocket mask is commonly used as a barrier device.*

To perform rescue breathing:

1. Pinch the patient's nose closed with your fingers. Cover the mouth with the barrier device.

2. Give two slow breaths. Deliver one breath every 3 seconds. In adults, deliver each breath over 1 to 2 seconds. Take a deep breath between ventilations. Watch the patient's chest rise with each breath. The correct volume for each breath is the amount that causes the chest to rise.

3. In infants and children, deliver each breath over 1 to 1.5 seconds. Take a deep breath between ventilations. The volume and pressure that causes the chest to rise will vary depending on the patient's size. All that may be required to ventilate a newborn is to empty the air from your mouth when your cheeks are inflated. Avoid using too much pressure in an infant or child. Ventilations that are too aggressive, forceful, or rapid can cause gastric distention. This impairs the tidal volume in the lungs.

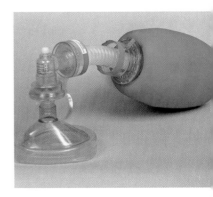

Figure B.7 *Bag-valve mask device.*

4. For all patients, if the first ventilation attempt is unsuccessful, reposition the airway and try again. If still unsuccessful, begin the foreign body airway obstruction (FBAO) sequence. This is described later in this appendix.

External Chest Compressions

After assisting with the breathing as necessary, determine whether the patient has a pulse. Check an adult's carotid pulse for 5 to 10 seconds (see Fig. B.8). Locate the carotid artery by placing two fingers on the larynx, or Adam's apple. Slide your fingers laterally into the groove between the trachea and the muscles on the same side of the neck. Press lightly so that you do not compress the artery. Do not use your thumb. Establish pulselessness in an infant by checking the brachial pulse on the inside of the upper arm, between the armpit and elbow. Grasp the outside of the upper arm with your thumb. Palpate for a pulse with your index and middle fingers on the inside of the arm (see Fig. B.9).

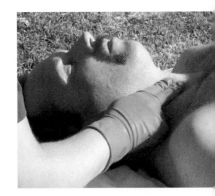

Figure B.8 *Whenever possible, avoid reaching across the patient's face to check the carotid pulse.*

Figure B.9 *An infant's brachial artery is larger than other arteries, and therefore easier to find for a pulse.*

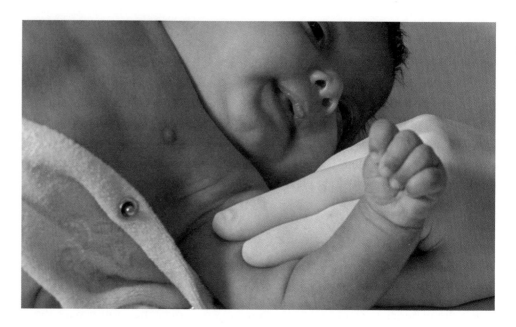

If the patient has a pulse and is not breathing, continue to provide artificial ventilations once every 5 seconds. Recheck the pulse every few minutes. If the pulse is absent, begin chest compressions. External chest compressions are repeated depressions of the lower half of the sternum. They increase the pressure in the chest, forcing blood to circulate. Combined with artificial ventilation, this will sustain life for a short period. Table B.1 summarizes chest compressions and artificial ventilation for adult, child, and infant patients.

Table B.1 • SUMMARY OF CPR METHODS

Procedure	Adult	Child (1 to 8 Years Old)	Infant (Under 1 Year)
Hand Position	Two hands on lower half of sternum	One hand on lower third of sternum	Two fingers on lower third of sternum (one finger width below nipple line)
Chest Compressions	80 to 100 per minute 1.5 to 2 inches deep	100 per minute 1 to 1.5 inches deep	At least 100 per minute .5 to 1 inch deep
Ventilations	1.5 to 2 seconds each 12 per minute	1 to 1.5 seconds each About 20 per minute	1 to 1.5 seconds each About 20 per minute
Ratio of Compressions to Ventilations in a CPR Cycle	15:2 (one rescuer) 5:1 (two rescuers)	5:1	5:1

Procedures for External Chest Compressions

Correct hand position on the chest wall is very important (see Fig. B.10). Proper hand position increases the effectiveness of chest compressions and reduces the risk of injury. Improper hand placement can cause:

• Fractured ribs or sternum

• Liver laceration or hemorrhage

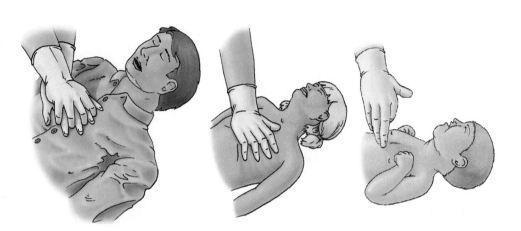

Figure B.10 *Correct hand positions for external chest compressions on an adult, a child, and an infant.*

- Severe damage to underlying organs, such as the spleen, lungs, or heart
- Ineffective compressions
- Fat embolism

Chest compressions can injure a person with a heartbeat. Make sure that the patient is pulseless before beginning.

Adult Patient. Follow these steps to perform external chest compressions for an adult:

1. Kneel alongside the patient, between the shoulders and lower ribs. Spread your knees about as far apart as your shoulders.

2. Using your hand closest to the patient's feet, locate the patient's lower rib margin on the side on which you are working. Run the fingers of your gloved hand up the rib margin until you reach the xiphoid process, the landmark for CPR. This is the notch where the ribs join the lower sternum. Keep two fingers directly over this to mark the location.

3. Place the heel of your other hand in the center of the chest, next to your fingers. It should be approximately two finger-widths above the notch (see Fig. B.11).

4. Place your first hand on top of the one on the chest. Your fingers may be extended or interlaced, but keep them off the chest wall. An alternate position is to grasp the wrist of the hand that is over the sternum with your free hand. This position is helpful for rescuers with arthritic hands and wrists. Again, be sure that your fingers are not in contact with the chest wall.

5. Position your shoulders directly over an imaginary line running between the patient's nose and navel. Lock your elbows so they do not bend. Bend at your hips to compress, using a straight, downward thrust (see Fig. B.12). Depress the sternum 1 to 2 inches.

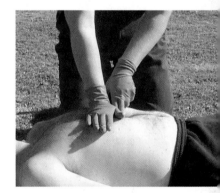

Figure B.11 *Use two fingers to measure the correct distance from the xiphoid process.*

Figure B.12 *Locking your arms causes you to push straight down on the sternum and provides the best blood flow.*

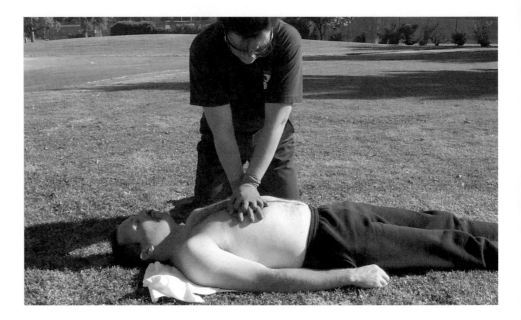

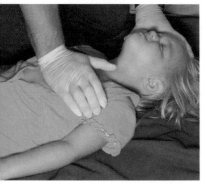

Figure B.13 *One-hand compressions exert the appropriate pressure on child's small frame.*

6. While maintaining contact with the chest wall, release pressure completely after each compression. Do not move your hand position. If direct contact with the chest wall is lost, stop and locate the landmark again. Then, repeat the procedure for finding the correct hand position.

7. Perform compressions at a rate of 80–100 per minute. Count each compression aloud. This helps others to time ventilations and to keep track of the number of cycles completed. Movements should be smooth and not jerky. Compression and relaxation time should be equal. Effective compressions will produce a carotid pulse.

Child Patient. Follow these steps to perform external chest compressions for a child aged 1 to 8 years:

1. Kneel beside the child's chest as you would for an adult. Use one hand to maintain the correct head and airway position.

2. Locate the correct hand position with your other hand. Slide your middle finger along the lower edge of the ribs until you reach the sternal notch. Place your middle and index finger over the lower sternum. Move the heel of that same hand to the spot just above your index finger. Do not rest your fingers on the chest. Use one hand for chest compressions in a child (see Fig. B.13).

3. Keep your shoulders directly over your hand. Push straight down. Depress the sternum 1 to 1.5 inches. This is roughly one-third to one-half the total depth of the chest. Use a smooth up-and-down movement. Release the pressure on the chest completely between compressions. Do not lift your hand from the chest.

4. Perform compressions at a rate of 100 per minute. Pause for ventilation for 1 to 1.5 seconds after every fifth compression. The compression-to-ventilation ratio is 5:1 for one or two rescuers.

5. If you are alone, keep one hand on the child's forehead to maintain head position during compressions (see Fig. B.14). After ventilating, return your hand to the previous position on the sternum and resume compressions. Try to visualize this location. Do not repeat the full procedure for finding the correct hand position, because this is too time-consuming.

Infant Patient. If you do not have the proper size barrier device for an infant, an adult collapsible face mask can be turned upside down to fit the infant's face. The nose portion of the mask fits over the chin. The rest of the mask covers the face. The strap can be tightened around the head to keep the mask in place.

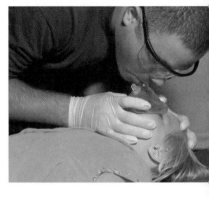

Figure B.14 *Depending on the size of the child, one rescuer may be able to seal the mask while maintaining an open airway.*

Follow these steps to perform external chest compressions for an infant aged less than 1 year:

1. Place the infant face up on a hard, flat surface. If possible, raise the shoulders slightly with a folded towel or blanket, or use your hand, palm up. This position provides a slight head-tilt, keeping the airway patent. Stand or kneel beside the infant's chest. Use one hand to maintain the head position (unless it is under the infant's back).

2. Find the correct position for chest compressions with your other hand (see Fig. B.15). Draw an imaginary line between the nipples. Place your index finger directly below that line in the center of the chest. Place your ring and middle fingers just below, directly over the sternum. Lift the index finger off the chest wall.

3. Perform chest compressions using your middle and ring fingers over the lower half of the sternum. Avoid compressing the xiphoid process. Depress the sternum .5 to 1 inch. This is roughly one-third to one-half the total depth of the chest. Compress with a smooth movement. Release pressure completely. However, do not lose contact with the chest wall between compressions.

Figure B.15 *Adequate compression can be delivered to an infant using two fingers.*

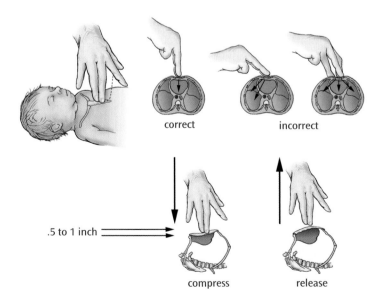

correct   incorrect

.5 to 1 inch

compress   release

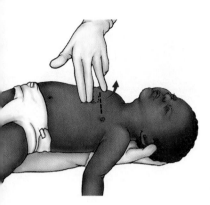

Figure B.16 *By cradling an infant in one arm, an EMT-B can support the head, deliver compressions, and ventilate quickly.*

4. Perform compressions at a rate of at least 100 per minute. Pause for ventilation for 1 to 5 seconds after every fifth compression. The compression-to-ventilation ratio is 5:1 for one or two rescuers.

For infants, there is an alternate method to deliver chest compressions (see Fig. B.16). If you are alone, using this method allows you to move the infant while you activate the EMS system.

1. Place the infant supine on your forearm. Your hand supports the head and neck. The torso is supported by your forearm. This tilts the head back slightly, which helps to maintain airway patency. Avoid excessive hyperextension of the neck. This could obstruct the airway. Avoid lifting the infant's head higher than the rest of the body.

2. Perform compressions with your other hand. Lift the infant to ventilate. This allows you to perform CPR with the infant on your forearm without changing hands or removing your fingers from the sternum.

When to Stop CPR

Continue CPR until one of the following occurs:

- Heart and lung function is restored
- Care is transferred to someone of equal or higher training
- A physician assumes care or determines that CPR should be stopped
- You are too exhausted to continue
- Environmental hazards endanger the rescuer or others ·
- A valid do not resuscitate (DNR) order is presented to the rescuers

Foreign Body Airway Obstruction

Airway obstruction is a common respiratory emergency. When the airway is blocked, the patient cannot breathe. As you can imagine, this condition quickly leads to loss of consciousness. If uncorrected, biological death will occur. Suspect airway obstruction in any person who suddenly stops breathing or becomes unconscious for no apparent reason. To treat airway obstruction successfully, you must recognize it early.

Foreign body airway obstruction (FBAO) may be caused by:

- Choking on food
- Foreign objects
- Vomit
- Blood in the airway
- Teeth in the airway from facial trauma

The airway may also be blocked by soft tissue swelling. Common causes are anaphylaxis, infection, or trauma. In unconscious patients such as those in cardiac arrest, the most common cause of airway obstruction is the tongue. When a person is unconscious, the tongue and soft tissues at the back of the throat relax and fall back. This blocks the upper airway.

Airway obstructions fall into two general categories—partial and complete. Complete airway obstruction occurs when the airway is completely blocked. No air can pass to the lungs. A patient with a partial airway obstruction has limited air movement in and out of the lungs.

With partial airway obstruction, the patient's air exchange may be adequate or poor. Determine whether air movement is adequate by observing the following:

- Level of responsiveness
- Ability to cough forcefully
- Ability to speak
- Ability to make audible sounds
- Presence of wheezing as air moves through the narrowed airway

If there is a partial airway obstruction with good air exchange, do not interfere with the person's attempts to clear the airway. Encourage him or her to continue coughing. Monitor the patient closely. If obstruction persists, activate the EMS system. If the obstruction worsens, be prepared to act. A patient with partial airway obstruction and good air exchange may progress to poor air exchange or complete obstruction.

Treatment for partial airway obstruction with poor air exchange is the same as for complete airway obstruction. A patient with poor air exchange will have:

- A weak, ineffective cough
- A high-pitched noise upon inhaling, called stridor
- Increased respiratory distress
- Cyanosis

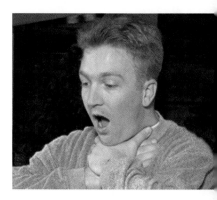

Figure B.17 *The universally recognized sign for choking.*

With complete airway obstruction, the patient is unable to breathe, cough, speak, or cry. He or she may clutch the throat with one or both hands (see Fig. B.17). This position is called the universal sign for choking. Air movement is absent or insufficient to support life. Begin emergency FBAO procedures immediately.

Special Considerations: Infants and Children

More than 90 percent of childhood deaths from FBAO occur in children under the age of 5. Sixty-five percent of these are infants. Suspect an airway obstruction in infants and children who demonstrate a sudden onset of respiratory distress associated with coughing, gagging, stridor, or wheezing.

In children, foreign body airway obstruction may be caused by:

- Small parts of toys
- Balloons
- Food such as hot dogs, round candies, nuts, and grapes

Airway obstruction may also be caused by infection, such as epiglottitis. If the obstruction is accompanied by congestion, lethargy, fever, or drooling, suspect infection as the cause. Children with this type of obstruction should be transported immediately to the nearest emergency facility.

As for adults, encourage children with a partial obstruction and good air exchange to continue coughing, if the cough is forceful. Attempt to clear the airway only if it is completely obstructed or partially obstructed with poor air exchange.

Procedures for FBAO

The specific procedure for clearing a foreign body airway obstruction depends on the patient's size and his or her position during the maneuver.

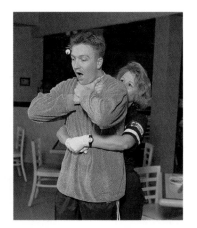

Figure B.18 *Proper hand positions for abdominal thrusts.*

Sitting or Standing Patient. A conscious patient with an obstructed airway is often found in a sitting or standing position. For both adults and children, check for scene safety, apply the principles of BSI and standard precautions, then:

1. Determine if the person is choking. He or she may clutch the throat with one or both hands. Ask, "Are you choking?"

2. Stand behind the patient. Wrap your arms around his or her waist. Place the thumb side of one fisted hand against the patient's abdomen in the middle, above the navel, but well below the xiphoid process. Grasp your fist with the other hand (see Figs. B.18 and B.19).

Figure B.19 *Locate the correct thrusting location with a fist.*

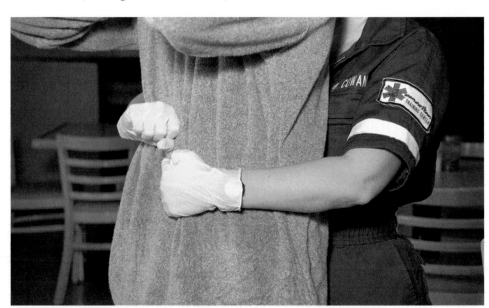

3. Give a series of up to five quick, upward thrusts into the abdomen. Avoid touching the xiphoid process or lower ribs. Each thrust is delivered as a distinct attempt to dislodge the object.

4. Repeat the abdominal thrusts until the material is dislodged, the patient begins coughing forcefully, or he or she becomes unconscious.

Patient Lying Down. Use this sequence to clear a foreign body obstruction from the airway of an adult or child who is found lying down. He or she may be conscious or unconscious. Check for scene safety, apply the principles of standard precautions, and then follow these steps:

1. Establish unresponsiveness. Pinch the patient gently or shout. If the patient is unresponsive, activate the EMS system.

2. Position the patient. The patient should be supine on a firm, flat surface. If he or she is prone, carefully roll the patient so that the head, shoulders, and torso move as a unit, without twisting. Keep the neck and back in a straight line.

3. Open the airway. Use the head-tilt/chin-lift or jaw-thrust maneuver. Avoid overextending the neck of a child.

4. Establish breathlessness. Look, listen, and feel for breathing for 3 to 5 seconds. If the patient is not breathing, proceed to the next step.

5. Provide two slow breaths. If the first attempt is unsuccessful, reposition the airway and try again.

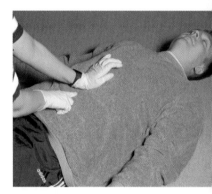

Figure B.20 *The proper position for the heel of the hand is just above the navel.*

6. Give five abdominal thrusts. Straddle the victim's thighs. Place the heel of one hand against the middle of the abdomen, just above the navel. Stay well below the xiphoid process (see Fig. B.20). Place the other hand on top of the first. Press into the abdomen with a series of up to five quick upward thrusts (see Fig. B.21). Each thrust is a distinct movement with the intent of dislodging the object.

Figure B.21 *Deliver a series of quick upward thrusts.*

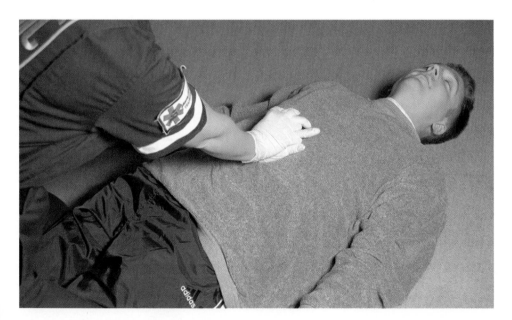

Figure B.22 *Hook a finger around the object and sweep it out.*

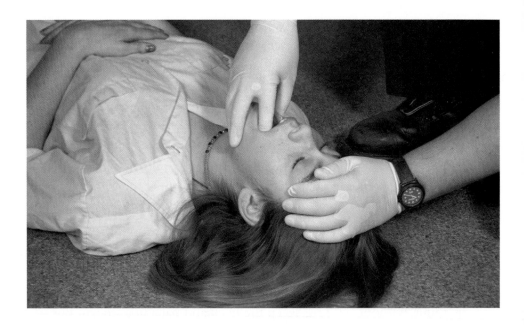

7. Do a finger sweep of the mouth (see Fig. B.22). Grasp the tongue and jaw between your thumb and fingers. Lift the jaw. Slide your finger down the side of the cheek to the base of the tongue. Attempt to remove any foreign body. This maneuver is done only for an unconscious patient. Avoid blind finger sweeps in children. Only do a finger sweep if you can see the foreign object.

8. Open the airway and give two slow breaths. If the breaths go in, check for a pulse and spontaneous breathing. If the patient has a pulse but is not breathing, provide artificial ventilation and monitor the pulse. If the pulse is absent, begin CPR.

9. If the first attempt is unsuccessful, reposition the airway and attempt to ventilate. If the breaths still do not go in, repeat the sequence until the obstruction is removed, or the person starts breathing or coughing.

Obese Patient or Late Pregnancy. Use the chest thrust when there is no room between the abdomen and the rib cage in which to do abdominal thrusts. The procedure is used for obese patients or women in the late stages of pregnancy. First check for scene safety and apply the principles of BSI and standard precautions.

Stand behind the patient. Place your arms under the patient's armpits and around the chest. Place the thumb side of one fist against the center of the sternum. Avoid pressing on the ribs or xiphoid process. Grab your fist with your other hand. Thrust inward repeatedly until the object is dislodged or the patient loses consciousness.

For an unconscious patient, kneel beside the patient. Place the heel of one hand on the center of the sternum. Position the other hand on top of it. Deliver up to five quick thrusts, each 1 to 2 inches deep. Then do a finger sweep, followed by two slow breaths. If the first attempt is unsuccessful, reposition the airway and attempt to ventilate again. If the breaths still do not go in, repeat the sequence until the obstruction is removed or the person starts to breathe or cough.

Infant Patient. This sequence is used to clear a foreign body obstruction from an infant's airway. Check for scene safety, apply the principles of standard precautions, and then follow these steps:

1. Establish unresponsiveness. Shake or tap the infant gently.

2. Position the infant face down on your forearm. If he or she is prone, carefully roll so that the head, shoulders, and torso move as a unit, without twisting. If possible, have others help you. Keep the neck and back in a straight line.

3. Open the airway. Use the head–tilt/chin–lift or jaw–thrust maneuver. Avoid overextending the neck of an infant, since this could collapse the airway.

4. Establish breathlessness. Look, listen, and feel for breathing (3 to 5 seconds).

5. If the infant is not breathing, provide two slow breaths. If the first attempt is unsuccessful, reposition the airway and try again. If the second attempt is unsuccessful, consider the airway to be completely blocked and continue with the FBAO procedure.

6. Position the infant prone on your forearm (see Fig. B.23). Keep the head lower than the body. Support the infant's head by firmly holding the jaw. Avoid blocking the airway with your hand. Place your forearm against your thigh for stability during back blows. Deliver five forceful back blows between the infant's shoulder blades with the heel of your hand. Each blow is a distinct movement with the intent of dislodging the object. Elevate the hand, doing the back blows about 4 to 5 inches from the infant's back. Each back blow should increase in strength to help dislodge the object.

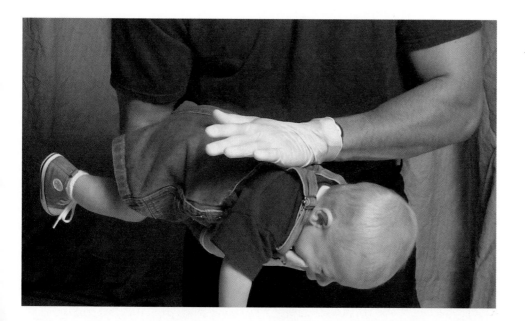

Figure B.23 *Deliver five forceful blows between the shoulder blades.*

7. If the object is not dislodged, support the infant's back with your free hand. Roll him or her to a supine position on your forearm. Rest your forearm and the infant on your thigh. The infant's head must remain lower than the body. Deliver five quick upward chest thrusts, compressing the lower sternum .5 to 1 inch. Each blow is a distinct movement with the intention of dislodging the object. The correct position is the same as for chest compressions, one finger width below the line between the nipples. Keep your fingers off the xiphoid process.

8. Do a finger sweep. Grasp the tongue and jaw between your thumb and fingers and lift the jaw. If you see an object, slide your little finger down the side of the cheek to the base of the tongue. Attempt to remove the object. Never do a blind finger sweep on an infant.

9. Open the airway and give two slow breaths. If the first attempt is unsuccessful, reposition the airway and attempt to ventilate again. If the breaths still do not go in, repeat the back blows and chest thrusts until the obstruction is removed or the infant starts to breathe, cough, or cry.

10. If the breaths go in, check for pulse and spontaneous breathing. If the patient has a pulse but is not breathing, provide artificial ventilation and monitor the pulse. If the pulse is absent, begin CPR.

Self-Administered FBAO. If you are alone and choking, you can do abdominal thrusts by placing your fist, thumb side in, on your upper abdomen, above the navel. Stay well below the xiphoid process. Apply quick upward thrusts. If this does not work, press your abdomen firmly over a flat surface, such as the back of a chair, the side of a table, or a sink.

If your EMS system has enhancement features, dial 9-1-1 while you are choking. An enhanced system instantly lists the caller's address on the dispatcher's screen. Dial and leave the phone connected. You should receive help quickly.

APPENDIX

C

Infection Control

Infection control has become one of the most important aspects of health care, especially for those who provide emergency medical care. Emergency medical professionals often encounter patients with severe illnesses or injuries. You may not know that a patient had an infectious disease until days or weeks after providing care. Therefore, it is extremely important to keep abreast of the latest infection control standards and techniques.

Adequate infection control is an essential step in caring for both your patients and yourself. Failing to practice proper infection control can lead to added illness for yourself and for your patients. Imagine if a trauma patient from your shift today was exposed to an infection from a sick child you transported yesterday. Infection often seriously compromises a patient's recovery. Practicing effective infection control is an essential responsibility of every EMT-Basic.

Effective infection control precautions combine effective work-practice, administrative, and engineering controls with personal protective equipment, medical management techniques, and education. Standard precautions should be utilized for all patient contact, and transmission-based precautions should be used when appropriate.

INFECTION CONTROL IN EMS

Although infection control is a relatively new addition to EMS training, the concept of preventing the spread of diseases has existed since the 1800s. The Centers for Disease Control and Prevention (commonly referred to as the CDC) are agencies of the federal government. The CDC are branches of the Department of Health and Human Services. They are responsible for research related to infectious disease, focusing primarily on treating and preventing the spread of these diseases. In 1970, the CDC issued the first guidelines for hospitals to help combat the spread of infectious disease. These guidelines continue to be revised and updated as knowledge advances.

In 1985, the infection control strategy known as universal precautions was developed in response to the HIV epidemic. Healthcare providers were greatly concerned after initial reports of hospital personnel contracting the disease through accidental needlesticks and skin contamination. Prior to implementation of universal precautions, patients were not considered infectious until a diagnosis had been made in the hospital setting. These guidelines recommended handling all blood and certain body fluids as if they were potentially infectious.

In 1987, the concept of body substance isolation (BSI) was adopted by numerous hospitals, based on research done at Harborview Medical Center in Seattle and the University of California at San Diego. BSI, which is the infection control concept presented in the 1994 EMT-B curriculum, assumed that all moist and potentially infectious body substances from all patients should be isolated from the healthcare provider.

Although BSI and universal precautions had many similar features, each had strengths and weaknesses. Many hospitals and agencies combined aspects of both into their infection control programs. This led to widely varying interpretations of the standards. The standards did not address the fact that airborne droplets transmit some infectious diseases, like tuberculosis. Also, some infectious diseases can be transmitted by contact with unbroken, dry skin.

The lack of unified guidelines that addressed each system's weaknesses was very distressing to the CDC and infection control personnel. In view of these problems and concerns, a revised set of guidelines regarding isolation precautions in hospitals was established in 1996. The revised guidelines were developed to meet the following objectives of an infection control system:

- The system is epidemiologically sound. This means the system is developed, studied, and tested by qualified scientists.

- The system recognizes the role of all body fluids (except sweat), secretions, excretions, mucous membranes, and non-intact skin in the transmission of pathogens. The most common are bacteria and viruses.

- The system contains adequate precautions for infections spread by airborne, droplet, and contact routes of transmission.

- The system is simple and as user-friendly as possible.

- The system uses new terms to avoid confusion with existing systems.

The revised guidelines contain two levels of precautions. The first level, known as standard precautions (SP), is designed to apply to all patients, regardless of diagnosis or presumed infections. The second level, known as transmission-based precautions, applies to patients with symptoms of a disease that can be transmitted by air, droplet, or contact methods. The system relies on the healthcare worker's judgment, rather than a medical diagnosis, to assess risk and identify necessary protective steps.

Following the publication of *Standard and Transmission-Based Precautions* in early 1996, and the release of *Draft Guidelines for Infection Control for Health Care Personnel* by the CDC in 1997, standard precautions became part of the CDCs' overall infection control plan. Emergency medical professionals are specifically addressed in this document. The guidelines set a new, higher standard for infection control for all healthcare providers.

Besides these guidelines for preventing transmission of infection, legislation was passed in 1990 to ensure that emergency response employees are notified of potentially fatal infectious diseases that they are exposed to while caring for patients. This legislation is known as the *1990 Ryan White Comprehensive AIDS Resources Emergency Act*. It encompasses all emergency response employees, including EMTs, firefighters, and policemen.

Infectious Disease Basics

In order for a disease to be transmitted, there are certain events that must occur. This process is called the chain of infection. First, a person must be carrying, or hosting, a pathogen. Pathogens are the agents that cause infection. Two of the most common pathogens are viruses and bacteria; others include parasites, fungi, and protozoa. Second, there has to be enough of the pathogen present to be transmitted to another person (a reservoir). There also must be a way for the pathogen to exit the host. This can involve a cough, bleeding, or a secretion of the body.

Once an exit route has been established for the pathogen, it is available for transmission to others. Common routes of transmission include direct and indirect contact with the patient's secretions, or breathing pathogens carried in the air. Impeding transmission of pathogens is the most important goal of standard precautions.

Simply being exposed to a pathogen does not guarantee that you will become infected with the disease. After transmission, the pathogen must have a way to get into your body. Common entry sites include the mucous membranes, non-intact skin, and the respiratory system. Once a pathogen has entered your body, several other factors influence whether or not you will contract the disease. A person's natural ability to resist disease is called immunity. Factors that can affect your immunity include diet, age, underlying illness, medications, previous exposures to or immunizations against the disease, and even your stress level.

Interrupting the chain of infection at any point greatly reduces your chances of catching an infectious disease. The best way is to interrupt the transmission of the disease. Most pathogens cannot survive outside a host for very long.

Pathogen Transmission

Pathogens are transmitted by five distinct methods:

- Contact
- Droplet
- Air
- Common vehicle
- Vector

Contact transmission occurs in two distinct ways, directly or indirectly. Direct contact transmission refers to contact between body surfaces that results in the physical transfer of a pathogen from one person to another. It usually occurs through nonintact skin or through the mucous membranes of the eyes, nose, or mouth. For example, direct contact may occur when examining, moving, or treating a patient who has external bleeding. Another common example is exposure to sputum or saliva when establishing an airway in a patient. Indirect contact takes place when one person touches an object contaminated by another, such as a dressing soaked with blood or an airway covered with oral secretions. Perhaps the most obvious and worrisome example of contact transmission is the bloodborne route. Bloodborne transmission can occur by either direct contact, such as blood squirting into your eye or onto an open cut on your arm, or indirect contact, such as a stick from a contaminated needle.

Droplet transmission occurs when tiny droplets containing a pathogen are expelled by the patient by a cough, a sneeze, or speech. Droplets can also be generated when performing tasks such as suctioning or endotracheal intubation. When these droplets come in contact with the mucous membranes of the eyes, nose, or mouth, the provider can become infected. Some pathogens are truly airborne. These pathogens may originally be expelled in droplet form, but they can remain airborne for long periods of time and may be widely dispersed by air currents. Some pathogens can be suspended in dust particles, as well. The nucleus or core of these pathogens is very small and can be carried great distances.

Common-vehicle transmission occurs when the pathogen is transmitted by contaminated items such as food, water, medications, devices, or equipment. Vector-borne pathogens are transmitted by animal bites, insects, and rodents.

Controlling the Spread of Infections

There are five major components to every comprehensive infection control program. The essential elements are:

- Administrative controls
- Engineering controls
- Work-practice controls
- Medical management practices
- Provider education

How each agency controls the risk of exposure to infectious disease should be outlined in an exposure control plan. In many agencies, this plan only addresses exposure to bloodborne pathogens.

Administrative controls are policies and procedures that are set for an agency. They ensure that all employees with the potential for exposure to pathogens are treated equally. Administrative controls include policies for new employee training, immunization requirements, and post-exposure plans. One administrative control that is often overlooked in EMS is a proactive stance towards employee illness. Some agencies encourage employees to stay out of work when they have an infectious disease such as the flu, so that the illness is not transmitted to other employees or patients.

Engineering controls are designed to reduce the exposure to pathogens by removing hazards or isolating the worker from hazards whenever possible. Providing personal protective equipment (PPE) such as gloves, goggles, and respirators is an essential engineering control. Respirators must be approved by the National Institute of Occupational Safety and Health (NIOSH). Examples include the N95, PFR95, and high-efficiency particulate air (HEPA) respirators. HEPA respirators are capable of filtering out the tuberculosis bacterium, something an ordinary face mask cannot do. A HEPA respirator should be worn whenever treating a patient with suspected or known tuberculosis. Other engineering controls found in EMS include the placement of sharps containers in the ambulance and the availability of self-capping needles or needleless administration systems.

Work-practice controls are ways in which tasks are altered to minimize or eliminate the exposure to a pathogen. One of the first work-practice controls implemented was to eliminate the recapping of needles. Proper disposal of contaminated linen and biohazardous materials are also work-practice controls. Another example is handwashing.

Medical management practices are designed to reduce the risk of developing an infection in the event an exposure occurs. Annual tuberculosis skin testing and physical exams for providers are examples of proactive medical management. Providing immunizations when available is also essential. Post-exposure therapy with antibiotics or antiviral agents is a crucial medical management tool.

Perhaps the single most important aspect of infection control is continuing education. Infection control is a rapidly changing area of study. Standard precautions, which are outlined below, represent a dramatic departure from previous guidelines, but they have been developed in less than two years. It is very important for EMS providers to maintain a current knowledge of the local infection control standards.

Standard Precautions

Standard precautions are designed to interrupt the chain of infection. They are sufficient to prevent the transmission of most common diseases. Standard precautions include:

• Handwashing

• Gloves

• Limiting the placement and transportation of patients

- Use of masks, respiratory protection, eye protection and face shields, gowns, and protective apparel
- Safe handling of patient equipment and soiled linen and laundry
- Cleaning or disinfecting procedures

Standard precautions apply to blood; to all body fluids, secretions, and excretions (except sweat) regardless of whether blood is visible; to nonintact skin; and to mucous membranes.

Handwashing

Handwashing is the single most important measure for reducing the risk of transmitting microorganisms from one person to another. Handwashing should be performed immediately before donning gloves and after removing gloves. Handwashing should be performed after contact with body substances or equipment contaminated by such substances. If handwashing is not feasible, an alcohol-based hand cleaner or disinfectant is recommended. Handwashing should be thorough and complete, including your wrists, forearms, between the fingers, and around the nail cuticles. Remove any jewelry from your hands. Using plain soap, lather and scrub for a minimum of 10 to 15 seconds. This should be sufficient to remove most contaminants.

Personal Protective Equipment

Gloves serve three basic purposes. First, they create a barrier between the provider and patient, preventing contamination when touching body substances. This reduces the chance of a pathogen reaching the provider. Second, gloves prevent pathogens from traveling from the provider to the patient. Third, they prevent pathogens from one patient being transmitted to another patient when being cared for by the same provider. However, wearing gloves is not a substitute for handwashing.

Some basic rules for glove use are:

- Change gloves frequently, especially before and after patient contact
- Change gloves when they are grossly contaminated with body substances
- Replace torn or damaged gloves immediately
- Replace soiled gloves before performing invasive or sterile procedures
- Change gloves before caring for different sites on the same person (i.e., moving from open wounds to airway management)
- Change gloves immediately before contact with nonintact skin and mucous membranes
- Remove gloves (and wash hands) promptly after use and before touching uncontaminated objects

There are several devices designed to protect the mucous membranes of the eyes, nose, and mouth. These include masks, eye protection, and face shields. Any time a procedure is likely to generate splashes or sprays of blood, body fluids, secretions, or excretions, protection must be given to the provider's mucous membranes. Airway management procedures are situations in which such protection is advisable. If a patient has a very active, productive cough, consider placing a mask on the patient as well, to limit dispersal of any pathogens. Remember that a mask may be worn without protective eyewear, but eyewear should not be worn without a mask.

If the patient's signs or symptoms make you suspect tuberculosis, be sure to use specialized respiratory protection. The pathogens responsible for tuberculosis are so small that a normal mask does not filter out the particles. You should use either a high-efficiency particulate air (HEPA) mask or a mask certified to meet the NIOSH N95 standard. There is a picture of a HEPA mask in Chapter 2 (Figure 2.8).

Numerous articles of clothing are available to protect EMS providers. Wear a gown or another protective garment to reduce the chance of contaminating your clothing or exposing nonintact skin to pathogens. The use of these protective garments is necessary when splashing may be anticipated, or when large quantities of infectious material may be present.

Limiting the Placement and Transport of Patients

Although more applicable to the hospital environment, EMS providers must consider appropriate placement and transportation of patients. Placing a sick, potentially infectious patient in the same vehicle as a healthy patient is an infection control hazard.

Patient Care Equipment

Whenever possible, the use of single-patient, disposable equipment is recommended. Care must be taken to dispose of such items properly. All used sharps (needles, scalpels, or other sharp instruments) should be placed in a puncture-resistant container immediately after use. Do not recap used needles. Other items should be placed in an appropriate container and disposed of in accordance with your agency's policy and procedures.

Care must be taken when handling soiled patient linen. In many cases, pathogens are present after patient contact. If handled, transported, and laundered appropriately, there is little danger of disease transmission. Many organizations now utilize disposable sheets, blankets, and towels to minimize laundry costs and patient risk. Always wear gloves when handling soiled linen. Your agency's exposure control plan should provide instructions on the handling of soiled linen or laundry items.

All disposable supplies and equipment should be discarded as soon as practical after patient use. All other materials should be cleaned using disinfection, high-level disinfection, or sterilization. Cleaning of EMS equipment is discussed in more detail in Chapter 24.

Transmission-Based Precautions

Standard precautions are meant to be used on all patients. In some cases, the EMS provider may identify certain signs and symptoms that warrant steps in addition to standard precautions. The CDC have identified three additional levels of isolation for certain patients to prevent airborne, droplet, and contact transmissions. Called transmission-based precautions, the EMS provider will most likely encounter these during interfacility transports or in extended care facilities. In these environments, you may be informed of specific transmission-based precautions to take by patient care staff or by a sign on a patient's door. The need for these precautions may be based on a known diagnosis of an infectious process, or simply on the signs and symptoms the patient is exhibiting. Some examples are shown in Table C.1. Note that certain infections require more than one type of precaution.

Airborne precautions are designed to inhibit the transmission of pathogens through the air. Airborne pathogens can be widely dispersed and may present a threat to providers in the same room or the same house as the patient. Airborne precautions center on the use of respiratory protection, notably N95 or HEPA respirators. Examples of conditions that require airborne precautions are measles, varicella (chicken pox), and tuberculosis.

Droplet precautions are necessary when patients are coughing, sneezing, or talking. Droplet transmission is especially likely during airway management procedures. Providers working within 3 feet of the patient should utilize masks, eye protection, or shields to protect their mucous membranes. Use droplet precautions in cases of:

- Epiglottitis (Haemophilus influenzae type b)
- Meningitis (Neisseria meningitidis, Haemophilus influenzae type b)
- Diphtheria (pharyngeal)
- Pertussis (whooping cough)
- Streptococcal (group A) pharyngitis, pneumonia, or scarlet fever in infants and young children
- Serious viral infections spread by droplet transmission, including influenza, mumps, and respiratory syncytial virus (RSV)

Table C.1 • SPECIFIC TRANSMISSION-BASED PRECAUTIONS

Sign, Symptom, or Complaint	Isolation Guidelines
Diarrhea in an incontinent or diapered patient	Contact precautions
Diarrhea in an adult with a recent history of antibiotic use	Contact precautions
History of high fever and neck pain or stiffness	Droplet precautions
Rash, cause unknown, with fever	Airborne, droplet, and contact precautions
Adult with persistent cough, fever, weight loss	Airborne precautions
Child with history of respiratory infections, specifically bronchiolitis or croup	Contact precautions
History of antibiotic-resistant infections	Contact precautions
Skin, wound, or urinary infection, together with a recent stay in a hospital or extended care facility where antibiotic-resistant infections are present	Contact precautions
Skin or wound infection with drainage	Contact precautions

Contact precautions reduce the risk of transmission of pathogens by direct or indirect contact. Often, this occurs during the transfer of a patient from a stretcher to a bed or vice versa. In addition to standard precautions, the use of gowns and disposable patient equipment is recommended. Contact precautions should be used for:

- Hepatitis A or diarrheal diseases (for diapered or incontinent patients)
- Respiratory syncytial virus (RSV)
- Rubella (German measles)
- Skin infections
- Diphtheria (cutaneous)
- Herpes simplex virus (neonatal or mucocutaneous)
- Impetigo (Strep or Staph)
- Major (noncontained) abscesses, skin infections, or decubiti
- Lice (Pediculosis)
- Scabies
- Staphylococcal (boils)
- Zoster (shingles)

Table C.2 summarizes important properties of many infectious diseases that are of concern to EMS personnel.

Table C.2 • COMMON INFECTIOUS DISEASES

Disease or Pathogen	Types of Transmission	Infection Risk to EMS Providers	Exposure, Infection, Follow-Up
Chicken pox (Varicella)	Contact Airborne	Low if immune; high if not immunized	Avoid contact with susceptible populations for days 10–21 after exposure. An exposed person who develops chicken pox is contagious from 2 days prior to rash until all lesions are dry and crusted.
Common Cold	Droplet	Unknown; possibly significant	None
Conjunctivitis	Contact	Moderate	If infected, avoid patient contact until discharge ceases.
Cytomegalovirus	Contact Droplet	Low	None
Diarrheal Diseases	Contact Common-vehicle Airborne (possible)	Low to moderate	Follow up with personal physician if symptoms develop. Avoid patient care until symptoms resolve.
Diphtheria	Contact Droplet	Low	Contact infection control officer. Maintain 10-year vaccination (Td, tetanus-diphtheria). If exposed, prophylaxis may be indicated and suggest a 5-year vaccine. If infected, no patient care until treated and medically cleared.
Epiglottitis	Droplet	Unknown; probably low	Refers to Haemophilus influenzae type b. Contact infection control officer. Prophylaxis may be indicated.
German Measles (Rubella)	Droplet	Unknown; at risk if not immune	Avoid contact with susceptible populations for days 7–21 after exposure, or for 5 days after rash appears. Pregnant women should contact their obstetrician.
Hepatitis A	Oral-fecal contact Common-vehicle	Minimal	Contact infection control officer. Prophylaxis may be indicated. Avoid patient care and food handling for 7 days after onset of illness.
Hepatitis B, C, D, E	Bloodborne contact	Significant unless immunized (only available for hepatitis B)	Hepatitis B immune globulin and hepatitis B vaccine if not previously immunized. Contact infection control officer in all cases.
Herpes Simplex	Contact	Unknown; probably significant	None
Herpes Zoster (Shingles)	Contact Airborne, if widely disseminated	Localized risk	Same virus as chicken pox. If susceptible to chicken pox, avoid contact with susceptible populations for days 10–21 after exposure. If chicken pox develops, follow exposure guidelines given earlier.
HIV/AIDS	Bloodborne contact	Low	Wash exposed area. Prophylaxis medications if significant exposure (i.e., needlestick or mucous membrane splash) from blood or body fluid of high-risk patient. Contact infection control officer in all cases.

Table C.2 • **COMMON INFECTIOUS DISEASES** *(cont.)*

Disease or Pathogen	Types of Transmission	Infection Risk to EMS Providers	Exposure, Infection, Follow-Up
Influenza	Airborne Droplet	Unknown; probably significant	Annual immunization if possible. If unvaccinated and community outbreak, consider antiviral post-exposure prophylaxis. If symptomatic, avoid contact with high-risk patients until acute symptoms resolve.
Lice (Head, Body, Pubic)	Contact (close contact required)	Unknown; probably significant if contact is intimate	Observe for signs of infestation. Contact physician for prescription of prophylactic shampoo. If infected, avoid patient contact until treated and free of adult and immature lice.
Measles	Droplets Airborne (possible)	Unknown; probably significant	Check immunity status. If susceptible, administer vaccine within 72 hours, and avoid susceptible people from 5 days after first exposure to 21 days after last exposure or for 7 days after rash appears.
Meningitis	Contact Droplet	Unknown; probably low	Refers to meningococcal disease; other pathogens possible. Prophylaxis medication if significant exposure. If infected, avoid patient contact until 24 hours after effective treatment started.
Mumps	Contact	Low	Immunize (if possible) if no documented immunity. Avoid patient contact for days 12 through 25 after exposure or for 9 days after onset of symptoms.
Pertussis (Whooping Cough)	Contact Droplet	Moderate	Contact infection control officer. If symptomatic, avoid patient care for 5 days after treatment started.
Scabies	Contact (close contact required)	Unknown; probably significant if contact is intimate	Observe for signs of infestation. Contact physician for prescription of prophylactic shampoo. If infested, avoid patient contact until treated and medically cleared.
Respiratory Syncytial Virus (RSV)	Contact Droplet	Moderate	If community outbreak, avoid contact with susceptible populations (most notably infants and children) for days 2–16 after exposure, or until symptoms resolve.
Staphylococcus (Staph)	Contact (major route) Droplet Airborne (possible)	Moderate	If skin lesions are actively draining, avoid contact until appropriate antibiotic treatment and lesions have resolved.
Streptococcus, Group A Infection (Strep)	Contact Droplet Airborne (possible)	Moderate	If infected, avoid contact until 24 hours after antibiotic therapy begins.
Tuberculosis	Airborne	Moderate	Follow-up evaluations after exposure. If active disease, exclude from duty until proven noninfectious.

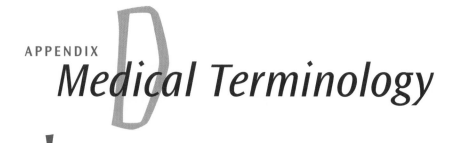

APPENDIX
Medical Terminology

In this Appendix you will be introduced to word elements that make up many medical terms commonly used in the EMS profession. At first glance, medical terminology may seem to be a highly technical and rather complex vocabulary to learn. But the understanding of many medical terms can actually be quite simple. Medical terms, more often than not, adhere to just a few fairly straight-forward laws of pronunciation and meaning in the English language.

Most medical terms are combinations of word elements or combining forms known as prefixes, roots, and suffixes. Use of these elements builds recognition from one term to the next. Since the elements are usually based on Latin or Greek roots, you will see remarkable overlap between many medical terms in different languages. For example, *pericarditis* has exactly the same spelling and meaning in Spanish as in English (although it has a different pronunciation).

Medical word prefixes, roots, and suffixes are often used interchangeably and common patterns exist. Consequently, your ability to decipher unfamiliar medical words will improve as you study and apply the information in this appendix. Once you learn the major medical words and word parts, you will be able to understand many terms used throughout the medical professions.

Table D.1 shows an example of how medical terms depend on combining forms. Three combining forms are used to make the word *pericarditis*. Not all medical terms include a prefix, root, and suffix; some terms are just roots, some contain prefix and root combining forms, and some have only root and suffix combining forms.

History of Medical Terminology

At one time, the study of Latin and Greek was prerequisite to the study of medicine. Perhaps 75 percent of scientific vocabulary originated from these languages. The earliest recorded clinicians, Hippocrates, Galen, and Aristotle

Table D.1 • ELEMENTS OF A MEDICAL TERM

Combining Form	Example	Meaning
Prefix	peri-	around
Root	cardi/o	heart
Suffix	-itis	inflammation
Term	pericarditis	inflammation around the heart

(460 BC to 201 AD) wrote in Greek. *Bronchus, carcinoma, coccyx, diastole, emphysema, erythema, glaucoma, herpes, meninges, pancreas, thorax,* and *urethra* are just a few examples of words still used 2000 years later. Terms that appeared in ancient Latin medical writing (30 to 79 AD) include *abdomen, cancer, delirium, fistula, hernia, patella,* and *pus.*

Medical terms have also evolved from familiar words. Many terms find their origins in words for weapons, household items, living creatures, vegetables, and fruits. Ancient misconceptions have also left their mark: *artery* means air carrier and *melancholia* was thought to be caused by black bile. Throughout the ages, words and phrases have been continuously added from every language as new discoveries, concepts, and theories have necessitated new words to describe and define them.

Table D.2 lists combining forms that comprise common medical terms used by EMS professionals. This is not a complete reference for learning general medical terminology. For students who are interested in expanding their knowledge of medical terminology, *Med Terms–Illustrated* is an interactive, multimedia course on CD-ROM published by Victory Technology, Inc. The added feature of sound provides a key tool for mastering proper pronunciation, a vital skill for medical professionals. You can find more information on ordering it on the Internet at www.MedCollege.com.

Table D.2 • COMMON MEDICAL TERMINOLOGY

Combining Form	Definition	Example
ab-	away; from	abduct (movement of a limb away from the body)
ad-	toward; to	adduction (movement of a limb towards the body)
aden/o	gland	adenoids
adip/o	fat; lipid (also lip/o)	adipose (fatty tissue)
-algia	pain (also -dynia)	myalgia (muscle pain)
angi/o	vessel (also vas/o)	angiogram (radiographic technique to visualize the vessels)
anti-	against (also contra-)	antibiotic (a drug that fights microscopic pathogens) anti-inflammatory (something that reduces inflammation)
a-; an-	no; none	anuria (no urine output)
brachi/o	upper arm	brachial pulse
brady-	slow	bradycardia (slow heart rate)
carcin/o	cancer	carcinogen (a substance that causes cancer)
cardi/o	heart	cardiovascular (pertaining to the heart and vessels)
chem/o	chemical; drug	chemotherapy
contra-	against (also anti-)	contraindicated (not advisable)

Table D.2 • **COMMON MEDICAL TERMINOLOGY** (cont.)

Term	Definition	Example
crani/o	skull	cranium
cutane/o	skin (also cuti)	subcutaneous (under the skin)
cyan/o	blue	cyanosis (lack of oxygen causes purple/blue color in tissues)
dis-	remove; absence	disinfect (remove pathogens)
-emesis	vomiting	antiemetic (drug that reduces the likelihood of vomiting)
-emia	blood or blood condition	anemia (reduced hemoglobin or blood)
encephal/o	brain	encephalitis (an inflammation of the brain)
endo-	in; within (also en-, ento-)	endocarditis (inflammation of the innermost layer of the heart)
gastr/o	stomach	gastrointestinal (referring to stomach and intestines)
hem/o	blood (also hemat/o)	hemoglobin (blood protein that carries oxygen)
hemat/o	blood (also hem/o)	hematoma (blood clot)
hemi-	half	hemiplegia (paralysis of half of the body)
hepat/o	liver	hepatitis (inflammation of the liver)
hyper-	over; abnormally high	hypertension (abnormally increased blood pressure)
hypo-	under; abnormally low	hypothermia (abnormally low body temperature)
idi/o	unknown	idiopathic (disease of unknown origin)
inter-	between	intercostal (between the ribs)
intra-	within	intramuscular (within the muscle) intravenous (within a vein)
-itis	inflammation	pharyngitis (inflammation of the pharynx)
leuk/o	white (also alb/o)	leukocyte (white blood cell)
-ology	study of	cardiology (medical specialty relating to the study of the heart)
mast/o	breast	mastectomy (surgical removal of a breast)
mega-	huge; enlarged	megadose (large dose)
mening/o	meninges	meningitis (inflammation of the membrane covering the brain)
my/o	muscle	myocardial (the muscle of the heart)
neur/o	nerve	neurology (the study of the nervous system)
-oma	tumor (also onc/o)	carcinoma (a type of cancer)
ot/o	ear	otitis (inflammation of the ear)
path/o	disease	pathogen (an organism that causes disease)
-pathy	disease	cardiomyopathy (a disease of the muscle of the heart)
ped	child	pediatrics (medical specialty that deals with children)
peri-	around	pericardium (the membrane that surrounds the heart)

Table D.2 • **COMMON MEDICAL TERMINOLOGY** *(cont.)*

Term	Definition	Example
pharyng/o	pharynx	pharyngitis (inflammation of the pharynx)
-phasia	speech	aphasia (inability to speak)
phleb/o	vein	phlebitis (inflammation of a vein)
-phobia	abnormal fear	arachnophobia (fear of spiders)
-plegia	paralysis	quadriplegia (paralysis of all four limbs)
pleur/o	pleura	pleuritis (inflammation of the lining of the lungs)
-pnea	breathe; air	apnea (inability to breath)
pneum/o	lung; breathe; air (also pneumon/o, pulmon/o)	pneumonia (infection of the lungs)
post-	after; behind	posterior (back)
pre-	before; forward	prehospital care
primi-	first (also prot/o)	primigravida (a woman in her first pregnancy)
psych/o	mind	psychogenic (originating in the mind rather than the body)
-ptysis	spitting	hemoptysis (spitting up blood)
pulmon/o	lung; air; breathe (also pneum/o, pneumon/o)	pulmonary edema (fluid in the lungs)
quadri-	four	quadriplegia (paralysis of all four limbs)
rhin/o	nose	rhinitis (inflammation of the mucous membrane of the nose)
-rrhage	excessive or unusual discharge; profuse flow	hemorrhage (excessive bleeding)
-rrhea	flow	diarrhea (loose, watery stool)
-somnia	sleep	insomnia (inability to sleep)
son/o	sound	sonogram (diagnostic imaging test which uses sound waves)
stomat/o	mouth	stomatitis (inflammation of the mouth)
-stomy	surgical opening	colostomy (surgical opening in the bowel)
sub-	under (also hypo-)	subcutaneous (under the skin) sublingual (under the tongue)
tachy-	fast	tachycardia (rapid heart rate) tachypnea (rapid respiration rate)
therm/o	hot; temperature	hypothermia (abnormally low body temperature)
-tomy	incision	tracheotomy (incision in the windpipe)
trache/o	windpipe	tracheostomy (surgical opening in the windpipe)
uni-	one (also mono-)	unilateral (pertaining to one side)
ur/o	urine	uremia (excessive waste products in the blood)

APPENDIX

E
Answers to Review Questions

Following are the correct answers to the odd-numbered Review Questions.

1 | Introduction to Emergency Medical Care

1 D
3 C
5 C
7 A
9 B
11 C

2 | The Well-Being of the EMT-Basic

1 D
3 D
5 C
7 A
9 A
11 C
13 B

3 | Medical, Legal, and Ethical Issues

1 C
3 D
5 C
7 D
9 D
11 D
13 D
15 A

4 | The Human Body

1 B
3 D
5 C
7 D
9 B
11 B
13 B
15 D
17 B

5 | Vital Signs and SAMPLE History

1 A
3 A
5 B
7 B
9 A
11 B
13 B
15 D
17 B
19 D
21 C

6 | Lifting and Moving Patients

1 B
3 A
5 D
7 C
9 D
11 D
13 C
15 D
17 B

7 | Airway Management

1 B
3 D
5 C
7 A
9 C
11 C
13 C
15 C
17 D
19 B
21 B

8 | Scene Size-Up and Initial Assessment

1 A
3 D
5 B
7 A
9 B
11 B
13 B

9 | Patient Assessment

1 B
3 A
5 A
7 D
9 D
11 A

10 | Communications and Documentation

1 D
3 C
5 C
7 A
9 B
11 B
13 C
15 B
17 C
19 B

11 | General Pharmacology

1 C
3 C
5 B
7 D
9 B
11 A

12 | Respiratory Emergencies

1 C
3 A
5 C
7 A
9 C
11 C
13 B
15 D

13 | Cardiovascular Emergencies

1 A
3 D
5 B
7 C
9 C
11 C

14 | Neurological, Diabetic, and Behavioral Emergencies

1 A
3 C
5 B
7 A
9 A
11 D
13 B
15 C

15 | Allergic Reactions

1 B
3 B
5 C
7 B
9 A
11 A
13 C
15 D

16 | Poisoning and Overdose

1 B
3 C
5 D
7 A
9 A
11 D
13 D

17 | Environmental Emergencies

1 D
3 B
5 B
7 C
9 C
11 D
13 D

18 | Obstetrics and Gynecology

1 C
3 D
5 D
7 D
9 A
11 B
13 C
15 A

19 | Bleeding and Shock

1 C
3 A
5 A
7 B
9 A
11 A
13 A
15 B

20 | Soft Tissue Injuries

1 B
3 B
5 C
7 B
9 B

11 A
13 B
15 A

21 | Musculoskeletal Injuries

1 C
3 B
5 B
7 A
9 D
11 A
13 C

22 | Head and Spine Injuries

1 A
3 C
5 A
7 C
9 A
11 B
13 A
15 A

23 | Infants and Children

1 B
3 D
5 A
7 B
9 B
11 B
13 A
15 B

24 | Operations

1 B
3 A
5 C
7 A
9 B
11 C
13 B
15 D

APPENDIX F
D.O.T. Objectives

1 | Introduction to Emergency Medical Care

Cognitive Objectives

1-1.1 Define Emergency Medical Services (EMS) systems.

1-1.2 Differentiate the roles and responsibilities of the EMT-Basic from other prehospital care providers.

1-1.3 Describe the roles and responsibilities related to personal safety.

1-1.4 Discuss the roles and responsibilities of the EMT-Basic towards the safety of the crew, the patient and bystanders.

1-1.5 Define quality improvement and discuss the EMT-Basic's role in the process.

1-1.6 Define medical direction and discuss the EMT-Basic's role in the process.

1-1.7 State the specific statutes and regulations in your state regarding the EMS system.

Affective Objectives

1-1.8 Assess areas of personal attitude and conduct of the EMT-Basic.

1-1.9 Characterize the various methods used to access the EMS system in your community.

2 | The Well-Being of the EMT-Basic

Cognitive Objectives

1-2.1 List possible emotional reactions that the EMT-Basic may experience when faced with trauma, illness, death and dying.

1-2.2 Discuss the possible reactions that a family member may exhibit when confronted with death and dying.

1-2.3 State the steps in the EMT-Basic's approach to the family confronted with death and dying.

1-2.4 State the possible reactions that the family of the EMT-Basic may exhibit due to their outside involvement in EMS.

1-2.5 Recognize the signs and symptoms of critical incident stress.

1-2.6 State possible steps that the EMT-Basic may take to help reduce/alleviate stress.

1-2.7 Explain the need to determine scene safety.

1-2.8 Discuss the importance of body substance isolation (BSI).

1-2.9 Describe the steps the EMT-Basic should take for personal protection from airborne and bloodborne pathogens.

1-2.10 List the personal protective equipment necessary for each of the following situations:
- Hazardous materials
- Rescue operations
- Violent scenes
- Crime scenes
- Exposure to bloodborne pathogens
- Exposure to airborne pathogens

Affective Objectives

1-2.11 Explain the rationale for serving as an advocate for the use of appropriate protective equipment.

Psychomotor Objectives

1-2.12 Given a scenario with potential infectious exposure, the EMT-Basic will use appropriate personal protective equipment. At the completion of the scenario, the EMT-Basic will properly remove and discard the protective garments.

1-2.13 Given the above scenario, the EMT-Basic will complete disinfection/ cleaning and all reporting documentation.

3 | Medical, Legal, and Ethical Issues

Cognitive Objectives

1-3.1 Define the EMT-Basic scope of practice.

1-3.2 Discuss the importance of Do Not Resuscitate [DNR] (advance directives) and local or state provisions regarding EMS application.

1-3.3 Define consent and discuss the methods of obtaining consent.

1-3.4 Differentiate between expressed and implied consent.

1-3.5 Explain the role of consent of minors in providing care.

1-3.6 Discuss the implications for the EMT-Basic in patient refusal of transport.

1-3.7 Discuss the issues of abandonment, negligence, and battery and their implications to the EMT-Basic.

1-3.8　State the conditions necessary for the EMT-Basic to have a duty to act.

1-3.9　Explain the importance, necessity and legality of patient confidentiality.

1-3.10　Discuss the considerations of the EMT-Basic in issues of organ retrieval.

1-3.11　Differentiate the actions that an EMT-Basic should take to assist in the preservation of a crime scene.

1-3.12　State the conditions that require an EMT-Basic to notify local law enforcement officials.

Affective Objectives

1-3.13　Explain the role of EMS and the EMT-Basic regarding patients with DNR orders.

1-3.14　Explain the rationale for the needs, benefits and usage of advance directives.

1-3.15　Explain the rationale for the concept of varying degrees of DNR.

4 | The Human Body

Cognitive Objectives

1-4.1　Identify the following topographic terms: Medial, lateral, proximal, distal, superior, inferior, anterior, posterior, midline, right and left, mid-clavicular, bilateral, mid-axillary.

1-4.2　Describe the anatomy and function of the following major body systems: Respiratory, circulatory, musculoskeletal, nervous and endocrine.

5 | Vital Signs and SAMPLE History

Cognitive Objectives

1-5.1　Identify the components of vital signs.

1-5.2　Describe the methods to obtain a breathing rate.

1-5.3　Identify the attributes that should be obtained when assessing breathing.

1-5.4　Differentiate between shallow, labored and noisy breathing.

1-5.5　Describe the methods to obtain a pulse rate.

1-5.6　Identify the information obtained when assessing a patient's pulse.

1-5.7　Differentiate between a strong, weak, regular and irregular pulse.

1-5.8　Describe the methods to assess the skin color, temperature, condition (capillary refill in infants and children).

1-5.9　Identify the normal and abnormal skin colors.

1-5.10　Differentiate between pale, blue, red and yellow skin color.

1-5.11　Identify the normal and abnormal skin temperature.

1-5.12　Differentiate between hot, cool and cold skin temperature.

1-5.13　Identify normal and abnormal skin conditions.

1-5.14　Identify normal and abnormal capillary refill in infants and children.

1-5.15　Describe the methods to assess the pupils.

1-5.16　Identify normal and abnormal pupil size.

1-5.17　Differentiate between dilated (big) and constricted (small) pupil size.

1-5.18　Differentiate between reactive and non-reactive pupils and equal and unequal pupils.

1-5.19　Describe the methods to assess blood pressure.

1-5.20　Define systolic pressure.

1-5.21　Define diastolic pressure.

1-5.22　Explain the difference between auscultation and palpation for obtaining a blood pressure.

1-5.23　Identify the components of the SAMPLE history.

1-5.24　Differentiate between a sign and a symptom.

1-5.25　State the importance of accurately reporting and recording the baseline vital signs.

1-5.26　Discuss the need to search for additional medical identification.

Affective Objectives

1-5.27　Explain the value of performing the baseline vital signs.

1-5.28　Recognize and respond to the feelings patients experience during assessment.

1-5.29　Defend the need for obtaining and recording an accurate set of vital signs.

1-5.30　Explain the rationale of recording additional sets of vital signs.

1-5.31　Explain the importance of obtaining a SAMPLE history.

Psychomotor Objectives

1-5.32　Demonstrate the skills involved in assessment of breathing.

1-5.33　Demonstrate the skills associated with obtaining a pulse.

1-5.34　Demonstrate the skills associated with assessing the skin color, temperature, condition, and capillary refill in infants and children.

1-5.35　Demonstrate the skills associated with assessing the pupils.

1-5.36　Demonstrate the skills associated with obtaining blood pressure.

1-5.37 Demonstrate the skills that should be used to obtain information from the patient, family, or bystanders at the scene.

6 | Lifting and Moving Patients

Cognitive Objectives

1-6.1 Define body mechanics.

1-6.2 Discuss the guidelines and safety precautions that need to be followed when lifting a patient.

1-6.3 Describe the safe lifting of cots and stretchers.

1-6.4 Describe the guidelines and safety precautions for carrying patients and/or equipment.

1-6.5 Discuss one-handed carrying techniques.

1-6.6 Describe correct and safe carrying procedures on stairs.

1-6.7 State the guidelines for reaching and their application.

1-6.8 Describe correct reaching for log rolls.

1-6.9 State the guidelines for pushing and pulling.

1-6.10 Discuss the general considerations of moving patients.

1-6.11 State three situations that may require the use of an emergency move.

1-6.12 Identify the following patient carrying devices:
- Wheeled ambulance stretcher
- Portable ambulance stretcher
- Stair chair
- Scoop stretcher
- Long spine board
- Basket stretcher
- Flexible stretcher

Affective Objectives

1-6.13 Explain the rationale for properly lifting and moving patients.

Psychomotor Objectives

1-6.14 Working with a partner, prepare each of the following devices for use, transfer a patient to the device, properly position the patient on the device, move the device to the ambulance and load the patient into the ambulance:
- Wheeled ambulance stretcher
- Portable ambulance stretcher
- Stair chair
- Scoop stretcher
- Long spine board
- Basket stretcher
- Flexible stretcher

1-6.15 Working with a partner, the EMT-Basic will demonstrate techniques for the transfer of a patient from an ambulance stretcher to a hospital stretcher.

7 | Airway Management

Cognitive Objectives

2-1.1 Name and label the major structures of the respiratory system on a diagram.

2-1.2 List the signs of adequate breathing.

2-1.3 List the signs of inadequate breathing.

2-1.4 Describe the steps in performing the head-tilt chin-lift.

2-1.5 Relate mechanism of injury to opening the airway.

2-1.6 Describe the steps in performing the jaw thrust.

2-1.7 State the importance of having a suction unit ready for immediate use when providing emergency care.

2-1.8 Describe the techniques of suctioning.

2-1.9 Describe how to artificially ventilate a patient with a pocket mask.

2-1.10 Describe the steps in performing the skill of artificially ventilating a patient with a bag-valve-mask while using the jaw thrust.

2-1.11 List the parts of a bag-valve-mask system.

2-1.12 Describe the steps in performing the skill of artificially ventilating a patient with a bag-valve-mask for one and two rescuers.

2-1.13 Describe the signs of adequate artificial ventilation using the bag-valve-mask.

2-1.14 Describe the signs of inadequate artificial ventilation using the bag-valve-mask.

2-1.15 Describe the steps in artificially ventilating a patient with a flow restricted, oxygen-powered ventilation device.

2-1.16 List the steps in performing the actions taken when providing mouth-to-mouth and mouth-to-stoma artificial ventilation.

2-1.17 Describe how to measure and insert an oropharyngeal (oral) airway.

2-1.18 Describe how to measure and insert a nasopharyngeal (nasal) airway.

2-1.19 Define the components of an oxygen delivery system.

2-1.20 Identify a nonrebreather face mask and state the oxygen flow requirements needed for its use.

2-1.21 Describe the indications for using a nasal cannula versus a nonrebreather face mask.

2-1.22 Identify a nasal cannula and state the flow requirements needed for its use.

Affective Objectives

2-1.23 Explain the rationale for basic life support artificial ventilation and airway protective skills taking priority over most other basic life support skills.

2-1.24 Explain the rationale for providing adequate oxygenation through high inspired oxygen concentrations to patients who, in the past, may have received low concentrations.

Psychomotor Objectives

2-1.25 Demonstrate the steps in performing the head-tilt chin-lift.

2-1.26 Demonstrate the steps in performing the jaw thrust.

2-1.27 Demonstrate the techniques of suctioning.

2-1.28 Demonstrate the steps in providing mouth-to-mouth artificial ventilation with body substance isolation (barrier shields).

2-1.29 Demonstrate how to use a pocket mask to artificially ventilate a patient.

2-1.30 Demonstrate the assembly of a bag-valve-mask unit.

2-1.31 Demonstrate the steps in performing the skill of artificially ventilating a patient with a bag-valve-mask for one and two rescuers.

2-1.32 Demonstrate the steps in performing the skill of artificially ventilating a patient with a bag-valve-mask while using the jaw thrust.

2-1.33 Demonstrate artificial ventilation of a patient with a flow restricted, oxygen-powered ventilation device.

2-1.34 Demonstrate how to artificially ventilate a patient with a stoma.

2-1.35 Demonstrate how to insert an oropharyngeal (oral) airway.

2-1.36 Demonstrate how to insert a nasopharyngeal (nasal) airway.

2-1.37 Demonstrate the correct operation of oxygen tanks and regulators.

2-1.38 Demonstrate the use of a nonrebreather face mask and state the oxygen flow requirements needed for its use.

2-1.39 Demonstrate the use of a nasal cannula and state the flow requirements needed for its use.

2-1.40 Demonstrate how to artificially ventilate the infant and child patient.

2-1.41 Demonstrate oxygen administration for the infant and child patient.

8 | Scene Size-Up and Initial Assessment

Cognitive Objectives

3-1.1 Recognize hazards/potential hazards.

3-1.2 Describe common hazards found at the scene of a trauma and a medical patient.

3-1.3 Determine if the scene is safe to enter.

3-1.4 Discuss common mechanisms of injury/nature of illness.

3-1.5 Discuss the reason for identifying the total number of patients at the scene.

3-1.6 Explain the reason for identifying the need for additional help or assistance.

3-2.1 Summarize the reasons for forming a general impression of the patient.

3-2.2 Discuss methods of assessing altered mental status.

3-2.3 Differentiate between assessing the altered mental status in the adult, child and infant patient.

3-2.4 Discuss methods of assessing the airway in the adult, child and infant patient.

3-2.5 State reasons for management of the cervical spine once the patient has been determined to be a trauma patient.

3-2.6 Describe methods used for assessing if a patient is breathing.

3-2.7 State what care should be provided to the adult, child and infant patient with adequate breathing.

3-2.8 State what care should be provided to the adult, child and infant patient without adequate breathing.

3-2.9 Differentiate between a patient with adequate and inadequate breathing.

3-2.10 Distinguish between methods of assessing breathing in the adult, child and infant patient.

3-2.11 Compare the methods of providing airway care to the adult, child and infant patient.

3-2.12 Describe the methods used to obtain a pulse.

3-2.13 Differentiate between obtaining a pulse in an adult, child and infant patient.

3-2.14 Discuss the need for assessing the patient for external bleeding.

3-2.15 Describe normal and abnormal findings when assessing skin color.

3-2.16 Describe normal and abnormal findings when assessing skin temperature.

3-2.17 Describe normal and abnormal findings when assessing skin condition.

3-2.18 Describe normal and abnormal findings when assessing skin capillary refill in the infant and child patient.

3-2.19 Explain the reason for prioritizing a patient for care and transport.

Affective Objectives

3-1.7 Explain the rationale for crew members to evaluate scene safety prior to entering.

3-1.8 Serve as a model for others explaining how patient situations affect your evaluation of mechanism of injury or illness.

3-2.20 Explain the importance of forming a general impression of the patient.

3-2.21 Explain the value of performing an initial assessment.

Psychomotor Objectives

3-1.9 Observe various scenarios and identify potential hazards.

3-2.22 Demonstrate the techniques for assessing mental status.

3-2.23 Demonstrate the techniques for assessing the airway.

3-2.24 Demonstrate the techniques for assessing if the patient is breathing.

3-2.25 Demonstrate the techniques for assessing if the patient has a pulse.

3-2.26 Demonstrate the techniques for assessing the patient for external bleeding.

3-2.27 Demonstrate the techniques for assessing the patient's skin color, temperature, condition and capillary refill (infants and children only).

3-2.28 Demonstrate the ability to prioritize patients.

9 | Patient Assessment

Cognitive Objectives

3-3.1 Discuss the reasons for reconsideration concerning the mechanism of injury.

3-3.2 State the reasons for performing a rapid trauma assessment.

3-3.3 Recite examples and explain why patients should receive a rapid trauma assessment.

3-3.4 Describe the areas included in the rapid trauma assessment and discuss what should be evaluated.

3-3.5 Differentiate when the rapid assessment may be altered in order to provide patient care.

3-3.6 Discuss the reason for performing a focused history and physical exam.

3-4.1 Describe the unique needs for assessing an individual with a specific chief complaint with no known prior history.

3-4.2 Differentiate between the history and physical exam that are performed for responsive patients with no known prior history and responsive patients with a known prior history.

3-4.3 Describe the needs for assessing an individual who is unresponsive.

3-4.4 Differentiate between the assessment that is performed for a patient who is unresponsive or has an altered mental status and other medical patients requiring assessment.

3-5.1 Discuss the components of the detailed physical exam.

3-5.2 State the areas of the body that are evaluated during the detailed physical exam.

3-5.3 Explain what additional care should be provided while performing the detailed physical exam.

3-5.4 Distinguish between the detailed physical exam that is performed on a trauma patient and that of the medical patient.

3-6.1 Discuss the reasons for repeating the initial assessment as part of the on-going assessment.

3-6.2 Describe the components of the on-going assessment.

3-6.3 Describe trending of assessment components.

Affective Objectives

3-3.7 Recognize and respect the feelings that patients might experience during assessment.

3-4.5 Attend to the feelings that these patients might be experiencing.

3-5.5 Explain the rationale for the feelings that these patients might be experiencing.

3-6.4 Explain the value of performing an on-going assessment.

3-6.5 Recognize and respect the feelings that patients might experience during assessment.

3-6.6 Explain the value of trending assessment components to other health professionals who assume care of the patient.

Psychomotor Objectives

3-3.8 Demonstrate the rapid trauma assessment that should be used to assess a patient based on mechanism of injury

3-4.6 Demonstrate the patient assessment skills that should be used to assist a patient who is responsive with no known history.

3-4.7   Demonstrate the patient assessment skills that should be used to assist a patient who is unresponsive or has an altered metal status.

3-5.6   Demonstrate the skills involved in performing the detailed physical exam.

3-6.7   Demonstrate the skills involved in performing the on-going assessment.

10 | Communications and Documentation

Cognitive Objectives

3-7.1   List the proper methods of initiating and terminating a radio call.

3-7.2   State the proper sequence for delivery of patient information.

3-7.3   Explain the importance of effective communication of patient information in the verbal report.

3-7.4   Identify the essential components of the verbal report.

3-7.5   Describe the attributes for increasing effectiveness and efficiency of verbal communications.

3-7.6   State legal aspects to consider in verbal communication.

3-7.7   Discuss the communication skills that should be used to interact with the patient.

3-7.8   Discuss the communication skills that should be used to interact with the family, bystanders, individuals from other agencies while providing patient care and the difference between skills used to interact with the patient and those used to interact with others.

3-7.9   List the correct radio procedures in the following phases of a typical call:
- To the scene.
- At the scene.
- To the facility.
- At the facility.
- To the station.
- At the station.

3-8.1   Explain the components of the written report and list the information that should be included in the written report.

3-8.2   Identify the various sections of the written report.

3-8.3   Describe what information is required in each section of the prehospital care report and how it should be entered.

3-8.4   Define the special considerations concerning patient refusal.

3-8.5   Describe the legal implications associated with the written report.

3-8.6   Discuss all state and/or local record and reporting requirements.

Affective Objectives

3-7.10   Explain the rationale for providing efficient and effective radio communications and patient reports.

3-8.7   Explain the rationale for patient care documentation.

3-8.8   Explain the rationale for the EMS system gathering data.

3-8.9   Explain the rationale for using medical terminology correctly.

3-8.10   Explain the rationale for using an accurate and synchronous clock so that information can be used in trending.

Psychomotor Objectives

3-7.11   Perform a simulated, organized, concise radio transmission.

3-7.12   Perform an organized, concise patient report that would be given to the staff at a receiving facility.

3-7.13   Perform a brief, organized report that would be given to an ALS provider arriving at an incident scene at which the EMT-Basic was already providing care.

3-8.11   Complete a prehospital care report.

11 | General Pharmacology

Cognitive Objectives

4-1.1   Identify which medications will be carried on the unit.

4-1.2   State the medications carried on the unit by the generic name.

4-1.3   Identify the medications with which the EMT-Basic may assist the patient with administering.

4-1.4   State the medications the EMT-Basic can assist the patient with by the generic name.

4-1.5   Discuss the forms in which the medications may be found.

Affective Objectives

4-1.6   Explain the rationale for the administration of medications.

Psychomotor Objectives

4-1.7   Demonstrate general steps for assisting patient with self-administration of medications.

4-1.8   Read the labels and inspect each type of medication.

12 | Respiratory Emergencies

Cognitive Objectives

4-2.1   List the structure and function of the respiratory system.

4-2.2   State the signs and symptoms of a patient with breathing difficulty.

4-2.3   Describe the emergency medical care of the patient with breathing difficulty.

4-2.4   Recognize the need for medical direction to assist in the emergency medical care of the patient with breathing difficulty.

4-2.5   Describe the emergency medical care of the patient with breathing distress.

4-2.6   Establish the relationship between airway management and the patient with breathing difficulty.

4-2.7   List signs of adequate air exchange.

4-2.8   State the generic name, medication forms, dose, administration, action, indications and contraindications for the prescribed inhaler.

4-2.9   Distinguish between the emergency medical care of the infant, child and adult patient with breathing difficulty.

4-2.10   Differentiate between upper airway obstruction and lower airway disease in the infant and child patient.

Affective Objectives

4-2.11   Defend EMT-Basic treatment regimens for various respiratory emergencies.

4-2.12   Explain the rationale for administering an inhaler.

Psychomotor Objectives

4-2.13   Demonstrate the emergency medical care for breathing difficulty.

4-2.14   Perform the steps in facilitating the use of an inhaler.

13 | Cardiovascular Emergencies

Cognitive Objectives

4-3.1   Describe the structure and function of the cardiovascular system.

4-3.2   Describe the emergency medical care of the patient experiencing chest pain/discomfort.

4-3.3   List the indications for automated external defibrillation (AED).

4-3.4   List the contraindications for automated external defibrillation.

4-3.5   Define the role of EMT-B in the emergency cardiac care system.

4-3.6   Explain the impact of age and weight on defibrillation.

4-3.7   Discuss the position of comfort for patients with various cardiac emergencies.

4-3.8   Establish the relationship between airway management and the patient with cardiovascular compromise.

4-3.9   Predict the relationship between the patient experiencing cardiovascular compromise and basic life support.

4-3.10   Discuss the fundamentals of early defibrillation.

4-3.11   Explain the rationale for early defibrillation.

4-3.12   Explain that not all chest pain patients result in cardiac arrest and do not need to be attached to an automated external defibrillator.

4-3.13   Explain the importance of prehospital ACLS intervention if it is available.

4-3.14   Explain the importance of urgent transport to a facility with Advanced Cardiac Life Support if it is not available in the prehospital setting.

4-3.15   Discuss the various types of automated external defibrillators.

4-3.16   Differentiate between the fully automated and the semiautomated defibrillator.

4-3.17   Discuss the procedures that must be taken into consideration for standard operations of the various types of automated external defibrillators.

4-3.18   State the reasons for assuring that the patient is pulseless and apneic when using the automated external defibrillator.

4-3.19   Discuss the circumstances which may result in inappropriate shocks.

4-3.20   Explain the considerations for interruption of CPR, when using the automated external defibrillator.

4-3.21   Discuss the advantages and disadvantages of automated external defibrillators.

4-3.22   Summarize the speed of operation of automated external defibrillation.

4-3.23   Discuss the use of remote defibrillation through adhesive pads.

4-3.24   Discuss the special considerations for rhythm monitoring.

4-3.25   List the steps in the operation of the automated external defibrillator.

4-3.26 Discuss the standard of care that should be used to provide care to a patient with persistent ventricular fibrillation and no available ACLS.

4-3.27 Discuss the standard of care that should be used to provide care to a patient with recurrent ventricular fibrillation and no available ACLS.

4-3.28 Differentiate between the single rescuer and multi-rescuer care with an automated external defibrillator.

4-3.29 Explain the reason for pulses not being checked between shocks with an automated external defibrillator.

4-3.30 Discuss the importance of coordinating ACLS trained providers with personnel using automated external defibrillators.

4-3.31 Discuss the importance of post-resuscitation care.

4-3.32 List the components of post-resuscitation care.

4-3.33 Explain the importance of frequent practice with the automated external defibrillator.

4-3.34 Discuss the need to complete the Automated Defibrillator: Operator's Shift Checklist.

4-3.35 Discuss the role of the American Heart Association (AHA) in the use of automated external defibrillation.

4-3.36 Explain the role medical direction plays in the use of automated external defibrillation.

4-3.37 State the reasons why a case review should be completed following the use of the automated external defibrillator.

4-3.38 Discuss the components that should be included in a case review.

4-3.39 Discuss the goal of quality improvement in automated external defibrillation.

4-3.40 Recognize the need for medical direction of protocols to assist in the emergency medical care of the patient with chest pain.

4-3.41 List the indications for the use of nitroglycerin.

4-3.42 State the contraindications and side effects for the use of nitroglycerin.

4-3.43 Define the function of all controls on an automated external defibrillator, and describe event documentation and battery defibrillator maintenance.

Affective Objectives

4-3.44 Defend the reasons for obtaining initial training in automated external defibrillation and the importance of continuing education.

4-3.45 Defend the reason for maintenance of automated external defibrillators.

4-3.46 Explain the rationale for administering nitroglycerin to a patient with chest pain or discomfort.

Psychomotor Objectives

4-3.47 Demonstrate the assessment and emergency medical care of a patient experiencing chest pain/discomfort.

4-3.48 Demonstrate the application and operation of the automated external defibrillator.

4-3.49 Demonstrate the maintenance of an automated external defibrillator.

4-3.50 Demonstrate the assessment and documentation of patient response to the automated external defibrillator.

4-3.51 Demonstrate the skills necessary to complete the Automated Defibrillator: Operator's Shift Checklist.

4-3.52 Perform the steps in facilitating the use of nitroglycerin for chest pain or discomfort.

4-3.53 Demonstrate the assessment and documentation of patient response to nitroglycerin.

4-3.54 Practice completing a prehospital care report for patients with cardiac emergencies.

14 | Neurological, Diabetic, and Behavioral Emergencies

Cognitive Objectives

4-4.1 Identify the patient taking diabetic medications with altered mental status and the implications of a diabetes history.

4-4.2 State the steps in the emergency medical care of the patient taking diabetic medicine with an altered mental status and a history of diabetes.

4-4.3 Establish the relationship between airway management and the patient with altered mental status.

4-4.4 State the generic and trade names, medication forms, dose, administration, action, and contraindications for oral glucose.

4-4.5 Evaluate the need for medical direction in the emergency medical care of the diabetic patient.

4-8.1 Define behavioral emergencies.

4-8.2 Discuss the general factors that may cause an alteration in a patient's behavior.

4-8.3 State the various reasons for psychological crises.

4-8.4   Discuss the characteristics of an individual's behavior which suggests that the patient is at risk for suicide.

4-8.5   Discuss special medical/legal considerations for managing behavioral emergencies.

4-8.6   Discuss the special considerations for assessing a patient with behavioral problems.

4-8.7   Discuss the general principles of an individual's behavior which suggests that he is at risk for violence.

4-8.8   Discuss methods to calm behavioral emergency patients.

Affective Objectives

4-4.6   Explain the rationale for administering oral glucose.

4-8.9   Explain the rationale for learning how to modify your behavior toward the patient with a behavioral emergency.

Psychomotor Objectives

4-4.7   Demonstrate the steps in the emergency medical care for the patient taking diabetic medicine with an altered mental status and a history of diabetes.

4-4.8   Demonstrate the steps in the administration of oral glucose.

4-4.9   Demonstrate the assessment and documentation of patient response to oral glucose.

4-4.10 Demonstrate how to complete a prehospital care report for patients with diabetic emergencies.

4-8.10 Demonstrate the assessment and emergency medical care of the patient experiencing a behavioral emergency.

4-8.11 Demonstrate various techniques to safely restrain a patient with a behavioral problem.

15 | Allergic Reactions

Cognitive Objectives

4-5.1   Recognize the patient experiencing an allergic reaction.

4-5.2   Describe the emergency medical care of the patient with an allergic reaction.

4-5.3   Establish the relationship between the patient with an allergic reaction and airway management.

4-5.4   Describe the mechanisms of allergic response and the implications for airway management.

4-5.5   State the generic and trade names, medication forms, dose, administration, action, and contraindications for the epinephrine auto-injector.

4-5.6   Evaluate the need for medical direction in the emergency medical care of the patient with an allergic reaction.

4-5.7   Differentiate between the general category of those patients having an allergic reaction and those patients having an allergic reaction and requiring immediate medical care, including immediate use of epinephrine auto-injector.

Affective Objectives

4-5.8   Explain the rationale for administering epinephrine using an auto-injector.

Psychomotor Objectives

4-5.9   Demonstrate the emergency medical care of the patient experiencing an allergic reaction.

4-5.10 Demonstrate the use of epinephrine auto-injector.

4-5.11 Demonstrate the assessment and documentation of patient response to an epinephrine injection.

4-5.12 Demonstrate proper disposal of equipment.

4-5.13 Demonstrate completing a prehospital care report for patients with allergic emergencies.

16 | Poisoning and Overdose

Cognitive Objectives

4-6.1   List various ways that poisons enter the body.

4-6.2   List signs/symptoms associated with poisoning.

4-6.3   Discuss the emergency medical care for the patient with possible overdose.

4-6.4   Describe the steps in the emergency medical care for the patient with suspected poisoning.

4-6.5   Establish the relationship between the patient suffering from poisoning or overdose and airway management.

4-6.6   State the generic and trade names, indications, contraindications, medication form, dose, administration, actions, side effects and reassessment strategies for activated charcoal.

4-6.7   Recognize the need for medical direction in caring for the patient with poisoning or overdose.

Affective Objectives

4-6.8   Explain the rationale for administering activated charcoal.

4-6.9   Explain the rationale for contacting medical direction early in the prehospital management of the poisoning or overdose patient.

Psychomotor Objectives

4-6.10 Demonstrate the steps in the emergency medical care for the patient with possible overdose.

4-6.11 Demonstrate the steps in the emergency medical care for the patient with suspected poisoning.

4-6.12 Perform the necessary steps required to provide a patient with activated charcoal.

4-6.13 Demonstrate the assessment and documentation of patient response.

4-6.14 Demonstrate proper disposal of the equipment for the administration of activated charcoal.

4-6.15 Demonstrate completing a prehospital care report for patients with a poisoning/overdose emergency.

17 | Environmental Emergencies

Cognitive Objectives

4-7.1 Describe the various ways that the body loses heat.

4-7.2 List the signs and symptoms of exposure to cold.

4-7.3 Explain the steps in providing emergency medical care to a patient exposed to cold.

4-7.4 List the signs and symptoms of exposure to heat.

4-7.5 Explain the steps in providing emergency care to a patient exposed to heat.

4-7.6 Recognize the signs and symptoms of water-related emergencies.

4-7.7 Describe the complications of near drowning.

4-7.8 Discuss the emergency medical care of bites and stings.

Psychomotor Objectives

4-7.9 Demonstrate the assessment and emergency medical care of a patient with exposure to cold.

4-7.10 Demonstrate the assessment and emergency medical care of a patient with exposure to heat.

4-7.11 Demonstrate the assessment and emergency medical care of a near drowning patient.

4-7.12 Demonstrate completing a prehospital care report for patients with environmental emergencies.

18 | Obstetrics and Gynecology

Cognitive Objectives

4-9.1 Identify the following structures: Uterus, vagina, fetus, placenta, umbilical cord, amniotic sac, perineum.

4-9.2 Identify and explain the use of the contents of an obstetrics kit.

4-9.3 Identify predelivery emergencies.

4-9.4 State indications of an imminent delivery.

4-9.5 Differentiate the emergency medical care provided to a patient with predelivery emergencies from a normal delivery.

4-9.6 State the steps in the predelivery preparation of the mother.

4-9.7 Establish the relationship between body substance isolation and childbirth.

4-9.8 State the steps to assist in the delivery.

4-9.9 Describe care of the baby as the head appears.

4-9.10 Describe how and when to cut the umbilical cord.

4-9.11 Discuss the steps in the delivery of the placenta.

4-9.12 List the steps in the emergency medical care of the mother post-delivery.

4-9.13 Summarize neonatal resuscitation procedures.

4-9.14 Describe the procedures for the following abnormal deliveries: Breech birth, prolapsed cord, limb presentation.

4-9.15 Differentiate the special considerations for multiple births.

4-9.16 Describe special considerations of meconium.

4-9.17 Describe special considerations of a premature baby.

4-9.18 Discuss the emergency medical care of a patient with a gynecological emergency.

Affective Objectives

4-9.19 Explain the rationale for understanding the implications of treating two patients (mother and baby).

Psychomotor Objectives

4-9.20 Demonstrate the steps to assist in the normal cephalic delivery.

4-9.21 Demonstrate necessary care procedures of the fetus as the head appears.

4-9.22 Demonstrate infant neonatal procedures.

4-9.23 Demonstrate post delivery care of infant.

4-9.24 Demonstrate how and when to cut the umbilical cord.

4-9.25 Attend to the steps in the delivery of the placenta.

4-9.26 Demonstrate the post-delivery care of the mother.

4-9.27 Demonstrate the procedures for the following abnormal deliveries: vaginal bleeding, breech birth, prolapsed cord, limb presentation.

4-9.28 Demonstrate the steps in the emergency medical care of the mother with excessive bleeding.

4-9.29 Demonstrate completing a prehospital care report for patients with obstetrical/gynecological emergencies.

19 | Bleeding and Shock

Cognitive Objectives

5-1.1 List the structure and function of the circulatory system.

5-1.2 Differentiate between arterial, venous and capillary bleeding.

5-1.3 State methods of emergency medical care of external bleeding.

5-1.4 Establish the relationship between body substance isolation and bleeding.

5-1.5 Establish the relationship between airway management and the trauma patient.

5-1.6 Establish the relationship between mechanism of injury and internal bleeding.

5-1.7 List the signs of internal bleeding.

5-1.8 List the steps in the emergency medical care of the patient with signs and symptoms of internal bleeding.

5-1.9 List signs and symptoms of shock (hypoperfusion).

5-1.10 State the steps in the emergency medical care of the patient with signs and symptoms of shock (hypoperfusion).

5-2.23 Describe the steps in applying a pressure dressing.

Affective Objectives

5-1.11 Explain the sense of urgency to transport patients that are bleeding and show signs of shock (hypoperfusion).

Psychomotor Objectives

5-1.12 Demonstrate direct pressure as a method of emergency medical care of external bleeding.

5-1.13 Demonstrate the use of diffuse pressure as a method of emergency medical care of external bleeding.

5-1.14 Demonstrate the use of pressure points and tourniquets as a method of emergency medical care of external bleeding.

5-1.15 Demonstrate the care of the patient exhibiting signs and symptoms of internal bleeding.

5-1.16 Demonstrate the care of the patient exhibiting signs and symptoms of shock (hypoperfusion).

5-1.17 Demonstrate completing a prehospital care report for patient with bleeding and/or shock (hypoperfusion).

20 | Soft Tissue Injuries

Cognitive Objectives

5-2.1 State the major functions of the skin.

5-2.2 List the layers of the skin.

5-2.3 Establish the relationship between body substance isolation (BSI) and soft tissue injuries.

5-2.4 List the types of closed soft tissue injuries.

5-2.5 Describe the emergency medical care of the patient with a closed soft tissue injury.

5-2.6 State the types of open soft tissue injuries.

5-2.7 Describe the emergency medical care of the patient with an open soft tissue injury.

5-2.8 Discuss the emergency medical care considerations for a patient with a penetrating chest injury.

5-2.9 State the emergency medical care considerations for a patient with an open wound to the abdomen.

5-2.10 Differentiate the care of an open wound to the chest from an open wound to the abdomen.

5-2.11 List the classifications of burns.

5-2.12 Define superficial burn.

5-2.13 List the characteristics of a superficial burn.

5-2.14 Define partial thickness burn.

5-2.15 List the characteristics of a partial thickness burn.

5-2.16 Define full thickness burn.

5-2.17 List the characteristics of a full thickness burn.

5-2.18 Describe the emergency medical care of the patient with a superficial burn.

5-2.19 Describe the emergency medical care of the patient with a partial thickness burn.

5-2.20 Describe the emergency medical care of the patient with a full thickness burn.

5-2.21 List the functions of dressing and bandaging.

5-2.22 Describe the purpose of a bandage.

5-2.24 Establish the relationship between airway management and the patient with chest injury, burns, blunt and penetrating injuries.

5-2.25 Describe the effects of improperly applied dressings, splints and tourniquets.

5-2.26 Describe the emergency medical care of a patient with an impaled object.

5-2.27 Describe the emergency medical care of a patient with an amputation.

5-2.28 Describe the emergency care for a chemical burn.

5-2.29 Describe the emergency care for an electrical burn.

Psychomotor Objectives

5-2.29 Demonstrate the steps in the emergency medical care of closed soft tissue injuries.

5-2.30 Demonstrate the steps in the emergency medical care of open soft tissue injuries.

5-2.31 Demonstrate the steps in the emergency medical care of a patient with an open chest wound.

5-2.32 Demonstrate the steps in the emergency medical care of a patient with open abdominal wounds.

5-2.33 Demonstrate the steps in the emergency medical care of a patient with an impaled object.

5-2.34 Demonstrate the steps in the emergency medical care of a patient with an amputation.

5-2.35 Demonstrate the steps in the emergency medical care of an amputated part.

5-2.36 Demonstrate the steps in the emergency medical care of a patient with superficial burns.

5-2.37 Demonstrate the steps in the emergency medical care of a patient with partial thickness burns.

5-2.38 Demonstrate the steps in the emergency medical care of a patient with full thickness burns.

5-2.39 Demonstrate the steps in the emergency medical care of a patient with a chemical burn.

5-2.40 Demonstrate completing a prehospital care report for patients with soft tissue injuries.

21 | Musculoskeletal Injuries

Cognitive Objectives

5-3.1 Describe the function of the muscular system.

5-3.2 Describe the function of the skeletal system.

5-3.3 List the major bones or bone groupings of the spinal column; the thorax; the upper extremities; the lower extremities.

5-3.4 Differentiate between an open and a closed painful, swollen, deformed extremity.

5-3.5 State the reasons for splinting.

5-3.6 List the general rules of splinting.

5-3.7 List the complications of splinting.

5-3.8 List the emergency medical care for a patient with a painful, swollen, deformed extremity.

Affective Objectives

5-3.9 Explain the rationale for splinting at the scene versus load and go.

5-3.10 Explain the rationale for immobilization of the painful, swollen, deformed extremity.

Psychomotor Objectives

5-3.11 Demonstrate the emergency medical care of a patient with a painful, swollen, deformed extremity.

5-3.12 Demonstrate completing a prehospital care report for patients with musculoskeletal injuries.

22 | Head and Spine Injuries

Cognitive Objectives

5-4.1 State the components of the nervous system.

5-4.2 List the functions of the central nervous system.

5-4.3 Define the structure of the skeletal system as it relates to the nervous system.

5-4.4 Relate mechanism of injury to potential injuries of the head and spine.

5-4.5 Describe the implications of not properly caring for potential spine injuries.

5-4.6 State the signs and symptoms of a potential spine injury.

5-4.7 Describe the method of determining if a responsive patient may have a spine injury.

5-4.8 Relate the airway emergency medical care techniques to the patient with a suspected spine injury.

5-4.9 Describe how to stabilize the cervical spine.

5-4.10 Discuss indications for sizing and using a cervical spine immobilization device.

5-4.11 Establish the relationship between airway management and the patient with head and spine injuries.

5-4.12 Describe a method for sizing a cervical spine immobilization device.

5-4.13 Describe how to log roll a patient with a suspected spine injury.

5-4.14 Describe how to secure a patient to a long spine board.

5-4.15 List instances when a short spine board should be used.

5-4.16 Describe how to immobilize a patient using a short spine board.

5-4.17 Describe the indications for the use of rapid extrication.

5-4.18 List steps in performing rapid extrication.

5-4.19 State the circumstances when a helmet should be left on the patient.

5-4.20 Discuss the circumstances when a helmet should be removed.

5-4.21 Identify different types of helmets.

5-4.22 Describe the unique characteristics of sports helmets.

5-4.23 Explain the preferred methods to remove a helmet.

5-4.24 Discuss alternative methods for removal of a helmet.

5-4.25 Describe how the patient's head is stabilized to remove the helmet.

5-4.26 Differentiate how the head is stabilized with a helmet compared to without a helmet.

Affective Objectives

5-4.27 Explain the rationale for immobilization of the entire spine when a cervical spine injury is suspected.

5-4.28 Explain the rationale for utilizing immobilization methods apart from the straps on the cots.

5-4.29 Explain the rationale for utilizing a short spine immobilization device when moving a patient from the sitting to the supine position.

5-4.30 Explain the rationale for utilizing rapid extrication approaches only when they indeed will make the difference between life and death.

5-4.31 Defend the reasons for leaving a helmet in place for transport of a patient.

5-4.32 Defend the reasons for removal of a helmet prior to transport of a patient.

Psychomotor Objectives

5-4.33 Demonstrate opening the airway in a patient with suspected spinal cord injury.

5-4.34 Demonstrate evaluating a responsive patient with a suspected spinal cord injury.

5-4.35 Demonstrate stabilization of the cervical spine.

5-4.36 Demonstrate the four person log roll for a patient with a suspected spinal cord injury.

5-4.37 Demonstrate how to log roll a patient with a suspected spinal cord injury using two people.

5-4.38 Demonstrate securing a patient to a long spine board.

5-4.39 Demonstrate using the short board immobilization technique.

5-4.40 Demonstrate procedure for rapid extrication.

5-4.41 Demonstrate preferred methods for stabilization of a helmet.

5-4.42 Demonstrate helmet removal techniques.

5-4.43 Demonstrate alternative methods for stabilization of a helmet.

5-4.44 Demonstrate completing a prehospital care report for patients with head and spinal injuries.

23 | Infants and Children

Cognitive Objectives

6-1.1 Identify the developmental considerations for the following age groups:
- infants
- toddlers
- pre-school
- school age
- adolescent

6-1.2 Describe differences in anatomy and physiology of the infant, child and adult patient.

6-1.3 Differentiate the response of the ill or injured infant or child (age specific) from that of an adult.

6-1.4 Indicate various causes of respiratory emergencies.

6-1.5 Differentiate between respiratory distress and respiratory failure.

6-1.6 List the steps in the management of foreign body airway obstruction.

6-1.7 Summarize emergency medical care strategies for respiratory distress and respiratory failure.

6-1.8 Identify the signs and symptoms of shock (hypoperfusion) in the infant and child patient.

6-1.9 Describe the methods of determining end organ perfusion in the infant and child patient.

6-1.10 State the usual cause of cardiac arrest in infants and children versus adults.

6-1.11 List the common causes of seizures in the infant and child patient.

6-1.12 Describe the management of seizures in the infant and child patient.

6-1.13 Differentiate between the injury patterns in adults, infants, and children.

6-1.14 Discuss the field management of the infant and child trauma patient.

6-1.15 Summarize the indicators of possible child abuse and neglect.

6-1.16 Describe the medical legal responsibilities in suspected child abuse.

6-1.17 Recognize need for EMT-Basic debriefing following a difficult infant or child transport.

Affective Objectives

6-1.18 Explain the rationale for having knowledge and skills appropriate for dealing with the infant and child patient.

6-1.19 Attend to the feelings of the family when dealing with an ill or injured infant or child.

6-1.20 Understand the provider's own response (emotional) to caring for infants or children.

Psychomotor Objectives

6-1.21 Demonstrate the techniques of foreign body airway obstruction removal in the infant.

6-1.22 Demonstrate the techniques of foreign body airway obstruction removal in the child.

6-1.23 Demonstrate the assessment of the infant and child.

6-1.24 Demonstrate bag-valve-mask artificial ventilations for the infant.

6-1.25 Demonstrate bag-valve-mask artificial ventilations for the child.

6-1.26 Demonstrate oxygen delivery for the infant and child.

24 | Operations

Cognitive Objectives

7-1.1 Discuss the medical and non-medical equipment needed to respond to a call.

7-1.2 List the phases of an ambulance call.

7-1.3 Describe the general provisions of state laws relating to the operation of the ambulance and privileges in any or all of the following categories:
- Speed
- Warning lights
- Sirens
- Right-of-way
- Parking
- Turning

7-1.4 List contributing factors to unsafe driving conditions.

7-1.5 Describe the considerations that should by given to:
- Request for escorts
- Following an escort vehicle
- Intersections

7-1.6 Discuss "Due Regard For Safety of All Others" while operating an emergency vehicle.

7-1.7 State what information is essential in order to respond to a call.

7-1.8 Discuss various situations that may affect response to a call.

7-1.9 Differentiate between the various methods of moving a patient to the unit based upon injury or illness.

7-1.10 Apply the components of the essential patient information in a written report.

7-1.11 Summarize the importance of preparing the unit for the next response.

7-1.12 Identify what is essential for completion of a call.

7-1.13 Distinguish among the terms cleaning, disinfection, high-level disinfection, and sterilization.

7-1.14 Describe how to clean or disinfect items following patient care.

7-2.1 Describe the purpose of extrication.

7-2.2 Discuss the role of the EMT-Basic in extrication.

7-2.3 Identify what equipment for personal safety is required for the EMT-Basic.

7-2.4 Define the fundamental components of extrication.

7-2.5 State the steps that should be taken to protect the patient during extrication.

7-2.6 Evaluate various methods of gaining access to the patient.

7-2.7 Distinguish between simple and complex access.

7-3.1 Explain the EMT-Basic's role during a call involving hazardous materials.

7-3.2 Describe what the EMT-Basic should do if there is reason to believe that there is a hazard at the scene.

7-3.3 Describe the actions that an EMT-Basic should take to ensure bystander safety.

7-3.4 State the role the EMT-Basic should perform until appropriately trained personnel arrive at the scene of a hazardous materials situation.

7-3.5 Break down the steps to approaching a hazardous situation.

7-3.6 Discuss the various environmental hazards that affect EMS.

7-3.7 Describe the criteria for a multiple-casualty situation.

7-3.8 Evaluate the role of the EMT-Basic in the multiple-casualty situation.

7-3.9 Summarize the components of basic triage.

7-3.10 Define the role of the EMT-Basic in a disaster operation.

7-3.11 Describe basic concepts of incident management.

7-3.12 Explain the methods for preventing contamination of self, equipment and facilities.

7-3.13 Review the local mass casualty incident plan.

Affective Objectives

7-1.15 Explain the rationale for appropriate report of patient information.

7-1.16 Explain the rationale for having the unit prepared to respond.

Psychomotor Objectives

7-1.17 Given a scenario of a mass casualty incident, perform triage.

Appendix A | Advanced Airway Management (elective)

Cognitive Objectives

8-1.1 Identify and describe the airway anatomy in the infant, child and the adult.

8-1.2 Differentiate between the airway anatomy in the infant, child, and the adult.

8-1.3 Explain the pathophysiology of airway compromise.

8-1.4 Describe the proper use of airway adjuncts.

8-1.5 Review the use of oxygen therapy in airway management.

8-1.6 Describe the indications, contraindications, and technique for insertion of nasal gastric tubes.

8-1.7 Describe how to perform the Sellick maneuver (cricoid pressure).

8-1.8 Describe the indications for advanced airway management.

8-1.9 List the equipment required for orotracheal intubation.

8-1.10 Describe the proper use of the curved blade for orotracheal intubation.

8-1.11 Describe the proper use of the straight blade for orotracheal intubation.

8-1.12 State the reasons for and proper use of the stylet in orotracheal intubation.

8-1.13 Describe the methods of choosing the appropriate size endotracheal tube in an adult patient.

8-1.14 State the formula for sizing an infant or child endotracheal tube.

8-1.15 List complications associated with advanced airway management.

8-1.16 Define the various alternative methods for sizing the infant and child endotracheal tube.

8-1.17 Describe the skill of orotracheal intubation in the adult patient.

8-1.18 Describe the skill of orotracheal intubation in the infant and child patient.

8-1.19 Describe the skill of confirming endotracheal tube placement in the adult, infant and child patient.

8-1.20 State the consequence of and the need to recognize unintentional esophageal intubation.

8-1.21 Describe the skill of securing the endotracheal tube in the adult, infant and child patient.

Affective Objectives

8-1.22 Recognize and respect the feelings of the patient and family during advanced airway procedures.

8-1.23 Explain the value of performing advanced airway procedures.

8-1.24 Defend the need for the EMT-Basic to perform advanced airway procedures.

8-1.25 Explain the rationale for the use of a stylet.

8-1.26 Explain the rationale for having a suction unit immediately available during intubation attempts.

8-1.27 Explain the rationale for confirming breath sounds.

8-1.28 Explain the rationale for securing the endotracheal tube.

Psychomotor Objectives

8-1.29 Demonstrate how to perform the Sellick maneuver (cricoid pressure).

8-1.30 Demonstrate the skill of orotracheal intubation in the adult patient.

8-1.31 Demonstrate the skill of orotracheal intubation in the infant and child patient.

8-1.32 Demonstrate the skill of confirming endotracheal tube placement in the adult patient.

8-1.33 Demonstrate the skill of confirming endotracheal tube placement in the infant and child patient.

8-1.34 Demonstrate the skill of securing the endotracheal tube in the adult patient.

8-1.35 Demonstrate the skill of securing the endotracheal tube in the infant and child patient.

Reference

Glossary

Abandonment Termination of care without the patient's consent and without making any provisions for continuing care at the same or higher level

Abdominal Cavity The portion of the torso beneath the thorax and above the pelvis; contains the liver, gallbladder, stomach, pancreas, intestines, spleen, kidneys, and ureters

Abortion Delivery of the products of conception early in a pregnancy; may be spontaneous or medically induced

Abrasion A superficial scrape injury to the top layer of skin

Absorbed Poison A toxic substance taken into the body across unbroken skin or mucous membranes

Acromion *(ah-KRO-me-un)* The highest point of the shoulder

Action The desired effect of a medication or a treatment

Activated Charcoal Substance that hinders the absorption of ingested poisons and enhances their elimination from the body, preventing further damage

Acute Illness Illness with a severe, rapid onset

Acute Myocardial *(my-oh-KAR-de-ul)* **Infarction (AMI)** Sudden cardiac muscle death or injury due to lack of oxygen; a heart attack

Adolescent Child who is 12 to 18 years old

Adrenaline Another name for epinephrine

Advance Directive A legal statement of a patient's wishes regarding his or her health care; used in the event the patient becomes unable to make decisions

Agonal *(AY-gun-ul)* **Respirations** Occasional gasping breaths that may occur in the final stage of death

Airway Adjunct Device that helps keep the airway open by keeping the tongue away from the back of the throat

Allergen An antigen that causes an allergic reaction, such as dust, mold, or pollen

Allergic Reaction An exaggerated immune response to a substance that is normally harmless

Altered Mental Status (AMS) Broad term indicating a change in normal thinking or clarity of thought; behavior may range from mild confusion to complete unresponsiveness

Alveoli *(al-VEE-o-li)* Termination of the respiratory passages; the functional units of the lungs, across whose walls gas exchange occurs

Ambient Temperature The air temperature surrounding the patient

Amniotic *(am-nee-OT-ik)* **Sac** Sac which holds the fetus suspended in amniotic fluid; also called "bag of waters"

Amputation Removal of an extremity through trauma or surgery

Anaphylactic *(an-eh-feh-LAK-tik)* **Shock** Severe allergic reaction in which blood vessels dilate rapidly, causing a drop in blood pressure and respiratory distress

Anaphylaxis Another name for anaphylactic shock

Anatomy The study of the structures of the body and how they relate to one another

Angina Pectoris *(an-JI-nah pek-TOR-is)* Severe pain and constriction about the heart; also called angina or myocardial ischemia; often treated with nitroglycerin

Anterior Toward the front; front of the body; also called ventral

Antibody A protein produced by the immune system that combines with a specific antigen and helps to destroy it

Antidote An agent that blocks or reverses the effect of a poison

Antigen A foreign substance that enters the body and causes and immune response

Aorta *(ay-OR-tuh)* The main trunk of the arterial system of the body; it leaves the heart from the upper surface of the left ventricle

APGAR Score Method for assessing newborns based on five ratings: Appearance, Pulse, Grimace, Activity, and Respiration

Arteries Blood vessels that carry blood away from the heart

Arterioles *(ar-TEAR-ee-olz)* Smaller vessels that branch off the arteries and lead to the capillaries

Aspiration To draw foreign material, a foreign body, or fluid into the respiratory tract while inhaling

Assault Threatening or attempting to inflict offensive physical contact; physical contact is not necessary for assault to occur

Assessment Evaluation of a situation or patient; the information is used to determine priorities for management

Asthma *(AZ-muh)* Reactive airway disease caused by spasmodic contraction of the bronchi; characterized by recurrent attacks of dyspnea, coughing, and wheezing

Atrium *(AY-tree-um)* One of two upper chambers of the heart

Auscultation Listening for sounds with a stethoscope

Automated External Defibrillator (AED) Defibrillation equipment designed to analyze, shock, and re-analyze cardiac dysfunction after applying electrodes to patient

AVPU Memory aid used to help categorize a patient's level of unresponsiveness: A= Alert, V = responds to Verbal stimuli, P= responds to Pain, U= Unresponsive

Avulsion A tearing off or tearing away of a skin flap or body part

Bag-Valve Mask Device (BVM) An oxygen delivery device comprised of a self-inflating bag, face mask, one-way valve, and oxygen reservoir

Ball-and-Socket Joint Cup-shaped surface of a bone that joins with the ball-shaped head of a long bone

Bandage Holds a dressing in place (self-adherent, gauze rolls, triangular, air splint)

Barotrauma Ruptured lung resulting from over-aggressive ventilations

Base Station Radio used for central dispatch operations and coordination of emergency services in an EMS communication system

Battery Actual offensive physical contact or touching of another person without their consent; usually combined with a charge of assault, particularly if threatening words were exchanged between the parties

Battle's Sign Bruising behind the ears or mastoid process due to basilar skull fracture

Behavioral Emergency A situation in which the patient exhibits behavior that others consider unacceptable or intolerable

Bilateral On both sides of the midline (right and left sides)

Blood Pressure Force of the blood on the vessels; systolic pressure is the working pressure; diastolic pressure is the resting pressure

Blunt Trauma Injury caused by non-penetrating forces

Body Mechanics Moving your body correctly while lifting and moving to prevent injury

Body Substance Isolation (BSI) Precautions Equipment and standards designed to prevent the spread of communicable diseases

Brachial *(BRAY-kee-ul)* **Artery** Major artery of the upper arm

Brachial Pulse The flow of blood through the brachial artery, in the medial aspect of the upper arm

Bradycardia *(bray-deh-KAR-de-uh)* Slow heart rate

Breech Presentation Abnormal delivery in which the infant's buttocks or lower extremities are the presenting part; places infant at high risk for prolapsed cord and oxygen deprivation

Bronchi *(BRONG-kee)* Plural of bronchus; the two major subdivisions of the trachea

Bronchioles Subdivisions of the bronchi; terminate in the alveoli

Bronchoconstriction Narrowing of the air passageways due to constriction of the smooth muscle of the bronchi and bronchioles

Bronchodilator Drug that relaxes the smooth muscle of the bronchi and bronchioles, reversing bronchoconstriction

Calcaneus *(kal-KAY-ne-us)* The heel bone

Capillaries *(KA-pul-air-eez)* Tiny vessels that carry blood through the tissues; the network of capillaries in the tissues and organs is called the capillary bed

Capillary Refill Time Time required for the capillary beds to refill with blood after blanching; used for assessing perfusion in infants and children

Cardiac Compromise Any action or factor that reduces the functionality of the cardiac system

Cardiac Muscle Involuntary muscle tissue of the heart that is usually not under conscious control

Carina *(kah-REE-nuh)* A triangular projection of the lowest tracheal cartilage; forms the division of the primary bronchi

Carotid *(kah-RAH-tid)* **Artery** Major artery in the neck

Carpals *(KAR-pulz)* The eight bones of the wrist

Cavitation Tissue compression and cavity formation caused by the pressure of a projectile entering the body

Central Nervous System The brain and spinal cord

Cerebellum *(seh-reh-BEL-em)* Portion of the brain that coordinates voluntary muscular movements

Cerebrospinal Fluid (CSF) Fluid that fills the ventricles and cavities of the brain and surrounds the spinal cord

Cerebrovascular *(se-REE-bro-VAS-kyu-ler)* **Accident (CVA)** Stroke or brain attack; occurs when a blood vessel in the brain becomes blocked or ruptures

Cerebrum *(seh-REE-brem)* The largest part of the brain; consists of two hemispheres

Cervical *(SUR-vi-kul),* **Cervical Vertebrae** First 7 vertebrae; the neck

Chain of Survival Term used for the four interventions that provide the best chance for successful resuscitation of a patient in cardiac arrest: Early access, early CPR, early defibrillation, early ACLS

Chief Complaint Patient's self-described worst or most serious concern

Chronic Illness Long term illness

Chronic Obstructive Pulmonary Disease (COPD) Generic term for emphysema, chronic bronchitis, and other obstructive airway diseases

Circulation Flow of blood from the heart through arteries to capillaries and returning to the heart through veins

Clavicle *(KLA-vi-kul)* Bone of the shoulder girdle that joins the sternum to the scapula; collarbone

Closed Head Injury Trauma to the head in which the skull remains intact; scalp may or may not be lacerated

Closed Soft Tissue Injury Damage to muscle, vessels, or skin; outer skin remains intact

Coccyx *(KOK-siks),* **Coccygeal Bones** The last 4 vertebrae; the tailbone

Complex Access A rescue requiring specialized skills and equipment

Compression Injury Spinal injury caused when a strong force is transmitted up or down the length of the body

Concussion Temporary disruption of normal brain function, usually caused by blunt trauma to the head

Conduction Transfer of heat from a warmer object in contact with a colder object

Confidentiality An obligation to protect the patient's privacy by not disclosing information to unauthorized individuals

Conjunctiva *(kon-junk-TIE-vuh)* Membrane lining the eyelids and the surface of the sclera of the eye

Contraindication *(KON-trah-in-duh-KAY-shun)* Condition under which a specific medication or treatment should not be given

Contralateral On the opposite side of the body

Contusion Bruise; a wound in which the epidermis remains intact, but the cells and blood vessels in the dermis become damaged

Convection Transfer of heat from a warm object to cooler air moving past its surface

Coronary Artery Blood vessels that supply the heart with blood

Coronary Artery Disease (CAD) Condition of plaque accumulation causing narrowing within coronary artery walls; leads to decreased oxygen delivery to heart muscle

Cranium *(KRAY-nee-em)* The skull

Crepitation *(krep-eh-TAY-shun)* A crackling sensation felt and heard beneath the skin; caused by broken bone ends grating against each other or by subcutaneous air

Cricoid *(KRY-koyd)* **Cartilage** Ring of cartilage that forms the bottom of the larynx and is an anatomical landmark

Critical Incident Stress Debriefing (CISD) A meeting held after a critical incident that encourages emergency care workers to discuss their feelings openly with trained mental health professionals and peer counselors

Crowning The stage of delivery in which the head of the fetus is first visible as it stretches the vaginal opening

Crush Injury Open or closed soft tissue injury resulting from bilateral blunt trauma forces

Cyanosis *(Sy-uh-NO-sis)* Blue coloring of the skin; may indicate poor oxygen uptake or reduced perfusion

Decontamination The removal or cleansing of dangerous chemicals and other dangerous or infectious materials

Defibrillation Electrical shock or current delivered to the heart through the patient's chest wall to help the heart restore a normal rhythm

Dementia A loss of cognitive and intellectual functions caused by a variety of disorders

Dermis *(DER-mus)* Layer of skin located beneath the epidermis that supplies the skin with nutrients

Detailed Physical Exam A careful, comprehensive examination of the body performed on critical patients, usually while en route to the receiving facility

Diabetes Mellitus *(di-uh-BEE-teez muh-LEE-tus)* A disease characterized by inadequate production or use of insulin

Diaphragm Primary muscle of breathing; forms the bottom portion of the thoracic cavity

Diastolic *(di-uh-STALL-ik)* **Pressure** The pressure exerted on the walls of the arteries when the heart is at rest; when assessing blood pressure by auscultation, measured at point when the sound stops

Direct Force A force that causes injury to a body part at the site of impact

Disinfection Removal of germs, bacteria or other potentially infectious materials

Distal Farthest from head or source; opposite of proximal

Do Not Resuscitate (DNR) Orders Written physician's order directing healthcare providers to withhold lifesaving care from a patient in cardiac or respiratory arrest

Dorsal Pertaining to the back of the body; also called posterior

Dorsalis Pedis *(dor-SAL-is PEE-dis)* **Artery** Artery located on the upper surface of the foot; can be used to assess blood supply distal to a leg injury

Dosage Appropriate amount of a medication to administer; also dose

Dressing Protective covering applied directly to a soft tissue wound

Drowning Death resulting from suffocation or cardiac arrest while submerged in water

Durable Power of Attorney for Health Care (DPAC) A type of advance directive that assigns another person to make medical decisions on the patient's behalf; used only if an individual becomes unable to make decisions

Duty to Act A contractual or legal obligation to care for any patient who requests services; does not apply if caring for the patient endangers the EMT-Basic's life

Dysrhythmia *(dis-RITH-me-uh)* A disturbance in heart rate and/or rhythm; formerly called arrhythmia

Early Respiratory Distress Respiratory problem in which patient can compensate for decreased oxygenation or circulation by increasing breathing rate and effort

Edema *(eh-DEE-muh)* Abnormal accumulation of fluid in the tissues causing swelling

Emergency Medical Dispatchers (EMDS) Specially trained personnel who answer calls for help, gather essential information, and when indicated, provide prearrival instructions over the phone until EMS personnel arrive

Emergency Medical Services Systems (EMSS) Act The 1973 Congressional Act which provided federal dollars to begin EMS systems throughout the United States

Emergency Moves Specific extrication or lifting and moving techniques used when immediate danger threatens the EMT or the patient

EMT-Basic (EMT-B) Personnel trained in prehospital techniques including assessment and primary care for the ill or injured patient

EMT-Intermediate (EMT-I) An advanced EMT trained in intravenous lines, airway techniques, manual defibrillation and administration of some medications

EMT-Paramedic (EMT-P) The most highly trained EMT personnel; paramedics perform invasive field care

Endocrine System Collection of ductless glands that internally secrete hormones into the bloodstream

Endotrachael Intubation Advanced airway technique involving insertion of a tube through the mouth and into the trachea; also orotracheal intubation

Epidermis *(ep-i-DER-mus)* Outermost layer of skin

Epiglottis *(ep-i-GLOT-us)* A leaf-shaped, lid-like structure attached to the top of the larynx; closes during swallowing, preventing food or liquid from entering the respiratory tract

Epinephrine Hormone secreted in response to stress; causes tachycardia and vasoconstriction; used as an injected medication to relieve severe allergic reactions

Epistaxis *(ep-eh-STAK-ses)* Hemorrhage from the nose; a nosebleed

Esophagus *(eh-SOF-eh-gus)* Part of the gastrointestinal tract that joins the pharynx to the stomach

Evaporation The process of converting a liquid to a gas in which heat is lost

Evisceration *(eh-VIS-er-ay-shun)* Abdominal organs (viscera) protruding through an open wound

Expiration Expelling air from the lungs (exhalation)

Expressed Consent Permission for treatment from a patient who is of legal age and is able to make rational decisions; expressed consent is given after the patient is informed of procedures involved in a treatment in a language he or she understands

Face Consists of orbits, nasal bone, maxilla, mandible, zygomatic bones

Febrile *(FEE-bril)* Having a fever

Femoral *(FEM-or-ul)* **Artery** The major artery in the thigh

Femoral *(FEM-or-ul)* **Pulse** The flow of blood through the femoral artery in the upper thigh

Femur *(FEE-mer)* The thigh bone

Fetus Developing, unborn offspring in the uterus; called an embryo for the first eight weeks after conception

Fibula *(FIB-yuh-luh)* The lateral and smaller bone of the lower leg

First Responder One whose training emphasizes immediate care and scene control prior to the arrival of additional EMS services

Flexible Stretcher Carrying device made of flexible materials with large carrying handles; used for moving patients in narrow or confined spaces

Focused History and Physical Exam Assessment procedure used to identify conditions requiring emergency care; performed after initial assessment and life-saving interventions

Fowler's Position Supine position with the upper body elevated by a 45-60° bend at the hips

Full Thickness Burn Burn extending through all dermal layers; may involve the subcutaneous tissues, muscle, bone, or organs; third degree burn

General Impression The first step in initial assessment to quickly identify what is wrong and how serious it is; a time to use instinct and draw upon past experience

Generic Name Official, common name of a medication

Glasgow Coma Scale (GCS) A tool for assessing a patient's level of responsiveness

Glottis *(GLOT-is)* Space between the vocal cords; sound is produced when air passes through opening causing vocal cords to vibrate

Glucose A simple sugar that is the body's basic source of energy

Gynecology The medical specialty concerned with conditions of the female reproductive organs

Hazardous Material (HAZ-MAT) Substance that is potentially harmful or that presents an unreasonable risk for injury, health problems, or significant property damage if not properly controlled

HAZ-MAT Team Personnel specially trained to manage emergencies involving hazardous materials

Head-Tilt/Chin-Lift Maneuver The preferred method for opening and maintaining an airway in a patient without suspected neck injury

Heart Organ located in the thoracic cavity that receives blood from the veins and pumps it to the arteries

Hematoma *(hee-muh-TOE-muh)* Swelling or mass of blood caused by breaking of a blood vessel

Hemoglobin *(HEE-muh-glow-ben)* Protein in red blood cells responsible for oxygen transport

Hemorrhagic *(hem-or-AJ-ik)* **Shock** Hypoperfusion syndrome caused by excessive blood loss; a type of hypovolemic shock; the most common cause of shock in a trauma patient

High Efficiency Particulate Air (HEPA) Respirator A specially filtered mask that is worn when caring for patients suspected or diagnosed with tuberculosis and other diseases caused by airborne pathogens

Hinge Joint Joint that allows movement in one plane, forward and backward

Hives Raised, red blotches associated with allergic reactions

Hormones Biologically active substances secreted by an endocrine gland; travel through the bloodstream to exert an influence on distant organs or body tissues

Humerus *(HYU-me-rus)* The upper arm bone

Hydrocephalus *(high-dro-SEF-il-is)* Excessive fluid accumulation inside the brain

Hyperextension Extension of a joint beyond its normal limit during movement

Hyperglycemia *(high-per-gly-SEE-me-uh)* Condition in which blood sugar is too high; results from inadequate insulin in the blood for glucose metabolism

Hypertension Abnormally high blood pressure

Hyperthermia Abnormally high core body temperature

Hypoglycemia *(high-po-gly-SEE-me-uh)* Condition in which blood sugar is too low; results from too much insulin or not enough glucose in the blood

Hypoperfusion *(HY-po-per-few-zhun)* Shock; inadequate cardiac output causing a decrease in the delivery of oxygen and clearance of carbon dioxide

Hypothermia Abnormally low core body temperature

Hypovolemic Shock Shock caused by inadequate circulatory volume; may be due to loss of blood or depletion of other body fluids

Hypoxia *(high-POKS-e-uh)* Deficiency of oxygen

Iliac *(ILL-e-ak)* **Crest** Upper part of the pelvis

Immune Response A series of reactions that are the body's defense mechanism against invading viruses, bacteria, and toxins

Impaled Object An object that pierces the skin

Implied Consent Used for unconscious or mentally incompetent patients requiring emergency intervention; based on the assumption that the patient would give permission to treat life-threatening conditions

Incident Management System (IMS) A system designed to control, direct, and coordinate emergency responders and resources in case of a disaster

Indication A sign, symptom, or condition for which a specific medication or treatment is given

Indirect Force A transmitted force that causes injury some distance away from the point of impact

Inferior Below or beneath another structure

Ingested Poison A liquid or solid toxic substance that is swallowed

Inhaled Poison A toxic substance such as a gas, fumes, vapor, or spray that is breathed in

Initial Assessment Conducted after scene size-up in order to find and manage any life-threatening conditions

Injected Poison A toxic substance that enters the body through a puncture in the skin; injection may be by needle, animal bite, or insect sting

Inspiration Taking air into the lungs (inhalation)

Insulin Hormone secreted by the pancreas that regulates blood sugar levels

Intercostal Muscles Muscles located between the ribs; involved in breathing

Interventions Procedures done in an effort to improve the patient's condition

Involuntary Muscles Muscles that carry out the automatic muscular functions of the body

Ischium *(ISH-e-em)* One of the bones forming the pelvis

Jaundice *(JAWN-dis)* Yellow deposits in skin and whites of the eyes caused by increased bilirubin in the blood; indication of liver abnormality

Jaw-Thrust Maneuver The preferred method for opening and maintaining an airway in a patient with suspected spinal injury

Joint A place where bones connect

Jugular Venous Distention *(JUG-yuh-ler VEE-nus di-STEN-shun)* **(JVD)** Abnormal bulging of the jugular veins indicating injury to the heart or chest

Labor Physical processes of childbirth; begins with uterine contractions and leads to delivery of the fetus and the placenta

Laceration Wound or irregular tear of the skin

Laryngectomy *(lair-en-JEK-tuh-mee)* Removal of the larynx

Laryngoscope An instrument with a light and interchangeable blades, used for holding the tongue out of the way for intubation

Larynx *(LAIR-inks)* Part of respiratory tract between the pharynx and the trachea, responsible for the production of voice; also called the voice box

Lateral Away from the midline, to the sides

Lateral Recumbent Position Lying on one side

Lens Refracting structure of the eye located directly behind the pupil

Limb Presentation Abnormal delivery in which a limb of the infant is the initial part to deliver through the birth canal

Localized Cold Injury A cold injury confined to a limited area of the body; more severe cases are called frostbite

Long Backboard Device used for full spinal immobilization

Lumbar *(LUM-bar)*, **Lumbar Vertebrae** The 5 vertebrae forming the lower back

Lungs Respiratory organs that exchange oxygen, carbon dioxide, and water between the blood and the outside atmosphere

Malleolus *(ma-LEE-oh-lus)* The surface landmark of the ankle

Mandible *(MAN-di-bul)* The lower jaw bone

Manubrium *(ma-NEW-bre-um)* Superior portion of the sternum

Maxillae *(mak-SIL-ee)* The two fused bones that form the upper jaw

Mechanism of Injury (MOI) The forces involved or factors influencing an injury

Meconium *(meh-KO-ne-um)* Dark green fetal waste material that passes into the amniotic fluid; if inhaled, it will cause fetal distress

Medial Toward the middle of a body or region

Medical Director Physician experienced and knowledgeable in all aspects of emergency care who delegates emergency medical practice to non-physician providers, such as EMT-Basics and other EMS personnel

Metacarpals *(met-uh-KAR-pulz)* The hand bones

Metatarsals *(met-uh-TAR-sulz)* Foot bones

Metered Dose Inhaler (MDI) Hand-held inhalation device for delivering liquid or powdered medication in pre-measured doses

Mid-Axillary *(mid-AKS-ul-eh-ree)* **Line** Imaginary line drawn vertically through the side of the body, extending from the middle of the armpit to the ankle, dividing the body into front and back sides

Mid-Clavicular *(mid-kluh-VIK-yu-ler)* **Line** Imaginary line drawn through the middle of the clavicle (or collar bone), dividing the body into unequal right and left sides

Midline An imaginary vertical line that divides the body into equal right and left sides

Minimum Data Set Patient and administrative information required to be included in a prehospital care report

Miscarriage Delivery of an embryo or fetus prior to viability; spontaneous abortion

Mobile Radio Two-way radios that are usually built into emergency vehicles

Multiple Casualty Incident (MCI) Response that can involve a few serious injuries or several hundred patients; can place great demands on a local EMS system

Musculoskeletal System Consists of the muscular system and the skeletal system. A human body functions through the actions and interactions of these systems

Nasal Bone Bone of the nose

Nasal Cannula *(NAY-zul KAN-yuh-luh)* A tube inserted into the nose to deliver low-flow oxygen

Nasogastric (NG) Tube Tube inserted into the nasal passage for decompression of the stomach or proximal bowel or for gastric lavage

Nasopharyngeal *(NAY-zoh-fair-en-GEE-ul)* **Airway (NPA)** A soft rubber airway device inserted through the nose; designed to maintain an open airway by displacing the tongue off the pharynx

Nasopharynx *(nay-zo-FAIR-inks)* Part of pharynx above the level of the soft palate

Nature of Illness The type of condition or complaint a medical patient has

Near Drowning An immersion situation from which the patient is resuscitated and survives for at least 24 hours

Nebulizer Device for administering vaporized liquid medication

Negligence Failure to act as a reasonable, prudent, similarly trained person would act under similar circumstances

Nitroglycerin (NTG) Medication that dilates blood vessels and decreases the workload of the heart; taken sublingually by tablet or by spray for relief of chest pain

Non-Rebreather Mask High-flow oxygen delivery device characterized by an inflatable oxygen reservoir bag and a one-way valve that prevents exhaled air from being reinhaled

Non-Urgent (Routine) Moves Lifting and moving patients when there is no immediate threat to life

Obstetrics *(ob-STET-rics)* The medical specialty concerned with the care of women during pregnancy and child birth

Occlusive Dressing A dressing that forms an airtight seal; often applied to open neck, chest or abdominal wounds; items commonly used include defibrillation pads or thick plastic wrap

Olecranon *(oh-LEK-re-non)* Elbow bone; tip of the elbow

Ongoing Assessment Frequent reevaluation of a patient after initial assessment and primary interventions; to identify changes in patient condition and ensure appropriate care

Open Head Injury A severe traumatic head injury in which the skull is fractured

Open Soft Tissue Injury Open wound in which muscle, vessels, and/ or skin is damaged

Oral Mucosa Pink membrane lining the inside of the mouth

Orbit Eye socket

Oropharyngeal *(or-oh-FAIR-en-GEE-ul)* **Airway (OPA)** A curved plastic device with a flange inserted in the patient's mouth; used to keep the tongue from blocking the pharynx

Oropharynx *(or-oh-FAIR-inks)* Part of pharynx between the soft palate and upper end of epiglottis

Orotracheal Intubation Technique involving insertion of a tube through the mouth and into the trachea; also endotracheal intubation

Palmar Ventral surface of the hand; the palm of the hand

Palpation Assessment by touch or feel

Paradoxical Motion Chest movement during breathing in which one section of the chest moves in the opposite direction from the rest; indicates multiple rib fractures (flail chest)

Paresthesia *(pair-as-THEEZ-e-uh)* Abnormal sensations of tingling, numbness, burning, coldness, pain, or tightness in the extremities

Partial Thickness Burn Burn involving both the epidermis and the dermis, but not involving underlying tissue; second degree burn

Patella *(pa-TELL-uh)* The kneecap

Patent *(PAY-tent)* Open; accessible

Pathogen *(PATH-oh-jen)* Microorganism that causes disease

Pelvis The massive cup-shaped ring of bone at the lower end of the trunk; formed by the hip bones

Penetrating Trauma An injury caused by an object that pierces the skin or other body structure

Perfusion *(per-FEW-zhun)* Microcirculation of blood within the organs and tissues, when oxygen and nutrients are delivered to the cells and their waste products are removed

Perineum *(pair-eh-NEE-em)* The area of skin between the vagina and anus in females and between the scrotum and anus in males

Peripheral Nervous System The sensory and motor nerves that extend from the spinal cord throughout the body

Personal Protective Equipment (PPE) Equipment used by an emergency rescuer to protect against injury and infectious disease

Phalanges *(fuh-LAN-jeez)* Small bones of the fingers and toes

Pharynx *(FAIR-inks)* The throat

Physiology The study of the normal functions of the human body

Placenta Organ that enables the exchange of nutrients, oxygen, and metabolic wastes between the maternal and fetal circulatory systems

Plantar Pertaining to the sole of the foot

Plasma The serum, or fluid component, of blood

Platelets Component of blood essential for clotting

Pneumothorax *(NU-mo-THOR-aks)* Air in the chest cavity between the lung and chest wall

Poison A food, plant, chemical, or drug that has an adverse effect on the body

Portable Stretcher Light, collapsible stretcher useful in small spaces

Posterior Toward the back of the body; also called dorsal

Postictal *(post-IK-tul)* **State** A patient's condition after a seizure, during which the patient may appear sleepy, confused, or unresponsive

Power Grip Gripping items with palms and fingers in complete contact with the object; fingers bent at the same angle and hands 10 inches apart

Power Lift A specialized lifting and moving technique that uses the large muscles of the legs to lift and carry the weight

Prehospital Care Report (PCR) Documentation of the assessment and treatment of a patient in the field

Preschooler Child who is 3 to 6 years old

Presenting Part The part of a newborn that comes out of the birth canal first

Pressure Point A place where an artery passes near the surface of the body and over a bone; pressure here can stop or reduce bleeding

Prolapsed Cord Presentation of the umbilical cord before the infant's head at delivery; may cause fetal death due to constriction of blood flow through the cord

Prone (Position) Lying on the stomach, face down

Protocols Medical orders designed by a physician for a given list of procedures or medications; protocols will vary among localities

Proximal Nearer to the head, trunk, or point of origin

Pubis *(PEW-bis)* Bony structure forming anterior part of hip bone

Pulmonary Artery Originates in the right ventricle and enters the lungs where it branches off and follows the bronchi of the lungs

Pulse Pressure caused by contraction of the heart; can be palpated where an artery lies close to an underlying bone; an indication of cardiac output

Pupil Circular opening in the iris that allows passage of light into the eye

Quality Improvement (QI) Component of an EMS system that identifies the program's strengths and weaknesses and guarantees that the public receives the highest caliber of prehospital care

Radial Artery Major artery of the forearm

Radial Pulse The flow of blood through the radial artery; palpated on the anterior lateral surface of the wrist, proximal to the thumb

Radiation Heat released by an object into the surrounding air as waves of infrared radiation

Radius Bone forming the lateral side of the forearm

Rapid Extrication Specialized techniques for quickly removing a patient from a vehicle without compromising the cervical spine

Rapid Medical Assessment A physical exam designed to quickly determine the nature and severity of an illness and identify necessary interventions

Rapid Trauma Assessment A physical exam designed to quickly identify critical injuries and emergency interventions

Recovery Position Standard transportation position for a patient without spinal injury; patient is rolled onto one side, usually the left

Red Blood Cells Components of blood that contain hemoglobin; transport oxygen to the body's cells and remove carbon dioxide

Repeaters Communications devices that receive a low-power transmission and rebroadcast the signal at higher power

Respiration *(res-per-AY-shun)* Breathing; process through which air enters and leaves the lungs

Respiratory *(RES-pruh-tor-ee)* **Rate** Breathing rate; measured in breaths per minute

Respiratory Arrest A complete lack of respiratory drive or pulmonary function

Respiratory Distress Difficulty breathing; increased effort necessary to breathe due to impaired respiratory function

Respiratory Failure When the respiratory system cannot deliver an adequate supply of oxygen to meet the body's current demand

Retraction Depressions in the neck, above the shoulder blades, between and below the ribs; indicates extensive muscle use during breathing due to respiratory distress

Right Mainstem Intubation Placement of an endotracheal tube beyond the carina and into the right mainstem bronchus; results in ventilation of the right lung only

Rigid Suction Catheter Nonflexible catheter used to suction an unresponsive patient

Route of Administration Pathway by which a medication is administered: sublingual, oral ingestion, injection, inhalation, etc

Sacrum, Sacral Vertebrae The 5 fused vertebrae that form the rigid part of the posterior side of the pelvis

SAMPLE History Mnemonic used to summarize a patient's relevant medical history (Signs/Symptoms, Allergies, Medications, Past history, Last oral intake, Events leading to injury or illness)

Scapula *(SKA-pyu-luh)* The shoulder blade

Scene Size-Up The process of determining scene safety, the nature of the problem, total number of patients, and need for additional resources

School Aged Child who is 6 to 12 years old

Sclera Outermost layer of the eyeball; whites of the eyes

Scoop Stretcher Device used to move patients with no suspected spinal injuries from confined areas

Scope of Practice A description of the specific care and actions expected and allowed by law

Seizure Chaotic electrical activity in the brain that can lead to a momentary break in the stream of thought, muscular spasms, or a complete loss of consciousness

Self-Contained Breathing Apparatus (SCBA) Equipment that provides clean air to a rescuer and protects him or her from hazardous vapors

Sellick's Maneuver Pressure applied directly over the cricoid cartilage; also cricoid pressure

Shock Position See Trendelenburg Position

Short Backboard Device for immobilizing the upper part of the spine when a long board cannot be used

Show Discharge of small amount of blood-tinged mucus from the vagina at the onset of labor; also bloody show

Side Effect Unwanted effects of a medication

Sign An observable indication of illness or injury

Simple Access A rescue that does not require sophisticated equipment

Skull Cranium; the bones that comprise and protect the head

Soft Suction Catheter A soft catheter used for suctioning the nasopharynx and in other situations where a rigid catheter cannot be used

Sphygmomanometer *(sfig-mo-mah-NOM-eh-ter)* Blood pressure cuff

Spinal Column Vertebral column; consists of the cervical, thoracic, and lumbar vertebrae

Splint Equipment used to prevent or reduce movement of body joints or injured tissue

Stair Chair Specialized device used for transportation of patients down stairs or through narrow spaces; may have wheels

Standard Anatomical Position Reference position in which the body is standing upright, facing the EMT with feet flat, arms at the side, palms forward

Standard of Care The minimum acceptable level of care provided in an EMS system

Standard Precautions The first level of the Centers for Disease Control's revised set of guidelines regarding isolation precautions established in 1996. Replaces BSI and universal precautions

Standing Orders Preexisting written plans for treatment of specific complaints, interventions, or medications allowed by protocol without direct contact with medical direction

Status Epilepticus *(STA-tus ep-uh-LEP-ti-kus)* A state of prolonged seizures or multiple seizures between which the patient does not regain consciousness

Sterile Free of microorganisms (bacteria, viruses, spores) that can cause infection

Sternum Flat bone in the center of the anterior chest; the breastbone

Stoma A surgically created opening into a body cavity

Stress Natural emotional or physical reaction to threatening or challenging situations

Stridor Harsh, high-pitched sound during inspiration

Stroke Common term for a cerebrovascular accident

Subcutaneous *(sub-kew-TAY-ne-is)* **Layer** Third layer of skin located under the dermis; attaches the skin to underlying structures

Sudden Infant Death Syndrome (SIDS) Crib death; cause unknown

Superficial Burn Burn involving only the top layer of the skin (epidermis); first degree burn

Superior Above another structure

Supine (Position) Lying on the back

Supine Hypotensive Syndrome Maternal hypotension caused when the mother is lying on her back and the weight of the fetus compresses her inferior vena cava

Symptom Condition described by the patient that can't be observed

Syncope *(sin-KO-pee)* Sudden onset of a temporary loss of consciousness caused by low blood pressure in the brain; fainting

Systolic *(sis-TALL-ik)* **Pressure** The pressure in the arterial system when the left ventricle contracts; first sound heard when assessing blood pressure by auscultation

Tachycardia *(tak-eh-KAR-de-uh)* An unusually rapid heart rate

Tarsal *(TAR-sul)* The ankle bone

Thoracic *(tho-RAS-ik)* **Cavity** Body cavity enclosed by the sternum, ribs, and vertebral column

Thorax Part of the body between the neck and abdomen

Tibia *(TIB-e-uh)* The shin bone

Tidal Volume The amount of air inhaled and exhaled in a single breath

Toddler Child who is 1 to 3 years old

Torso The trunk of a body, not including the head or limbs

Tourniquet A device that is wrapped around an extremity to prevent blood flow to or from the distal area

Toxin A substance that is poisonous to cells or tissues

Trachea *(TRAY-kee-uh)* The windpipe; main air passage, arising from larynx and dividing into bronchi

Tracheal Deviation *(TRAY-kee-ul dee-vee-AY-shun)* A shifting of the trachea to either side of the midline caused by the pressure of air trapped in the chest cavity

Tracheostomy *(tray-kee-AHS-tuh-mee)* Surgical opening of the trachea

Tracheostomy Tube A specialized airway device for surgical placement into a tracheal stoma; used to maintain an airway passage

Trade Name Manufacturer's brand name for a medication

Transient Ischemic *(is-KEE-mik)* **Attack (TIA)** A sudden loss of neurological functions that clears up within 24 hours; the symptoms are similar to a CVA; also called a ministroke

Trauma A serious injury to the body or a severe emotional shock

Trauma Centers Regional facilities having specialized physicians and equipment necessary for treating trauma injuries

Trendelenburg Position The supine position inclined with the feet elevated about a foot above the head level

Triage The process of prioritizing patients to receive the appropriate level of care or transportation

Tripod Position Position that helps keep the airway open and maximizes respiratory effort: sitting, leaning forward with hands on the knees

Twisting Force Occurs when one part of an extremity remains in place while the rest moves or twists

Ulna Bone forming the medial side of the forearm

Umbilical *(um-BILL-ik-ul)* **Cord** Structure that connects the fetus to the placenta; contains arteries and veins responsible for the exchange of materials between fetal and maternal circulations

Unilateral On one side of the body

Urgent Moves Techniques for moving a patient whose condition is life-threatening; cervical spine procedures are taken

Uterus Female reproductive organ in which menstruation and fetal development occur; also womb

Uvula *(YEW-vyu-luh)* The small structure that hangs from the roof of the mouth just in front of the oropharynx; made of connective tissue

Vagina Female genital structure; the lower portion of the birth canal

Vagus Nerve Tenth cranial nerve; controls smooth muscles of the lungs, heart, and abdominal viscera

Valves Structures within the heart and circulatory system that prevent backflow of blood

Veins Vessels carrying blood back to the heart

Vena Cava *(VEE-nuh KAY-vuh)* Inferior and superior; the final vein of the systemic circulation; it empties into the right atrium of the heart

Ventilation Exchange of air between lungs and ambient air

Ventral Front of the body; also called anterior

Ventricles The two lower chambers of the heart

Ventricular Fibrillation *(ven-TRIK-yu-ler fi-bri-LAY-shun)* **(VF)** Rapid, uncoordinated movements of the ventricle walls that replace the normal contraction; treated with defibrillation methods

Venules The smallest branches of the veins

Vertebrae *(VER-te-bray)* Plural of vertebra *(VER-te-bruh)*; block-like bones that stack upon one another to form the spinal column

Vest-Type Extrication Device A flexible device used to help immobilize the spine in confined spaces

Vital Signs Pulse rate and quality, breathing rate and quality, blood pressure, skin color, skin temperature, skin condition, pupil size and quality, and capillary refill in children

Voluntary Muscles Muscles that are under conscious control

Wheeled Stretcher Most commonly used ambulance stretcher; may be rolled on smooth surfaces; adjustable height

White Blood Cells Cells in the blood responsible for controlling disease conditions, such as infections caused by microorganisms

Wind Chill The combined cooling effect of wind speed and ambient temperature

Wire Basket Stretcher (Stokes Litter) Carrying device used for patient transport over rough or irregular terrain

Xiphoid *(ZY-foyd)* **Process** The inferior tip of the sternum; it is prominent and easy to palpate

Zygomatic *(ZI-go-MA-tik)* **Bones** The cheek bones

Spanish Terms and Phrases

THE BASICS

Yes | Si *(See)*

No | No *(Noh)*

INITIAL PATIENT CONTACT

Phrases used to identify the EMT-Basic

My name is _____ | Mi nombre es _____
(Mee / nOHm-breh / ehs _____)

I am an EMT. | Yo soy un EMT. *(Joh / soee / oon / EMT.)*

And other alternatives:

I am a rescuer. | Pertenezco al cuerpo de rescate. *(Pehr-teh-nEHs-koh / ahl / coo-EHR-poh / deh / rehs-kAH-teh.)*

I am an ambulance driver. | Soy un chofer de ambulancia. *(Soee / oon / choh-FEHR / deh / ahm-boo-lAHn-see-ah.)*

I am here to help | Estoy aquí para ayudarle *(Ehs-tOHee / ah-kEE / pAH-ra / ah-yoo-dAHr-leh)*

Phrases used to ask permission to begin treatment

Can I help you? | ¿Le puedo ayudar? *(Leh / pooEH-doh / ah-yoo-dAHr?)*

Can I take care of you? | ¿Me permite atenderlo? *(Meh / pehr-mEE-teh / ah-tehn-dEHr-lo?)*

May I have permission to treat your injuries? | ¿Me da permiso de tratar sus lesiones? *(Meh / dah / pehr-mEE-soh / deh / trah-tAHr / zoos / leh-see-OH-nehs?)*

Do you speak English? | ¿Habla usted Inglés? *(AH-blah / oos-TEHD / een-glEHS?)*

Phrases used to obtain patient information

What is your name? | ¿Cómo se llama? *(KOH-moh / seh / yAH-mah?)*

Please write your name. | Por favor escriba su nombre. *(Pohr / fah-vOHr / ehs-krEE-bah / zoo / nOHm-breH.)*

Please write your address. | Por favor escriba su dirección. *(Pohr / fah-vOHr / ehs-krEE-bah / zoo / dee-rehk-ze-eOHn.)*

Please write your age. | Por favor escriba su edad. *(Pohr / fah-vOHr / ehs-krEE-bah / zoo / eh-dAHd.)*

Please write your date of birth. | Por favor escriba su fecha de nacimiento. *(Pohr / fah-vOHr / ehs-krEE-bah / zoo / fEH-chah / deh / nah-see-meeEHNto.)*

Please write your phone number. | Por favor escriba su número de teléfono. *(Pohr / fah-vOHr / ehs-krEE-bah / zoo / nOO-meh-roh / deh / teh-lEH-foh-noh.)*

OBTAINING PERMISSION TO TREAT

Asking permission to transport to the hospital

Can the ambulance take you to the hospital? | ¿Desea que la ambulancia lo lleve al hospital? *(Deh-sEHah / keh / lah / ahm-boo-lAHn-see-ah / loh / yEH-veh / ahl / hohs-pee-tAHL?)*

Asking permission to administer oxygen

Can we give you oxygen through this mask? | ¿Le podemos dar oxígeno por medio de la máscara? *(Leh / poh-dEH-mohs / dahr / ohks-sEE-geh-noh / pohr / mEH-deeoh / deh / lah / mAHs-cah-rah?)*

Asking permission to immobilize the patient and patient instructions

We need to put you on this board to carry you to the hospital. | Necesitamos colocarlo en esta camilla para llevarlo al hospital. *(Neh-ceh-si-tAH-mohs / koh-loh-cAHr-loh / ehn / EHs-ta / cah-mEE-yah / pAH-rah / yeh-vAHr-loh / ahl / hohs-pee-tAHL.)*

Your neck might have been injured in the accident. | Puede ser que su cuello se haya lastimado en el accidente. *(PooEH-deh / sehr / keh / zoo / coo-EH-yoh / seh / hAH-ya / lahs-tee-mAH-doh / ehn / ehl / ax-cee-dEHn-te.)*

May we do that? | ¿Nos permite hacer eso? *(Nohs / pehr-mEE-teh / hah -sEHr / EH-soh?)*

Please hold your head still. | Por favor no mueva su cabeza. *(Pohr / fah-vOHr / noh / moo-EH-vah / zoo / ka-bEH-sah.)*

Answer my questions verbally. Don't try to shake your head. | Conteste mis preguntas verbalmente. No intente mover su cabeza. *(Kohn-tEHs-teh / mees / preh-gOOn-tahs / vehr-bAHL-mehn-teh. / Noh / een-tEHn-teh / moh-vEHr / zoo / cah-bEH-sah.)*

We are going to put this collar around your neck to keep it safe. | Por seguridad, vamos a poner este collar alrededor de su cuello. *(Pohr / seh-goo-ree-dAHd /, vAH-mohs / ah / poh-nEHr / EHsteh / koh-yAHr / ahl-reh-deh-dOHr / deh / zoo / koo-EH-yoh.)*

This will be uncomfortable, but it is to protect you. | Esto será incomodo, pero es por su seguridad. *(Ehs-toh / seh-rAH / een-kOH-moh-doh,/ pEH-roh / ehs / pohr / zoo / seh-goo-ree-dAHd.)*

We are going to put some straps over you to keep your back from moving. | Vamos a amarrarlo con las cintas de seguridad para prevenir que se mueva su espalda. *(VAH-mohs / ah / ah-mah-trAHr-loh / kohn / lahs / sEEn-tahs / deh / seh-goo-ree-dAHd / pAH-rah / preh-veh-nEEr / keh / seh / moo-EH-vah / zoo / ehs-pAHL-da.)*

This will keep from making your injuries worse. | Esto le ayudará a prevenir que sus heridas se agraven. *(Ehs-toh / leh / ah-yoo-dah-rAH / ah / preh-veh-nEEr / keh / zoos / eh-rEE-dahs / seh / ah-grAH-vehn.)*

USE OF SAMPLE HISTORY-TAKING QUESTIONS

Phrases related to signs and symptoms

Where is the pain? | ¿En dónde le duele? *(Ehn / dOHn-deh / leh / dooEH-leh?)*

Point to where it hurts. | Señale donde siente dolor. *(Seh-neeAH-leh / dOHn-deh / see-EHn -teh / doh-lOHr.)*

Are you having chest pain? | ¿Tiene dolor en el pecho? *(Tee-EH-neh / doh-lOHr / ehn / ehl / pEH-cho?)*

Did you pass out (lose consciousness)? | ¿Perdió la conciencia? *(Pehr-dee-OH / lah / kohn-see-EHn-see-ah?)*

Are you having trouble breathing? | ¿En este momento, tiene problemas para respirar? *(Ehn / ehs-teh / moh-mEHn-toh, / tee-EH-neh / proh-blEH-mahs / pah-rah / rehs-pee-rAHr?)*

Are you having trouble walking? | ¿En este momento, tiene problemas para caminar? *(Ehn / ehs-teh / moh-mEHn-toh, / tee-EH-neh / proh-blEH-mahs / pAH-ra / cah-mee-nAHr?)*

Are you having trouble moving? | ¿En este momento, tiene problemas para moverse? *(Ehn / ehs -teh / moh-mEHn-toh, / tee-EH-neh / proh-blEH-mahs / pAH-ra / moh-vEHr-seh?)*

Do you have a sugar problem? | ¿Es usted dia-bético? *(Ehs / oos-tEHd / dee-ah-bEH-tee-koh?)*

Have you had seizures? | ¿Ha tenido usted ataques? *(Ah / teh-nee-doh / oos-tEHd / ah-TAH-kehs?)*

Do you feel like you have to throw up (vomit)? | ¿Siente la necesidad de vomitar? *(See-EHn-teh / lah / neh-seh-see-dAHd / deh / voh-mee-tAhr?)*

Have you been running a fever? | ¿Ha estado con fiebre? *(Ah / ehs-tAH-doh / kohn / fee-EH-breh?)*

Phrases related to allergies

Are you allergic to any medicine? | ¿Es alérgico a alguna medicina? *(Ehs / ah-lEHr-hee-koh / ah / ahl-gOO-nah / meh-dee-sEE-nah?)*

Are you allergic to any foods? | ¿Es alérgico a alguna comida? *(Ehs / ah-lEHr-hee-koh / ah / ahl-gOO-na / koh-mEE-dah?)*

Are you allergic to bee stings? | ¿Es alérgico a piquetes de abeja? *(Ehs / ah-lEHr-hee-koh / ah / pee-kEH-tehs / deh / ah-bEH-hah?)*

Phrases related to medications

Do you take any medicines? | ¿Toma usted alguna medicina? *(TOH-mah / oos-tEHd / ahl-gOO-nah / meh-dee-sEE-nah?)*

Have you taken any medicine today? | ¿Ha tomado alguna medicina hoy? *(Ah / toh-mAH-doh / ahl-gOO-nah / meh-dee-sEE-nah / Oee?)*

Please show me the medicine bottles | Por favor enséñeme los frascos de medicina *(Pohr / fah-vOHr / ehn-sEH-nyeh-meh / lohs / frAHs-kohs / deh / meh-dee-sEE-nah)*

Phrases related to past medical history

Did you ever have this problem before? | ¿Ha tenido este problema antes? *(Ah / teh-nEE-doh / ehs-teh / proh-blEH-mah / AHn-tehs?)*

Do you have heart disease? | ¿Padece de alguna enfermedad del corazón? *(Pah-dEH-seh / deh / ahl-gOO-nah / ehn-fehr-meh-dAHd / dehl / koh-rah-sOHn?)*

Have you ever had a heart attack? | ¿Ha tenido algún ataque al corazón (infarto)? *(Ah / teh-nEE-doh / ahl-gOOn / ah-tAH-keh / ahl / koh-rah-sOHn / (een-fAHr-toh)?)*

Do you have any breathing problems? | ¿Tiene algún problema para respirar? *(Tee-EH-neh / ahl-gOOn / proh-blEH-mah / pAH-rah / rehs-pee-rAHr?)*

Have you ever had a stroke? | ¿Alguna vez ha tenido un infarto? *(Ahl-gOO-nah / vehz / ah / teh-nEE-doh / oon / een-fAHr-toh?)*

Have you ever been told you have diabetes? | ¿Alguna vez ha sido diagnosticado con diabetes? *(Ahl-gOO-nah / vehz / ah / sEE-doh / dee-ahg-nohs-tee-cAH-doh / kohn / dee-ah-bEH-tehs?)*

Do you have blood pressure problems? | ¿Tiene problemas de hipertensión? *(Tee-EH-neh / proh-blEH-mahs / deh / ee-pehr-tehn-seeOHn?)*

Have you ever had mental problems? | ¿Alguna vez ha sufrido de problemas mentales? *(Ahl-gOO-nah / vehz / ah / zoo-frEE-doh / deh / proh-blEH-mahs / mehn-tAH-lehs?)*

Do you have cancer? | ¿Padece de cáncer? *(Pah-dEH-seh / deh / kAHn-sehr?)*

Do you have a terminal illness? | ¿Padece de alguna enfermedad terminal? *(Pah-dEH-seh / deh / ahl-gOO-nah / ehn-fehr-meh-dAHd / tehr-mee-nAHL?)*

Are you pregnant? | ¿Esta embarazada? *(Ehs-tAH / ehm-bah-rah-sAH-dah?)*

Phrases related to last oral intake

What time did you last eat solid food? | ¿Cuándo fue la última vez que comió comida sólida? *(Koo-AHn-doh / foo-EH / lah / OOL-tee-mah / vehz / keh / koh-mee-OH / koh-mEE-dah / sOH-lee-dah?)*

What time did you last drink any liquid? | ¿Cuándo fue la última vez que tomó algo líquido? *(Koo-AHn-doh / fooEH / lah / OOL-tee-mah / vehz / keh / toh-mOH / AHl-goh / lEE-kee-doh?)*

What was it? | ¿Qué fue lo que comió o bebió? *(Keh / fooEH / loh / keh / koh-mee-OH / oh / beh-bee-OH?)*

How much did you eat? | ¿Cuánto comió? *(Koo-AHn-toh / koh-meeOH?)*

How much did you drink? | ¿Cuánto tomó? *(Koo-AHn-toh / toh-mOH?)*

Did you vomit? | ¿Vomitó? *(Voh-mee-tOH?)*

Have you had any alcoholic drinks today? | ¿Ha tomado hoy bebidas alcohólicas? *(Ah / toh-maH-doh / oee / beh-bee-dahs / ahl-koh-OH-lee-cahs?)*

Phrases related to an event history

Has this ever happened before? | ¿Le ha sucedido antes? *(Leh / ah / soo-seh-dEE-doh / AHn-tehs?)*

What makes your condition worse? | ¿Qué hace que su condición empeore? *(Keh / hAHh-seh / keh / zoo / kohn-dee-see-Ohn / ehm-peh-OH-reh?)*

USE OF OPQRST HISTORY-TAKING QUESTIONS

Phrases related to onset

What time did the problem start? | ¿Cuándo comenzó el problema? *(Koo-AHn-doh / koh-mehn-zOH / ehl / proh-blEH-mah?)*

Phrases related to provocation

Did it start when you were doing something hard or exciting? | ¿Comenzó al hacer algo difícil o estimulante? *(Koh-mehn-sOH / ahl / ah-sehr / AHL-go / dee-fEE-seel / oh / ehs-tee-moo-lAHn-teh?)*

Does it get better when you move a certain way? | ¿Se siente mejor al moverse de alguna manera? *(Seh / see-EHn-teh / meh-hOHr / ahl / moh-vEHr-seh / deh / ahl-gOO-nah / mah-nEH-rah?)*

Have you been under a lot of stress? | ¿Ha estado bajo mucha presión? *(Ah / ehs-tAH-doh / bAH-hoh / mOO-chah / preh-see-OHn?)*

Phrases related to quality

Is the pain sharp? | ¿Es el dolor agudo? *(Ehs / ehl / doh-lOHr / ah-gOO-doh?)*

Is the pain dull? | ¿Es el dolor leve? *(Ehs / ehl / doh-lOHr / LEH-veh?)*

Does the pain feel like a constant pressure on your chest? | ¿Se siente el dolor como una constante presión en el pecho? *(Seh / see-EHn-teh / ehl / doh-lOHr / cOH-moh / OO-nah / kohns-tAHn-teh / preh-seeOHn / ehn / ehl / pEH-choh?)*

Is the pain constant? | ¿Es el dolor constante? *(Ehs / ehl / doh-lOHr / kohns-tAHn-teh?)*

Does the pain come and go? | ¿Es el dolor constante o intermitente (viene y se va)? *(Ehs / ehl / doh-lOHr / kohns-tAHn-teh / oh / een-tehr-mee-tEHn-teh / (vee-EH-neh / ee / seh / vah)?)*

Phrases related to radiation

Does the pain go anywhere else? | ¿El dolor se le corre para algún lado? *(Ehl / doh-lOHr / seh / leh / koh-treh / pAH-rah / ahl-gOOn / lAH-doh?)*

Using your hand, show me how the pain moves. | Usando su mano, muéstreme cómo se mueve el dolor. *(OO-sAHn-doh / zoo / mAH-noh, / mooEHs-treh-meh / cOH-moh / seh / moo-EH-veh / ehl / doh-lOHr.)*

Phrases related to severity

Rate the pain for me. 0 is no pain, 10 is great pain. Give me a number that tells how you feel. | Clasifíqueme el dolor. Zero es un dolor muy leve, diez es un dolor muy intenso. Deme un número que indique como se siente. *(Klah-see-fEE-keh-meh / ehl / doh-lOHr. / zeh-roh / ehs / oon / doh-lOHr / moo-ee / lEH-veh, / deeEHs / ehs / oon / doh-lOHr / moo-ee / een-tEHn-soh. /DEH-meh / oon / nOO-meh-roh / keh / een-dEE-keh / kOH-moh / seh / see-EHn-teh.)*

Phrases related to time

How long have you had the problem? | ¿Desde cuándo ha tenido este problema? *(DEHs-deh / koo-AHn-doh / hah / teh-nEE-doh / EHs-teh / proh-blEH-mah?)*

How long does it last? | ¿Cuánto tiempo le dura? *(Koo-AHn-toh / teeEHm-poh / leh / dOO-rah?)*

OBSTETRICAL QUESTIONING & PHRASES

Are you pregnant? | ¿Esta embarazada? *(Ehs-tAH / ehm-bah-rah-zAH-dah?)*

When is the baby due? | ¿Cuándo es la fecha aproximada de su parto? *(Koo-AHn-doh / ehs / lah / fEH-chah / ah-proh-xee-mAH-dah / deh / zoo / pAHr-toh?)*

Has your water broken? | ¿Se le ha roto la fuente? *(Seh / leh / ah /rOH-toh / lah /foo-EHn-teh?)*

Do you need to push? | ¿Siente deseos de pujar? *(See-EHn-teh / deh-seh-ohs / deh / poo-hAHr?)*

Do not push. | No puje. *(Noh / poo-heh.)*

How many times have you been pregnant? | ¿Cuántos embarazos ha tenido? *(Koo-AHn-tohs / ehm-bah-rAH-sohs / ah / teh-nEE-doh?)*

How many children do you have? | ¿Cuántos hijos tiene? *(Koo-AHn-tohs / EE-hohs / tee-EH-neh?)*

Have you ever had a miscarriage? | ¿Ha sufrido algún aborto espontáneo? *(Ah / soo-frEE-doh / ahl-gOOn / ah-bOHr-toh / ehs-pohn-tAH-neh-oh?)*

Have you ever had an abortion? | ¿Ha tenido algún aborto? *(Ah / teh-nEE-doh / ahl-gOOn / ah-bOHr-toh?)*

Have you had any problems during the pregnancy? | ¿Ha tenido algún problema durante su embarazo? *(Ah / teh-nEE-doh / ahl-gOOn / proh-blEH-mah / doo-rAHn-teh / zoo / ehm-bah-rAH-soh?)*

MENTAL STATUS QUESTIONS

Do you know where you are? | ¿Sabe en qué lugar está? *(SAH-beh / ehn / keh / loo-gAHr / eh-stAH?)*

Do you know what day it is? | ¿Sabe qué día es hoy? *(SAH-beh / keh / dEE-ah / ehs / oee?)*

OTHER PHRASES AND TERMS ESSENTIAL TO THE EMT-BASIC

We need to splint this. | Necesitamos inmovilizar esto (Necesitamos enyesarlo). *(Neh-seh-see-tAH-mohs / een-moh-vee-lee-sAHr / EHs-toh / [Neh-seh-see-tAH-mohs / ehn-yeh-sAHr-loh].)*

Can you help us lift this? | ¿Nos puede ayudar a levantar esto? *(Nos / pooEH-deh / ah-yoo-dAHr / ah / leh-vahn-tAHr / EHs-toh?)*

Please be still. | Por favor manténgase quieto. *(Pohr / fah-vOHr / mahn-tEHn-gah-seh / keeEH-toh.)*

Does this feel better? | ¿Con esto se siente mejor? *(Kohn / EHs-toh / seh / see-EHn-teh / meh-hOHr?)*

Do you feel worse? | ¿Se siente peor? *(Seh / see-EHn-teh / peh-OHr?)*

Reassurance

We will be at the hospital shortly. | Llegaremos al hospital muy pronto. *(Yeh-gah-rEH-mohs / ahl / hohs-pee-tAHl / mooee / prOHn-toh.)*

We will be at the hospital in _____ minutes. | Llegaremos al hospital en _____ minutos. *(Yeh-gah-rEH-mohs / ahl / hohs-pee-tAHl / ehn / _____ / mee-nOO-tohs.)*

We are taking good care of you. | Lo estamos atendiendo muy bien. *(Loh / ehs-tAH-mohs / ah-tehn-deeEHn-doh / mooee / bee-EHn.)*

You're very sick, but we are doing everything we can for you. | Usted está grave, pero haremos todo lo posible. *(Oos-tEHd / ehs-tAH / grAH-veh, / pEH-roh / ah-rEH-mohs / tOH-doh / loh / poh-sEE-bleh)*

BASIC ANATOMICAL TERMS

Abdomen | Abdomen *(Ab-dOH-mehn)*

Ankle | Tobillo *(Toh-bEE-lloh)*

Anus | Ano *(AH-noh)*

Arm | Brazo *(BrAH-soh)*

Back | Espalda *(Ehs-pAHl-dah)*

Breast | Senos *(SEH-nohs)*

Buttock | Nalgas *(NAHl-gahs)*

Chest | Pecho *(PEH-choh)*

Ear | Oreja *(Oh-rEH-hah)*

Eye | Ojo *(OH-hoh)*

Face | Cara *(KAH-rah)*

Finger | Dedo *(DEH-doh)*

Foot | Pie *(Pee-EH)*

Hand | Mano *(MAH-noh)*

Head | Cabeza *(Cah-bEH-sah)*

Heart | Corazón *(Coh-rah-sOHn)*

Hip | Cadera *(Cah-dEH-rah)*

Knee | Rodilla *(Roh-dEE-yah)*

Leg | Pierna *(PeeEHr-nah)*

Lung | Pulmón *(Pool-mOHn)*

Mouth | Boca *(BOH-cah)*

Neck | Cuello *(Koo-EH-yoh)*

Nose | Nariz *(Nah-rEEs)*

Penis | Pene *(PEH-neh)*

Spine | Espina dorsal, columna vertebral *(Ehs-pEE-nah / dohr-sAHl, / koh-lOOm-nah / vehr-teh-brAHl)*

Stomach | Estómago *(Ehs-tOH-mah-goh)*

Teeth | Diente *(Dee-EHn-teh)*

Thigh | Muslo *(MOOs-loh)*

Throat | Garganta *(Gahr-gAHn-tah)*

Toe | Dedo del pie *(DEH-doh / dehl / pee-EH)*

Tongue | Lengua *(LEHn-gooah)*

Vagina | Vagina *(Vah-hEE-nah)*

QUANTITATIVE TERMS

Better | Mejor *(Meh-hORr)*

Worse | Peor *(Peh-OHr)*

Dead | Muerto *(Moo-EHr-toh)*

Sleep | Dormido *(Dohr-mEE-doh)*

Unconscious | Inconciente *(Een-kohn-cee-EHn-teh)*

DAYS OF THE WEEK

Monday | Lunes *(LOO-nehs)*

Tuesday | Martes *(MAHr-tehs)*

Wednesday | Miércoles *(MeeEHr-koh-les)*

Thursday | Jueves *(HooEH-vehs)*

Friday | Viernes *(Vee-EHr-nehs)*

Saturday | Sábado *(SAH-bah-doh*

Sunday | Domingo *(Doh-mEEn-goh)*

NUMBERS

One | Uno *(Oonoh)*

Two | Dos *(Dohs)*

Three | Tres *(Trehs)*

Four | Cuatro *(Koo-AH-troh)*

Five | Cinco *(CEEn-koh)*

Six | Seis *(SEHees)*

Seven | Siete *(SeeEH-teh)*

Eight | Ocho *(OH-choh)*

Nine | Nueve *(NooEH-veh)*

Ten | Diez *(DeeEHs)*

Metric Conversions

UNITS OF LENGTH

meters (m)

1 meter = 39.4 inches

1 meter = 3.28 feet

centimeters (cm)

1 cm = 3/8 inch

1 inch = 2.54 cm

millimeters (mm)

1 mm = 1/10 cm

1 cm = 10 mm

UNITS OF VOLUME

liters (l)

1 liter = 1.06 quarts

1 quart = 0.946 liters

milliliters (ml)

cubic centimeters (cc)

1 liter = 1000 ml = 1000 cc

1 quart = 946 ml

1 tsp. = 5 cc = 5 ml

1 Tbsp. = 15 cc =15 ml

UNITS OF MASS

grams (g)

1 oz = 28 grams

1 lb = 454 grams

kilograms (kg)

1 kg = 1000 grams = 2.2 pounds

UNITS OF TEMPERATURE

Celsius / Centigrade

$C = (F - 32)/1.8$

Fahrenheit

$F = C (1.8) + 32$

METRIC BODY TEMPERATURE CONVERSIONS

°F	°C	°F	°C	°F	°C	°F	°C	°F	°C	°F	°C	°F	°C	°F	°C
107	41.7	101	38.3	96	35.6	90	32.2	84	28.9	78	25.6	72	22.2	66	18.9
106	41.1	100	37.8	95	35.0	89	31.7	83	28.3	77	25.0	71	21.7	65	18.3
105	40.6	99	37.2	94	34.4	88	31.1	82	27.8	76	24.4	70	21.1	64	17.8
104	40.0	98.6	37.0	93	33.9	87	30.6	81	27.2	75	23.9	69	20.6	63	17.2
103	39.4	98	36.7	92	33.3	86	30.0	80	26.7	74	23.3	68	20.0	62	16.7
102	38.9	97	36.1	91	32.8	85	29.4	79	26.1	73	22.8	67	19.4	61	16.1

METRIC WEIGHT CONVERSIONS

lbs	kg	lbs	kg	lbs	kg	lbs	kg	lbs	kg	lbs	kg	lbs	kg	lbs	kg
400	182	320	145	240	109	160	73	80	36	48	21.8	32	14.5	16	7.3
395	180	315	143	235	107	155	70	75	34	47	21.4	31	14.1	15	6.8
390	177	310	141	230	105	150	68	70	32	46	20.9	30	13.6	14	6.4
385	175	305	139	225	102	145	66	65	30	45	20.5	29	13.2	13	5.9
380	173	300	136	220	100	140	64	60	27.3	44	20.0	28	12.7	12	5.5
375	170	295	134	215	98	135	61	59	26.8	43	19.5	27	12.3	11	5.0
370	168	290	132	210	95	130	59	58	26.4	42	19.1	26	11.8	10	4.5
365	166	285	130	205	93	125	57	57	25.9	41	18.6	25	11.4	9	4.1
360	164	280	127	200	91	120	55	56	25.5	40	18.2	24	10.9	8	3.6
355	161	275	125	195	89	115	52	55	25.0	39	17.7	23	10.5	7	3.2
350	159	270	123	190	86	110	50	54	24.5	38	17.3	22	10.0	6	2.7
345	157	265	120	185	84	105	48	53	24.1	37	16.8	21	9.5	5	2.3
340	155	260	118	180	82	100	45	52	23.6	36	16.4	20	9.1	4	1.8
335	152	255	116	175	80	95	43	51	23.2	35	15.9	19	8.6	3	1.4
330	150	250	114	170	77	90	41	50	22.7	34	15.5	18	8.2	2	0.9
325	148	245	111	165	75	85	39	49	22.3	33	15.0	17	7.7	1	0.5

Index

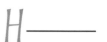

Other Titles of Interest

EMT-B Computerized Student Review

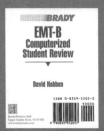

Habben, 1998, 3.5" diskette ISBN 0-8359-5205-3

This IBM-compatible review software covers all major DOT topics with 750 multiple choice, fill-in-the-blank and True/False questions. Each correct answer is followed by a rationale to help you understand why it is correct.

EMT-Basic Exam Review

Cherry, 1999, 240 pp., ISBN 0-8359-5182-0

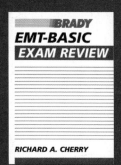

Brady's newest EMT review book helps students prepare for EMT-B certification exam with 1,000 questions. This text provides a rationale for each correct answer and an opening chapter on improving classroom performance.

Pocket Reference for the EMT-Basic and First Responder

Elling, 1999, 144 pp. ISBN 0-8359-5191-X

This handy pocket-sized field reference includes a skills performance check list, and covers topics like vital signs, common medications, abbreviations and acronyms, airway management, immobilization skills, CPR, anatomy charts, and important phone numbers. This guide is a must-have for every EMT-B and First Responder!

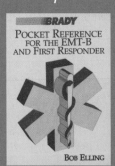

MedReview for EMT-B

Elling, 2000, 400 pp. ISBN 0-8385-6388-0

This workbook resource is a companion to *MedEMT: A Learning System for Prehospital Care*. It provides 1000 new multiple choice questions, over 150 new case scenarious, plus labeling diagrams, terminology matching exercises, and a summary of key chapter content. Links to the *MedEMT CD-ROM* are provided throughout. Answers to all questions and exercises are provided in the back of the book.

MedWorks–Anatomy & Physiology

Victory Technology, 1997, CD-ROM, ISBN 0-8385-6377-5

This IBM-compatible CD-ROM is a 50-hour college-level course in human anatomy and physiology. Each lesson includes 2D and 3D color illustrations, text, and exercises that include multiple choice, true/false, and fill-in questions. *MedWorks–A&P* includes an on-line dictionary with over 2,500 terms and definitions, covering all body systems. Every term is pronounced by a human voice, quickly building your vocabulary of anatomy and physiology terms.

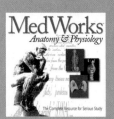

Burnout to Balance: EMS Stress

Hopson, et al, 2001, 256 pp., ISBN 0-13-007806-9

This must-have guide offers helpful advice for coping with stress and educates readers on how to find more options and make wise choices in the midst of difficult situations.

EMT-B National Standards Review Self-Test

Miller, 1998, 387 pp., ISBN 0-8359-5155-3

This review manual uses a self-test format to help you identify the areas you need to study further and helps you prepare for any local, county, state or national exam. A section on preparing for the National Registry Exam, and an Elective Test Section covering advanced airway techniques, ALS-Assist Skills and Infectious Diseases are also included.

To order any of these titles, call Brady Publishing at 800-374-120